NEW AVENUES IN DEVELOPMENTAL CANCER CHEMOTHERAPY

BRISTOL-MYERS CANCER SYMPOSIA

Series Editor
MAXWELL GORDON
Science and Technology Group
Bristol-Myers Company

NEW AVENUES IN DEVELOPMENTAL CANCER CHEMOTHERAPY

Edited by

KENNETH R. HARRAP
The Institute of Cancer Research
Royal Cancer Hospital
Sutton, Surrey, United Kingdom

THOMAS A. CONNORS
Medical Research Council Toxicology Unit
Carshalton, Surrey, United Kingdom

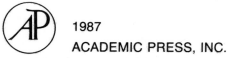

1987
ACADEMIC PRESS, INC.
Harcourt Brace Jovanovich, Publishers
Orlando   San Diego   New York   Austin
Boston   London   Sydney   Tokyo   Toronto

ACADEMIC PRESS, INC.
Orlando, Florida 32887

United Kingdom Edition published by
ACADEMIC PRESS INC. (LONDON) LTD.
24–28 Oval Road, London NW1 7DX

Library of Congress Cataloging in Publication Data

New avenues in developmental cancer chemotherapy.

(Bristol-Myers cancer symposia; 8)
Papers presented at the 8th annual Bristol-Myers
Symposium on Cancer Research, Sept. 1985, London,
England.
Includes index.
1. Cancer—Chemotherapy—Evaluation—Congresses.
2. Antineoplastic agents—Testing—Congresses.
Congresses. I. Harrap, K. R. II. Connors, Thomas A.,
Date . III. Bristol-Myers Symposium on Cancer
Research (8th : 1985 : London, England) IV. Series.
RC271.C5N46 1986   616.99'4061   86-17328
ISBN 0—12—326020—5 (alk. paper)

PRINTED IN THE UNITED STATES OF AMERICA

87 88 89 90   9 8 7 6 5 4 3 2 1

Contents

PART I MATHEMATICAL MODELING IN DRUG DESIGN AND UTILIZATION

Computer Simulation of the Effects of Antimetabolites on Metabolic Pathways
ROBERT C. JACKSON

v

PART II   BIOCHEMICAL MODULATION OF DRUG ACTIVITY

Does Modulation of 5-Fluorouracil by Metabolites or Antimetabolites Work in the Clinic?

JOSEPH R. BERTINO AND ENRICO MINI

PART III   INITIATION OF CELL DIFFERENTIATION

Induction of Cell Differentiation and Bypassing of Genetic Defects in Cancer Therapy

LEO SACHS

The Regulatory Role of Commitment in Gene Expression during Induction of Leukemic Cell Differentiation

ASTERIOS S. TSIFTSOGLOU, JACK HENSOLD, STEPHEN H. ROBINSON, AND WILLIE WONG

Cancer Chemotherapeutic Agents as Inducers of Leukemia Cell Differentiation

ALAN C. SARTORELLI, MICHAEL J. MORIN, AND KIMIKO ISHIGURO

The Role of Natural Differentiation Factors in Leukemic Cell Maturation Induced by Antineoplastic Agents

ALEXANDER BLOCH

PART IV TARGETING WITH MONOCLONAL ANTIBODIES

Targeted Therapy *in Vitro* and *in Vivo*: Probing the Limits

LEE D. LESERMAN, PATRICK MACHY, DENISE ARAGNOL, BERNT ARNOLD, AND SALVADOR ALINO

PART V NEW DRUGS IN DEVELOPMENT

Second-Generation Azolotetrazinones

MALCOLM F. G. STEVENS

5-Aminoanthrapyrazoles (CI-937; CI-941, CI-942): A Novel Class of DNA Binders with Broad Spectrum Anticancer Activity

LESLIE M. WERBEL, EDWARD F. ELSLAGER, DAVID W. FRY, ROBERT C. JACKSON, WILBUR R. LEOPOLD, AND H. D. HOLLIS SHOWALTER

PART VI   ONCOGENES AS A TARGET FOR DRUG DESIGN

Oncogene Function and Mechanism of Action

SYDONIA I. RAYTER, JOHN C. BELL, MICHAEL J. FRY, AND J. GORDON FOULKES

Major Histocompatibility Complex Class I Expression and Malignancy

MICHAEL J. CHORNEY, RAKESH SRIVASTAVA, YURI BUSHKIN, YVON CAYRE, JULIAN PAN, AND SHERMAN M. WEISSMAN

The Regulation of Cellular Transcription by Viral Transforming Proteins

BARBARA I. SKENE, NICHOLAS B. LA THANGUE, DAVID MURPHY, AND PETER W. J. RIGBY

Contributors

Numbers in parentheses indicate the pages on which the authors' contributions begin.

HERBERT ABELSON (503), Department of Pediatrics, University of Washington School of Medicine, Seattle, Washington 98195

Z. H. L. ABRAHAM (83), Cancer Research Campaign Biomolecular Structure Research Unit, The Institute of Cancer Research, Sutton, Surrey SM2 5PX, United Kingdom

SALVADOR ALINO[1] (299), Centre d'Immunologie INSERM-CNRS de Marseille-Luminy, Marseille, France

DENISE ARAGNOL (299), Centre d'Immunologie INSERM-CNRS de Marseille-Luminy, Marseille, France

BERNT ARNOLD (299), Deutsches Krebsforschungszentrum, Heidelberg, Federal Republic of Germany

THOMAS L. AVERY[2] (367), St. Jude Children's Research Hospital, Memphis, Tennessee 38101

R. BAER (485), Medical Research Council, Laboratory of Molecular Biology, Cambridge CB2 2QH, United Kingdom

R. W. BALDWIN (277), Cancer Research Campaign Laboratories, University of Nottingham, Nottingham NG7 2RD, United Kingdom

JOHN C. BELL (421), Laboratory of Eukaryotic Molecular Genetics, National Institute for Medical Research, Mill Hill, London NW7 1AA, United Kingdom

MICHAEL E. BERENS (387), Department of Biochemistry, Department of Obstetrics and Gynecology, and Oncology Research Center, Bowman Gray School of Medicine of Wake Forest University, Winston-Salem, North Carolina 27103

---

[1] Present address: Facultad de Medicine, Departamento de Histologia, Universidad del Pais Vasco, Leonja, Vizcaya, Spain.

[2] Present address: Nucleic Acid Research Institute, ICN Plaza, 3300 Hyland Avenue, Costa Mesa, California 92626

JOSEPH R. BERTINO (163), Departments of Pharmacology and Medicine, Yale University School of Medicine, New Haven, Connecticut 06510

ALEXANDER BLOCH (245), Department of Experimental Therapeutics, Grace Cancer Drug Center, Roswell Park Memorial Institute, Buffalo, New York 14263

YURI BUSHKIN (453), Laboratory of Molecular Immunology, Memorial Sloan-Kettering Cancer Center, New York, New York 10021

YVON CAYRE (453), Laboratory of Molecular Immunogenetics, Memorial Sloan-Kettering Cancer Center, New York, New York 10021

K.-C. CHEN (485), Department of Haematological Medicine, University of Cambridge, Clinical School, Cambridge CB2 2QH, United Kingdom

MICHAEL J. CHORNEY (453), Department of Human Genetics, Yale University School of Medicine, New Haven, Connecticut 06510-8005

TING-CHAO CHOU (37), Laboratory of Pharmacology, Sloan-Kettering Institute for Cancer Research, Cornell University Graduate School of Medical Sciences, New York, New York 10021

D. A. COLLIER (83), Cancer Research Campaign Biomolecular Structure Research Unit, The Institute of Cancer Research, Sutton, Surrey SM2 5PX, United Kingdom

JAMES CROOP (503), Dana-Farber Cancer Institute, Boston, Massachusetts

LARRY W. DANIEL (387), Department of Biochemistry, Department of Obstetrics and Gynecology, and Oncology Research Center, Bowman Gray School of Medicine of Wake Forest University, Winston-Salem, North Carolina 27103

EDWARD F. ELSLAGER (355), Departments of Chemistry and Chemotherapy, Warner-Lambert/Parke-Davis Pharmaceutical Research, Ann Arbor, Michigan 48105

ALEXANDRA H. FILIPOVICH (291), Bone Marrow Transplantation Program, Departments of Pediatrics, Medicine, and Therapeutic Radiology, University of Minnesota, Minneapolis, Minnesota 55455, and National Institutes of Health, Bethesda, Maryland 20205

A. FORSTER (485), Medical Research Council, Laboratory of Molecular Biology, Cambridge CB2 2QH, United Kingdom

J. GORDON FOULKES (421), Laboratory of Eukaryotic Molecular Genetics, National Institute for Medical Research, Mill Hill, London NW7 1AA, United Kingdom

DAVID W. FRY (355), Departments of Chemistry and Chemotherapy, Warner-Lambert/Parke-Davis Pharmaceutical Research, Ann Arbor, Michigan 48105

MICHAEL J. FRY (421), Laboratory of Eukaryotic Molecular Genetics, National Institute for Medical Research, Mill Hill, London NW7 1AA, United Kingdom

ELENA GIULOTTO (495), Imperial Cancer Research Fund, Lincoln's Inn Fields, London WC2A 3PX, United Kingdom

PHILIPPE GROS (503), Department of Biochemistry, McGill University, Montreal, Quebec, Canada H3A 2T5

WILLIAM J. HENNEN (367), Department of Chemistry, Brigham Young University, Provo, Utah 84602

JACK HENSOLD (205), Charles A. Dana Research Institute, Harvard-Thorndike Laboratory, Department of Medicine, Beth Israel Hospital, Harvard Medical School, Boston, Massachusetts 02215

DAVID HOUSMAN (503), Center for Cancer Research, Massachusetts Institute of Technology, Cambridge, Massachusetts 02139

DAVID HURD (291), Bone Marrow Transplantation Program, Departments of Pediatrics, Medicine, and Therapeutic Radiology, University of Minnesota, Minneapolis, Minnesota 55455, and National Institutes of Health, Bethesda, Maryland 20205

KIMIKO ISHIGURO (229), Department of Pharmacology and Developmental Therapeutics Program, Comprehensive Cancer Center, Yale University School of Medicine, New Haven, Connecticut 06510

S. A. ISLAM[3] (83), Cancer Research Campaign Biomolecular Structure Research Unit, The Institute of Cancer Research, Sutton, Surrey SM2 5PX, United Kingdom

ROBERT C. JACKSON (3, 355), Departments of Chemistry and Chemotherapy, Warner-Lambert/Parke-Davis Pharmaceutical Research, Ann Arbor, Michigan 48105

JOHN H. KERSEY (291), Bone Marrow Transplantation Program, Departments of Pediatrics, Medicine, and Therapeutic Radiology, University of Minnesota, Minneapolis, Minnesota 55455, and National Institutes of Health, Bethesda, Maryland 20205

TAE KIM (291), Bone Marrow Transplantation Program, Departments of Pediatrics, Medicine, and Therapeutic Radiology, University of Minnesota, Minneapolis, Minnesota 55455, and National Institutes of Health, Bethesda, Maryland 20205

NICHOLAS B. LA THANGUE[4] (473), Cancer Research Campaign, Eukaryotic Molecular Genetics Research Group, Department of Bio-

---

[3] Present address: Molecular Biology Laboratory, Birkbeck College, London WC1E 7HU, United Kingdom.

[4] Present address: Laboratory of Eukaryotic Molecular Genetics, National Institute for Medical Research, Mill Hill, London NW7 1AA, United Kingdom.

chemistry, Imperial College of Science and Technology, London SW7 2AZ, United Kingdom

M.-P. LEFRANC[5] (485), Medical Research Council, Laboratory of Molecular Biology, Cambridge CB2 2QH, United Kingdom

WILBUR R. LEOPOLD (355), Departments of Chemistry and Chemotherapy, Warner-Lambert/Parke-Davis Pharmaceutical Research, Ann Arbor, Michigan 48105

LEE D. LESERMAN (299), Centre d'Immunologie INSERM-CNRS de Marseille-Luminy, Marseille, France

PATRICK MACHY[6] (299), Centre d'Immunologie INSERM-CNRS de Marseille-Luminy, Marseille, France

DANIEL S. MARTIN (113), Department of Developmental Chemotherapy, Memorial Sloan-Kettering Cancer Institute, New York, New York 10021, and Department of Cancer Research, Catholic Medical Center of Brooklyn and Queens, Woodhaven, New York 11421

DAVID A. MATTHEWS (65), The Agouron Institute, La Jolla, California 92037

PHILLIP McGLAVE (291), Bone Marrow Transplantation Program, Departments of Pediatrics, Medicine, and Therapeutic Radiology, University of Minnesota, Minneapolis, Minnesota 55455, and National Institutes of Health, Bethesda, Maryland 20205

ENRICO MINI[7] (163), Departments of Pharmacology and Medicine, Yale University School of Medicine, New Haven, Connecticut 06510

EDWARD J. MODEST (387), Department of Biochemistry, Department of Obstetrics and Gynecology, and Oncology Research Center, Bowman Gray School of Medicine of Wake Forest University, Winston-Salem, North Carolina 27103

MICHAEL J. MORIN (229), Department of Pharmacology and Developmental Therapeutics Program, Comprehensive Cancer Center, Yale University School of Medicine, New Haven, Connecticut 06510

SUSAN MORRIS-NATSCHKE (387), Department of Medicinal Chemistry and Natural Products, University of North Carolina, Chapel Hill, North Carolina 27514

TAKETO MUKAIYAMA (503), Cancer Chemotherapy Center, Japanese Foundation for Cancer Research, Tokyo, Japan

[5] Present address: Laboratoire des Sciences et Techniques du Languedoc, 34060 Montpellier Cedex, France

[6] Present address: Department of Cell Biology, Smith Kline and French Laboratories, Philadelphia, Pennsylvania 19101.

[7] Present address: Dipartimento di Farmacologia Preclinica e Clinica, Universita degli Studi, Firenza 50100, Italy.

DAVID MURPHY[8] (473), Cancer Research Campaign, Eukaryotic Molecular Genetics Research Group, Department of Biochemistry, Imperial College of Science and Technology, London SW7 2AZ, United Kingdom

V. L. NARAYANAN (401), Drug Synthesis and Chemistry Branch, Developmental Therapeutics Program, Division of Cancer Treatment, National Cancer Institute, Bethesda, Maryland 20892

S. NEIDLE (83), Cancer Research Campaign Biomolecular Structure Research Unit, The Institute of Cancer Research, Sutton, Surrey SM2 5PX, United Kingdom

DAVID NEVILLE (291), Bone Marrow Transplantation Program, Departments of Pediatrics, Medicine, and Therapeutic Radiology, University of Minnesota, Minneapolis, Minnesota 55455, and National Institutes of Health, Bethesda, Maryland 20205

JULIAN PAN (453), Department of Human Genetics, Yale University School of Medicine, New Haven, Connecticut 06510-8005

CLAUDE PIANTADOSI (387), Department of Medicinal Chemistry and Natural Products, University of North Carolina, Chapel Hill, North Carolina 27514

T. H. RABBITTS (485), Medical Research Council, Laboratory of Molecular Biology, Cambridge CB2 2QH, United Kingdom

NORMA K. C. RAMSAY (291), Bone Marrow Transplantation Program, Departments of Pediatrics, Medicine, and Therapeutic Radiology, University of Minnesota, Minneapolis, Minnesota 55455, and National Institutes of Health, Bethesda, Maryland 20205

SYDONIA I. RAYTER (421), Laboratory of Eukaryotic Molecular Genetics, National Institute for Medical Research, Mill Hill, London NW7 1AA, United Kingdom

GANAPATHI R. REVANKAR (367), Nucleic Acid Research Institute, Costa Mesa, California 92626

PETER W. J. RIGBY[9] (473), Cancer Research Campaign, Eukaryotic Molecular Genetics Research Group, Department of Biochemistry, Imperial College of Science and Technology, London SW7 2AZ, United Kingdom

ROLAND K. ROBINS (367), Nucleic Acid Research Institute, Costa Mesa, California 92626

STEPHEN H. ROBINSON (205), Charles A. Dana Research Institute,

[8] Present address: Laboratory of Molecular Embryology, National Institute for Medical Research, Mill Hill, London NW7 1AA, United Kingdom.

[9] Present address: Laboratory of Eukaryotic Molecular Genetics, National Institute for Medical Research, Mill Hill, London NW7 1AA, United Kingdom.

Harvard-Thorndike Laboratory, Department of Medicine, Beth Israel Hospital, Harvard Medical School, Boston, Massachusetts 02215

IGOR RONINSON (503), Center for Genetics, University of Illinois at Chicago Circle, Chicago, Illinois 60680

LEO SACHS (187), Department of Genetics, Weizmann Institute of Science, Rehovot 76100, Israel

IZUMU SAITO (495), Imperial Cancer Research Fund, Lincoln's Inn Fields, London WC2A 3PX, United Kingdom

ALAN C. SARTORELLI (229), Department of Pharmacology and Developmental Therapeutics Program, Comprehensive Cancer Center, Yale University School of Medicine, New Haven, Connecticut 06510

H. D. HOLLIS SHOWALTER (355), Departments of Chemistry and Chemotherapy, Warner-Lambert/Parke-Davis Pharmaceutical Research, Ann Arbor, Michigan 48105

BARBARA I. SKENE[10] (473), Cancer Research Campaign, Eukaryotic Molecular Genetics Research Group, Department of Biochemistry, Imperial College of Science and Technology, London SW7 2AZ, United Kingdom

S. SMITH (485), Department of Pediatrics, Stanford University, Stanford, California 94305

RAKESH SRIVASTAVA (453), Department of Human Genetics, Yale University School of Medicine, New Haven, Connecticut 06510-8005

GEORGE R. STARK (495), Imperial Cancer Research Fund, Lincoln's Inn Fields, London WC2A 3PX, United Kingdom

MALCOLM F. G. STEVENS (335), Department of Pharmaceutical Sciences, Aston University, Birmingham B4 7ET, United Kingdom

G. T. STEVENSON (255), Lymphoma Research Unit, Tenovus Laboratory, General Hospital, Southampton S09 4XY, United Kingdom

M. A. STINSON (485), Medical Research Council, Laboratory of Molecular Biology, Cambridge CB2 2QH, United Kingdom

JEFFERSON R. SURLES (387), Department of Medicinal Chemistry and Natural Products, University of North Carolina, Chapel Hill, North Carolina 27514

PAUL TALALAY (37), Department of Pharmacology and Experimental Therapeutics, The Johns Hopkins University, School of Medicine, Baltimore, Maryland 21205

PHILIP E. THORPE (265), Drug Targeting Laboratory, Imperial Cancer Research Fund Laboratories, London WC2A 3PX, United Kingdom

[10] Present address: Heinrich-Pette-Institut für Experimentelle Virologie und Immunologie, an der Universität Hamburg, D-2000 Hamburg 20, Federal Republic of Germany.

ASTERIOS S. TSIFTSOGLOU (205), Charles A. Dana Research Institute, Harvard-Thorndike Laboratory, Department of Medicine, Beth Israel Hospital, Harvard Medical School, Boston, Massachusetts 02215

DANIEL VALLERA (291), Bone Marrow Transplantation Program, Departments of Pediatrics, Medicine, and Therapeutic Radiology, University of Minnesota, Minneapolis, Minnesota 55455, and National Institutes of Health, Bethesda, Maryland 20205

ELLEN S. VITETTA (265), Department of Microbiology, University of Texas Health Science Center at Dallas, Dallas, Texas 75235

ROBIN A. WEISS (413), The Institute of Cancer Research, Chester Beatty Laboratories, London SW3 6JB, United Kingdom

SHERMAN M. WEISSMAN (453), Department of Human Genetics, Yale University School of Medicine, New Haven, Connecticut 06510-8005

LESLIE M. WERBEL (355), Departments of Chemistry and Chemotherapy, Warner-Lambert/Parke-Davis Pharmaceutical Research, Ann Arbor, Michigan 48105

WILLIE WONG (205), Charles A. Dana Research Institute, Harvard-Thorndike Laboratory, Department of Medicine, Beth Israel Hospital, Harvard Medical School, Boston, Massachusetts 02215

ROBERT L. WYKLE (387), Department of Biochemistry, Department of Obstetrics and Gynecology, and Oncology Research Center, Bowman Gray School of Medicine of Wake Forest University, Winston-Salem, North Carolina 27103

RICHARD YOULE (291), Bone Marrow Transplantation Program, Departments of Pediatrics, Medicine, and Therapeutic Radiology, University of Minnesota, Minneapolis, Minnesota 55455, and National Institutes of Health, Bethesda, Maryland 20205

Editor's Foreword

It is fitting that The Institute of Cancer Research, London, was the host for the symposium reported in this volume, the eighth in the annual Bristol-Myers symposia on cancer research. The host institution, and Professor Kenneth Harrap in particular, were responsible for the clinical development of carboplatin, the new platinum anticancer drug which was approved for marketing in the United Kingdom while this volume was in press.

This symposium title was New Avenues in Developmental Cancer Chemotherapy. A broad range of cancer-related topics was covered including oncogenes as a basis for selective drug design, targeting with monoclonal antibodies, initiation of cell differentiation, biochemical modulation of drug activity, mathematical modeling in drug design, and, finally, new drugs in development.

The past year has seen a period of ferment in the field of cancer research, as reflected in this list of topics. In addition, for the first time biological response modifiers have been approved by the U.S. Food and Drug Administration. Alpha-interferon was approved for use in hairy cell leukemia, and its approval is pending for other tumors. The monoclonal antibody OKT-3 was approved for use in organ transplants, this being the first approval of a monoclonal antibody for therapeutic purposes. One can hope that the therapeutic application of monoclonal antibodies in cancer will not be far behind, used either alone or in targeting applications.

The use of interleukin-2 in producing lymphokine-activated killer cells (LAK) has elicited interest, and the newer discovery of tumor-infiltrating lymphocytes having greater cytotoxic effects than LAK cells is the subject of investigation. The area of AIDS infections is not directly relevant to the subject of this series, except that the relatively rare Kaposi's sarcoma has become commonplace and a serious clinical problem in

AIDS patients. The possible utility of alpha-interferon in this disease has been an interesting dividend of the lymphokine research. Tumor necrosis factor, mentioned in earlier volumes, has entered clinical trial.

Maxwell Gordon
Series Editor

Foreword

The past few years have seen many important advances in our understanding of basic biological science. Recent developments in molecular biology, genetic engineering, and related fields have brought with them exciting new possibilities for therapeutic progress.

But amid the excitement this research has generated, a compelling question remains: How far off is that future?

This question was explored at the eighth annual Bristol-Myers Symposium on Cancer Research, "New Avenues in Developmental Cancer Chemotherapy." Held in London in September 1985, it was organized by The Institute of Cancer Research and drew an audience from the United States, the United Kingdom, and a number of other European countries.

The symposium series is an example of scientific inquiry transcending national boundaries. The London symposium was the second in the Bristol-Myers series to be held in Europe. Future symposia will be held in Canada and Japan as well as in Europe and the United States.

The symposia are an important part of the program of unrestricted grants for cancer research our company initiated in 1977. To date, 19 grants totaling $9.34 million have been awarded to institutions in the United States, Canada, Europe, and Japan. The most recent grant recipients are Cold Spring Harbor Laboratory in Cold Spring Harbor, New York, and the Oncology Center at Johns Hopkins University School of Medicine in Baltimore, Maryland.

The program also includes the annual Bristol-Myers Award for Distinguished Achievement in Cancer Research. The ninth award was presented in April 1986 to Dr. Susumu Tonegawa of the Massachusetts Institute of Technology for his discovery of the genetic basis of how the immune system works.

As we enter the tenth year of the program, it is our hope that these proceedings will be helpful to scientists working around the world to expand our knowledge of cancer and how to treat it more effectively.

Richard L. Gelb
Chairman of the Board
Bristol-Myers Company

Preface

The eighth annual Bristol-Myers Symposium on Cancer Research was held in London, England, in September 1985, hosted by The Institute of Cancer Research. The subject, "New Avenues in Developmental Cancer Chemotherapy," embraced a discussion of recent laboratory advances in the design, evaluation, and utilization of anticancer agents. While the present generation of drugs is of value in the treatment of relatively rare malignancies, it has made little impact on the management of common cancers. There is an unequivocal need to discover more potent and selective anticancer drugs. Recent advances in knowledge of the biochemistry of the cancer cell, and of the mode of action of established drugs, provided a basis for the elaboration of the various topics. These included:

Mathematical modeling in drug design and utilization, addressing the role of mathematical models both in quantifying the integrated effects of drugs on multienzyme pathways and in elucidating the nature of interactions between combinations of drugs. Other contributions discussed the application of computer graphic-modeling techniques in the design of enzyme-targeted drugs and of intercalating agents directed at defined DNA sequences.

Biochemical modulation of drug activity: Many laboratory studies have exploited a knowledge of the biochemical mechanisms of established drugs in the design and scheduling of combination treatments. Much of this work is reviewed here, together with a discussion of clinical studies based on biochemical modulation.

Initiation of cell differentiation focused upon leukemic cells and the role of natural growth regulators and differentiation effectors in restricting their proliferation. Also discussed was the use of conventional anticancer drugs as inducers of cell differentiation.

Targeting with monoclonal antibodies explored the anticancer properties of monoclonal antibodies used either alone or conjugated to drug or other toxic species, notably plant lectins.

New drugs in development surveyed a number of new initiatives which are close to the clinical trials interface.

Oncogenes as a target for drug design: Intuitively it would seem that oncogene activation or expression in cancer cells must provide exploitable targets for new drug design. The role and function of oncogenes was explored from this viewpoint.

The editors wish to acknowledge the dedication and competence of the technical editor, Ann S. Robinson.

Kenneth R. Harrap
Thomas A. Connors

Abbreviations

abl, Abelson murine leukemia virus (A-MuLV)
ACIV, acivicin
ADP, adenosine diphosphate
ADR, doxorubicin (Adriamycin)
AEV, avian erythroblastosis virus
AIC, aminoimidazole carboxamide
AICR, aminoimidazole carboxamide riboside
ALL, acute lymphocytic leukemia
ALP, alkyl lysophospholipids
AMP, adenosine-5'-phosphate
6-AN, 6-aminonicotinamide
ANL, acute nonlymphocytic leukemia
anti-Id, anti-idiotype antibodies
ara-C, cytosine arabinoside (cytarabine)
ara-CTP, cytarabine triphosphate
ATP, adenosine triphosphate

BAU, benzylacyclouridine
BCNU, 1,3-bis-(2-chloroethyl) 1-nitrosourea
BHK, nontumorigenic cell line

CCRG, pro drug of MTIC (8-carbamoyl-3-methyl-imidazo-[5,1-d]-1, 2, 3, 5-tetrazin-4 (3H)one)
CD, cordycepin (3'-deoxyadenosine)
CDP, cytidine diphosphate
CF, carboxyfluorescein
CH, cycloheximide
CH_2-FH_4, 5,10-methylene tetrahydrofolate

CMFP, cyclophosphamide, methotrexate, 5-fluorouracil, prednisone
CML, chronic myelocytic leukemia
CMP, cytidine 5'-monophosphate
CSF, colony stimulating factor
CTL, cytotoxic T-lymphocytes
CTP, cytidine triphosphate

DG, diacylglycerol
DHFR, dihydrofolate reductase
DMSO, dimethyl sulfoxide
DNP-cap-PE, dinitrophenyl-caproyl-phosphatidylethanolamine
DPPC, dipalmitoyl phosphatidylcholine
dTHD, deoxythymidine
dTGuo, 6-thiodeoxyguanosine
DTIC, 5(3,3-dimethyl-1-triazenyl)-1H-imidazole-4-carboxamide (dacarbazine)

EGF, epidermal growth factor
ER, estrogen receptor
*erb*B oncogene, avian erythroblastosis virus (AEV)
ets oncogene, avian myeloblastosis virus (AMV)

FabIgG, chimeric univalent antibody
FAH_2, 7,8-dihydrofolate
FAH_4, 5,6,7,8-tetrahydrofolate
FcR, Fc receptor portion of IgG
FdUMP, fluorodeoxyuridine monophosphate
FdUrd, 5-fluorodeoxyuridine
FdUTP, fluorodeoxyuridine triphosphate
fes oncogene, Gardner-Arnstein feline sarcoma virus (GA-FeSV)
fes oncogene, Snyder-Theilin feline sarcoma virus (ST-FeSV)
fgr oncogene, Gardner-Rasheed feline sarcoma virus (GR-FeSV)
FH_2, dihydrofolate
FH_4, tetrahydrofolate
FITC, fluorescein isothiocyanate
fms oncogene, McDonough feline sarcoma virus (GR-FeSV)
fos oncogene, FBJ osteosarcoma virus
fps oncogene, Fujinami avian sarcoma virus (FSV)
fps oncogene, UR-1 virus, 16L virus, PRC11 virus
5-FUra, 5-fluorouracil
FUTP, fluorouridine triphosphate

GA-FeSV, Gardner-Arnstein feline sarcoma virus
GDP, guanosine diphosphate
GM-CSF, granulocyte/macrophage colony stimulating factor
GMP, guanosine-5'-phosphate
GTP, guanosine triphosphate
GVHD, graft versus host disease

Ha-*ras* oncogene, Harvey murine sarcoma virus (rat)
4-HC, 4-hydroperoxycyclophosphamide
10-HCO-FH-4, 10-formyl tetrahydrofolate
5-HETE, 5-hydroxyeicosatetraenoic acid
HGPRT, hypoxanthine-guanine phosphoribosyltransferase
HL, human leukemia cells
HL-60, cells from acute promyelocytic leukemia
HLA, human leukocyte antigens
HMBA, hexamethylene-*bis*-acetamide
HSA, human serum albumin
HTLV, human tumor leukemia virus (also called human
    T-cell lymphotropic virus)

IFN, interferon
IGF-1, insulin-like growth factor
IL-2, interleukin-2
IL-3, interleukin-3
ILS, increase in life-span
IMP, inosine-5'-monophosphate

Ki-*ras* oncogene, Kirsten murine sarcoma virus (rat)
kit oncogene, HZ 4 feline sarcoma virus
KLH, keyhole limpet hemocyanin

Lst, nonviral protein kinase
LTB$_4$, leukotriene B$_4$
LTR, long terminal repeat
LV, leucovorin (5-formyl tetrahydrofolate)

mAb, monoclonal antibody
m-AMSA, 9-(*p*-methylsulfonamido-*o*-methoxyphenyl)-aminoacridine or
    4'-(9-acridinylamino) methanesulfon-*m*-anisidide
M-CSF, multi-colony stimulating factor
MCTIC, 5-[3-(2-chloroethyl) triazen-1-yl]-imidazole-4-carboxamide

met oncogene, nonviral protein kinase
MeFH$_4$, 5-methyl tetrahydrofolate
MEL, murine erythroleukemia cells
MGI, macrophage and granulocyte inducers
MHC, major histocompatability complex
mil oncogene, MH2 avian virus
Mito C, mitomycin C
MLF, mean linear fluorescence
MMP, 6-methylmercaptopurine
6-MMPR, 6-methylmercaptopurine riboside
MMTV, mouse mammary tumor virus
MNase, micrococcal nuclease
mos oncogene, Moloney murine sarcoma virus
6-MP, 6-mercaptopurine
MTD, maximum tolerated dose
MTIC, 5-(3-methyl-1-triazenyl)-1H-imidazole-4-carboxamide
MTX, methotrexate
myb oncogene, avian myeloblastosis virus (AMV)
myc oncogene, MC29 myelocytomatosis virus

NADPH, nicotinamide adenine dinucleotide phosphate (reduced)
NBT, nitroblue tetrazolium
neu oncogene, nonviral protein kinase
NMR, nuclear magnetic resonance

ODSC, optimal differentiation-sensitizing concentration
*onc*D oncogene, nonviral protein kinase

PAF, platelet activating factor
PALA, *N*-(phosphonoacetyl)-L-aspartic acid
PC, phosphocholine
PDGF, platelet-derived growth factor
PE, phosphatidylethanolamine
PHA, phytohemagglutinin assay
PI, phosphatidyl inositol
poly(ADP-ribose), polyadenosine diphosphoribose
Polyoma middle T, polyoma tumor virus
PRPP, 5-phosphoribosyl-1-pyrophosphate

RA, retinoic acid
raf oncogene, murine sarcoma virus 3611
rel oncogene, reticuloendotheliosis virus

RES, reticuloendothelial system
RIP, ribosome inactivating protein
ros oncogene, UR-2 sarcoma virus
RSV, respiratory syncytial virus

SDS-PAGE, sodium dodecylsulfate polyacrylamide gel electrophoresis
sis oncogene, simian sarcoma virus
ski oncogene, avian SKV770 virus
SPDP, *N*-hydroxysuccinnimidyl-3(2-pyridyldithio) propionate
src oncogene, Rous sarcoma virus (RSV)

TCR, T-cell antigen receptor
TGua, 5-thioguanine
TGuo, 6-thioguanosine
TL, thymus leukemia antigen
TMP, thymidine monophosphate
TMP, trimethoprim
TPA, 12-*O*-tetradecanoyl-phorbol-13-acetate
TS, thymidylate synthase
TTP, thymidine triphosphate

UR, uridine
UTP, uridine triphosphate

VP-16, etoposide (Vepesid TM)

XMP, xanthine-5′-phosphate

yes oncogene, Esh sarcoma virus (ESV)
yes oncogene, Y73 virus

PART I

Mathematical Modeling in Drug Design and Utilization

1

Computer Simulation of the Effects of Antimetabolites on Metabolic Pathways

ROBERT C. JACKSON

Departments of Chemistry and Chemotherapy
Warner-Lambert/Parke-Davis Pharmaceutical Research
Ann Arbor, Michigan

I. Introduction: The Kinetics of Inhibition of Complex Pathways

The response of metabolic pathways to inhibition often cannot be understood intuitively, particularly where feedback effects occur. Moreover, effects of multiple inhibitors cannot be predicted by consideration of

NEW AVENUES IN DEVELOPMENTAL
CANCER CHEMOTHERAPY

3

the sequential or concurrent relationship of their sites of action (3,4) but are determined by the topographical and cybernetic configuration of the entire pathway. The order of administration of drugs may determine whether synergism or antagonism is obtained. Because the effects of inhibitors on complex pathways cannot be readily explained by a small number of general rules, the technique of kinetic modeling has been applied to specific problems. The first application of computer modeling to the biochemical pharmacology of antimetabolites was the pioneering work of Werkheiser and associates (4,22,23), which included studies of antifolates and ribonucleotide reductase inhibitors, two classes of antimetabolites that continue to be of great interest. Results obtained with some of these earlier models have been reviewed by Jackson and Harrap (5,12) and Grindey and Cheng (3). Although many early antimetabolites were primarily antileukemic agents with poor activity against solid tumors, newer antimetabolites (and new protocols for old drugs such as methotrexate) have shown more activity against solid tumors. Thus it seems likely that antimetabolites will continue to be a valuable class of anticancer agents. It is probable that the near future will see the development of novel antimetabolites that act as very specific inhibitors of regulatory molecules, including oncogene products (a possible example might be guanosine triphosphate (GTP) analogs that bind the GTP site of *ras*-p21). The understanding of antimetabolite action on cellular regulatory processes will therefore continue to be an important part of anticancer drug pharmacology.

In this chapter, some of the contributions of kinetic simulation to the understanding of anticancer drug effects will be illustrated by considering five specific questions that have been approached through this technique.

1. If methotrexate is a stoichiometric inhibitor of dihydrofolate reductase, why is free cellular methotrexate required for effective inhibition?

2. If sequential blockade does not cause synergism, why do sulfa drugs give synergistic interaction with trimethoprim?

3. Which is the more appropriate target for cancer chemotherapy: an enzyme whose activity is decreased in tumors, relative to normal tissues, or a proliferation and transformation-linked enzyme with elevated activity in tumors?

4. When purine nucleotide synthesis is blocked, why does the inhibition of DNA synthesis correlate more closely with depletion of the GTP pool than with depletion of the dGTP pool?

5. Can we explain the high antitumor selectivity, in sensitive systems, of inhibitors of inosine 5'-phosphate (IMP) dehydrogenase?

All these questions involve interesting features of the regulation of metabolic pathways that are not intuitively obvious but that are clearly illuminated by the technique of kinetic simulation. Finally, to enable the curious or skeptical reader to repeat some of the calculations, the Appendix gives an annotated listing of a simple program used to simulate the pathways studied in case study number 3.

II. Case Study Number 1: The Reversible Interaction of Methotrexate with Dihydrofolate Reductase

Early studies in which the kinetics of inhibition of dihydrofolate reductase by such compounds as methotrexate were examined in isolated enzyme systems resulted in several misunderstandings. The inhibition appeared to be noncompetitive with dihydrofolate; it appeared to be stoichiometric and essentially irreversible. However, these isolated enzyme studies did not appear to predict very accurately the behavior of methotrexate within intact cells. For example, if the activity of thymidylate synthase in cells is monitored by following incorporation of tritiated deoxyuridine into DNA, the reaction is inhibited by methotrexate, with a time course that corresponds to elimination of free dihydrofolate reductase in cells. If cells are then washed, however, incorporation of deoxyuridine into DNA resumes rapidly, showing that the inhibition is freely reversible. Moreover, effective inhibition by methotrexate appears to require the presence of free inhibitor (i.e., inhibitor that is not bound to dihydrofolate reductase) within the cells, which appears to be incompatible with a tight-binding inhibition mechanism. The apparent noncompetitive mechanism of methotrexate inhibition of dihydrofolate reductase was readily explicable by the fact that competitive, tight-binding inhibitors do not display the same close dependence on substrate concentration as do conventional competitive inhibitors. However, the other anomalies were less readily explained. Various hypotheses were advanced, such as the suggestion that dihydrofolate reductase might have different kinetic properties within the cell from those observed in purified preparations (or even in crude cell homogenates). The fact that inhibition of growth of cells by methotrexate correlated with the appearance of free inhibitor within cells was quoted as evidence that the true site of action of methotrexate was some enzyme other than dihydrofolate reductase; thymidylate synthetase appeared to be a favorite candidate, despite the fact that the K_i of methotrexate was about six orders of magnitude weaker than its K_i for dihydrofolate reductase. An early kinetic model of folate metabolism (11) showed that when the properties of the whole system were taken into account, the observed effects of methotrexate were compatible with its primary mechanism being its high-affinity interaction with dihydrofolate reductase. An important feature of the pathway in which dihydrofolate is oxidized and reduced is the fact that in all cells in which accurate measurements are available, activity of dihydrofolate reductase is in great excess over activity of the rate-limiting enzyme of the cycle, thymidylate synthetase. This non-rate-limiting role of dihydrofolate reductase determines the response of the thymidylate cycle to tight-binding inhibitors of dihydrofolate reductase. Some of the properties of the system are illustrated by Fig. 1. The system is initially in an uninhibited steady state such that the dihydrofolate concentration is very low, 10-HCO-FH_4 is fairly high, and the other folate cofactors have intermediate concentrations. When methotrexate (1 μM) is added to the system, it cannot equilibrate immediately within cells, because it requires facilitated transport. Consider the events of the first 15 min after addition of inhibitor. As methotrexate enters the cell, because of its high affinity for dihydrofolate reductase, it binds tightly to the enzyme, and at this stage intracellular methotrexate is almost entirely enzyme-bound. This titration of dihydrofolate reductase by methotrexate decreases the effective V_{max} of the enzyme. Since dihydrofolate is now being produced faster than it is reduced, the dihydrofolate pool starts to increase. However, at this point the dihydrofolate pool size is two or three orders of magnitude below the tetrahydrofolate pool size, so that the

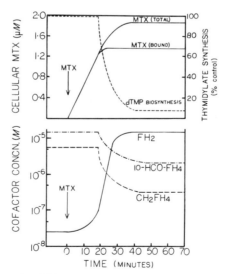

Fig. 1. The effect of addition of methotrexate (1 μM) to the medium on folate metabolism in L1210 cells. The upper figure shows enzyme-bound and total cellular methotrexate and the predicted rate of dTMP biosynthesis. The lower figure shows cellular concentrations of some folate cofactors.

accumulation of dihydrofolate has a negligible effect on the concentration of 5,10-methylenetetrahydrofolate, and the rate of thymidylate biosynthesis does not change. Despite the partial inhibition of dihydrofolate reductase, the rate of dihydrofolate reduction can still keep pace with the rate of tetrahydrofolate oxidation in the thymidylate synthetase reaction, i.e., the latter reaction remains rate-limiting. In many cell types it is possible to inhibit dihydrofolate reductase by 95% or more without altering the rate of biosynthesis of thymidylate (and hence of DNA). As dihydrofolate accumulates, the apparent K_i of methotrexate, $K_{i,app}$ which equals $K_{i,slope} \times (1 + S/K_m)$, becomes two to three orders of magnitude weaker. Eventually a stage is reached at which the dihydrofolate reductase has been inhibited to such an extent that it can no longer reduce dihydrofolate as fast as it is being produced in the thymidylate synthetase reaction. In other words, dihydrofolate reductase becomes rate-limiting for the cycle. In the simulation shown in Fig. 1, this occurred about 17 min after addition of methotrexate to the medium. At this point, the rate of dihydrofolate reduction, and consequently the tetrahydrofolate pools, begin to fall rapidly. The rates of thymidylate and purine biosynthesis also fall. The rate of accumulation of dihydrofolate accelerates. Dihydrofolate reductase is now more than 95% titrated by methotrexate, so the bound methotrexate in the cell does not increase much further. Instead, free methotrexate now appears inside the cell. When the free methotrexate has accumulated to such an extent that its rate of efflux from the cell equals the rate of uptake of extracellular methotrexate, the system settles at a new, inhibited steady state. This steady state is characterized by high cellular dihydrofolate, decreased pools of tetrahydrofolates, and decreased production of thymidylate and purines. Dihydrofolate reductase is almost entirely inhibited, although depending upon the value of the K_i and the degree of dihydrofolate accumulation, a small amount of free dihydrofolate reductase will be in equilibrium with the free methotrexate and the enzyme–inhibitor complex. A significant amount of free methotrexate will be present within the cell. For the system depicted in Fig. 1, this inhibited steady state was reached at about 40 min.

If extracellular methotrexate is now removed, the accumulated dihydrofolate, coupled with the fairly high "k_{off}" (inhibitor dissociation rate constant) results in rapid reactivation of the inhibited enzyme, and incorporation of deoxyuridine into DNA will resume. This reactivation continues until a point is reached at which dihydrofolate reductase activity again becomes greater than that of thymidylate synthetase. When this happens, dihydrofolate is now being used faster than it is produced, and its concentration starts to fall. The apparent K_i of methotrexate then becomes lower, and the net rate of loss of methotrexate from the cell suddenly decreases. The cell is now left with the so-called nonexchangeable methotrexate, which is almost entirely bound to dihydrofolate reductase. The cell also contains about 5% of uninhibited dihydrofolate reductase, so that thymidylate synthetase is rate-limiting for thymidylate production.

From this study (11) it may be concluded that the observed inhibition behavior, at the cellular level, is explained by a single high-affinity site of action of methotrexate. That free cellular inhibitor is necessary reflects the fact that in the inhibited steady state with excess dihydrofolate present, the inhibition of dihydrofolate reductase by methotrexate is not stoichiometric. In the absence of free inhibitor the system assumes a state in which there is sufficient free dihydrofolate reductase for the cell to resume DNA synthesis (11,24,25).

III. Case Study Number 2: Kinetics of the Synergistic Interaction of Sulfa Drugs with Trimethoprim

A number of reports from the early days of combination chemotherapy claimed that the use of pairs of drugs with sequential sites of action should result in synergistic drug effects, and a few mathematical studies using improbable and unrealistic assumptions and sometimes even erroneous mathematics, provided specious theoretical support for this misconception. The fact that sulfa drugs, which inhibit biosynthesis of dihydrofolate in bacteria, and trimethoprim, which inhibits reduction of dihydrofolate to the active tetrahydrofolate form, are in fact markedly synergistic reinforced the concept that sequential blockade was always an advantageous mode of drug combination. More rigorous experimental and mathematical studies, reviewed in Refs. 3–6, approached the questions: Does sequential blockade cause synergism? If not, why do sulfa drugs give synergistic interaction with trimethoprim? The major conclusions from these studies were as follows: (1) for an unbranched monolinear system, in an inhibited steady state, sequential use of inhibitors cannot result in inhibition greater than that caused by the inhibitor of the rate-limiting enzyme acting alone (3–5); (2) during the kinetic transient phase, combined effects of sequential inhibitors may be greater than the effects of the separate inhibitors (5); (3) in branched pathways, in which inhibitors straddle a divergent branch point, combined steady-state inhibitor effects may be independent (additive), antagonistic, or synergistic, depending upon parameter values (3–5); (4) in a simple, monolinear chain in which feedback regulation operates, the combined effects of sequential inhibitors could be antagonistic, additive, or synergistic (3,4); and (5) consideration of the system of a linear sequence feeding into a cycle predicted that inhibitors of the linear pathway should be synergistic with inhibitors of the cycle (3,4,6).

To demonstrate that the known kinetics of the multienzyme system were compatible with a synergistic interaction of sulfa drugs (such as sulfamethoxazole) and dihydrofolate reductase inhibitors (such as trimethoprim) the simplified pathway shown in Fig. 2 was modeled. In this model, dihydrofolate is cyclically reduced by dihydrofolate reductase (v_1) and oxidized by thymidylate synthase (v_3). Dihydrofolate is synthesized by a linear pathway feeding into the cycle (v_0). The v_0 reaction is inhibited by sulfamethoxazole, and v_1 is inhibited by trimethoprim. Dihydrofolate causes product inhibition of the v_0 reaction; this feature was introduced to model the effect of various constraints upon the input to the system, and its presence or absence did not affect the qualitative properties of the model. The divergent branch points at dihydrofolate and tetrahydrofolate (reactions v_4 and v_2, respectively) reflect the fact that a growing system is being modeled, so that folate cofactors are being constantly removed in the process of cell division. In the steady state, $v_2 + v_4 = v_0$, and without some "sink" for folates, no steady state would be possible for the system unless v_0 was also zero. The activity of the cycle was assessed by the rate of reaction v_3, which produces thymidylate, necessary for DNA synthesis and cell division. When concentrations of sulfamethoxazole and trimethoprim, singly or in combination, required to give 50% inhibition of v_3 were calculated, the results were compatible with synergistic interaction of the two drugs. These data are shown in isobologram form in Fig. 3.

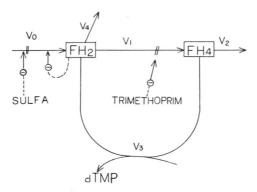

Fig. 2. Pathways of dihydrofolate biosynthesis and oxidoreduction in bacteria and sites of inhibitors as modeled by program SIM1 (see Appendix).

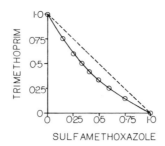

Fig. 3. Isobologram for interaction of trimethoprim and sulfamethoxazole, as modeled by program SIM1.

IV. Case Study Number 3: Key Enzymes as Targets for Selective Anticancer Agents

The target molecules for anticancer drugs are, in general, not qualitatively different between normal and malignantly transformed cells, and the selectivity of such drugs resides at a higher level of organization, namely, the regulation of the target pathways. For example, the dihydrofolate reductase of malignant cells is not different from that of untransformed cells, but the malignant cell reacts more drastically to inhibition of its dihydrofolate reductase by antifolate drugs such as methotrexate. Although activity of some enzymes appears to show random alterations in tumors, rate-controlling enzymes of several pathways are systematically increased or decreased in tumors (20,21). Thus, adenosine kinase activity tends to be low in many kinds of tumors, both murine and human (10,14), while activity of IMP dehydrogenase is frequently elevated (17).

There has been controversy over the predictive value of such transformation-linked enzyme activity changes for sensitivity to antimetabolites. Which is the more appropriate target for cancer chemotherapy: an enzyme whose activity is decreased in tumors, relative to normal tissues, or a proliferation and transformation-linked enzyme, with elevated activity in tumors? Two contradictory arguments have been extended: (a) if a particular enzyme has low activity in a certain tumor, relative to normal tissues, then inhibition of that enzyme should have a proportionately greater effect in the tumor, with resulting antitumor selectivity; and (b) proliferation and transformation-linked increases in enzyme activity indicate that the tumor has a particularly high requirement for that activity, so that enzyme should be a sensitive target for anticancer agents. Both these statements appear intuitively logical, but they are mutually contradictory. Which is correct?

As support for case (a), the example of N-(phosphonoacetyl)-L-aspartic acid (PALA) has been quoted (18). PALA inhibits the aspartate transcarbamylase reaction of the pyrimidine biosynthetic complex. The activity of this complex correlates with tumor growth rate, and PALA tends to be more active against some of the slowly growing tumors. Supporting case (b), one may cite such enzymes as ribonucleotide reductase, thymidylate synthase, and IMP dehydrogenase, all of which are particularly increased in rapidly growing tumors, and all of which are effective targets for anticancer drugs, even in rapidly growing tumors.

Attempting to study this question by kinetic simulation forces us first of all to define the problem more precisely. For case (a), what is meant by low activity of an enzyme in tumors? It is necessary to distinguish two situations: (1) the enzyme is a non-rate-limiting enzyme, whose activity decreases in tumors as compared to normal tissues, e.g., adenylate kinase; and (2) the enzyme is a rate-limiting enzyme, whose activity correlates with growth rate and is thus lower in slowly growing tumors than in rapidly growing tumors. Are slowly growing tumors more sensitive to inhibitors of this enzyme? Similarly, two situations may be distinguished for case (b): (1) the enzyme is a non-rate-limiting enzyme that is overproduced in certain tumors; this situation frequently arises in drug-resistant lines, e.g., overproduction of dihydrofolate reductase in methotrexate-resistant tumors, in which high target enzme activity is clearly associated with decreased drug sensitivity; and (2) the enzyme is a rate-limiting enzyme, whose activity is correlated with growth rate.

Consideration of the rate equation for simple competitive inhibition [Eq. (1)] shows that the molar enzyme concentration E does not appear in the equation

$$v_i = (V_{max} \cdot S/K_m)/(1 + S/K_m + I/K_i) \tag{1}$$

Thus, the percentage of inhibition at a given inhibitor concentration should be independent of the activity of the target enzyme. For tight-binding competitive inhibition, however, as described by the Morrison equation [Eq. (2)], the activity in the presence of an inhibitor is an explicit function of molar enzyme concentration. In Eqs. (1) and (2), v_0 refers to the uninhibited rate of an enzyme reaction at substrate concentration S, and v_i is the inhibited rate at inhibitor concentration I. E_t is the total molar concentration of enzyme. K_i refers to the $K_{i,slope}$ value for a competitive inhibitor, and V_{max} and K_m have their usual meaning. In Eq. (2) $K_{i,app}$ is defined as $K_{i,slope} \cdot (1 + S/K_m)$:

$$v_i = v_0/2E_t \left[(E_t - K_{i,app} - I) + \sqrt{(E_t - K_{i,app} - I)^2 + 4K_{i,app}E_t} \right] \tag{2}$$

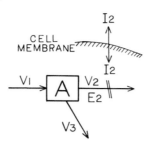

Fig. 4.   Inhibition of a rate-limiting enzyme by an inhibitor (I2) that requires membrane transport.

The validity of these suggestions that percentage of inhibition of the activity of a pathway should be independent of target enzyme concentration for a conventional competitive inhibitor but dependent upon target enzyme concentration for a tight-binding inhibitor was tested by kinetic simulation of the simple model pathway shown in Fig. 4. In this system, the enzyme E2 is the target for inhibitor I2. Substrate A is produced at rate v_1; substrate A is then utilized by two competing reactions, v_2 (catalyzed by E2) and v_3. The v_3 branch must be introduced into the model because without this branch, the rate of v_2 in the steady state would always equal v_1, even in the presence of a competitive inhibitor. Table I summarizes the results of a number of simulations with this model. Consider first simulations 1–3. In these calculations, v_1 was assumed to remain constant while E2 (and thus VM2, the V_{max} for reaction 2) increased. The rate of reaction 2 increased approximately fivefold for a tenfold increase in VM2, consistent with the rate-determining role of E2 for this pathway. Simulations 4–6 show the effect of the presence of a constant concentration of a competitive inhibitor of E1 on the system at different levels of E1. Note that the percentage of inhibition of v_2 was greater than when VM2 was lowest, contrary to what would have been expected from considering the rate equation for v_2 in isolation from the rest of the system. The reason for this is that, other things being equal, when VM2 is low, the ratio v_3/v_2 is greater, so that substrate A will accumulate less, giving less competition with I_2 and consequently more inhibition.

Simulations 1–6 considered the situation in which v_1 was constant. However, in many tumors, the activity of several enzymes in a pathway will show coordinate changes. This is the case in the pyrimidine *de novo* biosynthetic pathway. When aspartate transcarbamylase, the target enzyme for PALA, is increased, the initial enzyme of the pathway, carbamyl phosphate synthetase II (which is part of the same multienzyme complex) increases in proportion. This situation was modeled in simula-

TABLE I

Simulation of the Effects of a Single Inhibitor on a Branched Pathway at Different Levels of the Target Enzyme[a]

Simu- lation no.	v_1	VM2	I2 (total)	I2 (free)	Mechanism of inhibition[b]	v_2 Units	v_2 Percentage of control
1	3	2	0		—	0.44	100
2	3	8	0		—	1.28	100
3	3	20	0		—	2.00	100
4	3	2	3.012		Comp	0.19	42.5
5	3	8	3.012		Comp	0.64	50.0
6	3	20	3.012		Comp	1.23	61.4
7	0.75	2	0		—	0.13	100
8	3	8	0		—	1.28	100
9	7.5	20	0		—	4.72	100
10	0.75	2	3.012		Comp	0.05	39.1
11	3	8	3.012		Comp	0.64	50.0
12	7.5	20	3.012		Comp	2.90	61.5
13	3	2	0.424		TBI	0.16	36
14	3	8	0.424		TBI	0.64	50
15	3	20	0.424		TBI	1.46	73
16	0.75	2	0.424		TBI	0.043	33
17	3	8	0.424		TBI	0.64	50
18	7.7	20	0.424		TBI	3.36	71
19	3	2	0.3315	0.3012	TBI	0.19	42.5
20	3	8	0.424	0.3012	TBI	0.64	50.0
21	3	20	0.6144	0.3012	TBI	1.23	61.4
22	0.75	2	0.3337	0.3012	TBI	0.05	39.1
23	3	8	0.424	0.3012	TBI	0.64	50.0
24	7.5	20	0.5865	0.3012	TBI	2.90	61.5

[a] K_1 values were 1.5 nM (competitive inhibitor) and 0.15 nM (tight-binding inhibitor). Other variables were as shown in the program listing (see Appendix).
[b] Comp, conventional competitive inhibition; TBI, tight-binding inhibition.

tions 7–12. Once again, the degree of inhibition of the pathway was greatest for low values of VM2. The fact that the degree of inhibition of this pathway by a constant inhibitor concentration should vary with absolute enzyme activity even when the ratio of v_1 to VM2 is constant may seem contrary to intuition. However, it should be remembered that the K_m of E2 does not change in proportion with VM2. From these simulations we concluded that even a simple competitive inhibitor may have a proportionately greater inhibitory effect in tissues which contain relatively low activity of a key target enzyme.

Considering the situation in which I2 was a tight-binding inhibitor, simulations 13–15 (Table I) show inhibition of various levels of E2 by a constant amount of I2, with v_1 constant. Simulations 16–18 represent tight-binding inhibition of E2 when v_1 varies in proportion with VM2. In both instances, the percentage of inhibition was greater for a low level of E2. Note that the variation in v_2 in the presence of constant inhibitor concentration and varying values of VM2 was greater for a tight-binding inhibitor than for a conventional competitive inhibitor (i.e., the spread between percentage of control values of v_2 was greater between simulations 16 and 18 than it was between simulations 10 and 12).

Simulations 13–18 assumed a constant total concentration of inhibitor (i.e., free plus enzyme-bound inhibitor). However, if the situation within a cell is considered for an inhibitor that enters cells by passive diffusion or by a rapid, reversible transport mechanism, the system will reach a steady state when the free inhibitor within the cell (not the total inhibitor) equals the extracellular inhibitor concentration. Simulations 19–21 show the effects of tight-binding inhibitor at total concentrations such that the free inhibitor levels are constant in the presence of varying levels of E2. Note that the values of v_2 predicted by simulations 19–21 are exactly the same as predicted by simulations 4–6, respectively, for a corresponding amount of a conventional competitive inhibitor. Similarly, simulations 22–24, in which v_1 varied in proportion to VM2, gave identical results with simulations 10–12. Thus, although the kinetic effects of tight-binding inhibitors on isolated enzymes differ from the kinetics of conventional competitive inhibitors, when the whole system is considered, the effects of the two classes of inhibitors are identical.

A version of the model was also used to address the question of the effects of inhibitors on non-rate-limiting enzymes in relation to the activity of those enzymes. Functionally, non-rate-limiting enzymes are of two classes: those that catalyze a reversible reaction, and those that catalyze an irreversible reaction. An enzyme with high activity that catalyzes both directions of a reversible reaction will maintain a state close to thermodynamic equilibrium between its substrates (products). Clearly, moderate degrees of inhibition of such an enzyme will not alter the function of the pathway in any significant way. An example of this kind of enzyme is nucleoside diphosphokinase. The situation is different for those enzymes which, although not normally rate-limiting in their pathway, catalyze an irreversible reaction. The effects of inhibition of such an enzyme were studied using the model illustrated in Fig. 5. Results of some of these simulations are summarized in Table II. Simulations 1–3 show the steady-state rates of v_4 for the uninhibited system at three levels of E4. A tenfold increase in VM4 caused a less than 3% change in v_4, consistent with the

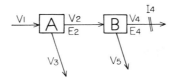

Fig. 5. Inhibition of a non-rate-limiting enzyme in a branched pathway.

non-rate-limiting role of E4 in this pathway. This was also demonstrated by the fact that, to give 50% inhibition of the flux through the pathway, a large excess of I4 was required, and this was associated with extensive accumulation of substrate B. In this system, a constant inhibitor concentration gave a proportionately greater effect when E4 was low (simulations 4–6, Table II). Dihydrofolate reductase is an example of a non-rate-limiting enzyme that catalyzes an essentially irreversible reaction; it shows that as predicted by the model, such enzymes may be effective targets for inhibition, that enzyme overproduction results in relative insensitivity to inhibition, and that low activity of such enzymes in target tissues confers partial selectivity upon inhibitors.

The conclusions of this study are thus: (1) both rate-limiting enzymes and those non-rate-limiting enzymes that catalyze irreversible reactions may be effective targets for inhibition; (2) for both conventional competitive inhibitors and tight-binding irreversible inhibitors, low activity of the target enzyme in a cell is associated with greater sensitivity to inhibition; and (3) the relationship between susceptibility to inhibition and target

TABLE II

Simulation of the Effects of an Inhibitor of a Non-Rate-Limiting Enzyme in a Branched Reaction Pathway[a]

| Simulation no. | VM4 | I4 | Steady-state levels of | | V4 | |
			A	B	Units	Percentage of control
1	20	0	0.954	0.199	1.242	100
2	80	0	0.954	0.048	1.272	100
3	200	0	0.954	0.019	1.278	100
4	20	200	0.954	5.125	0.251	19.6
5	80	200	0.954	3.232	0.636	50.0
6	200	200	0.954	1.847	0.912	73.4

[a] Calculations were performed using the program listed in the Appendix, with I2 set to zero.

enzyme activity is similar for conventional competitive inhibitors and tight-binding competitive inhibitors. The fact that the relatively slow-growing B16 melanoma and Lewis lung carcinoma are more sensitive to PALA than are the more rapidly growing murine leukemias may indeed be related to the activity of aspartate transcarbamylase being lower in more slowly dividing cells.

The question thus arises: Why are inhibitors of proliferation-linked enzymes such as ribonucleotide reductase, thymidylate synthase, and IMP dehydrogenase such effective drugs? Since these enzymes are rate-limiting for their respective pathways, clearly they are sensitive sites for inhibition. What is not so clear is why inhibitors of these enzymes tend to be particularly effective against rapidly growing cells. This question may perhaps not be answerable by consideration of enzyme kinetics alone. These enzymes are associated with the S-phase of the cell cycle, and their inhibitors tend to be selectively toxic to proliferating cells. However, normal tissues and slowly growing tumors often contain noncycling cells which are highly refractory to cell cycle phase-specific agents. The B16 and Lewis lung tumors happen to be relatively slow-growing tumors with a low noncycling cell fraction, and this may explain the selectivity of PALA toward these tumors.

V. Case Study Number 4: Shutdown of DNA Synthesis by Modulation of Ribonucleoside Diphosphate Pools

Several of the kinetic models of anticancer drug action have simulated the inhibition of key enzymes leading to synthesis of tumor cell DNA. The early model of Werkheiser, Grindey, and Moran (22,23) included expressions for the key enzymes DNA polymerase, ribonucleotide reductase, dCMP (deoxycytidine 5'-monophosphate) deaminase and thymidylate synthase and studied combinations of inhibitors of these enzymes. Many of the responses of nucleotide pools to inhibition, as predicted by this model, were unexpected; often, the response of the system to inhibition was determined primarily by the complex regulatory properties of ribonucleotide reductase. An almost identidal model studied by Nicolini et al. (19) confirmed many of the earlier conclusions. A model studied by Jackson et al. (7–9,16) included expressions for the same enzymes and, in addition, for several deoxyribonucleoside kinases. Besides the antimetabolite effects, this model was used to predict effects of nucleosides, such as thymidine, deoxyadenosine, and deoxyguanosine. Excess salvage deoxyribonucleosides, in general, tended to be more disruptive than noncompetitive inhibitors of ribonucleotide reductase. The latter, in moderate amounts, gave inhibited steady states, whereas even quite small amounts of the former often caused undamped oscillations and total shutdown (9).

Another way in which the deoxyribonucleoside triphosphate pools of cells and, hence, the rate of DNA synthesis may be modulated is through manipulation of the ribonucleoside diphosphate pools. The model indicated that, for moderate degrees of perturbation, the rate of DNA synthesis was relatively independent of the ribonucleoside diphosphate pool size. For example, a 45% reduction in cytidine diphosphate (CDP) was predicted to result in only 14% inhibition of DNA synthesis, and a 45% depletion of adenosine diphosphate (ADP) caused only 3% inhibition of DNA synthesis. When the effect of reducing the CDP pool to 46% of the normal level was simulated, the system did not reach a steady state but went into stable, undamped oscillations, with a period of 18 min (9). The rate of DNA synthesis varied from 45 to 92% of the control. When CDP was decreased further to 40% of the control, the system went into unstable oscillations and approached a shutdown state, with DNA synthesis close to zero. Similarly, decreasing the ADP pool to 40% of its normal value also resulted in unstable oscillations and shutdown.

Interest in the effect of decreasing guanosine diphosphate (GDP) on the rate of DNA synthesis was prompted by a report of Cohen et al. (2) that when purine nucleotide synthesis was blocked, e.g., with mycophenolic acid, inhibition of DNA synthesis correlated more closely with the pool size of GTP than with depletion of the dGTP pool. Cohen et al. speculated that GTP may have some as yet unknown function in the control of DNA synthesis. However, since GDP pools are likely to correlate closely with GTP, it is possible that an effect similar to that described by the model for depletion of CDP or ADP could be operating. If decreased GDP resulted in oscillations of the deoxyribonucleoside triphosphate pools and in decreased DNA synthesis, and since the oscillations, if not synchronized between cells, would not be detected by experimental measurement, the rate of DNA synthesis could appear to be unrelated to the oscillating dGTP pool but to follow the pool of GDP and, hence, that of GTP. Moreover, when the Michaelis constants of ribonucleotide reductase for ADP and GDP are compared with the respective pool sizes, it is seen that for Novikoff hepatoma cells, $ADP/K_m = 5.1$, and $GDP/K_m = 1.7$, so that the GDP reductase reaction is relatively much less saturated with its substrate than is the ADP reductase reaction. This could indicate that depletion of GDP may be even more likely to result in unstable oscillations and shutdown of DNA synthesis than would depletion of ADP. While this hypothesis remains an attractive possibility in that it would explain the effects of such compounds as mycophenolic acid and tiazo-

TABLE III

Effect of Modulation of the Cellular GDP Pool on Deoxyribonucleoside Triphosphate Pools and DNA Synthesis[a]

GDP		dGTP (μM)	dATP (μM)	dCTP (μM)	dTTP (μM)	DNA synthesis (% Control)
μM	(% Control)					
110	(100)	7.01	9.56	8.88	29.53	100
77	(70)	6.92	9.24	10.18	32.85	102
66	(60)	7.17	7.81	10.79	35.93	104
44	(40)	6.95	6.42	12.98	41.71	103
27.5	(25)	3.74	5.05	27.85	96.45	95
15	(14)	0.02	187.0	28.27	462.1	0.3
11	(10)	0.01	260.0	27.30	478.5	0.1

[a] Simulations were run using the model described previously (9).

furin on DNA synthesis in relation to nucleotide pool perturbations without the necessity of postulating unknown effects of GTP, this concept has not been supported by the simulation studies carried out to date.

The results of seven simulation runs are summarized in Table III. For these studies the model described in Ref. (9) was used. The system was assumed to be unihibited, and only the GDP concentration was varied. For decreases in GDP of up to 75%, the effect on the rate of DNA synthesis was not greater than 5%. Probably because dGTP is an obligatory activator of the ADP reductase reaction, decreased GDP reductase activity resulted in lower dATP concentrations. Since dATP is a general inhibitor of ribonucleotide reductase, this in turn caused greater activity of CDP reductase and uridine diphosphate (UDP) reductase and increased pools of deoxycytidine triphosphate (dCTP) and thymidine triphosphate (dTTP). Further depletion of GDP to 14% of the control level caused a dramatic qualitative change in the response of the system. As dGTP became rate-limiting for DNA synthesis, the adenosine triphosphate (dATP) pool, instead of declining further, began to accumulate. In this system, large upward changes in the dATP pool are invariably linked with shutdown of DNA synthesis (Table III).

Thus, according to the present model, decreasing the GDP pool to a certain threshold value causes little change either in dGTP or in DNA synthesis; beyond that threshold, dGTP drops rapidly, and DNA synthesis ceases. The extent to which the model faithfully represents the real situation in Novikoff cells and to which this behavior may vary between cell types must be determined by further study.

VI. Case Study Number 5: IMP Dehydrogenase Inhibitors and Multistability in the Purine Nucleotide Pathway

A number of recently developed antimetabolites, including tiazofurin and selenazofurin (1) are activated within target cells to analogs of nicotinamide adenine dinucleotide (NAD⁺) and in that form act as powerful inhibitors of IMP dehydrogenase. These drugs possess unusually high therapeutic indices against sensitive tumors; for example, tiazofurin is active against Lewis lung carcinoma at doses of 12.5 mg/kg (daily for 5 days), although the drug is tolerated at doses up to 1000 mg/kg (daily × 5). What is the explanation for this unusually high antitumor selectivity of IMP dehydrogenase inhibitors? Why are inhibitors of guanine nucleotide biosynthesis more effective antitumor agents than are inhibitors of adenine nucleotide biosynthesis? These questions were studied using a model of the key reactions and regulatory effects of purine nucleotide interconversions (Fig. 6) in the Novikoff rat hepatoma cell. Figure 6 shows the simplified model used in earlier studies, in which guanosine 5′-monophosphate (GMP) was considered to be produced from IMP in a single reaction. In a later, more detailed model, the xanthosine 5′-phosphate (XMP) pool was treated as a separate variable, and the IMP dehydrogenase and GMP synthetase reactions were modeled in detail. This later version of the model also included expressions for 5′-nucleotidase (AMP, XMP, and

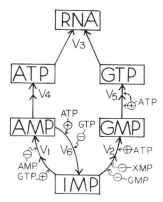

Fig. 6. Simplified model of purine ribonucleotide interconversions, showing sites of positive and negative regulation. The reactions are v_1, adenylosuccinate synthetase and adenylosuccinate lyase; v_2, IMP dehydrogenase and GMP synthetase; v_3, RNA polymerase; v_4, AMP kinase and ADP kinase; v_5, GMP kinase and GDP kinase; and v_6, AMP deaminase.

GMP phosphatases). The key regulatory features of this system are as follows: (1) GTP is a cosubstrate for adenylosuccinate synthetase, a rate-limiting enzyme of ATP biosynthesis; (2) ATP is a cosubstrate for GMP synthetase, a key enzyme of GTP synthesis; ATP is also required for the GMP kinase and GDP kinase reactions. This mutual requirement of ATP and GTP for the biosynthesis of each other constitutes a cross-catalytic relationship between the adenylate and guanylate branches; (3) In addition to this "cross-activation" there is "same-side" feedback inhibition of adenylosuccinate synthetase by AMP and of IMP dehydrogenase by GMP and XMP; (4) An additional regulatory feature of the pathway is the AMP deaminase reaction, which shows sigmoidal kinetics with respect to AMP. AMP deaminase is activated by ATP, which decreases the Hill coefficient for AMP, and is inhibited by GTP, which increases the Hill coefficient. In the model, all these regulatory features were included. Reactions were considered as taking place in homogeneous solution in a single cytosol compartment. The cell was treated as an open system that is normally at or near a steady state. The *de novo* purine biosynthetic pathway was considered as the source for the system, and nucleic acid biosynthesis was considered to be a purine sink.

Modeling this pathway, using kinetic parameters established experimentally for rat hepatoma cells, indicated a considerable rate of "futile cycling" of IMP to AMP via the adenylosuccinate synthetase and adenylosuccinase reactions and back to IMP through AMP deaminase. The latter enzyme, by virtue of its kinetic properties, tends to maintain a constant ratio of AMP to ATP (i.e., it is sensitive to adenylate energy charge), and it also regulates the ratio of adenylates to guanylates. Consider a cell in which the ratio of GTP to ATP is abnormally low: the release of AMP deaminase from GTP inhibition will cause increased breakdown of AMP to IMP (so less AMP will be available for ATP production). IMP is normally partitioned between production of adenylates and guanylates; however, conversion of IMP to AMP requires GTP, so at lower GTP concentration, proportionately more IMP is converted to guanylate. Conversely, under conditions of low ATP concentration, activation of AMP deaminase is less, and adenylates are conserved. The adenylate "futile cycle" and the regulatory sensitivity of AMP deaminase result in buffering of the adenylate pool and make it relatively difficult to block nucleic acid synthesis through selective inhibition of adenylate biosynthesis.

The steady-state behavior of the pathway is illustrated by Fig. 7. Consider first the upper portion of Fig. 7. The dashed line (marked $v_3 = v_4$) shows the steady-state rate of ATP production and utilization of ATP as a function of GTP concentration (the various rates of reactions shown in

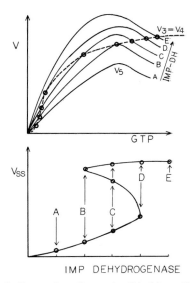

Fig. 7. Multistability in the purine ribonucleotide biosynthetic pathway. Upper figure: steady-state rates as a function of GTP concentration. Reaction rates are as defined in Fig. 6. Lower figure: steady states at different activities of IMP dehydrogenase.

Fig. 6). In the steady state, the ATP concentration will assume a value such that the rate of ATP production, v_4, is equal to the rate of ATP utilization, v_3. This line is a function of GTP concentration, because reaction v_4 depends upon reaction v_1, which is GTP dependent. The $v_3 = v_4$ line is sigmoidal, because of the effect of GTP on AMP deaminase; at low GTP concentration, AMP deaminase is relatively active and a high proportion of AMP will be deaminated. At higher GTP concentrations, AMP is produced more rapidly by v_1, and AMP deaminase is also inhibited, so that more AMP is converted to ATP. The dependence of ATP production on GTP concentration is thus higher order. The family of solid lines in Fig. 7 (top) marked v_5 represents the rate of GTP production. Reactions v_2 and v_5 are ATP dependent; however, since the steady-state ATP concentration is dependent upon GTP, v_5 can be plotted as a function of GTP. At high GTP concentrations, GMP is also high and causes product inhibition of v_2. Thus the v_5 curves pass through a maximum and decline at high GTP concentration. Figure 7 shows a family of such v_5 curves, representing different concentrations of IMP dehydrogenase. Where a v_5 curve intersects a $v_3 = v_4$ curve, both ATP and GTP are being produced and utilized at equal rates, so that the system as a whole is in a steady state (this simple model assumes that ATP and GTP are used in equal amounts for

RNA synthesis; changing this assumption would alter the details of the model but not the qualitative behavior). The steady-state points where $v_3 = v_4 = v_5$ are circled in Fig. 7 (top). The lower section of the figure plots these steady-state rates (v_{ss}) as a function of the IMP dehydrogenase activity. For a given activity of IMP dehydrogenase, there may be one, two, or three steady-state points. Where there are three, the middle one is unstable, for reasons that are explained in Ref. 9. Consider a cell with a high activity of IMP dehydrogenase: the system will be at point E (Fig. 7, bottom), so that only one steady state is possible, corresponding to a high rate of nucleic acid synthesis, v_{ss}. If IMP dehydrogenase is now inhibited, the system will move left along the upper limb of the curve, passing through the upper of the two points labeled D and the top one of the points labeled C and reaching the upper of the points marked B. Up to this point the rate of nucleic acid synthesis, v_{ss}, has not changed greatly. If IMP dehydrogenase is now inhibited further, the only way the system can achieve a steady state is by an abrupt transition to the lower limb of the curve, to the left of the lower point B. The rate of nucleic acid synthesis, v_{ss}, is now much lower. In this switching region, a small change in activity of IMP dehydrogenase has resulted in a dramatic decrease in synthesis of purines and nucleic acid. Further inhibition of IMP dehydrogenase will now result in the system moving left along the lower limb of the curve towards point A. Note that at these low levels of IMP dehydrogenase, only one steady state is possible for the system, corresponding to a low rate of nucleic acid synthesis. Now consider a system at the lower point B; if the activity of IMP dehydrogenase is increased, the system will move right along the lower limb of the curve, passing through the bottom of the three points marked C and reaching the lower point D. Up to this point, v_{ss} is comparatively low. If IMP dehydrogenase is now increased further, the only way the system can achieve a steady state is by an abrupt transition to the upper limb of the curve, with a resulting sudden increase in the rate of v_{ss}. Note that between points B and D, for a given activity of IMP dehydrogenase, the system may exist in either of two stable steady states, a "switched on" state, on the upper limb of the curve, or a "switched off" state, on the lower limb of the curve. This phenomenon is termed "multistability." Multistable systems have the following properties: (1) two or more stable steady states, separated by unstable steady states, (2) very high effective reaction orders in the switching regions, (3) they demonstrate hysteresis, and (4) they may exhibit oscillations. Requirements for multistability are autocatalysis or cross-catalysis, which is provided in the purine nucleotide pathway by the mutual requirements of ATP and GTP for synthesis of each other, and higher-order kinetics, which is introduced into this system by the properties of AMP deaminase.

It is clear from the preceding discussion that IMP dehydrogenase plays a critical role in the regulation of biosynthesis of purine nucleotides, according to the model. Experimental evidence for a regulatory role of IMP dehydrogenase is as follows: (1) IMP dehydrogenase has the lowest activity of all the enzymes of purine ribonucleotide biosynthesis in both resting and proliferating tissues; (2) IMP dehydrogenase shows the largest increase of all the purine ribonucleotide biosynthetic enzymes in hepatomas and regenerating liver, relative to normal liver; (3) unlike most other purine enzymes, IMP dehydrogenase correlates closely with growth rate in rat hepatomas (17); (4) in regenerating rat liver, IMP dehydrogenase activity increases earlier than any other enzyme studied, except for ornithine decarboxylase; and (5) IMP dehydrogenase inhibitors have an unusually high therapeutic index against some mouse tumors. The preceding analysis suggests that two kinds of steady states may be possible for the purine biosynthetic pathway in cells, a "switched off" state, with a low rate of purine biosynthesis sufficient for maintenance purposes in quiescent cells, and a "switched on" state, with a rapid rate of purine biosynthesis sufficient for cell proliferation in rapidly dividing cells. Quite small changes in the activity of IMP dehydrogenase may possibly trigger a quiescent cell into proliferation, as in the early stage of liver regeneration after partial hepatectomy. Conversely, a small degree of inhibition of IMP dehydrogenase may shut down a proliferating cell into the quiescent state. Note that in this scheme, the activity of IMP dehydrogenase controls not only the rate of guanylate nucleotides but also of adenylates.

To illustrate the properties of the purine model, a number of simulations were performed to examine the effects of inhibiting various enzymes in the pathway. Some results are shown in Figs. 8–12. When a metabolic network in a steady state is inhibited, there are three possible types of outcome: the system may achieve a new, uninhibited steady state; it may enter an inhibited steady state; or no steady state may be possible, and the system may oscillate or shut down. Figure 8 shows some data from a simulation of an abrupt, 50% inhibition of adenylosuccinate synthetase by an inhibitor such as alanosine or hadacidin. The model predicted a drop in concentration of AMP, with a resulting drop in ATP. This decrease in both substrate and activator of AMP deaminase resulted in inhibition of that enzyme, which tended to oppose further depletion of adenylates. There was essentially no change in adenylate charge. A minor, secondary drop in GTP and a moderate decrease in the rate of RNA synthesis occurred. Figure 9 shows a simulation of inhibition of AMP kinase. The model predicted a decrease in the pool of ATP and an increase in AMP, so that the adenylate charge was decreased, resulting in net depletion of adenylates. This caused increased IMP and XMP and an increase of the

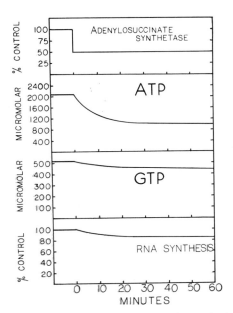

Fig. 8. Effect of a 50% decrease in activity of adenylosuccinate synthetase on pools of ATP and GTP and the rate of RNA synthesis.

GTP:ATP ratio, with resulting net inhibition of AMP deaminase. Thus AMP deaminase again had a buffering effect on the system. The rate of RNA synthesis was essentially unchanged. Tubercidin 5′-phosphate is an example of an inhibitor of AMP kinase which might be expected to produce such effects.

The predicted effects of inhibition of AMP deaminase are shown in Fig. 10. Coformycin 5′-phosphate is an example of an inhibitor of this enzyme. Inhibition of AMP deaminase resulted in increased AMP and ATP pools, which causes a compensatory activation of AMP deaminase (again demonstrating its great buffering power). A new steady state resulted with a slightly increased ATP:GTP ratio. The rate of RNA synthesis was essentially unaltered.

Figure 11 shows the predicted effect of 50% inhibition of GMP synthetase, as might be caused by inhibitors such as acivicin or oxanosine. The GTP pool was extensively depleted. The system contains some buffering capacity, because of buildup in the concentration of XMP, which is normally very low. However, the system was not completely buffered, since some conversion of XMP to xanthosine occurs. The extensive inhibition

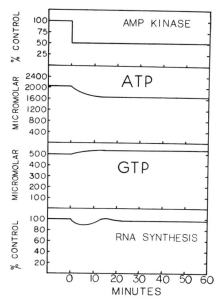

Fig. 9.   Effect of a 50% decrease in activity of AMP kinase on pools of ATP and GTP and the rate of RNA synthesis.

of GTP production caused a secondary drop in the ATP pool and a pronounced drop in RNA synthesis.

Inhibition of IMP dehydrogenase, e.g., by the active metabolite of tiazofurin, is illustrated in Fig. 12. Note that the degree of inhibition in this study was only 20%. The simulation predicted decreased XMP, GMP, and GTP, with a secondary drop in the steady-state ATP pool. The release of AMP deaminase from inhibition resulted in an elevated IMP pool. The great sensitivity of the system to inhibition of IMP dehydrogenase indicates that substoichiometric amounts of inhibitor may trigger a switch from the proliferating to the quiescent state. Excess inhibitor may make a steady state impossible.

In summary, the simulations illustrated in Figs. 8–12 showed that IMP dehydrogenase gave the most marked response to inhibitors. The results of inhibition of GMP synthetase were similar but less sensitive than inhibition of IMP dehydrogenase. Inhibition of adenylosuccinate sythetase was considerably less effective in shutting down nucleic acid synthesis, and inhibition of AMP kinase or AMP deaminase had very little effect on the rate of nucleic acid synthesis. Clearly the adenylate branch of the purine

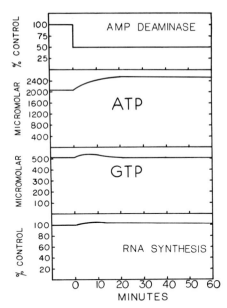

Fig. 10. Effect of a 50% decrease in activity of AMP deaminase on pools of ATP and GTP and the rate of RNA synthesis.

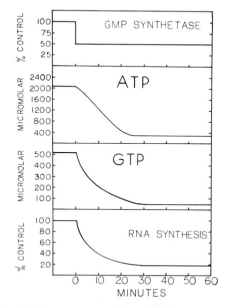

Fig. 11. Effect of a 50% decrease in activity of GMP synthetase on pools of ATP and GTP and the rate of RNA synthesis.

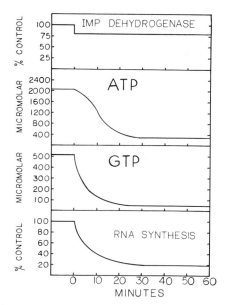

Fig. 12. Effect of a 20% decrease in activity of IMP dehydrogenase on pools of ATP and GTP and the rate of RNA synthesis.

pathway is much less sensitive to inhibition than the guanylate branch, and this is in large part due to the buffering effect of the AMP deaminase reaction. The potential for multistability in the purine pathways is also partly a consequence of AMP deaminase. As yet there is no convincing experimental evidence for the existence of multiple steady states in the purine ribonucleotide pools. However, the present study has shown that this behavior is kinetically possible, and the unusual sensitivity of certain tumor systems to inhibition of IMP dehydrogenase is consistent with the purine pathway being involved in the regulation of cell proliferation by this mechanism in at least some cell types.

VII. Conclusions: Kinetic Simulation as a Tool for Anticancer Drug Development

The case studies just presented exemplify the kind of problems that may be studied using kinetic stimulation. The technique can make helpful contributions at several stages of drug development. During the earliest stage of the drug design process, kinetic models may be used to predict answers to such questions as (1) In a particular metabolic pathway, which enzymes represent the most sensitive sites for inhibition? (2) For a particular site, how tightly need an inhibitor bind, to shut down the pathway? (3) For an enzyme with multiple ligand-binding sites (e.g., IMP dehydrogenase, ribonucleotide reductase), which site is the most effective one to block?

Most applications of kinetic simulation to date have been in the field of biochemical pharmacology. Such studies have included the prediction of effects of antimetabolites on precursor pools, the identification of control points and rate-limiting steps, and studies on the effects of salvage metabolites and on the optimization of drug selectivity (7). Where an inhibitor has multiple sites of action, kinetic modeling studies have been used to predict, for given metabolite pool sizes and kinetic parameters, which target enzyme will be the primary site of action (13) and at which point the rate-limiting site may shift when one target is overproduced because of gene amplification (15). In studies of antitumor drug resistance, kinetic models have been used to predict the quantitative effect of changes in drug transport parameters, the consequence of target enzyme overproduction, the quantitative results of changes in K_i values for target enzyme–drug interactions, and the effects of partial deletion of drug-activating enzymes (such as kinases or phosphoribosyltransferases).

Perhaps the most complex aspect of anticancer drug pharmacology is the prediction and understanding of the effects of combination chemotherapy. Computer simulation can make important contributions in suggesting effective combinations from the enormous number of possible combinations that could be selected from the available active agents. Modeling may assist in predicting and understanding synergistic and antagonistic drug–drug interactions. Other kinetic modeling studies that have been described have studied the time-sequence dependence of drug combinations and the optimization of rescue protocols (7). Because in clinical cancer chemotherapy anticancer agents are almost invariably used in combination, and because it is totally impractical to test more than a small fraction of all possible combination protocols even in experimental tumor systems, much less in clinical trials, the optimization of combination chemotherapy is likely to become one of the most important aspects of computer modeling of chemotherapy.

In many aspects of experimental chemotherapy, much misdirected effort could be avoided, misleading data interpretations prevented, and scarce resources more productively employed if major experimental projects were to be preceded by the rigorous definition of a problem required to create a computer model. The mental exercise involved in formulating a good model, coupled with the ability to conduct an almost unlimited number of "thought experiments" and the capacity of a computer model for predicting the consequences of perturbing highly interactive systems that defy grasp by human intuition, provide a degree of insight into biological phenomena that can probably not be obtained in any other way. If the predictions of a model are readily amenable to experimental verification, the model, by showing where experimental research resources can be most effectively employed, can optimize the productivity and cost-effectiveness of an experimental program. Conversely, better experimental values will improve the predictiveness of the model. Because of this synergistic interplay of theory and experiment, computer modeling is likely to become an increasingly essential aspect of the development of antimetabolite drugs.

APPENDIX: A BASIC Program for Simulation of Inhibition in a Branched Metabolic Pathway

SIM1 is a simple BASIC program for integrating the rate equations for the system shown in Fig. 2. With minor modification along the lines suggested below, it can be used for many simple simulation studies. It includes a library of subroutines that carry out fourth-order Runge-Kutta integration of six different rate equations.

Notes on the program listing:

Line 25:	The K$ array stores the output, in string format.
Line 100:	The 1100 subroutine defines the values of the enzyme kinetic parameters, time, and the two concentration variables, A ($=FH_2$) and B ($=FH_4$). It also defines starting values for the five rate variables, v_0, v_1, v_2, v_3, and v_4 (see Fig. 2).
Line 130:	DT is the time increment for the numerical integration.
Line 135:	F2 is the printer control flag (F2 = 0, printer off; F2 = 1, printer on).
Line 140:	A$ is a descriptive caption that will be reproduced on the printed output. If the first character is an asterisk, output will appear on both the screen and the printer.
Line 149:	This call to line 986 reads the concentrations of the two inhibitors.
Line 301:	This call to subroutine 2600 prints column headers on the screen.
Line 305:	The outer loop index I determines the number of lines of output printed.
Line 400:	The inner loop index J determines the number of integration cycles that will be run for each line of output. Thus if DT = 0.1 and J = 4, the program will print output for each 0.4 min of simulated time.

Lines 500–521:   These lines calculate the rate of reaction v_1. Subroutine 3600, which is called in line 520, requires a substrate concentration, a K_m value, a V_{max} value, and an inhibitor concentration, and these are defined in lines 500, 502, 504, and 505, respectively. Line 506 defines the complementary velocity for the substrate A, i.e., it provides an expression for all the reactions, other than the one being calculated, that produce or utilize A. In line 510, the molar enzyme concentration is defined. In line 521, the calculated rate, returned as W, is equated with v_1.

Lines 600–611:   In a similar process, v_2 is calculated, this time using a rate equation for a first-order nonenzymatic reaction.

Lines 650–661:   These lines calculate v_3, using a subroutine for a Michaelis-Menten-type rate equation with competitive inhibition. Lines 650, 652, and 654 define the substrate concentration, K_m, and V_{max}, respectively. This routine requires an expression for I/K_i for the competitive inhibitor, and this is defined in line 656.

Lines 700–709:   These lines calculate v_4, using a first-order nonenzymatic mechanism, again by a call to subroutine 3000.

Line 800:   This is the conservation equation for variable substrate A.

Line 810:   This is the conservation equation for variable substrate B.

Line 890:   This updates the time.

Line 908:   This call to subroutine 2500 packs the output variables into string form.

Lines 980–984:   At this point the program pauses to request further instructions. If A\$ = C, then the program will continue the current simulation. "N" will start a new simulation, and "S" will stop execution.

Rate equation subroutines:

Line 3000:   This will integrate the first-order nonenzymatic rate equation, $v = S * K$, where S (or S_0) is substrate concentration, and K is the first-order rate constant.

Line 3100:   Integrates the second-order rate equation, $v = S * T * K$, where S and T are substrates, and K is the rate constant.

Line 3200:   Integrates the Michaelis-Menten rate equation

$$v = V_{max}/(1 + I_{nc}/K_{i,nc})* S/(S + (K_m*(1 + I_c/K_{i,c})))$$

where S is substrate, K_m is the Michaelis constant, I_{nc} is the concentration of a noncompetitive inhibitor, and $K_{i,nc}$ is its K_i value, I_c is the concentration of a competitive inhibitor, and $K_{i,c}$ is its K_i value.

If a noncompetitive inhibitor is present, this routine must be called at line 3200. If no noncompetitive inhibitor is present, but competitive inhibitor is present, the routine should be called at line 3210. If no inhibitors are present, the equation reduces to the simple Michaelis equation, and the routine may be called at line 3200.

```
10 REM PROGRAM SIM1
20 REM VERSION 2; 15/7/85
25 DIM K$(22,32)
90 LET Z$="          "
100 GOSUB 1100
130 LET DT=.1
135 LET F2=0
140 PRINT "ENTER DESCRIPTION"
142 INPUT A$
143 IF A$(1)="*" THEN LET F2=1
144 IF F2 THEN LPRINT A$
149 GOTO 986
150 LET HD=DT/2
160 LET F1=1
300 CLS
301 GOSUB 2600
305 FOR I=1 TO 15
400 FOR J=1 TO 4
500 LET S0=A
502 LET K=KM1
504 LET V=VM1
505 LET IC=PALA
506 LET VS=V0-V2
508 LET KI=KI1
510 LET ET=E1
520 GOSUB 3600
521 LET V1=V
600 LET S0=A
602 LET K=K2
604 LET VS=V0-V1
610 GOSUB 3000
611 LET V2=V
650 LET S0=B
652 LET K=KM3
654 LET V=VM3
656 LET IC=AZAU/KI3
658 LET VS=V1-V4
660 GOSUB 3210
661 LET V3=V
700 LET S0=B
702 LET K=K4
704 LET VS=V1-V3
708 GOSUB 3000
709 LET V4=V
800 LET A=A+(V0-V1-V2)*DT
810 LET B=B+(V1-V3-V4)*DT
890 LET TIME=TIME+DT
899 NEXT J
908 GOSUB 2500
910 PRINT TIME;TAB 4;Q$
960 NEXT I
```

```
 970 IF F1 THEN LPRINT "TIME A
     B          V1          V3"
 972 IF F2 THEN LPRINT TIME;TAB
4;Q$
 974 PRINT
 975 IF PALA THEN PRINT "FREE IN
HIBITOR = ";PALA-(1-V1/VU)*E1
 980 INPUT A$
 981 IF A$="C" THEN LET F1=0
 982 IF A$="C" THEN GOTO 300
 983 IF A$="N" THEN GOTO 100
 984 IF A$="S" THEN GOTO 998
 985 IF F2 THEN LPRINT
 986 PRINT
 987 PRINT
 988 PRINT "ENTER PALA CONCN"
 989 IF F2 THEN LPRINT
 990 INPUT PALA
 991 PRINT "ENTER AZA-UR CONCN"
 992 INPUT AZAU
 994 IF F2 THEN LPRINT "PALA = "
PALA;"       AZA-UR = ";AZAU
 995 IF F2 THEN LPRINT
 996 GOSUB 1150
 997 GOTO 150
 998 IF F2 THEN LPRINT
 999 STOP
1120 LET VM1=8
1122 LET KM1=5
1124 LET KI1=.15
1125 LET TON=40
1126 LET E1=VM1/TON
1130 LET K2=1.8
1135 LET VM3=80
1136 LET KM3=3
1138 LET KI3=1.5
1140 LET K4=.2
1150 LET A=2.6039
1151 LET B=.05
1152 LET V0=3
1161 LET V1=2.63961
1162 LET V2=.26039
1165 LET V3=1.272
1170 LET V4=.009696
1198 LET TIME=0
1199 RETURN
2500 LET N$=STR$ A+Z$
2505 LET R$=STR$ B+Z$
2510 LET M$=STR$ V1+Z$
2520 LET P$=STR$ V3+Z$
2590 LET Q$=N$( TO 6)+"   "+R$( T
O 6)+"   "+M$( TO 6)+"   "+P$( TO 5
)
2599 RETURN
2600 CLS
2610 PRINT "TIME A         B
```

```
V1        V3"
2615 PRINT
2649 RETURN
3000 LET W0=S0*K
3010 LET S1=S0+(VS-W0)*HD
3020 LET W1=S1*K
3030 LET S2=S0+(VS-W1)*HD
3040 LET W2=S2*K
3050 LET S3=S0+(VS-W2)*HD
3060 LET W3=S3*K
3070 LET W=(W0+W1+W1+W2+W2+W3)/6
3080 RETURN
3100 LET W0=S0*T0*K
3110 LET S1=S0+(VS-W0)*HD
3120 LET T1=T0+(VT-W0)*HD
3125 LET W1=S1*T1*K
3130 LET S2=S0+(VS-W1)*HD
3140 LET T2=T0+(VT-W1)*HD
3145 LET W2=S2*T2*K
3150 LET S3=S0+(VS-W2)*HD
3160 LET T3=T0+(VT-W2)*HD
3165 LET W3=S3*T3*K
3170 LET W=(W0+W1+W1+W2+W2+W3)/6
3180 RETURN
3200 LET V=V/(1+IN)
3210 LET K=K*(1+IC)
3220 LET W0=V*S0/(S0+K)
3230 LET S1=S0+(VS-W0)*HD
3240 LET W1=V*S1/(S1+K)
3250 LET S2=S0+(VS-W1)*HD
3260 LET W2=V*S2/(S2+K)
3270 LET S3=S0+(VS-W2)*HD
3280 LET W3=V*S3/(S3+K)
3290 LET W=(W0+W1+W1+W2+W2+W3)/6
3299 RETURN

3600 LET S=S0
3610 GOSUB 3650
3612 LET W0=W
3614 LET S=S0+(VS-W0)*HD
3620 GOSUB 3650
3622 LET W1=W
3624 LET S=S0+(VS-W1)*HD
3630 GOSUB 3650
3632 LET W2=W
3634 LET S=S0+(VS-W2)*HD
3640 GOSUB 3650
3642 LET W=(W0+W1+W1+W2+W2+W)/6
3649 RETURN
3650 LET SP=S/K
3652 LET VU=V*SP/(1+SP)
3654 LET KIAP=KI*(1+SP)
3656 LET IO=ET-KIAP-IC
3658 LET W=VU/2*ET*(IO+SQR(IO+I
0+4*ET*KIAP))
3659 RETURN
```

References

1. Boritzki, T. J., Fry, D. W., Besserer, J., Cook, P. D., and Jackson, R. C. (1984). Inosine 5'-phosphate dehydrogenase as a target for cancer chemotherapy. Results with 3-deazaguanine, tiazofurin and 2-β-D-ribofuranosylselenazole-4-carboxamide. In "Cancer Chemotherapy and Selective Drug Development" (K. R. Harrap, A. H. Calvert, and W. Davis, eds.), pp. 315–320. Martinus Nijhoff, Boston, Massachusetts.
2. Cohen, M. B., Maybaum, J., and Sadee, W. (1981). Guanine nucleotide depletion and toxicity in mouse T-lymphoma (S-49) cells. J. Biol. Chem. **256**, 8713–8717.
3. Grindey, G. B., and Cheng, Y. C. (1979). Biochemical and kinetic approaches to inhibition of multiple pathways. Pharmacol. Ther. **4**, 307–327.
4. Grindey, G. B., Moran, R. G., and Werkheiser, W. C. (1975). Approaches to the rational combination of antimetabolites for cancer chemotherapy. In "Drug Design" (E. J. Ariens, ed.), Vol. 5, pp. 169–249. Academic Press, New York.
5. Harrap, K. R., and Jackson, R. C. (1975). Enzyme kinetics and combination chemotherapy: An appraisal of current concepts. Adv. Enzyme Regul. **13**, 77–96.
6. Harvey, R. J. (1978). Interaction of two inhibitors which act on different enzymes of a metabolic pathway. J. Theor. Biol. **74**, 411–437.
7. Jackson, R. C. (1980). Kinetic simulation of anticancer drug interactions. Int. J. Bio-Med. Comput. **11**, 197–224.
8. Jackson, R. C. (1983). Regulation of the deoxynucleoside triphosphate pool in relation to antimetabolite chemotherapy. Abstr. Int. Cancer Congr., 13th, 1982, p. 25.
9. Jackson, R. C. (1984). A kinetic model of regulation of the deoxyribonucleoside triphosphate pool composition. Pharmacol. Ther. **24**, 279–301.
10. Jackson, R. C., Goulding, F. J., and Weber, G. (1979). Enzymes of purine metabolism in human and rat renal cortex and renal cell carcinoma. JNCI, J. Natl. Cancer Inst. **62**, 749–754.
11. Jackson, R. C., and Harrap, K. R. (1973). Studies with a mathematical model of folate metabolism. Arch. Biochem. Biophys. **158**, 827–841.
12. Jackson, R. C., and Harrap, K. R. (1979). Computer models of anticancer drug interaction. Pharmacol. Ther. **4**, 245–280.
13. Jackson, R. C., Jackman, A. L., and Calvert, A. H. (1983). Biochemical effects of a quinazoline inhibitor of thymidylate synthetase (CB3717), on human lymphoblastoid cells. Biochem. Pharmacol. **32**, 2783–2790.
14. Jackson, R. C., Morris, H. P., and Weber, G. (1978). Adenosine deaminase and adenosine kinase in rat hepatomas and kidney tumours. Br. J. Cancer **37**, 701–713.
15. Jackson, R. C., and Niethammer, D. (1977). Acquired methotrexate resistance in lymphoblasts resulting from altered kinetic properties of dihydrofolate reductase. Eur. J. Cancer **13**, 567–575.
16. Jackson, R. C., Taylor, G. A., and Harrap, K. R. (1975). Optimization of antimetabolite chemotherapy by metabolic simulation. Abstr. Int. Cancer Congr., 11th, 1974, p. 427.
17. Jackson, R. C., Weber, G., and Morris, H. P. (1975). IMP dehydrogenase, an enzyme linked with proliferation and malignancy. Nature (London) **256**, 331–333.
18. Johnson, R. K., Inouye, T., Goldin, A., and Stark, G. R. (1976). Antitumor activity of N-(phosphonacetyl)-L-aspartic acid, a transition-state inhibitor of aspartate transcarbamylase. Cancer Res. **36**, 2720–2725.
19. Nicolini, C., Milgram, E., Kendall, F., and Giaretti, W. (1977). Mathematical models for drug action and interaction in vivo. In "Growth Kinetics and Biochemical Regulation of Normal and Malignant Cells" (B. Drewinko and R. M. Humphrey, eds.), pp. 411–433. Williams & Wilkins, Baltimore, Maryland.

20. Weber, G. (1977). Enzymology of cancer cells. Part 2. *N. Engl. J. Med.* **296,** 541–551.
21. Weber, G., Lui, M. S., Takeda, E., and Denton, J. E. (1980). Enzymology of human colon tumors. *Life Sci.* **27,** 293–799.
22. Werkheiser, W. C. (1971). Mathematical simulation in chemotherapy. *Ann. N.Y. Acad. Sci.* **186,** 343–358.
23. Werkheiser, W. C., Grindey, G. B., and Moran, R. G. (1973). Mathematical simulation of the interaction of drugs that inhibit deoxyribonucleic acid biosynthesis. *Mol. Pharmacol.* **9,** 320–329.
24. White, J. C. (1981). Methotrexate resistance in an L1210 cell line resulting from increased dihydrofolate reductase, decreased thymidylate synthetase activity and normal membrane transport: Computer simulations based on network thermodynamics. *J. Biol. Chem.* **256,** 5722–5727.
25. White, J. C., and Mikulecky, D. C. (1982). Application of network thermodynamics to the computer modeling of the pharmacology of anticancer agents: A network model for methotrexate action as a comprehensive example. *Pharmacol. Ther.* **15,** 251–291.

Applications of the Median-Effect Principle for the Assessment of Low-Dose Risk of Carcinogens and for the Quantitation of Synergism and Antagonism of Chemotherapeutic Agents

TING-CHAO CHOU

Laboratory of Pharmacology
Sloan-Kettering Institute for Cancer Research
Cornell University Graduate School of Medical Sciences
New York, New York

PAUL TALALAY

Department of Pharmacology and Experimental Therapeutics
The Johns Hopkins University
School of Medicine
Baltimore, Maryland

NEW AVENUES IN DEVELOPMENTAL
CANCER CHEMOTHERAPY

I. Introduction

Dose–effect relationships in biological systems are frequently far more complex than simple chemical or biochemical reactions involving only a few defined reactants. In each case, the basic principle of the mass action law remains a fundamental rule, though the details of each system may be very different. For example, different enzymes catalyze different chemical reactions with one, two, or more substrate(s) and product(s); with ordered, "ping-pong," or random interaction sequences; and with a variety of microscopic rate constants. However, the basic rates and behavior of these chemical reactions can be gainfully generalized and analyzed by the Michaelis-Menten equation (46) or the Hill equation (38), which are both governed by the principle of the mass action law. With this generalization serving as precedent, it is apparent that a simple, broadly applicable method for dose–response or dose–effect analysis also requires a basic, general principle rather than the delineation of detailed mechanisms of individual cases involving a large number of rate constants. It is well known that many simple enzyme reactions (28,29,54) contain numerous rate constants for forward, backward, and side reactions. The derivation of equations describing these reactions, though theoretically sound, often proves to be of little practical utility. For this reason, efforts have been made in our studies to deduce a generalized equation that can be easily used for dose–effect analysis: an equation that is applicable not only for substrate-type ligands but also for inhibitor-type ligands (14,16,21). Such a simplified, general equation would not only be useful for enzyme or receptor systems but also for cellular and animal systems. As is often the case, the prerequisite for an equation's broad applicability depends upon its simplicity.

II. The Median-Effect Principle

A. A Kinetic Approach

The changes of symbols in the Michaelis-Menten and Hill equations have given rise in the field of pharmacology to the receptor theory (36). One feature of the Michaelis-Menten and Hill equations is that they deal with substrates for enzymes or ligands for receptors. Consequently, their saturation curve is expressed relative to the V_{max}, or the maximal binding. Determination of the magnitude of this value requires extrapolation or approximation. An effective approach has been to analyze the dose–effect relationships of inhibitors using enzyme kinetic models whereby the equations for different reaction mechanisms, different substrates, and different types of inhibitors are systematically analyzed (14,23). After canceling out all kinetic constants and substrate concentrations, a simple formula describing the relationship of dose and effect emerges. This formula has been called the "median-effect equation" (16,24).

B. The Median-Effect Equation

The median-effect equation depicts the equality of two dimensionless ratios, doses (left) versus effects (right), in its simplest form:

$$f_a/f_u = (D/D_m)^m \tag{1}$$

where D is the dose, f_a and f_u are the fractions of the system affected and unaffected, respectively, by the dose D; D_m is the dose required to produce the median-effect (i.e., 50% affected), and m is a Hill-type coefficient signifying the sigmoidicity of the dose–effect curve ($m = 1$, hyperbola; $m>1$, sigmoidal; and m<1, negatively sigmoidal). Since by definition, $f_a + f_u = 1$, there are several other useful alternative forms of Eq. (1):

$$f_a = 1/[1 + (D_m/D)^m] \tag{2}$$

$$D = D_m[f_a/(1 - f_a)]^{1/m} \tag{3}$$

$$f_a/(1 - f_a) = [(f_a)^{-1} - 1]^{-1} = (f_u)^{-1} - 1 = (D/D_m)^m \tag{4}$$

C. The Median-Effect Plot

The logarithmic form of Eq. (1) or Eq. (4) becomes

$$\log(f_a/f_u) = m \log D - m \log D_m \tag{5}$$

or:

$$\log[(f_a)^{-1} - 1]^{-1} = m \log D - m \log D_m \tag{6}$$

Therefore, a plot of $y = \log(f_a/f_u)$ or its equivalents with respect to $x = \log D$ linearizes the dose–effect relationship with the slope m and the intercept of the x-axis at $\log D_m$. Thus, D_m can be conveniently calculated by

$$D_m = 10^{-(y\text{-intercept})/m} \tag{7}$$

This plot has been referred to as the "median-effect plot" (16,21,24,26). It will be used extensively in this paper for analytical and diagnostic purposes.

Equation (1) describes the equity of two basic ratios, the dose on the right and the effect on the left. The dose is relative to the median-effect dose, and the effect is relative to the unaffected (uninhibited) control. The control, unlike V_{max}, requires no extrapolation or approximation for its determination. The median-effect equation has been shown (16,19) to be a generalized form of not only the Michaelis-Menten and the Hill equations, but also the Henderson-Hasselbalch and the Scatchard equations.

The fact that the simple median-effect equation contains no conventional rate constants may be the basis for its broad applicability in biological systems, and because the median-effect equation is not limited to any one specific mechanism, its use can be extended into areas such as analysis of the antagonism/synergism of multiple drugs or assessments of low-dose risk of carcinogens and toxic substances.

D. Application of the Median-Effect Principle

The median-effect plot depicted by Eq. (5) or Eq. (6) has been used to obtain accurate values of IC_{50}, ED_{50}, LD_{50}, and the relative potencies of drugs or inhibitors in enzyme systems (8,9,16,23,24,26,32,37,42,48,50, 57,63), in cell culture systems (2,11,34,41,53), and in animals (15,21, 22,26,60). For the dose-effect data obtained from animals, the median-effect plot gives ED_{50} or LD_{50} values that are nearly identical to those obtained from statistical methods, such as the probit analysis (21,31). However, the median-effect equation is much simpler, more explicit (in terms of meaning of the slope and intercept), and easier to use than either the probit (7,31) or logit function (52). Comparisons of the median-effect equation with the probit and logit functions as well as with the power law have been carried out (18,21).

An alternative form of the median-effect equation (14) has also been used for calculating the dissociation constant (K_i or K_d) of ligands for pharmacological receptors (47,61,62). It has permitted the analysis of chemical carcinogenesis data and radiation effect data and has accurately predicted the risk at low-dose exposure (17,20–22). By using the median-effect principle, the general equation for describing a standard radioimmunological or ligand displacement curve has been recently derived by Smith (56). It has also been used to show that there is a marked synergism among chemotherapeutic agents in the treatment of hormone-responsive experimental mammary carcinomas (60). In our recent reports (25,26), we have shown that in conjunction with the multiple drug–effect equations (see Section III,A) the median-effect plot provides the basis for the determination of slope and intercept and permits diagnosis of sigmoidicity and quantitation of synergism, summation, and antagonism of multiple-drug effects. All of these operations can be performed by a personal computer (see Appendix).

III. Quantitation of Synergism and Antagonism

A. The Multiple Drug–Effect Equation

The median-effect principle has been extended to multiple drug–effect situations regardless of the number of drugs involved, the mechanism of action or kinetic constants, and whether the dose–effect curves are hyperbolic or sigmoidal (24,26). For the summation of effect of two drugs, we obtain

$$\left[\frac{(f_a)_{1,2}}{(f_u)_{1,2}}\right]^{1/m} = \left[\frac{(f_a)_1}{(f_u)_1}\right]^{1/m} + \left[\frac{(f_a)_2}{(f_u)_2}\right]^{1/m} + \left[\frac{\alpha(f_a)_1(f_a)_2}{(f_u)_1(f_u)_2}\right]^{1/m}$$

$$= \frac{(D)_1}{(D_m)_1} + \frac{(D)_2}{(D_m)_2} + \frac{\alpha(D)_1(D)_2}{(D_m)_1(D_m)_2} \tag{8}$$

where $\alpha = 0$ is for mutually exclusive drugs in which the median-effect plot gives parallel lines for the parent drugs and their mixtures. When

$\alpha = 1$, the effects of two drugs are mutually nonexclusive, and the median-effect plots are parallel for the parent drugs but give a concave, upward curve for the mixture of the two drugs (24).

B. The Derivation of the Fractional Product Equation

Equation (8) has recently been used (27) to derive the fractional product equation previously formulated by Webb (64):

$$(f_u)_{1,2} = (f_u)_1 \times (f_u)_2$$

or

$$[1 - (f_a)_{1,2}] = [1 - (f_a)_1][1 - (f_a)_2]$$

or

$$(f_a)_{1,2} = 1 - [1 - (f_a)_1][1 - (f_a)_2] \tag{9}$$

where f_a and f_u are the fractions that are affected and unaffected, respectively, by a drug (subscripted 1 or 2) or by two drugs (subscripted 1,2). If each of the two drugs inhibit an enzyme by 60%, then in combination the additive effect would be, $1 - (1 - 0.6)(1 - 0.6) = 0.84$, i.e., 84% inhibition. While this method has proved to be convenient and is widely used in complex pharmacological systems (3,6,40), it usually refers to single doses and does not take into consideration the shape of dose–effect curves. However, the serious limitations of this method were not revealed until recently when Eq. (9) was formally derived from enzyme kinetic models (24). As shown in Table I, the fractional product equation is not applicable in many of the kinetic models that have been used.

C. The Derivation of the Isobologram Equation from the Multiple Drug–Effect Equation

The concept of the isoeffective curve was first introduced over a century ago by Fraser and has been extensively studied and reviewed by Loewe (44,45), Berenbaum (4,5), and many other investigators (22,30,34,35,49,55,58,59). One of the most common uses of this concept is the ED_{50} isobologram, which depicts various combinations for drug 1 and drug 2 that produce a 50% effect. If $(ED_{50})_1$ and $(ED_{50})_2$ each are designated as unity, then for the additive effect of two drugs, the sum of the decimal fractions of the ED_{50}'s would also equal 1:

$$\frac{(D)_1}{(ED_{50})_1} + \frac{(D)_2}{(ED_{50})_2} = 1 \tag{10}$$

TABLE I

Applicability and Limitations of Different Methods of Enzyme Kinetic Systems[a]

	Applicable		Not applicable	
	Dose–effect relationship[e]	Exclusivity of effects of two drugs[f]	Dose–effect relationship[e]	Exclusivity of effects of two drugs[f]
Fractional product method[b]	First-order (hyperbolic)	Mutually nonexclusive	Non-first-order (sigmoidal)	Mutually exclusive
Isobologram method[c]	First-order or non-first-order	Mutually exclusive		Mutually nonexclusive
Multiple drug–effect equation based on the median-effect principle[d]	First-order or non-first-order	Mutually exclusive or nonexclusive		

[a] Mathematical derivations are given in Refs. 24 and 26.

[b] Reference *64;* also see Eq. (9).

[c] References 26, 44, 45; also see Eqs. (10) and (11).

[d] References 24, 26; also see Eqs. (8) and (13).

[e] The first-order dose–effect relationship gives a hyperbolic curve on arithmetic scales, or a slope of 1 ($m = 1$) in the median-effect plot. The non-first-order dose–effect relationship gives a sigmoidal curve on arithmetic scales or a slope greater than or less than 1 ($m \neq 1$) in the median-effect plot.

[f] Mutually exclusive drugs in a mixture give a parallel median-effect plot with respect to those of the parent drugs. Mutually nonexclusive drugs in a mixture give a concave upward dose–effect curve with respect to those of the parent drugs.

If the sum of the decimal fractions is lesser or greater than 1, synergism or antagonism, respectively, is indicated.

In employing the kinetic approach and the principle of the mass action law to explore this theoretical problem, we were led to the explicit derivation of the generalized isobologram equation (26). Of particular interest is that the isobologram equation is, in fact, a special case of the multiple drug–effect equation (see Appendix of Ref. 26). It has been shown that the isobologram equation is not applicable in the case of models in which the effects of two drugs are mutually nonexclusive (Table I). However, the multiple drug–effect equation based on the median-effect principle has no such restrictions.

A generalized equation for the dose-oriented isobologram for mutually exclusive drugs has been derived (24). It is given by

$$\frac{(D)_1}{(D_x)_1} + \frac{(D)_2}{(D_x)_2} = 1 \tag{11}$$

where D_x is the dose that is required to affect a system $x\%$. However, for mutually nonexclusive drugs this equation has an additional term:

$$\frac{(D)_1}{(D_x)_1} + \frac{(D)_2}{(D_x)_2} + \frac{(D)_1(D)_2}{(D_x)_1(D_x)_2}\left[\frac{f_a}{f_u}\right] = 1 \tag{12}$$

that *cannot* be represented by a conventional isobologram. It should be noted that Eq. 12 is valid for $m_1 = m_2 = 1$. For $m_1 \neq m_2$ and for $m_1 \neq m_2 \neq m_{1,2}$ (i.e., the slopes for drug 1, drug 2, and their mixtures are different for the corresponding median-effect plots), the analysis for mutually nonexclusive cases becomes exceedingly complex (see Appendix F of this chapter) and requires a practical simplification as proposed below.

D. Combination Index and f_a–CI Plot

"Combination index" (CI) has been proposed for quantitation of synergism, summation, and antagonism of effects (26):

$$CI = \frac{(D)_1}{(D_x)_1} + \frac{(D)_2}{(D_x)_2} + \frac{\alpha(D)_1(D)_2}{(D_x)_1(D_x)_2} \tag{13}$$

where $\alpha=0$ is for mutually exclusive drugs and $\alpha=1$ is for mutually nonexclusive drugs. CI values that are smaller, equal to, or greater than unity represent synergism, summation, and antagonism of drug effects, respectively. Eq. 13 is valid at the median-effect doses of each drug and their mixtures regardless of the m_1, m_2, and $m_{1,2}$ values.

E. A Step-by-Step Procedure for Synergism/Antagonism Analysis

1. Conduct a preliminary study by arbitrarily varying drug concentration (usually, 10^{-3}, 10^{-4}, 10^{-5}, 10^{-6}, 10^{-7}, 10^{-8} M) or by obtaining information from the scientific literature to estimate approximate potency (D_m value) for each drug and for the slope of the dose–effect curve.
2. Design the dose range (e.g., four doses above and two doses below D_m) and dose density (e.g., two- to fivefold serial dilution from the highest dose) for each drug of the experiment.
3. Make a mixture of D_1 and D_2 so that two components will be equipotent [i.e., the dose ratio at $D_1/D_2 = (D_m)_1/(D_m)_2$]. It is important that

D_1 and D_2 are varied at a constant ratio. (This condition can be satisfied by a mixture being serially diluted.) For more detailed studies, make two or three more mixtures so that the potency ratio of D_1 and D_2 will be approximately $0.2:1$, $5:1$, etc.

4. Measure the dose and effect relationships for each drug alone and for their mixture(s).

5. Graph the data obtained in step 4 with the median-effect plot and measure their parameters, m_1, $(D_m)_1$, r_1, m_2, $(D_m)_2$, r_2, $(m)_{1,2}$, $(D_m)_{1,2}$, and $r_{1,2}$, etc.

6. Calculate the dose $(D_x)_1$, $(D_x)_2$, and $(D_x)_{1,2}$ at each given effect level $(f_a)_x$ with the use of Eq. (3), $D=D_m [f_a/(1-f_a)]^{1/m}$, and the corresponding m and D_m values obtained in step 5. Note that $(D_x)_1$, $(D_x)_2$, and $(D_x)_{1,2}$ are doses of drug 1, drug 2, and their mixture which are required to affect a given system by $x\%$.

7. Calculate the contribution of D_1 and D_2 in the mixture $(D_x)_{1,2}$ from the known dose ratio of two drugs. For example, if $(D)_1/(D)_2 = P/Q$, then $(D)_1=(D_x)_{1,2}$, $\times P/(P + Q)$, and $(D)_2 = (D_x)_{1,2} \times Q/(P + Q)$, where $(D_x)_{1,2} = (D)_1 + (D)_2$.

8. Substitute $(D)_1$, $(D)_2$, $(D_x)_1$, and $(D_x)_2$ values in Eq. (13) in order to calculate the combination index:

$$CI = \frac{(D)_1}{(D_x)_1} + \frac{(D)_2}{(D_x)_2} + \frac{\alpha(D)_1(D)_2}{(D_x)_1(D_x)_2}$$

If the effects of two drugs are mutually exclusive (i.e., the median-effect plots for D_1, D_2, and $D_{1,2}$ are parallel or if D_1 and D_2 have similar modes of action), then $\alpha = 0$ [i.e., the last term of Eq. (13) is dropped]. If the effects of two drugs are mutually nonexclusive (i.e., the median-effect plots for D_1 and D_2 are parallel but $D_{1,2}$ is upwardly concave, or if D_1 and D_2 have independent modes of action), then $\alpha=1$. If the exclusivity of two drugs is not clear, it is suggested that the CI value be determined with both mutually exclusive ($\alpha=0$) and mutually nonexclusive ($\alpha=1$) assumptions. Note that a mutually nonexclusive assumption always predicts less synergism or more antagonism than the mutually exclusive assumption.

9. When the CI value is equal to, less than, or greater than 1, then summation, synergism, or antagonism of effects is suggested, respectively.

Note that computer software for Apple II series and IBM-PC is available for semiautomated analysis and graphing from steps 5 to 9. (See Ref. 12 and Appendix of this chapter.) This analysis can also be done manually with a pocket calculator that has logarithmic and power functions.

F. An Improved Method for Constructing Isobolograms

The median-effect plot of dose–effect relationships gives the parameters m and D_m, which according to Eq. (2) can then be used for calculating doses of drug 1, drug 2 and their mixtures at several different proportions required to produce a given level of effects. This provides a convenient way of constructing isobolograms (e.g., ED_{50}, ED_{70}, and ED_{90} isobolograms,). Equation (3) in conjunction with Eq. (11) provides an algorithm for computer-assisted construction of isobolograms. Examples 2 and 3 in Section IV,B and IV,C illustrate this procedure.

It is interesting to note that a single plot of the CI with respect to the fractional effect (f_a) directly provides information about synergism (CI<1), summation (CI = 1), or antagonism (CI>1) at all effect levels. In contrast, each isobologram represents a single effect level only, and a full analysis of the degree of synergism, summation, or antagonism requires the construction of multiple graphs (see Fig. 4). Furthermore, as already mentioned (Table I), whereas the median-effect plot and the multiple drug–effect equation distinguish mutually exclusive $(\alpha=0)$ and mutually nonexclusive $(\alpha=1)$ drug effects, the conventional isobologram cannot do so, and its use is theoretically justifiable only for mutually exclusive agents. The computer program of a new type of isobologram for mutually nonexclusive drugs, based on Equation (3) and Equation (12) [or Equation (13), $\alpha=1$] has been developed. This software has been incorporated in Ref. 12 for the IBM-PC Computers.

IV. Examples of Applications

A. Example 1. Low-Dose Risk Assessment of Carcinogens: Tumorigenic Effect of Polycyclic Hydrocarbons in Mice

1. Varied Single-Dose Studies

Bryan and Shimkin (10) studied the dose–effect relationships for tumorigenic effects of 3-methylcholanthrene, dibenz[a,h]anthracene and benzo[a]pyrene in mice, following single subcutaneous injections. Experimental procedures and data are described in Table II. The median-effect plot parameters ($m, r,$ and D_m) are given in the last two columns of Table II. These data obtained *in vivo* showed excellent linear regression coefficients ($r > .997$) for the median-effect plot of the dose–effect relationships. This animal system, therefore, closely conforms to the basic principle of the mass action law (Fig. 1). Even at low doses, there is no apparent tendency for systematic deviation from linearity. This conformity to the median-effect principle provides a rationale for low-dose risk assessment

TABLE II

Dose–Effect Relationships of Carcinogenic Hydrocarbons in Mice after Single Dose, s.c.: An Analysis by the Median-Effect Equation[a]

Carcinogen	Dose (μg/mouse) (D)	Fraction affected (f_a)	$\log \dfrac{f_a}{1 - f_a}$	Slope[b] (m)	Median-effect dose[b] (μg/mouse) (D_m)
3-Methylchol-	125	0.973	1.5567	1.9330	20.663
anthrene	62	0.881	0.8694	±0.040	
	31	0.668	0.3036		
	15.6	0.379	−0.2145	(r = .9992)	
	7.8	0.146	−0.7671		
	3.9	0.036	−1.4278		
Dibenz	62.5	0.912	1.0155	1.7720	16.208
[a,h]anthra-	31.2	0.748	0.4725	±0.0502	
cene	15.6	0.494	−0.0104		
	7.81	0.242	−0.4959	(r = .9984)	
	3.90	0.083	−1.0433		
	1.95	0.019	−1.7129		
Benzo[a]pyrene	2000	0.988	1.9155	1.3879	98.857
	1000	0.960	1.3802	±0.0455	
	500	0.888	0.8992		
	250	0.756	0.4911	(r = .9973)	
	125	0.565	0.1136		
	62	0.358	−0.2537		
	31	0.186	−0.6411		

[a] Statistically calculated values obtained by Bryan and Shimkin (10) are used. Tumor incidences of 100% and <1% have been excluded from analysis. For more detailed analysis see Ref. 21.

[b] The median-effect plot was carried out by plotting $\log[f_a/(1-f_a)]$ versus $\log D$, in which m is the slope and $\log D_m$ is the intercept of the plot at the median-effect axis (i.e., at $\log[f_a/(1-f_a)] = 0$). Both m and D_m are obtained from least-square regression analysis and $D_m = $ antilog($-y$ intercept/m). The range of m value is given by ±S.E., and r is a linear regression coefficient.

by using the slope m and intercept ($\log D_m$) for extrapolation. This type of assessment is given in Table III in the column, "acute experiments."

2. Chronic Exposure Studies

In chronic experiments, Peto *et al.* (51) exposed the skin of mice to benzo[a]pyrene for a period of up to 100 weeks. The experimental results were previously analyzed with the median-effect plot (21). The parameters and risk assessment are given in Table III in the column "chronic experiments." These two modes of exposure resulted in a marked difference in risk at low doses, as assessed by these procedures. The factor which contributed most significantly to this difference was apparently the

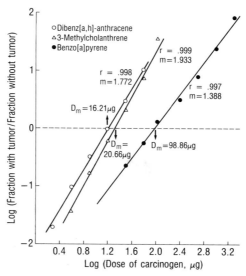

Fig. 1. The median-effect plot of the dose–effect relationship of carcinogenic poly-cyclic hydrocarbons in mice. Data from Table II have been used. The m and D_m values have been substituted in Eq. (2) for low-dose risk assessment, as shown in Table III.

much steeper slope of the dose–effect curve of the chronic exposure experiments. Whereas the carcinogenic potency (dose required to cause 50% of animals to have tumors) for single injections ($D_m = 98.86 \, \mu g$) is higher than for chronic applications (cumulative $D_m = 1579 \, \mu g$), the slope of the median-effect plot is more than three times higher for the chronic experiments ($m = 4.569$) than for the acute experiments ($m = 1.388$). These findings have interesting and divergent implications for risk at low and high doses. For a given low total dose of carcinogen, chronic expo-sure is much less hazardous than a single injection. Thus at $0.1D_m$ and $0.01D_m$, chronic exposure is 10^{-3} and 10^{-6} times less hazardous, respec-tively. In contrast, extrapolation to high cumulative or single doses indi-cates that chronic exposure is more hazardous than single injections. From the property of the median-effect plot (16) it can be expected that the D_m values will be affected by the route of administration. The m value, however, which describes the increment of dose versus the increment of effect, is a reflection of the basic characteristics of the dose–effect rela-tion, which is not expected to be affected by the difference in absorption or metabolic factors (16,21). Although these analyses have been carried out for single carcinogens only, similar methods utilizing the multiple-drug equation are clearly applicable to the effects of multiple carcinogens (including cocarcinogens) and the analysis of their interactions.

TABLE III

Influence of the Mode of Exposure on the Low-Dose Carcinogenic Risk Assessment of Benzo[a]pyrene in Mice[a]

Parameters of the median-effect plot[b]	Acute experiments[c]	Chronic experiments[d]
m	1.388 ± 0.046	4.569 ± 0.063
D_m (μg)	98.86	1579.0[e]
r	.9973	.9981

Calculated risk at a given dose	Acute experiments		Chronic experiments	
	Dose (μg)	f_a	Dose (μg)	f_a
$0.5D_m$	49.43	2.77×10^{-1}	789.5	4.03×10^{-2}
$0.1D_m$	9.886	3.93×10^{-2}	157.9	2.70×10^{-5}
$0.01D_m$	0.988	1.67×10^{-3}	15.79	7.28×10^{-10}
$0.001D_m$	0.0988	1.85×10^{-5}	1.579	1.96×10^{-14}

[a] Risk (f_a) at a given dose was calculated from Eq. (2).

[b] Parameters are calculated as illustrated previously (21). A sample calculation for the acute experiments is given in Fig. 1 and Table II.

[c] Data from Bryan and Shimkin (10) are used. C3H male mice were injected subcutaneously with a single dose of benzo[a]pyrene. Tumor incidence at the site of injection was histologically confirmed, spindle-cell sarcoma. Statistically calculated values reported by the original authors are used. Tumor incidence of 100% and <1% has been excluded from analysis.

[d] Data from Peto et al. (51) are used. Benzo[a]pyrene, 20 μg in 0.25 ml acetone, twice a week, was applied to the skin of Swiss albino female mice at 10 weeks old, treated for 100 weeks. Mice with epithelial tumors exceeding 10 mm in diameter were killed for histological examinations. The raw tumor incidence data were refined by the original authors (51) in accordance with the "life-table" procedure.

[e] The total cumulated doses over a period of 39.47 weeks as calculated previously (21).

B. Example 2. The Median-Effect Plot, the f_a–CI Plot, and the Construction of the Isobologram: Lethal Effect of Rotenone and Pyrethrins on Houseflies

About 50 years ago, Le Pelley and Sullivan (43) reported a set of very carefully measured data for the lethality of rotenone, pyrethrins, and their mixtures (at 1 : 5 and 1 : 15 ratios) on houseflies. Adult houseflies were sprayed with an alcoholic solution of these insecticides (900–1000 flies at each of the five dose levels), and mortality was scored on day 3 after exposure. These data are of historical interest, since five different laboratories, including ours (26), have attempted to answer the question of whether or not there is synergism among these insecticides, and, if so, how much synergism.

The numerical results (Table IV) were retrieved by Finney (31) and have been subjected to the computer analysis based on the median-effect plot (Fig. 2) and the multiple drug–effect equation (Figs. 3 and 4). The dose–effect parameters such as slope m, the median-effect dose D_m, and

TABLE IV

Toxicity of Rotenone and Pyrethrins to Houseflies[a]

Compound or mixture	Concentration (μg/ml)	% Kill[b]	Parameters[c]
Rotenone (R)	0.1	26.0	m: 2.626
	0.15	47.5	r: .997
	0.2	67.5	D_m: 0.151 μg/ml
	0.25	81.5	ED_{70}: 0.209 μg/ml
	0.35	89.5	ED_{90}: 0.349 μg/ml
			ED_{95} 0.463 μg/ml
Pyrethrins (P)	0.5	21.5	m: 2.404
	0.75	39.5	r: .996
	1.0	54.0	D_m: 0.890 μg/ml
	1.5	75.0	ED_{70}: 1.266 μg/ml
	2.0	89.0	ED_{90}: 2.220 μg/ml
			ED_{95}: 3.029 μg/ml
Mixture (1R : 5P)	0.3	27.0	m: 2.519
	0.45	53.0	r: .994
	0.6	64.0	D_m: 0.450 μg/ml (0.075 + 0.375)
	0.875	82.0	ED_{70}: 0.630 μg/ml (0.105 + 0.525)
	1.175	93.0	ED_{90}: 1.077 μg/ml (0.180 + 0.897)
			ED_{95}: 1.448 μg/ml (0.241 + 1.207)
Mixture (1R : 15P)	0.4	23.0	m: 2.513
	0.6	48.0	r: .983
	0.8	61.0	D_m: 0.652 μg/ml (0.041 + 0.611)
	1.2	76.0	ED_{70}: 0.911 μg/ml (0.057 + 0.854)
	1.6	93.0	ED_{90}: 1.552 μg/ml (0.097 + 1.455)
			ED_{95}: 2.085 μg/ml (0.130 + 1.955)

[a] Data from Le Pelley and Sullivan (43), as retrieved by Finney (31). Mortality was scored on day 3 after exposure.

[b] Data from rotenone or pyrethrins alone were the average of two series of experiments.

[c] The terms m, r, and D_m are the slope, regression coefficient, and the median-effect dose (antilog of $-y$ intercept/m) of the median-effect plot, respectively (see Fig. 2). ED_{70}, ED_{90}, and ED_{95} are calculated from Eq. (3).

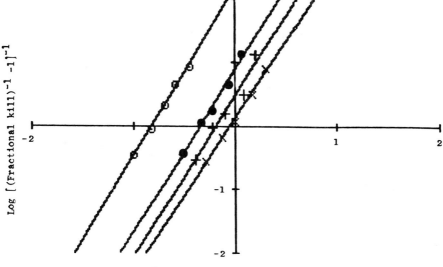

Fig. 2. The median-effect plot showing lethality of rotenone and pyrethrins to houseflies. Experimental data from Table IV have been used. The parameters of the plots are given in Table IV. Rotenone alone (O—O), pyrethrins alone (x—x), rotenone plus pyrethrins (1 : 5) (●—●), and rotenone plus pyrethrins (1 : 15) (+—+). Parallel plots of the mixtures with respect to the parent drugs indicate that the lethal effect of rotenone and pyrethrins are mutually exclusive. The graph was generated by a micro-computer using a program by Chou and Chou (12).

the linear regression coefficient r are also given in Table IV and are illustrated in Fig. 2. The following conclusions have been drawn:

1. Excellent linearity of the plot (r, .983–.997) indicates that the dose–effect relationships conform to the median-effect principle.
2. The dose–effect relationships give a sigmoidal curve on the arithmetic scales (i.e., $m > 1$).
3. The parallel median-effect plots (m values, 2.52 ± 0.12) suggest that the effects of two insecticides are mutually exclusive with respect to the end point of the measurement (lethality).

Because the insecticides are mutually exclusive drugs, the isobol method can be used. A computer program (12, 13) based on Eq. (3) was employed for the calculation of ED_{50}, ED_{70}, ED_{90}, and ED_{95}, etc., and thus greatly facilitated the construction of isobolograms (Fig. 4). The analysis based on Eq. (11) showed moderate synergism between rotenone and pyrethrins at different effect levels for two combinations. The com-

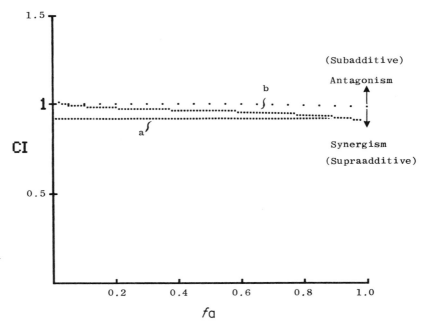

Fig. 3. Computer-generated graphical presentation of the combination index (CI) with respect to the fraction kill (f_a) of houseflies by mixtures of rotenone and pyrethrins (a) at a ratio of 1 : 5 and (b) at a ratio of 1 : 15. Equations (3) and (13) ($\alpha=0$) are the bases for a computer program (12) that has been used for this plot.

puter program (12, 13) based on Eq. (13) (in this case $\alpha=0$ for mutually exclusive drugs) allows for an automated analysis of synergism/antagonism at different combination ratios and at all effect levels (Fig. 3). The plot of CI with respect to fractional kill (f_a) (Fig. 3) is extremely efficient, since each dot in the plot is equivalent to an isobologram. The result showed moderate synergism at all effect levels when the 1:5 mixture (rotenone to pyrethrins) was used. For the 1:15 mixture, a similar degree of synergism was also observed. However, higher effect levels gave more synergism than lower effect levels. The preceding quantitative analysis used the pooled data for rotenone alone and for the pyrethrins alone. The results are qualitatively consistent and quantitatively similar to our previous studies (25,26) which used segregated data for two series of experiments.

The original authors interpreted the results to mean that there was no striking antagonistic or synergistic effect of the mixture. Richardson used a predictive method for the mixture equivalent to the "similar action law"

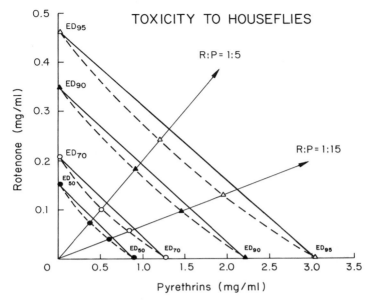

Fig. 4. ED_{50}, ED_{70}, ED_{90} and ED_{95} isobolograms for toxicity of rotenone (R) and pyrethrins (P) to houseflies. Calculated results in the last column of Table IV have been used (- - -). Arrows indicate combination ratios of rotenone to pyrethrins in the experimental systems. The solid lines (—) are calculated for summation of effects. Each of these isobols showed moderate synergism of insecticidal effects.

(31) and asserted that there was pronounced synergism. Bliss supported Richardson's conclusion, and Finney, after a new analysis of the data, also agreed that there was evidence of synergism (31). This chapter has used a new approach and presents additional information, as shown in Fig. 3, and provides a facile method for constructing isobolograms (Fig. 4), a method which in the past was a tedious undertaking.

C. Example 3. Constant Dose-Ratio Concept for Experimental Design and the Optimal Combination Ratio for Maximal Synergism: *In Vitro* Purging of Leukemia Cells by 4-HC and VP-16 for Autologous Bone Marrow Transplantation

Autologous stem cell transplantation using cryopreserved bone marrow offers the opportunity to rescue the hematopoietic system from the toxicity of intensive chemotherapy. This approach is potentially useful for high-risk leukemias as well as other malignancies. Normal bone marrow is often contaminated with malignant cells. The development of suitable *in vitro* methods for purging these cells will offer a better chance of success for autologous bone marrow transplantation. Chang *et al.* (11) recently used 4-hydroperoxycyclophosphamide (4-HC) and a semisynthetic congener of podophylotoxin (VP-16), either alone or in combination, to treat HL-60 (acute promyelocytic leukemia) cell lines and normal human bone marrow. Cytotoxicity was assayed by fractional cell kill or by the reduction of colony-forming units (CFU-c) for bone marrow cells. Experimental data (11) available in a tabulated form were subjected to analysis with the median-effect plot [Eq. (5) (Table V)] and doses (singly and in combination) required for various fractional kills were calculated according to Eq. (3) (Table VI).

Figure 5 gives the effect-oriented graph for combined effects of 4-HC and VP-16 using computer simulation (12) based on Eq. (13). The CI at various effect levels ($f_a = 0.2$–0.999) of two drug combinations is shown. The CI values, <1, $=1$, and >1, represent synergism, summation, and antagonism, respectively. It becomes obvious that at the desired high effect levels ($f_a > 0.99$), the combination of 4-HC and VP-16 shows marked synergism against HL-60 leukemic cells and marked antagonism against normal bone marrow cells. It is also clear that a $1:0.342$ ratio of 4-HC to VP-16 shows a more favorable result than the $1:0.856$ ratio.

The ED_{50}, ED_{65} (or ED_{75}), ED_{80}, ED_{85}, and ED_{90} isobolograms for the combined effects of VP-16 are given in Figs. 6A and 6B for HL-60 and bone marrow cells, respectively. It becomes obvious that these isobolograms exhibit drastically different shapes and the curves themselves deviate asymmetrically around the corresponding isoeffect lines representing summation. The ED_{50} isobol for CFU-c shows a marked antagonism. For practical purposes, the killing effect on the leukemic cells should be $>99\%$. In addition, it is preferable that the combined effects of 4-HC and VP-16 show synergism against leukemic cells but antagonism against normal bone marrow cells and thus gain superior selectivity which could not be obtained with a single drug. The contours of the ED_{90} isobol for HL-60 cells show that synergism occurs at high 4-HC and low VP-16 concentrations, whereas the contours of the ED_{90} isobol for CFU-c show that antagonism occurs at high 4-HC and VP-16 concentrations. It appears that a higher concentration of 4-HC over VP-16 is preferred in order to gain a more favorable therapeutic index.

In conclusion, the present method provides a useful quantitative way of measuring interactions of drug effects in molecular, enzymatic, cellular, and animal systems. Requiring a small number of data points, the method is highly efficient and readily adaptable to automated computer analysis.

TABLE V

Dose–Effect Parameters of 4-HC and VP-16[a]

Parameter	HL-60 cells				Bone marrow CFU-c[b]			
			4-HC + VP-16				4-HC + VP-16	
	4-HC	VP-16	1:0.342	1:0.856	4-HC	VP-16	1:0.342	1:0.856
m	2.463	1.516	3.122	2.539	1.566	0.987	0.886	0.588
D_m	2.232	2.074	2.567	3.719	10.63	9.160	4.872	3.792
(µg/ml)			(1.913 + 0.654)	(2.004 + 1.715)			(3.630 + 1.242)	(2.038 + 1.754)
r	.994	.965	.985	.958	.955	.972	.992	.996

[a] Experimental procedure and dose–effect analysis were carried out as described in Ref. 21. The values for m, D_m, and r are obtained from the median-effect plots.

[b] CFU-c: colony forming units.

TABLE VI

The Doses (μg/ml) of 4-HC and/or VP-16 That Are Needed for the Various Expected Cytotoxicity of HL-60 Cells or CFU-c of Normal Bone Marrow[a]

	Single drug				Combinations			
	4-HC alone		VP-16 alone		4-HC + VP-16 (1:0.342)[b]		4-HC + VP-16 (1:0.856)[b]	
	HL-60	CFU-c	HL-60	CFU-c	HL-60	CFU-c	HL-60	CFU-c
ED_{50}	2.23	10.63	2.07	9.16	1.91 + 0.65	3.63 + 1.24	2.00 + 1.72	2.04 + 1.75
ED_{65}	2.87	15.85	3.12	17.14	2.33 + 0.80	7.30 + 2.50	2.56 + 2.19	5.84 + 5.00
ED_{80}	3.92	26.08	5.17	37.31	3.00 + 1.00	17.36 + 5.94	3.46 + 2.96	21.51 + 18.41
ED_{85}	4.52	32.75	6.51	52.93	3.33 + 1.14	25.72 + 8.80	3.97 + 3.40	38.88 + 33.28
ED_{90}	5.45	44.37	8.83	85.04	3.87 + 1.32	43.36 + 14.83	4.76 + 4.08	85.36 + 73.07

[a] Doses were calculated using parameters listed in Table V. The doses needed were calculated by the computer program developed by Chou and Chou (12), using Eq. (3). The m and D_m values for each drug and combinations were obtained as showed in Charts 2 and 3 of Ref. 10, using the median-effect plot.

[b] Combination ratios of 4-HC/VP-16.

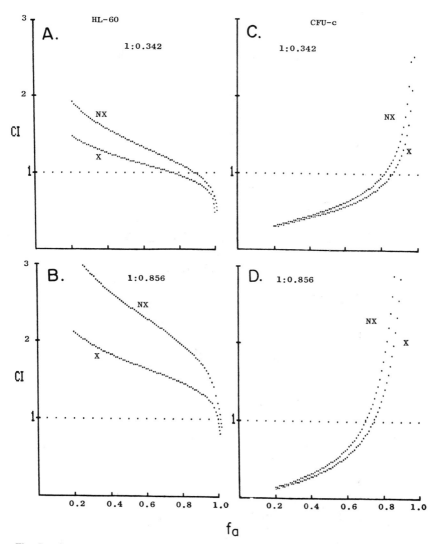

Fig. 5. Computer-generated graphical presentation of CI with respect to the fraction affected (f_a) for the cytotoxicity to HL-60 leukemia cells and normal bone marrow cells of mixtures of 4-HC and VP-16 at the ratios of 1 : 0.342 and 1 : 0.856. Equations (3) and (13) have been used for the computer programs (12), in which ($\alpha=0$) is for mutually exclusive assumptions (X) and $\alpha=1$ is for mutually nonexclusive assumptions (NX). Parameters given in Table V have been used for the computations. Note that for the purging of leukemic cells $f_a=0.999$ may be required. Since the slopes of the median-effect plot for 4-HC and VP-16 alone are not parallel, both mutually exclusive and nonexclusive assumptions have been used for analysis.

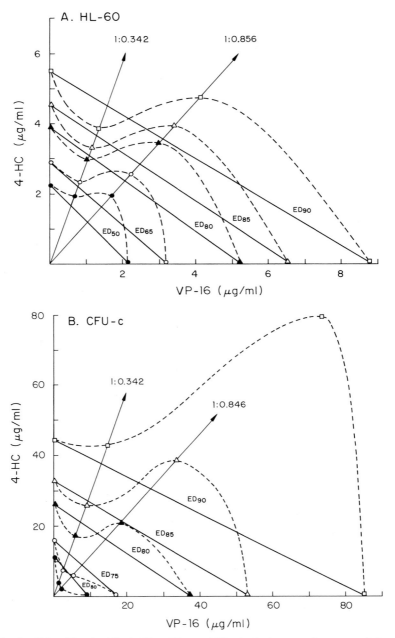

Fig. 6. ED$_{50}$, ED$_{65}$ (or ED$_{75}$), ED$_{80}$, ED$_{85}$ and ED$_{90}$ isobolograms for cytotoxicity of 4-HC and VP-16 to (A) HL-60 leukemic cells and (B) CFU-c of normal bone marrow cells. Data reported in Ref. 11 (Tables I and II) have been used. Calculated doses required for a given effect based on parameters given in Table V are listed in Table VI. Arrows indicate combination ratios of 4-HC to VP-16 used in the experiments. See text for details.

V. Summary

A generalized method, easier to use and more efficient in data utilization than the isobologram, has been developed for quantitation of synergism, summation, and antagonism of the effects of multiple drugs. This method combines a generalized equation (the median-effect equation), a simplified experimental design, a diagnostic plot, and computer analysis (26). The equation was derived from the median-effect principle of the mass action law and from enzyme kinetic models. The isobologram and the fractional product methods are special cases of this equation. Hyperbolic and sigmoidal dose–effect curves in enzymatic, cellular, and animal systems can usually be linearized by the median-effect plot (16,24). The plot determines (1) the relative potency of each drug alone and of drug combinations (ED_{50}, LD_{50}, IC_{50}, ED_{90}, ED_{95}, etc); (2) the sigmoidicity of the dose–effect curve; and (3) whether the effect of two drugs are mutually exclusive or nonexclusive. The slope and intercept of the median-effect plot can then be used for (1) determination of the dose required to produce a given effect and (2) determination of effect or risk generated by a given dose, e.g., assessment of low-dose-risk carcinogens or other toxic substances. When the median-effect equation is extended to multiple drugs, quantitation of synergism, summation, or antagonism of these agents becomes possible. Furthermore, synergism or antagonism can be determined for any desired effect level. Published data that provide dose-effect relationships for each drug alone (39) can be used for calculating individual CI values with the present method (Eqs. 11 and 12) even though two drugs in combination are not varied at a constant ratio.

As a model for the purging of neoplastic cells from bone marrow for autologous transplantation, the effects of combinations of 4-hydroperoxycyclophosphamide (4-HC) and etoposide (VP-16) on human leukemic cells (HL-60) and normal bone marrow have been analyzed in culture (11). Drug combination ratios and dose levels have been optimized by computerized application of the median-effect and multiple-drug equations to achieve a maximum synergistic kill of neoplastic cells while obtaining antagonism of cytotoxicity on normal bone marrow cells. Examples of carcinogenic effects of single and multiple doses of polycyclic aromatic hydrocarbons in mice have also been analyzed by the median-effect principle. The excellent regression coefficient for the entire dose range in the median-effect plot allows low-dose risk assessment for each carcinogen. The proposed method thus paves the way for analyzing synergistic, additive, or antagonistic interactions of carcinogens and cocarcinogens.

Acknowledgments

These studies were supported by National Institutes of Health Grants CA 27569, CA 18856, and AM 07422; the Elsa U. Pardee Foundation; and the American Cancer Society (SIG-3).

Appendix: Computerized Data Analysis

A. Dose–Effect Analysis with Microcomputers

After drawing the linear regression line with the median-effect plot, certain statistical, graphical, and repetitive procedures can be greatly facilitated by the use of a computer. For instance, the linear regression coefficient (r), the standard error of the mean of the slope ($m \pm$ S.E.), the y-intercept, and the graphs of the median-effect plot or f_a–CI plot can all be obtained almost instantly with microcomputers (12,26).

B. Determination of LD_{50}, ED_{50}, and IC_{50}

Depending on the system that is used for a given experiment (e.g., animal, cellular, and molecular systems) as well as on the end point of measurement (e.g., lethality, toxicity, or inhibition) LD_{50}, ED_{50}, and IC_{50} can be readily calculated by the antilog $-(y\text{-intercept}/m)$, e.g., $ED_{50} = 10^{-(y\text{-intercept})/m}$. The standard errors of the y-intercept and m value allow for the calculation of 95% confidence limits. In the case of calculating LD_{50}, the present method is far more convenient to use than the empirical probit function (7,31), as has been shown in example 2.

C. Assessment of Low-Dose Risk of Carcinogens and Toxic Substances

The present method treats different ligands in the same way, regardless of their nature. Thus, carcinogens or noncarcinogenic chemical agents, toxic substances, or relatively nontoxic pharmacological drugs are analyzed in the same way with the mass action law principle.

This rationale has been supported by numerous experimental observations, as indicated in Section II,D. Equation (3) has been used for computerized estimation of low-dose risk of carcinogens, as shown in example 1 (Fig. 1, and Tables II and III).

D. Software for the Median-Effect Plot

Computer software for calculating parameters of the median-effect equation (m and D_m) and their standard error and for presenting the median-effect plot in graphics (including x- and y-intercepts and linear regression coefficient) has been developed for both the Apple II microcomputers and the IBM-PC (12). Some examples of its application have been given in Section IV.

E. Software for the f_a–CI Plot for Synergism/Antagonism Analysis

Computer software for automated analysis of synergism/antagonism has also been developed for the Apple II and IBM-PC microcomputers (12). CI values at different effect levels (f_a's) can be calculated and presented either graphically or in a diagnostic table. The computer entries are (1) doses and effects for drug 1, drug 2, and their mixtures (if m and D_m values are already known, they can be entered directly for computing); (2) whether the effects of two drugs are mutually exclusive or nonexclusive (exclusivity can be diagnosed by the median-effect plot); (3) the dose ratio of drug 1 to drug 2 in the mixtures; and (4) the selection of scales for graphics or the increment of f_a in the synergism/antagonism diagnostic table. Several examples of its applications are given in Section IV.

F. Complexity of Mutually Nonexclusive Cases

Due to the upward concave curvature of the median-effect plots for mixtures involving mutually nonexclusive drugs (24) or other complications arising from the experimental determinations of (1) $m_1 \neq m_2$, (2) $m_1 \neq m_2 \neq m_{1,2}$, and (3) mutual depletion of reactants (such as formation of precipitate or tight-binding (titrating) type of interactions), a simple, exact identification of nonexclusivity is not yet feasible. The third term on the right side of Eq. (13) is attributed to the conservative estimation for synergism when compared with the conventional isobologram as depicted in Eq. (11). At the median-effect doses of each drug and their mixtures, the general equation for $m_1 \neq m_2 \neq m_{1,2}$ becomes:

$$\frac{(D)_1}{(D_x)_1}\left[\frac{f_a}{f_u}\right]^{\frac{1}{m_1}-\frac{1}{m_{1,2}}} + \frac{(D)_2}{(D_x)_2}\left[\frac{f_a}{f_u}\right]^{\frac{1}{m_2}-\frac{1}{m_{1,2}}}$$
$$+ \frac{(D)_1\,(D)_2}{(D_x)_1(D_x)_2}\left[\frac{f_a}{f_u}\right]^{\frac{1}{m_1}+\frac{1}{m_2}-\frac{1}{m_{1,2}}} = 1 \tag{14}$$

which can be reduced to Eq. (12) when $f_a = f_u$.

References

1. Ariens, E. J., and Simonis, A. M. (1961). Analysis of the action of drugs and drug combinations. *In* "Quantitative Methods in Pharmacology" (H. De Jonge, ed.), pp. 286–311, 318–327. Interscience, New York.
2. Bennett, B. M., Tam, G. S., Van Alstyne, K., Brien, J. F., Nakatsu, K., and Marks, G. S. (1985). Effect of 5-isosorbide mononitrate on isosorbide dinitrate-induced relaxation of rabbit aortic rings. *Can. J. Physiol. Pharmacol.* **62,** 1194–1197.

3. Benz, C., Cadman, E., Gwin, J., Wu, T., Amara, J., Eisenfeld, A., and Dannies, P. (1983). 5-Fluorouracil in breast cancer: Cytotoxic synergism *in vitro*. *Cancer Res.* **43,** 5298–5305.
4. Berenbaum, M. C. (1977). Synergy, additivism and antagonism in immunosuppression: A critical review. *Clin. Exp. Immunol.* **28,** 1–18.
5. Berenbaum, M. C. (1985). The expected effect of a combination of agents: The general solution. *J. Theor. Biol.* **114,** 413–431.
6. Bergerat, J., Green, C., and Drewinko, B. (1979). Combination chemotherapy *in vitro*. IV. Response of human colon carcinoma cells to combinations using cis-diamminedichloroplatinum. *Cancer Biochem. Biophys.* **3,** 173–180.
7. Bliss, C. I. (1967). "Statistics in Biology." McGraw-Hill, New York.
8. Bounias, M. (1980). Correlations between glucose-inhibition and control parameters of α-glucosidase kinetics in *Apis mellifica* haemolymph. *Experientia* **36,** 157–159.
9. Bounias, M. (1982). Kinetic study of the inhibition of the honeybee α-glucosidase *in vitro* by BAYe 4609, BAYg 5421 and BAYn 5595. *Biochem. Pharmacol.* **31,** 2769–2775.
10. Bryan, W. R., and Shimkin, M. B. (1943). Quantitative analysis of dose-response data obtained in strain C3H mice. *J. Natl. Cancer Inst. (U.S.)* **3,** 503–531.
11. Chang, T. T., Gulati, S. C., Chou, T.-C., Vega, R., Gandola, L., Ibrahim, S., Yopp, J., Colvin, M., and Clarkson, B. (1985). Synergistic effect of 4-hydroperoxycyclophosphamide and etoposide on HL-60 myelogenous leukemia cell line as demonstrated by computer analysis. *Cancer Res.* **45,** 2434–2439.
12. Chou, J., and Chou, T.-C. (1985). "Dose-Effect Analysis with Microcomputers: Quantitiation of ED_{50}, LD_{50}, Synergism, Antagonism, Low-Dose Risk, Receptor Ligand Binding and Enzyme Kinetics," Manual and Software Disk for Apple II or IMB PC Series. Elsevier-Biosoft, Cambridge, U.K.
13. Chou, J., Chou, T.-C., and Talalay, P. (1983). Computer simulation of drug effects: Quantitation of synergism, summation and antagonism of multiple drugs. *Pharmacologist* **25,** 175.
14. Chou, T.-C. (1974). Relationships between inhibition constants and fractional inhibition in enzyme-catalyzed reactions with different numbers of reactants, different reaction mechanisms, and different types and mechanisms of inhibition. *Mol. Pharmacol.* **10,** 235–247.
15. Chou, T.-C. (1975). A general procedure for determination of median-effect doses by a double logarithmic transformation of dose-response relationships. *Fed. Proc., Fed. Am. Soc. Exp. Biol.* **34,** 228.
16. Chou, T.-C. (1976). Derivation and properties of Michaelis-Menten type and Hill type equations for reference ligands. *J. Theor. Biol.* **59,** 253–276.
17. Chou, T.-C. (1977). Analysis of dose-effect relationships of carcinogens with a median-effect principle. *Fed. Proc., Fed. Am. Soc. Exp. Biol.* **36,** 304.
18. Chou, T.-C. (1977). Comparison of the mass-action law with the power law, the probit law and the logit law in dose-effect analysis. *Pharmacologist* **19,** 165.
19. Chou, T.-C. (1977). On the determination of availability of ligand binding sites in steady-state systems. *J. Theor. Biol.* **65,** 345–356.
20. Chou, T.-C. (1978). Estimation of low-risk carcinogens by the median-effect equation of the mass-action law. *Proc. Am. Assoc. Cancer Res.* **19,** 162.
21. Chou, T.-C. (1980). Comparison of dose-effect relationships of carcinogens following low-dose chronic exposure and high-dose single injection: An analysis by the median-effect principle. *Carcinogenesis (N.Y.)* **1,** 203–213.
22. Chou, T.-C. (1981). Carcinogenic risk assessment by a mass-action law principle: Application to large scale chronic feeding experiment with 2-acetylaminofuorene (2-AAF). *Proc. Am. Assoc. Cancer Res.* **22,** 141.

23. Chou, T.-C., and Talalay, P. (1977). A simple generalized equation for the analysis of multiple inhibitors of Michaelis-Menten kinetic systems. *J. Biol. Chem.* **252,** 6438–6442.

24. Chou, T.-C., and Talalay, P. (1981). Generalized equations for the analysis of inhibitions of Michaelis-Menten and higher-order kinetic systems with two or more mutually exclusive and nonexclusive inhibitors. *Eur. J. Biochem.* **115,** 207–216.

25. Chou, T.-C., and Talalay, P. (1983). Analysis of combined drug effects: A new look at a very old problem. *Trends Pharmacol. Sci.* **4,** 450–454.

26. Chou, T.-C., and Talalay, P. (1984). Quantitative analysis of dose-effect relationships: The combined effects of multiple drugs or enzyme inhibitors. *Adv. Enzyme Regul.* **22,** 27–55.

27. Chou, T.-C., Chou, J., and Talalay, P. (1984). Conservation of laboratory animals by improved experimental design, generalized equations and computer analysis. *Fed. Proc., Fed. Am. Soc. Exp. Biol.* **43,** 576.

28. Cleland, W. W. (1963). The kinetics of enzyme catalyzed reactions with two or more substrates or products. *Biochim. Biophys. Acta* **67,** 173–196.

29. Dixon, M., and Webb, E. C., eds. (1980). "Enzymes," 3rd ed., pp. 332–381. Academic Press, New York.

30. Elion, G. B., Singer, S., and Hitchings, G. H. (1954). Antagonists of nucleic acid derivatives. VIII. Synergism in combinations of biochemically related antimetabolites. *J. Biol. Chem.* **208,** 477–488.

31. Finney, D. J. (1952). "Probit Analysis," 2nd ed., pp. 146–153. Cambridge Univ. Press, London and New York.

32. Finotti, P., and Palatini, P. (1981). Canrenome as a partial agonist at the digitalis receptor site of sodium-potassium-activated adenosine triphosphatase. *J. Pharmacol. Exp. Ther.* **217,** 784–790.

33. Friedman, S. J., and Skehan, P. (1980). Membrane-active drugs potentiate the killing of tumor cells by D-glucosamine. *Proc. Natl. Acad. Sci. U.S.A.* **77,** 1172–1176.

34. Goldin, A., and Mantel, N. (1957). The employment of combinations of drugs in the chemotherapy of neoplasia: A review. *Cancer Res.* **17,** 635–654.

35. Goldin, A., Venditti, J. M., Mantel, N., Kline, I., and Gang, M. (1968). Evaluation of combination chemotherapy with three drugs. *Cancer Res.* **28,** 950–960.

36. Goldstein, A., Aronow, L., and Kalman, S. M. (1968). "Principles of Drug Action: The Basis of Pharmacology." Harper & Row, New York.

37. Hata, K., Hayakawa, M., Abiko, Y., and Takiguchi, H. (1981). Purification and properties of γ-glutamyl transpeptidase from bovine parotid gland. *Int. J. Biochem.* **13,** 681–692.

38. Hill, A. V. (1913). The combinations of hemoglobin with oxygen and carbon monoxide. *Biochem. J.* **7,** 471–480.

39. Institute for Scientific Information (1983). "Permutation Index, under the Titles of Synergism, Synergistic, Synergistically and Synergy." Current Contents, Life Sciences, Philadelphia, Pennsylvania.

40. Kobayashi, S., and Hoshino, T. (1983). Combined cytotoxic effect of low-dose 5-fluorouracil and hydroxyurea on 9L cells *in vitro. Cancer Res.* **43,** 5309–5313.

41. Kopelovich, L., and Chou, T.-C. (1984). The proliferative response of low density human cell cultures to tumor promoters and its relevance to carcinogenic mechanisms *in vitro. Int. J. Cancer* **34,** 781–788.

42. Kremer, A. B., Egan, R. M., and Sable, H. Z. (1980). The active site of transketolase: Two arginine residues are essential for activity. *J. Biol. Chem.* **255,** 2405–2410.

43. Le Pelley, R. H., and Sullivan, W. N. (1936). Toxicity of rotenone and pyrethrins alone and in combination. *J. Econ. Entomol.* **29,** 791–797.

44. Loewe, S. (1928). Die quantitation probleme der pharmakologie. *Ergeb. Physiol.* **27**, 47–187.
45. Loewe, S. (1953). The problem of synergism and antagonism of combined drugs. *Arzneim. Forsch.* **3**, 285–320.
46. Michaelis, L., and Menten, M. L. (1913). Die kinetik der invertinwirkung. *Biochem. Z.* **49**, 333–369.
47. Murphy, K. M. M., and Snyder, S. H. (1982). Heterogeneity of adenosine A, receptor binding in brain tissue. *Mol. Pharmacol.* **22**, 250–257.
48. Nakamura, C. E., and Abeles, R. H. (1985). Mode of interaction of β-hydroxy-β-methylglutaryl coenzyme A reductase with strong binding inhibitors: Compactin and related compounds. *Biochemistry* **24**, 1364–1376.
49. Nichol, C. A., Grindey, G. B., Moran, R. G., and Werkheiser, W. C. (1972). Combinations of drugs which interact as inhibitors of DNA biosynthesis. *Adv. Enzyme Regul.* **10**, 63–80.
50. Penning, M., Mukharji, I., Barrows, S., and Talalay, P. (1984). Purification and properties of a 3α-hydroxysteroid dehydrogenase of rat liver cytosol and its inhibition by anti-inflammatory drugs. *Biochem. J.* **222**, 601–611.
51. Peto, R., Roe, F. J. C., Levy, L., and Clark, J. (1975). Cancer and aging in mice and men. *Br. J. Cancer* **32**, 411–426.
52. Reed, L. J., and Berkson, J. (1929). The application of the logistic function to experimental data. *J. Phys. Chem.* **33**, 760–779.
53. Rosenberg, R. (1981). A kinetic analysis of L-tryptophan transport in human red blood cells. *Biochim. Biophys. Acta* **649**, 262–268.
54. Segel, I. H. (1975). Multiple inhibition analysis. *In* "Enzyme Kinetics," pp. 465–503. Wiley, New York.
55. Skipper, H. E. (1974). Combination therapy: Some concepts and results. *Cancer Chemother. Rep.* **5**, 137–146.
56. Smith, S. M. (1982). A model of labelled-ligand displacement assay resulting in logit-log relationships. *J. Theor. Biol.* **98**, 475–499.
57. Steckel, J., Robert, J., Philips, F. S., and Chou, T.-C. (1983). Kinetic properties and inhibition of Acinetobacter glutaminase-asparaginase. *Biochem. Pharmacol.* **32**, 971–977.
58. Steel, G. G., and Peckham, M. J. (1979). Exploitable mechanisms in combined radiotherapy-chemotherapy: The concept of additivity. *Int. J. Radiat. Oncol.* **5**, 85–91.
59. Stock, C. C., Reilly, H., Buckley, S. M., Clarke, D. A., and Rhoads, C. P. (1955). Azaserine, a tumor inhibitory antibiotic. *Acta Unio Int. Cancrum* **11**, 186–193.
60. Teller, M. N., Stock, C., Bowie, M., Chou, T.-C., and Budinger, J. M. (1982). Therapy of DMBA-induced rat mammary carcinomas with combinations of 5-fluorouracil and 2α-methyldihydrotestosterone propionate. *Cancer Res.* **42**, 4408–4412.
61. Vanderheyden, P., Andre, C., De Backer, J.-P., and Vauquelin, G. (1984). Agonist mediated conformational changes of solubilized calf forebrain muscarinic acetylcholine receptors. *Biochem. Proc.* **33**, 2981–2987.
62. Vauquelin, G., Andre, C., De Backer, J.-P., Lauduron, P., and Strosberg, A. D. (1982). Agonist-mediated conformational changes of muscarinic receptors in rat brain. *Eur. J. Biochem.* **125**, 117–124.
63. Viswanathan, T., and Alworth, W. F. (1981). Effects of 1-arylpyrroles and naphthoflavones upon cytochrome P-450 dependent monooxygenase activities. *J. Med. Chem.* **24**, 822–830.
64. Webb, J. L. (1963). Effect of more than one inhibitor. *In* "Enzyme and Metabolic Inhibitors," Vol. 1, pp. 66–79, 488–512. Academic Press, New York.

3

Stereochemical Determinants of Enzyme Inhibition

DAVID A. MATTHEWS

The Agouron Institute
La Jolla, California

I. The Principle of Receptor-Based Design of Therapeutic Agents

Chemotherapy is a contrived mechanism for biological intervention whereby specific pharmaceutical compounds are induced to interact with key cellular components in order to achieve some desired clinical effect. Drug development has usually followed a classical approach involving the empirical testing of more or less random chemicals. Especially in the case of antiinfectives, many of the most useful compounds are enzyme inhibitors. These antimetabolites are in effect poisons, and therefore a crucial and fundamental problem for efficacious chemotherapy is how to obtain selectivity of action.

The old methods of randomly screening compounds for desired phar-

NEW AVENUES IN DEVELOPMENTAL
CANCER CHEMOTHERAPY

macological activity that in the past have led to the discovery of many antiinfectives of varying degrees of efficacy are simply not providing the new leads required to meet this problem head-on. The difficulties lie not only with fundamental uncertainties having to do with whether compounds with the desired activity can ever be uncovered by such random methods, but also, past history tells us that the vast majority of compounds discovered in this manner have had dangerous toxicities which have led to their demise as useful therapeutic agents. Recently there have been significant major advances in molecular biology, X-ray crystallographic protein structure determination, computational methods, and computer graphics which now make it possible to think in terms of rationally designing drugs based on complementarity to the detailed molecular structures of selected essential proteins of the target parasites (9). Focusing on appropriately chosen enzymes it should be possible to engineer compounds that will selectively shut down key metabolic pathways of an invading organism, having the desired clinical effect while at the same time reducing the chances of unanticipated host toxicity.

In order to assess the practicality of this approach for drug design and to gain further insight into how subtle structural differences between homologous proteins can modulate inhibitor selectivity, we have used high-resolution X-ray diffraction methods to determine the molecular structures of four species of dihydrofolate reductase (DHFR) and various complexes of these enzymes with substrates, cofactors, and inhibitors. DHFR is an attractive target for design of antimicrobial agents, both because of its essential role in cell replication and its structural variability among evolutionarily divergent organisms. Thus the clinical importance of trimethoprim (TMP) and pyrimethamine as antibacterial and antimalarial agents, respectively, is a direct consequence of their remarkable selectivity for specific microbial DHFRs.

Almost 35 years ago in an insightful and prophetic analysis of their studies of 2,4-diaminoheterocycles as folic acid antagonists, George Hitchings and collaborators foresaw that "the successful application of antimetabolites to problems of chemotherapy is dependent for success on a differential affinity of antimetabolite for the receptor of the parasite owing to details of structure in parasite and host which are largely indefinable and unpredictable" (12). The "indefinable" nature of structural differences among isofunctional enzymes from different species (tissues) remains a primary impediment to the full realization of "rational" design of highly specific chemotherapeutic agents. It will be seen, however, that for DHFR, based on painstaking X-ray diffraction studies, we now have a plausible stereochemical hypothesis to explain inhibitor selectivity—a model that for the first time permits a detailed accounting to be made of the structural basis underlying the selectivity of a drug (TMP in this case). A demonstration of the potential power of these crystallographic methods for understanding selective inhibition of isofunctional proteins may encourage molecular biologists working with oncogenes and proto-oncogenes to overproduce the corresponding gene products so that they can be subjected to similar kinds of comparative structural analyses for the purpose of rationally designing novel selective antitumor agents with chemotherapeutic potential.

II. Dihydrofolate Reductase as a Target for Antimetabolites

DHFR is a very widely occurring enzyme that catalyzes the NADPH-dependent reduction of 7,8-dihydrofolate (FAH_2) to 5,6,7,8-tetrahydrofolate (FAH_4).

$$FAH_2 + NADPH + H^+ \rightleftharpoons FAH_4 + NADP^+$$

DHFR plays a vital role in the metabolism of proliferating cells, because it is required for the maintenance of adequate levels of fully reduced folates. Tetrahydrofolate in its various derivative forms is an important carrier of one-carbon units needed in the biosynthesis of thymidylate, purines, methionine, and other essential metabolites. In the reaction catalyzed by thymidylate synthase, 5,10-methylenetetrahydrofolate undergoes an unusual internal oxidation–reduction in which one molecule of tetrahydrofolate is oxidized to dihydrofolate for each molecule of thymidylate produced. Inhibition of DHFR in a line of rapidly multiplying cells blocks the re-reduction of dihydrofolate and thereby results in stasis or death due to depletion of the metabolic pool of tetrahydrofolate.

From the perspective of the scientist interested in unraveling the intricacies of ligand binding to macromolecules, it would be difficult to envision a more appealing and potentially informative protein for study than the enzyme DHFR. Inhibitors of DHFR include compounds such as methotrexate (MTX) (Fig. 1) that are close structural analogs of folate but act as extremely potent competitive inhibitors of chromosomal DHFRs, binding as much as 10^6 times more tightly to the reductase than folate itself. A second group of inhibitors comprises compounds that bear no obvious structural relationship to folate or dihydrofolate other than that they contain a 2,4-diaminoheterocycle, analogous to the 2-amino-4-oxopyrimidine portion of the substrate's pteridine ring. What makes this class of structurally diverse molecules so interesting is that individual compounds act as species-selective inhibitors of DHFR, with each partic-

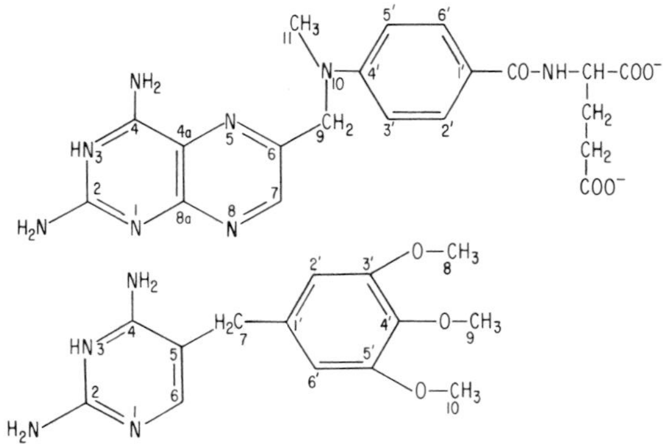

Fig. 1. Covalent structure and atom numbering for methotrexate (top) and tri-methoprim.

ular enzyme species exhibiting characteristic sensitivity to the exact electronic and geometrical properties of the inhibitor's ring substituents. TMP (Fig. 1), for example, binds about 3000 times more strongly to the *Escherichia coli* enzyme than to the vertebrate enzyme (1).

In what follows we begin by discussing the molecular architecture of bacterial DHFR and the details of its interaction with MTX and then go on to compare this structure with that of chicken DHFR. Finally, we contrast high-resolution refined X-ray structures for TMP and other 2,4-diaminoheterocyclic inhibitors bound to both *E. coli* and chicken DHFR and from these results develop a stereochemical hypothesis to account for DHFR inhibitor selectivity.

III. X-Ray Diffraction Studies of Dihydrofolate Reductase

A. Bacterial Enzymes

Backbone folding for the *Lactobacillus casei* DHFR : NADPH : MTX ternary complex (15) is indicated in Fig. 2 and may be taken as representative of all known chromosomal DHFR structures. The central architectural feature is an eight-stranded, mixed beta sheet with a single antiparallel strand leading to the carboxy terminus. This sheet shows the usual twist between adjacent strands amounting to approximately 130° from one edge to the other. Four alpha helices pack against the central beta sheet while the remaining residues make up loops, some quite lengthy, connect-

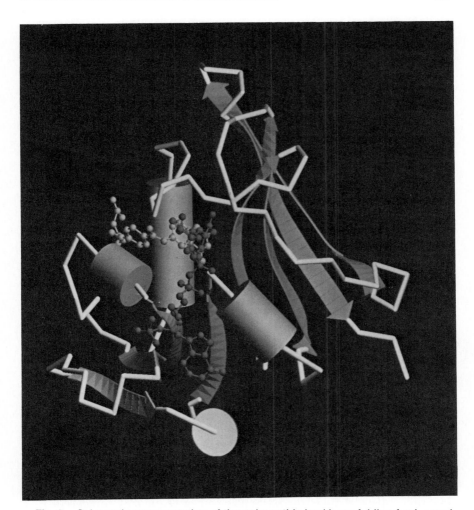

Fig. 2. Schematic representation of the polypeptide backbone folding for *L. casei* dihydrofolate reductase containing bound NADPH and methotrexate. Individual strands of the central beta sheet and the four helical regions are indicated by arrows and cylinders, respectively. [Adapted from a drawing by Dr. Jane Burridge, U.K. Scientific Centre of the IBM Corporation.]

ing the elements of secondary structure. The active site containing MTX is seen as a 15-Å-deep cavity cutting across one whole face of the enzyme while the cofactor binds in an open conformation along a shallow cleft with its nicotinamide ring tucked underneath and in close proximity to the pteridine portion of MTX. In subsequent discussions, individual strands of beta sheet are referred to as beta A through beta H, beginning with the amino-terminal strand. Each alpha helical segment, alpha A, alpha C, alpha E, or alpha F, is lettered according to the beta strand immediately following it in the linear amino acid sequence.

Although differing in total number of residues by only three, DHFRs from *E. coli* and *L. casei* have an amino acid sequence homology of less than 30%. In contrast to this variation in primary sequence, X-ray diffraction investigations reveal that overall backbone geometrics for the two bacterial reductases are almost identical, despite the presence of a bound cofactor molecule in the *L. casei* ternary complex that is not present in crystals of the *E. coli* DHFR : MTX binary complex (14,15). Thus when 142 of 159 alpha-carbon coordinates in *E. coli* DHFR are matched by least squares to structurally equivalent alpha-carbon coordinates for the *L. casei* enzyme, the root mean square deviation is only 1.07 Å (4). In three instances a single amino acid insertion or deletion occurs in *L. casei* DHFR, relative to the *E. coli* enzyme. These differences appear in loops connecting elements of secondary structure, and it is in these turns that one finds the greatest structural variability between the two bacterial reductases. A two-residue insertion in the *L. casei* molecule provides an extra half-turn of helix at the carboxyl end of alpha E, as compared with the corresponding alpha helix in *E. coli* DHFR.

B. Chicken Enzyme

The five vertebrate reductases of known sequence (chicken, mouse, cow, pig, and human) are highly homologous, having 75–95% amino acid identities, depending on the particular pair of sequences compared. As a group they differ from their bacterial counterparts in various physical and chemical properties, with respect to their relative sensitivities toward inhibitors and in terms of their molecular weights—vertebrate DHFRs being some 25–30 amino acids larger than the typical bacterial enzyme. Crystallographic studies of chicken DHFR were begun in the early 1980s in the anticipation that structural comparisons between it and the bacterial enzymes would reveal exactly how the additional residues in vertebrate DHFR are accommodated in the enzyme's overall tertiary structure, thus perhaps suggesting stereochemical mechanisms by which different species of DHFR modulate inhibitor selectivity. As we shall see later, with only a single exception the "extra" amino acids characteristic of vertebrate DHFRs occur in loops connecting individual pieces of secondary structure, and moreover, these insertions are far removed spatially from the enzyme's active site (21). This suggests that the influence of these additional residues, if any, on the characteristic inhibitor-binding properties of vertebrate DHFRs is probably indirect, in the sense that the geometric consequences of such insertions must be propogated to the active site over distances of 15 Å or more.

The overall backbone folding of chicken DHFR is very similar to that observed in the *E. coli* and *L. casei* enzymes (21). All four alpha helices and seven of the eight beta strands present in bacterial enzymes are conserved in the chicken reductase. It is notable, however, that the precise relative positioning of these elements of secondary structure in vertebrate DHFRs differs by as much as 1–3 Å from their relative positioning in the bacterial DHFRs, particularly in the neighborhood of the substrate binding site (21). This curious observation will be discussed further in a later section on inhibitor binding. Except for six residues that simply lengthen the amino and carboxy termini of chicken DHFR relative to those of *E. coli* and *L. casei,* over 70% of the extra residues in the chicken enzyme occur in three loops that are far removed from the active site. The

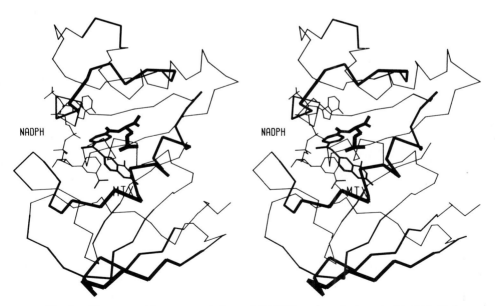

Fig. 3. Stereographic representation of NADPH and methotrexate binding to *L. casei* dihydrofolate reductase.

conformations of all insertions present in the chicken enzyme can be seen in Fig. 3, in which the extra loops are added onto a schematic drawing of the polypeptide backbone folding of *L. casei* DHFR.

IV. Stereochemistry of Inhibitor Binding

A. Methotrexate

We begin our discussion of inhibitor binding to DHFR with MTX, a potent, tight-binding inhibitor that is closely related structurally to folate itself. Although in the present context our principal interest is in providing structural insights into the mechanism of DHFR selectivity, MTX binding represents an important preliminary consideration, because it establishes the "ground rules" for potent inhibition of any DHFR. Thus we find that for all tight-binding 2,4-diaminoheterocyclic inhibitors of *E. coli* or chicken DHFR examined to date, including pteridines, pyridopyrimidines, quinazolines, pyrimidines, and triazines, the polar interactions between enzyme and inhibitor are indistinguishable from those observed for the 2,4-diaminopyrimidine portion of MTX (16,17). MTX binds to DHFR in an open conformation (Fig. 4), with its pteridine ring nearly perpendic-

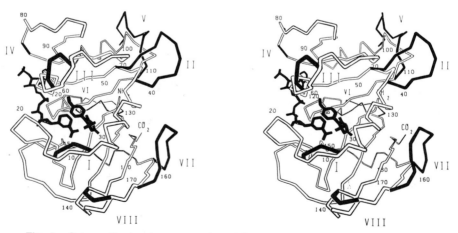

Fig. 4. Schematic drawing comparing alpha carbon backbone folding for ternary complexes of chicken dihydrofolate reductase (enzyme : NADPH : phenyltriazine) and *L. casei* dihydrofolate reductase (enzyme : NADPH : MTX). Backbone conformation is for the bacterial enzyme with "insertions" present in the chicken enzyme shown in black. [Adapted from Volz *et al.* (21).]

ular to the aromatic ring of its *p*-aminobenzoyl group. The inhibitor-binding cleft is a 15-Å-deep crevice formed primarily by residues from helix alpha B, the central beta strands beta A and beta F, and the loops connecting beta A to alpha B and alpha C to beta C. The pyrimidine portion of MTX is deeply buried in a portion of the pocket that is formed by highly conserved residues, including a key acidic amino acid (aspartate or glutamate, depending on the enzyme species) that is positioned at the amino-terminal end of alpha B. The *p*-aminobenzoylglutamate moiety leads away from the interior of the protein to the surface where its alpha carboxylate interacts with the guanidinium side chain of an invariant arginine residue. Anticipating subsequent discussion we will now consider in more detail protein–MTX interactions at the pteridine binding site.

A variety of evidence, namely, spectroscopic (11), calorimetric (20), and theoretical (18), strongly suggests that N-1 is protonated when MTX binds to DHFR. In an elegant series of experiments, Cocco, Blakley and co-workers have monitored the ^{13}C-NMR signal for MTX enriched at the 2 position of the pteridine ring when bound to DHFR from *L. casei* (6), *Streptococcus faecium* (7), and bovine liver (8). They find that the ^{13}C chemical shift for enzyme-bound MTX does not change as the pH is raised from 6 to 10, indicating that the pK_a for N-1 must be over 10—that is, 5 pH units above its value in free MTX. By elementary thermodynamic arguments, this must also mean that the protonated species of MTX binds to the enzyme (the latter in its COO$^-$ state—see next paragraph) with an association constant more than 10^5 times greater than that for the unprotonated species (7).

The crystallographic studies provide a structural explanation for this observation. When MTX binds to DHFR, a pair of hydrogen bonds is found between the carboxyl side chain of Asp-26 (*L. casei* DHFR numbering, lc) on the one hand and the pteridine ring N-1 and 2-amino group of the inhibitor on the other (see Fig. 5). Moreover, the carboxyl group is nearly coplanar with the bound pteridine ring. It appears very probable, in light of the evidence just cited, that the pteridine ring of bound MTX is protonated at N-1, and that the side chain of Asp-26 is in the ionized, anionic state. Thus if bound MTX is deprotonated at N-1, it would make one less hydrogen bond with the enzyme in its COO$^-$ state and would make no charge–charge interaction, thereby accounting for the factor of 10^5 just mentioned. It should be emphasized at this point that the foregoing analysis of MTX binding says nothing directly about a comparison with binding of dihydrofolate in the E : S complex, which is orders of magnitude weaker, since it is thought that Asp-26 is unionized in the E : S complex. Moreover, the pteridine ring of dihydrofolate is oriented differ-

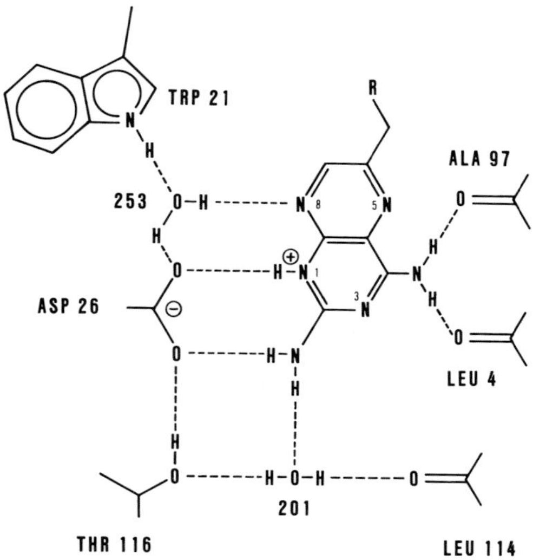

Fig. 5. Hydrogen bonding between *L. casei* dihydrofolate reductase and the pteridine portion of methotrexate. [From Bolin *et al.* (4).]

ently in the active site and has a 4-oxo group where MTX has a 4-amino group.

To continue with our description of protein–ligand interactions at the pteridine binding site, a second hydrogen bond exists between the 2-amino group of MTX and a fixed water molecule, which is in turn hydrogen-bonded to the side chain hydroxyl of Thr-116,1c. Since this threonine is strictly conserved in all DHFR sequences, the bridging water molecule is almost certainly an invariant feature of the enzyme structure (4).

Other than N-1, the only endocyclic ring nitrogen involved in hydrogen bonding is N-8. A structurally conserved fixed water molecule, Wat-253,1c, lies 3.3 Å from N-8 directly in line with its lone pair orbital. In turn, this water molecule can hydrogen-bond with two side chains and a second molecule of fixed solvent.

The inhibitor's 4-amino group donates hydrogen bonds to the backbone carbonyl oxygens of Leu-4,lc and Ala-97,lc (4,15). Corresponding backbone carbonyls exist in geometrically analogous locations in both the *E. coli* and chicken DHFRs (4,14,21). Notwithstanding the apparently fortuitous location of the carbonyl of residue 97,lc for hydrogen bonding to the 4-amino group of MTX, which is, of course, an artificial inhibitor with no role in biology, it would appear that the observed geometry in this region of the molecule is probably important for enzyme function.

B. Trimethoprim

1. Binding to E. coli DHFR

An interesting characteristic of the interaction between DHFR and its inhibitors is the high degree of species selectivity exhibited by some types of inhibitors. Such species selectivity is one of the important factors underlying TMP's value as an antibacterial agent. In light of the overall similarity in molecular architecture between *E. coli, L. casei,* and chicken DHFRs just noted, an intriguing question is to what extent species differences in binding affinity for TMP can be understood in terms of the molecular structures of the respective enzyme–inhibitor complexes. From a structure–function viewpoint we would like to have a geometrical description of TMP binding to a bacterial and vertebrate DHFR, some idea of which binding differences are most crucial in modulating selectivity, and some understanding of how subtle species-dependent differences in enzyme structure can account for observed inhibitor binding properties. In what follows, we examine the results of recent research designed to address some of these topics.

A model for TMP binding to *L. casei* DHFR in solution was first proposed by Cayley *et al.* (5), based on NMR transfer of saturation experiments which permitted identification of certain proton resonances of the bound inhibitor. Subsequent crystallographic studies by Baker *et al.* (2) revealed that for the TMP binary complex with *E. coli* DHFR, the inhibitor's two aromatic rings were held in a nearly perpendicular conformation closely resembling one of two possible conformers predicted from the magnetic resonance investigation. Shortly thereafter, Matthews and Volz (13) demonstrated that the geometry of TMP binding to chicken DHFR is significantly different from that reported earlier for the bacterial enzyme. Recently the crystallographic structures just cited have been refined and analyzed at high resolution in order to facilitate a detailed comparison of TMP binding to a bacterial and vertebrate DHFR (16,17).

The geometry of TMP binding to *E. coli* DHFR closely resembles that of MTX binding, especially at their respective 2,4-diaminopyrimidine moieties, which interact identically with the enzyme (Fig. 6). As in the case of MTX binding, the side chain of Asp-27,ec closely approaches both N-1 and the 2-amino group of TMP in a geometry that is consistent with the existence of a hydrogen-bonded salt bridge. Evidence from NMR experiments indicates that the pK_a of TMP is increased from about 7.5 in solution to over 10 upon binding to DHFR (8,19) the effect presumably occurring at N-1. Thus N-1 is probably protonated, and Asp-27 deprotonated in the complex. A further point of similarity between the MTX and TMP complexes is that a tightly bound solvent molecule mediates a

DAVID A. MATTHEWS

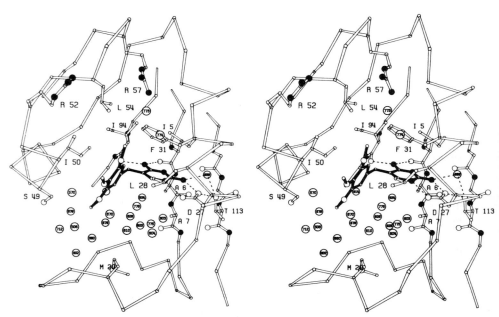

Fig. 6. Binding of trimethoprim to *E. coli* dihydrofolate reductase. Trimethoprim is indicated by solid bonds, and protein by open bonds. Carbon atoms are represented by smaller open circles, oxygen atoms by larger open circles, and nitrogen items by blackened circles. Large numbered circles represent fixed solvent molecules. Hydrogen bonds are indicated by dashed lines. [From Matthews *et al.* (16).]

second hydrogen bond between the 2-amino group and the side chain hydroxyl of the conserved residue Thr-113,ec. Finally, to complete the comparison between the environment of the pyrimidine rings in bound MTX and TMP, the same pair of backbone carbonyl oxygens (Ile-5 and Ile-94,ec) lies in the plane of the pyrimidine ring, positioned to accept hydrogen bonds from the 4-amino group. The active-site region below the pyrimidine ring is open to solvent and contains several bound water molecules. Structural comparison with the *L. casei* DHFR : NADPH : MTX ternary complex (10) suggests that in the presence of bound cofactor, many of these fixed solvent molecules will be displaced in order to accomodate the nicotinamide ring.

The crystallographic evidence suggests that an important factor underlying the strong affinity of TMP for *E. coli* DHFR is the favorable van der Waals interaction between the trimethoxybenzyl group of TMP and protein residues on two helices, alpha B and alpha C, at the entrance to the active site cleft. Ser-49 and Ile-50 are located at the C-terminal end of alpha C where they form a wall, composed of both main chain and side chain atoms, against which the trimethoxybenzene ring of TMP rests. On the opposite side of the active site cleft, Leu-28, in the middle of alpha B, provides the major protein contacts with the side chain of TMP.

2. Weak Binding to Chicken DHFR Results from Loss of a Crucial Hydrogen Bond

Structural comparison of chicken and *E. coli* DHFR complexes containing TMP reveals several notable differences in inhibitor binding geometry. The most obvious differences involve (1) hydrogen bonding at the 4-amino substituent of the pyrimidine ring, (2) enzyme-inhibitor interactions at the trimethoxybenzyl group, (3) inhibitor side chain torsion angles, and (4) a large swinging movement of the side chain of Tyr-31 when TMP binds to the chicken enzyme (16).

As would be expected, the pyrimidine binding site in chicken DHFR is analogous to the corresponding site in bacterial DHFRs (Fig. 7). How-

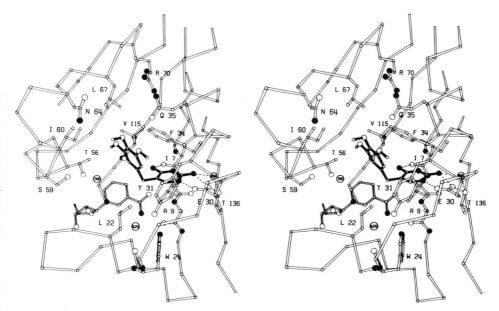

Fig. 7.   Binding of TMP and NADPH to chicken dihydrofolate reductase. Trimethoprim is indicated by solid bonds, protein by open bonds, and a portion of the NADPH molecule by striped bonds. Carbon atoms are represented by smaller open circles, oxygen atoms by larger open circles, and nitrogen atoms by blackened circles. Large numbered circles represent fixed solvent molecules. Hydrogen bonds are indicated by dashed lines. [From Matthews *et al.* (16).]

ever, an important finding is that there are certain peculiarities about the way TMP binds to the chicken enzyme. One such observation is that the pyrimidine ring is inserted almost 1 Å more deeply into the active site cleft than are the pyrimidines of TMP or MTX bound to the *E. coli* enzyme. Thus, whereas the 4-amino group of TMP participates in two hydrogen bonds with backbone carbonyl oxygens of *E. coli* DHFR, only one of the corresponding hydrogen bonds remains intact in the chicken DHFR : NADPH : TMP ternary complex—that between the 4-amino group of TMP and the backbone carbonyl of Ile-7,cl. Other hydrogen bonds between the pteridine ring and chicken DHFR are analogous to those previously discussed for TMP binding to *E. coli* DHFR, including the important hydrogen bond–mediated salt linkage between the active-site carboxylate (Glu-30 in chicken DHFR) and the N-1 and 2-amino group of TMP. Recent NMR data are also consistent with the notion that at least for TMP and MTX, interaction between the inhibitor's protonated N-1 and the active-site carboxylate group is very similar for DHFRs from three bacterial and two vertebrate species (3,8).

For TMP bound to *E. coli* DHFR the inhibitor's benzyl side chain is positioned low in the active site pocket, pointing down toward the nicotinamide binding site (the "down" conformation which positions the inhibitor side chain in the "lower" cleft), whereas in chicken DHFR the benzyl group is accommodated in a side channel running upward and away from the cofactor (the "up" conformation which positions the inhibitor side chain in the "upper" cleft). Clearly, interactions between the benzyl group and the enzyme are quite different in these two cases. Birdsall *et al.* (3) and Cocco *et al.* (8) have made similar inferences from their NMR studies and have gone on to propose that specific differences in the way a particular DHFR interacts with the TMP side chain is the major factor modulating inhibitor selectivity.

In a series of different Fourier analyses of inhibitor binding to chicken DHFR, Matthews *et al.* (17) have shown that this is probably not the major factor influencing TMP selectivity, since the trimethoxybenzyl group of TMP binds to chicken DHFR in the same hydrophobic pocket that accomodates the side chains of various other pyrimidine and triazine inhibitors that, unlike TMP, are extremely potent inhibitors of vertebrate DHFRs. Moreover, these authors were able to show that conformational changes accompanying TMP binding to chicken DHFR and torsional differences about the benzyl carbon for TMP bound to *E. coli* and chicken DHFRs are most likely of little importance in explaining TMP's poor affinity for vertebrate DHFRs. What was very clear from these crystallographic investigations, however, was that only for inhibitors that are weakly bound to chicken DHFR did Matthews *et al.* (16) observe an altered binding geometry wherein the 2,4-diamino heterocycle occupies a position approximately 1 Å closer to alpha B where it can no longer hydrogen-bond to the carbonyl of Val-115 (Ile-94,ec). Thus, the crystallographic evidence strongly suggests that loss of this hydrogen bond is a significant factor in TMP's low affinity for chicken DHFR and, therefore, must be an important determinant of the drug's selectivity.

C. Active Site Structural Differences and Inhibitor Selectivity

In attempting to explain why TMP binds differently to *E. coli* and chicken DHFR, Matthews *et al.* (17) have pointed out that residues on opposite sides of the active site cleft in chicken DHFR are about 1.5–2.0 Å further apart than are structurally equivalent residues in the *E. coli* enzyme. Because of this increased width across the cavity bound by alpha B and alpha C in chicken DHFR and because of the presence of Tyr or Phe at position 31 in vertebrate DHFRs (instead of Leu-28 in *E. coli* DHFR), model-building experiments conclusively demonstrate that the TMP side chain cannot be favorably accommodated in the lower cavity of vertebrate DHFR. Specifically, if hydrophobic interactions on the left side of the cleft of chicken DHFR between the side chain of Ile-60 and a hypothetical trimethoxybenzyl group of TMP in the down conformation are required to be similar to the corresponding interactions found for the *E. coli* DHFR : TMP binary complex, then it is not possible to position the side chain of Tyr-31,cl (or the corresponding Phe side chain of other vertebrate DHFRs) to provide favorable hydrophobic contacts on the right side of the cleft analogous to those provided by Leu-28 in the *E. coli* enzyme. In other words, a gap would be left between the benzyl group and the enzyme. The upshot of these considerations is that for chicken DHFR, the trimethoxybenzyl group of TMP can only be adequately accommodated in an alternate binding site (the upper cleft) which simultaneously results in a disruption of hydrogen bonding to the 2,4-diaminopyrimidine, thus reducing the binding of TMP to vertebrate DHFR.

V. Conclusions

What conclusions can be drawn from these studies and what have we learned that may be helpful in guiding future work on receptor-based design of selective chemotherapeutic agents? One important conclusion is that subtle structural differences among isofunctional proteins can significantly alter the geometry of inhibitor binding, leading to pronounced differences in enzyme–inhibitor association constants. Furthermore, it is unlikely that these structural differences could have been anticipated or predicted at some intermediate stage in the overall investigation, such as the point at which the vertebrate DHFR primary amino acid sequence could have been mapped onto the known three-dimensional structure of bacterial DHFR. In retrospect, the detailed structural arguments just presented as a stereochemical rationalization of the selectivity of TMP could only have been developed following painstaking X-ray diffraction studies of relevant enzyme–inhibitor complexes. Nevertheless these results lend welcome encouragement to the belief that similar structure-based methods can be successful in other arenas in which a need exists for engineering novel selective inhibitors with chemotherapeutic potential.

Acknowledgments

I am indebted to Dr. J. Kraut for his encouragement and advice throughout the course of this work. I also would like to acknowledge Drs. J. Bolin, D. Filman, and K. Volz, who as graduate students at the University of California, San Diego, made important contributions, particularly in the area of protein structure refinement, to the overall success of this research.

References

1. Baccanari, D. P., Daluge, S., and King, R. W. (1982). Inhibition of dihydrofolate reductase: Effect of reduced nicotinamide adenine dinucleotide phosphate on the selectivity and affinity of diaminobenzylpyrimidines. *Biochemistry* **21**, 5068–5975.
2. Baker, D. J., Beddell, C. R., Champness, J. N., Goodford, P. J., Norrington, F. E. A., Smith, D. R., and Stammers, D. K. (1981). The binding of trimethoprim to bacterial dihydrofolate reductase. *FEBS Lett.* **126**, 49–52.
3. Birdsall, B., Roberts, G. C. K., Feeney, J., Dann, J. G., and Burgen, A. S. V. (1983). Trimethoprim binding to bacterial and mammalian dihydrofolate reductase: A comparison by proton and carbon-13 nuclear magnetic resonance. *Biochemistry* **22**, 5597–5604.
4. Bolin, J. T., Filman, D. J., Matthews, D. A., Hamlin, R. C., and Kraut, J. (1982). Crystal structures of *Escherichia coli* and *Lactobacillus casei* dihydrofolate reductase refined a 1.7 Å resolution. I. General features and binding of methotrexate. *J. Biol. Chem.* **257**, 13650–13662.
5. Cayley, P. J., Albrand, J. P., Feeney, J., Roberts, G. C. K., Piper, E. A., and Burgen, A. S. V. (1979). Nuclear magnetic resonance studies of the binding of trimethoprim to dihydrofolate reductase. *Biochemistry* **18**, 3886–3894.
6. Cocco, L., Temple, C., Jr., Montgomery, J. A., London, R. E., and Blakley, R. L. (1981). Protonation of methotrexate bound to the catalytic site of dihydrofolate reductase from *Lactobacillus casei. Biochem. Biophys. Res. Commun.* **100**, 413–419.
7. Cocco, L., Groff, J. P., Temple, C., Jr., Montgomery, J. A., London, R. E., Matiwyoff, N. A., and Blakley, R. L. (1981). Carbon-13 nuclear magnetic resonance study of

protonation of methotrexate and aminopterin bound to dihydrofolate reductase. *Biochemistry* **20**, 3972–3978.

8. Cocco, L., Roth, B., Temple, C., Jr., Montgomery, J. A., London, R. E., and Blakley, R. L. (1983). Protonated state of methotrexate, trimethoprim and pyrimethamine bound to dihydrofolate reductase. *Arch. Biochem. Biophys.* **226**, 567–577.

9. Cohen, S. S. (1979). Comparative biochemistry and drug design for infectious disease. *Science* **205**, 964–971.

10. Filman, D. J., Bolin, J. T., Matthews, D. A., and Kraut, J. (1982). Crystal structures of *Escherichia coli* and *Lactobacillus casei* dihydrofolate reductase refined at 1.7 Å resolution. II. Environment of bound NADPH and implication for catalysis. *J. Biol. Chem.* **257**, 13663–13672.

11. Gready, J. E. (1980). Dihydrofolate reductase: Binding of substrates and inhibitors and catalytic mechanism. *Adv. Pharmacol. Chemother.* **17**, 37–102.

12. Hitchings, G. H., Falco, E. A., Vanderwerff, H., Russell, P. B., and Elion, G. B. (1952). Antagonists of nucleic acid derivatives. *J. Biol. Chem.* **199**, 43–56.

13. Matthews, D. A., and Volz, K. W. (1982). Structure of avian dihydrofolate reductase and its complexes with pyrimidine and triazine inhibitors. *In* "Molecular Structure and Biological Activity" (J. Griffin and W. Duax, eds.), pp. 13–25. Am. Elsevier, New York.

14. Matthews, D. A., Alden, R. A., Bolin, J. T., Freer, S. T., Hamlin, R., Xuong, N., Kraut, J., Poe, M., Williams, M., and Hoogsteen, K. (1977). Dihydrofolate reductase: X-ray structure of the binary complex with methotrexate. *Science* **197**, 452–455.

15. Matthews, D. A., Alden, R. A., Bolin, J. T., Filman, D. J., Freer, S. T., Hamlin, R., Hol, W. D. J., Kisliuk, R. L., Pastore, E. J., Plante, L. T., Xuong, N.-H., and Kraut, J. (1978). Dihydrofolate reductase from *Lactobacillus casei:* X-ray structure of the enzyme-methotrexate-NADPH complex. *J. Biol. Chem.* **253**, 6949–6954.

16. Matthews, D. A., Bolin, J. T., Burridge, J. M., Filman, D. J., Volz, K. W., Kaufman, B. T., Beddell, C. R., Champness, J. N., Stammers, D. K., and Kraut, J. (1985). Refined crystal structures of *Escherichia coli* and chicken liver dihydrofolate reductase containing bound trimethoprim. *J. Biol. Chem.* **260**, 381–391.

17. Matthews, D. A., Bolin, J. T., Burridge, J. M., Filman, D. J., Volz, K. W., and Kraut, J. (1985). Dihydrofolate reductase: The stereochemistry of inhibitor selectivity. *J. Biol. Chem.* **260**, 392–399.

18. Perault, A.-M., and Pullman, B. (1961). Electronic structure and mode of action of the antimetabolites of folic acid. *Biochem. Biophys. Acta* **52**, 266–280.

19. Roberts, G. C. K., Feeney, J., Burgen, A. S. V., and Daluge, S. (1981). The charge state of trimethoprim bound to *Lactobacillus casei* dihydrofolate reductase. *FEBS Lett.* **131**, 85–88.

20. Subramanian, S., and Kaufman, B. T. (1978). Interaction of methotrexate, folates, and pyridine nucleotides with dihydrofolate reductase: Calorimetric and spectroscopic binding studies. *Proc. Natl. Acad. Sci. U.S.A.* **75**, 3201–3205.

21. Volz, K. W., Matthews, D. A., Alden, R. A., Freer, S. T., Hansch, C., Kaufman, B. T., and Kraut, J. (1982). Crystal structure of avian dihydrofolate reductase containing phenyltriazine and NADPH. *J. Biol. Chem.* **257**, 2528–2536.

Application of Computer-Assisted Modeling to Structure–Activity Studies with Intercalating Drugs

S. NEIDLE, Z. H. L. ABRAHAM, D. A. COLLIER, AND S. A. ISLAM

Cancer Research Campaign Biomolecular Structure Research Unit
The Institute of Cancer Research
Sutton, Surrey, United Kingdom

I. Introduction

The majority of both current and envisaged clinically useful anticancer drugs are DNA-reactive compounds. They may be divided into two principal categories: (1) the covalently binding DNA alkylators (69), typified by the nitrosoureas, *cis*-platinum, and mitomycin; and (2) DNA intercalators that interact noncovalently and reversibly, prominent among which are daunorubicin, doxorubicin, amsacrine, and actinomycin D (23,45,66). This latter group has consistently been the subject of fundamental studies aimed at elucidating the nature of the activity, *in vitro* and *in vivo*, shown by these compounds. Indeed, the intercalation phenomenon has emerged

NEW AVENUES IN DEVELOPMENTAL
CANCER CHEMOTHERAPY

as a classic drug-receptor system at the detailed molecular level, primarily because of the very large body of information on DNA structure and molecular biology. Most recently, X-ray crystallographic methods have determined the three-dimensional molecular structures of a number of intercalating compounds complexed with short lengths of double-helical oligonucleotides that can serve as models for DNA itself (44). Combined with computerized molecular-modeling methods, this enables rationalizations of structure–activity data to be made for particular series of compounds. This chapter describes such approaches with particular reference to two classes of drugs (Fig. 1). Both are synthetic in nature and are the subject of very considerable current interest. The anthraquinones are structurally related to the anthracycline drugs daunorubicin and doxorubicin (14); one anthraquinone derivative, mitoxantrone (20), is showing promising clinical activity against breast cancer, with diminished cardiotoxicity compared to the anthracyclines. Acridine compounds were among the first to have established antitumor activity. Only recently, as the result of extensive structure–activity studies, has an acridine com-

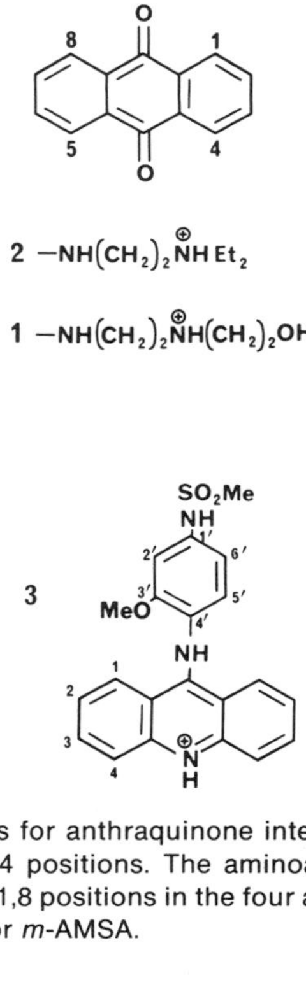

Fig. 1. (a) Structural formulas for anthraquinone intercalators. Mitoxantrone has the side chain (1) in the 1 and 4 positions. The aminoalkylamino side chain (2) is substituted at the 1; 1,4; 1,5; and 1,8 positions in the four anthraquinones discussed in the text. (b) Structural formula for *m*-AMSA.

pound demonstrated useful activity in humans. Amsacrine [*m*-AMSA (4'-(9-acridinylamino)methanesulphon-*m*-anisidide)] is showing promising activity against acute leukaemia.

The computer modeling approach is directed to describing drug–DNA interactions in molecular terms; such information may be of use in the rational design of new analogs. It is, however, important to realize that this approach to drug design does not consider other factors involved in the response of a cell or an animal to a foreign compound, critical though receptor interactions may be. Of particular importance are the factors involved in transport through the cell to reach nuclear DNA and metabolism by tissue-specific enzyme systems (55).

II. Fundamental Aspects of Intercalation

The intercalation process of drug–DNA interaction results in a number of well-documented physicochemical effects on DNA (23,40):

1. Elongation of the DNA double helix.
2. Stabilization of the helix against thermal denaturation.
3. A typical equilibrium constant of 10^5–10^6 mole^{-1} for the binding, which can be estimated from study of the drugs' spectral changes upon binding to DNA.
4. Unwinding of the double helix by an amount per bound drug molecule that appears to depend on the structural nature of the drug. Ethidium, the standard, unwinds by 20° compared to values that range from 11° for daunorubicin, 17° for proflavine, to the much higher values of 47–48° found for the bis-intercalating peptide antibiotic echinomycin and its analogs (66).

The classic model for intercalation, attributed to Lerman (31), provides a first-order explanation for these findings. The model (Fig. 2) indicates that the planar aromatic chromophore of an intercalating drug can become inserted inbetween adjacent DNA base pairs and thus extends the base pairs at a binding site from a 3.4-Å separation to one of 6.8 Å. The major biochemical consequences of drug binding also find a ready conceptual basis in the Lerman hypothesis. Frameshift mutagenesis can be explained in terms of shifts in the reading frame of the genetic code to produce altered gene products. Inhibition of events in the DNA replication and transcription pathway may be the result of intercalating drugs blocking crucial enzymes, such as the RNA polymerase system, as well as inhibiting DNA strand separation at and close to the replication fork. However, even though these are relevant factors, they are probably insufficient to

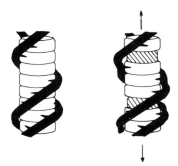

Fig. 2. The Lerman model for drug–DNA intercalation, with bound drug molecules shown schematically as shaded discs.

explain the antitumor effect of some intercalating compounds (55). As yet, it is not known whether selective action in some manner on critical DNA sequences is a relevant factor (43) (even though the declared aim of much current research on new intercalating drugs is to produce sequence-specific compounds). Lipophilicity differences have been discounted as major factors (for example, 5,17). Recent evidence has implicated the involvement of DNA topoisomerase II in mammalian cells with intercalative drug action (35,47,61,71). It had earlier been found that intercalating agents exposed to DNA in L1210 cells induced both single and double-strand breaks, as well as DNA–protein cross-links (53,54). The circumstantial evidence is strong (though at present not overwhelming) that the perturbations in DNA structure produced by an intercalator induce the topoisomerase II enzyme to make double-strand DNA breaks, which are reversible, and that these relate to the cytotoxicity of certain intercalators (50). Consistent with these hypotheses is the finding that the active anticancer compound *m*-AMSA is an effective inducer of these DNA breaks, whereas the inactive isomer *o*-AMSA (which is at least as effective an intercalator) does not produce significant DNA cleavage.

Relationships between DNA-binding ability and biological activities, both *in vitro* and *in vivo,* have been the subject of study for a number of classes of intercalating drugs. It would in principle be unwarranted for correlations between DNA binding and cellular effect to be consistently high, in part because factors such as drug transport and metabolism are often involved, as well as the possibility that non-DNA receptors and mechanisms not involving intercalation may play some role in the overall biological response (this is especially so for the anthracyclines). In addition, the relevance of particular methodologies for measuring the DNA interaction has rarely been explored. Factors to be considered include (1) whether thermodynamic or kinetic parameters of binding (or dissociation of the resulting complex) are more relevant to cytotoxicity, and (2) whether drug binding at particular DNA control sequences (such as promotors or transcription enhancers) are critical events. If so, measured association constants with calf thymus DNA are inappropriate.

It has nevertheless been established that in the AMSA series of acridine compounds, DNA binding as measured by overall association constants with poly(dA-dT), are the best single indicators of anticancer potency in experimental tumors (6–8). This property is then a necessary one, though in itself insufficient to ensure significant cytotoxicity and/or antitumor effect. Recent attempts to optimize aspects of DNA-intercalative ability in this series (4,5) have met with some success in the development of acridine 4-carboxamides, for which DNA kinetic factors may well be implicated as well.

The possibility that intercalators are at least selective for particular DNA sequences has long been a subject of controversy. The structurally more complex intercalators do have established sequence specificity. Actinomycin D has an almost absolute requirement for a guanine residue at the 5' side of the intercalation site (68), which is explicable in terms of specific hydrogen bonds between the N-2 guanine atom and peptide residues of the drug (59). The technique of DNA footprinting is a powerful one for examining sequence effects of DNA–ligand interactions (43). It has shown that the bis-intercalator echinomycin has a marked preference for sites containing the sequence 5'-CG-3' in between the two intercalated drug chromophores (32,63), and that neighboring sequences are also directly affected by drug binding. Structurally simple intercalators such as the acridines and anthracyclines do not appear to markedly prefer some intercalation sites over others, at least on the basis of footprinting. However, this may be a kinetic consequence of the rapid dissociation rate of their DNA complexes compared to that of, say, echinomycin– and actinomycin–DNA complexes. There are some other lines of evidence for sequence selectivity for the simpler drugs: (1) the 3.4–6.8 Å opening-up of adjacent base pairs significantly favors the sequence pyrimidine-3',5'-purine (13); (2) NMR studies (10,21) have indicated CG sequence preferences for many of these simple intercalators. It is perhaps insufficiently widely realized that the standard methods for estimating the thermodynamics and kinetics of drug–DNA interactions, using random-sequence polymeric DNA, produce results averaged over all binding sites and geometries. Even the use of defined-sequence polynucleotides does not readily answer all sequence-dependent questions, partly since they may adopt peculiar conformations that are not relevant to genomic DNA, and partly because the question of neighborhood sequence dependence cannot be readily addressed.

III. Molecular Structures of Intercalation Complexes

The Lerman model cannot explain these subtler aspects of the intercalation process. It also does not provide a detailed molecular structural picture of the changes produced in the tertiary structure of DNA itself, which increasingly is believed to display aspects of sequence-dependent microstructure, even without interacting molecules (19). A number of approaches have been employed to provide deeper structural information on defined-sequence short lengths of duplex DNA with bound drug; X-ray crystallography can provide the most detailed picture, but is necessarily restricted to defining conformation in the solid state. NMR methods can complement this with solution information but to date have not provided an equivalent level of information on intercalation complexes.

The shortest length of double-helical nucleic acid that may represent, at least in part, characteristics of the natural molecule is a dinucleoside. A number of drug–dinucleoside complexes have been subject to crystallographic examination. The majority have self-complementary dinucleotides with, for example, one C-3',5'-G molecule interacting with another by means of Watson-Crick base-pair hydrogen bonding (12,29,52,56). These structures, typified in Fig. 3, have a simple intercalator molecule (ethidium, proflavine, 9-aminoacridine, ellipticine) in the classically expected position midway between base pairs. This arrangement has also been found when the two base-paired strands are non-self-complementary, in the ternary proflavine–CpA–UpG complex (3), where the drug is flanked by a CG and an AU base pair. Detailed comparative analyses of

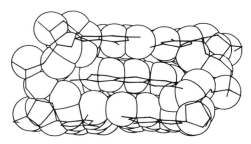

Fig. 3.   The molecular structure of the proflavine–dCpG complex.

these structures (9,11,44) have established several general principles for these structures that have been relevant to subsequent molecular modeling studies.

1. The backbone conformations of the dinucleosides in the duplex intercalated complexes are relatively invariant and can all be placed in the same conformational class. Regardless of the intercalated molecule, precise pyrimidine-3′,5′-purine sequence or even whether derived from duplex RNA or DNA, the only conformational angles that vary significantly from corresponding uncomplexed right-handed nucleic acid fragments are those around the O5′-C5′ and 3′-end glycosidic bonds, which are higher by some 50° and 60°, respectively (Fig. 4). This is perhaps contrary to expectation, in that the well-documented mobility of nucleotide conformation (60) might be predicted to lead to a general rearrangement of the total backbone structure upon drug binding. However, at present, it is not possible to provide a theoretical framework for these findings, largely because of the lack of reliable drug-base potential-energy functions (60). The overall effect of drug binding is clearly to ''stiffen'' the otherwise considerable conformational flexibility of nucleic acids; a recent study of

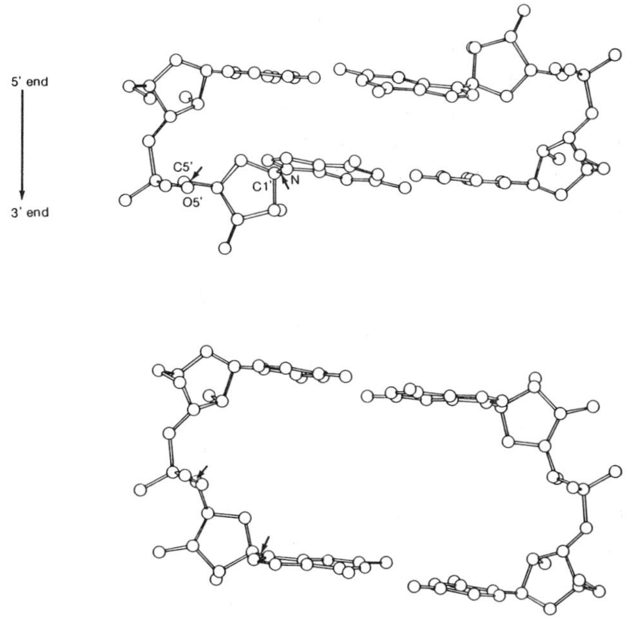

Fig. 4. Computer-modeling simulation of the opening-up of an intercalative binding site in a dinucleoside duplex.

molecular motion in the crystal structure of the proflavine–CpG complex (2) has shown that flexibility occurs primarily in the base-pair region, with concerted opening-up of the two base pairs towards the major groove direction. The intercalated drug itself has some motion within its binding site, principally in the intercalation plane.

2. In general, parameters of precise sugar pucker and unwinding angle are of only secondary importance at the dinucleoside level.

It is not directly known at present how relevant these structures are to intercalation into longer sequences in which the drug site is surrounded by a significant number of base pairs on both 3' and 5' sides. The structures of daunorubicin (51) and echinomycins (62,64) complexed to duplex hexanucleotides unfortunately do not provide information on this important issue, even though they are illuminating in other respects. Molecular modeling studies (9) that have attempted to build base-paired residues on either site of a crystallographic intercalation complex have shown that pronounced backbone asymmetry and distortion in these adjacent residues would be a necessary consequence of the geometry. This is suggestive of the induction of enzyme recognition sites, such as for DNA topoisomerase II. Clearly there is a need for further crystallographic studies on longer sequence complexes in order to verify theories such as these.

The observation of consistently closely similar dinucleoside conformations in a number of complexes with differing intercalated drugs has indicated that the structure of the drug itself would not have a major effect on the geometry of its receptor site. It also suggests that the effects of crystal packing forces in the different structures on conformation are relatively unimportant. Analysis of the water molecules present in the crystal structure of the proflavine–dCpG complex (46) has shown that these waters form a structured hydrogen-bonded network surrounding the complex and play an important role in maintaining the integrity of the network's conformation, without intimately involving the drug molecule.

The pattern of conformational conservation throughout the data base of intercalated duplex dinucleoside complexes has enabled an averaged consensus intercalation geometry to be defined that is based on the dCpG structure in its proflavine complex (56). This consensus structure (Fig. 5) has been employed as a first-order, yet well-defined, model for simulation studies with "simple" intercalators for which no crystallographic data are available. Drug design with this as a model receptor is thus in effect concentrating on a single, high-affinity intercalation site and necessarily ignores others that may be of equal importance but for which structural data are at present unavailable.

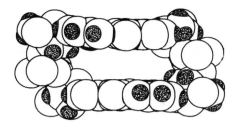

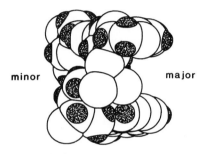

minor   major

Fig. 5. Two views of the dCpG consensus structure used for drug-receptor computer modeling, drawn in van der Waals space-filling representation. Major and minor nucleic acid grooves are labeled.

IV. Molecular Modeling Methodology

Computerized modeling procedures have been utilized in a number of laboratories to study drug–DNA interactions. In principle, they offer the possibility of examining the thermodynamics, kinetics, and molecular structures of complexes in low-energy and less stable states. In practice, approximating and simplifying methods have had to be used, which at the present time do not enable intercalation to be well understood in these terms. The complexes themselves, even when taken as dinucleoside models, are far too large for meaningful, *ab initio* quantum-mechanical calculations to be performed. More approximate molecular mechanics approaches can still only examine a small number of possible structures, since each nucleotide unit has a large number of degrees of conformational freedom. It is therefore unsurprising that several distinct yet plausible molecular structures for intercalation have been proposed on the basis of either simple minimization of nonbonded contacts or more elaborate molecular mechanics force fields (34,36–38). The number of apparently energetically plausible alternative structures increases sharply as systems larger than dinucleoside complexes become considered; it is, however, a measure of the current theoretical impasse that even at this level, no study has as yet fully rationalized the crystallographically observed dinucleoside conformations. Thus, attention has increasingly focused on using these structures as starting points for further theoretical analyses. These have rationalized the preference shown both in the crystal and in solution for simple intercalators to bind to a pyrimidine-3′,5′-purine site in a duplex dinucleoside (13,49). A semiempirical molecular orbital study has mapped the total electrostatic potential and charge distribution in an ethidium intercalated dinucleoside (15) and has shown that the field in the intercalation plane itself is both electron-rich and relatively constant, apart from the immediate neighborhood of the backbone phosphate groups. This finding has particular relevance to the design of new intercalating molecules, both as novel ones and as analogs of existing ones.

The procedure adopted in this laboratory for computerized molecular modeling uses interactive computer graphics together with molecular mechanics calculations. The intergrated system of graphics hardware and software enables docking maneuvers between drug and receptor (dCpG) to be performed and torsion angles to be altered, with the simultaneous and near real-time calculation of interaction energies (41). This procedure enables large areas of conformational and energy space to be rapidly explored and low-energy regions to be easily located, although it is not possible to be certain that some have not been overlooked.

Since the molecular assemblies being examined are relatively modest in size compared to proteins, it is possible to estimate net charges in a reasonably reliable manner. Rather than employ an electrostatic potential surface representation (67), individual Mulliken net atomic charges have been calculated, using the CNDO/2 molecular orbital method for large overlapping molecular fragments. This has the advantage of considerable computational speed over even minimal basis-set *ab initio* calculations and has been shown (48) to compare well in estimations of net charges with those obtained *ab initio*.

The force field used in these calculations is a summation of discrete, noninteracting energy contributions (30), which may be subjected to a minimization procedure:

$$E_{\text{Total}} = E_{\text{NB}} + E_{\text{ES}} + E_{\text{HB}} + E_{\text{Torsion}}$$

Where the nonbonded van der Waals term E_{NB} is defined as

$$\frac{-A}{r^6} + \frac{B}{r^{12}}$$

The parameters A and B have been detailed elsewhere (25). These have been chosen so as to have "soft" values that allow atoms to come slightly closer together than the sum of their van der Waals radii, thus largely compensating for bond length and angle rigidity. Explicit inclusion of energy terms for these could significantly increase the time taken to compute E_{Total}.

The electrostatic term E_{ES} has been taken as the classical coulombic expression $Q_iQ_j/\varepsilon r_{ij}$ relating charges Q_i and Q_j with a simple distance-dependent formalism for the dielectric constant (16). The hydrogen bonding and torsional contributions are as used previously in these studies (25,26).

This formalism and parameterization have been found to accurately reproduce the translational and rotational dispositions of proflavine as found in the crystal structure of its dinucleoside complexes (26) and accordingly have been subsequently used in a number of modeling studies for which no crystallographic data are available. The calculated energies are inherently less reliable than the indications of low-energy geometry and structure and can only be taken as relative values, of most use in a ranking order for a particular series of intercalators. Experience has shown the inadvisability of comparing calculated energies for complexes of structurally distinct drugs and analogs.

V. Anthraquinone–DNA Interactions

The evaluation of aminoalkylamino-substituted anthraquinones (14,39,72) for antitumor potency has led directly to the 1,4-bis-substituted compound mitoxantrone (Fig. 1), which is showing early clinical promise (58) in the treatment of breast cancer. This drug is a DNA intercalator *in vitro* and effectively inhibits nucleic acid synthesis, although there is some evidence that its *in vivo* activity is due to other factors as well (20).

In contrast to other "simple" intercalators, the anthraquinones do not have a formal positive charge residing on the chromophore. Calculations show that the chromophore itself interacts only relatively weakly in a dCpG intercalation site, compared to proflavine (27), because of the lack of significant electrostatic contribution (42) (Table I). Addition of a 1-amino group does not alter this situation, and the mitoxantrone precursor 1,4-diamino-5,8-dihydroxyl anthraquinone has only marginally improved interaction, due to a slight increase in attractive nonbonded interactions. Addition of the (aminoalkyl)aminoalkyl side chain at the 1-position to anthraquinone results in a significant improvement in the nonbonded energy; this is due to attractive interactions between the side-chain atoms

TABLE I

Calculated Energies of Interaction of Substituted Anthraquinones with dCpG, in kcal · mole^{-1} [a]

Substituted AQ[b]	E_{NB}	E_{ES}	E_{Total}
AQ	−60	4	−56
1-amino-AQ	−61	−1	−62
1,4-diamino-5,8-AQ	−66	−1	−67
AQ$_m$	−80	−12	−92
AQ^+_m	−86	−83	−169
Proflavine	−59	−64	−123

[a] The convention used is that a negative energy term is an attractive one. Energies are for the lowest-energy geometries. AQ$_m$, AQ^+_m carry the [(aminoethyl)amino]diethyl side chain, the latter with a protonated terminal nitrogen atom.
[b] AQ, anthraquinone.

and the bases, especially with the 06 atom of guanine in the major groove. The small net charges on the side-chain atoms also make a contribution to the total energy. Imposition of a formal proton charge on this side chain at the terminal nitrogen atom results in a dramatic increase in the electrostatic term, and the total interaction energy is now lower than for the proflavine cation. It may thus be concluded that the side chain in a substituted anthraquinone, provided it carries a formal positive charge, can more than compensate for the lack of charge on the chromophore itself. A more detailed study (28; S. A. Islam and S. Neidle, unpublished result) of the spacial requirements of both chromophore and the side chain itself has shown

1. That the 1-position amino group is involved in an intramolecular hydrogen bond with the anthraquinone carbonyl oxygen atom. This decreases the conformational mobility of the first few atoms of the side chain.

2. Side-chain mobility increases along its length; the low-energy conformations of the molecule in isolation do not altogether coincide with those when intercalated. Thus, the computer-modeling problem is increased by these extra degrees of freedom.

3. The number of intervening carbon atoms between the 1-amino nitrogen and the protonated nitrogen atom is crucial to optimal interaction. Altering this number from two renders it impossible for the charged nitro-

gen to participate in as effective electrostatic interactions with the dCpG bases.

4. The chromophore has a ± 0.5-Å and $\pm 10°$ motion in the intercalation plane with only small (<1 kcal·mole^{-1}) energy changes, in general accord with the librational and translation motions calculated from temperature-factor data (2).

A detailed study of the effects of varying positions of [(amino-ethyl)amino]diethyl side chain (Fig. 1) disubstituted on an anthraquinone has been made (28). The imposition of two sidechains at the 1,4; 1,5; or 1,8 positions results in severe constraints on the geometries of the calcu-lated low-energy complexes, with, for example, steric hindrance disallow-ing minor groove entry for both 1,4- and 1,8-derivatives. A very recent nuclear magnetic resonance (NMR) study has been interpreted in terms of major groove binding for mitoxantrone itself (33), in agreement with these predictions. The 1,5-compound interacts in an enhanced manner com-pared to others in the series (Table II) due to favorable nonbonded disper-sion forces. However, it cannot intercalate in a conventional mode, since the van der Waals dimensions of the side chains are greater than the possible maximum separation of the base pairs at the intercalation site. It is thus suggested that this compound initially interacts with a transiently non-base-paired (i.e., A-T-rich) region of DNA and stabilizes it. Dissocia-tion of the resulting complex would be slow in comparison with the others in the series, as indicated (Table II) by the measured kinetic data (24). The

TABLE II

Interactions of Anthraquinones Having [(Diethylamino)ethylamino] Substitution with DNA[a]

Substitution pattern	ΔT_m (°C)[b]	K ($10^{-6}M^{-1}$)[c]	K_{diss} (sec^{-1})[d]	Unwinding (degrees)[e]	Cell kill (%)[f]	E_{Tot} (kcal · mole^{-1})[g]
1	8.8	1.5	>150	11	92	−285
1,4	20.0	3.2	7.5	14	88*	−321
1,5	25.1	4.0	1.8	14	64*	−331
1,8	9.5	1.7	7.3	14	84*	−311

[a] From Islam et al. (28).
[b] Extent of thermal stabilization of the DNA helix → coil transmission.
[c] Determined spectrophotometrically.
[d] Determined by a SDS-induced stopped-flow technique (24).
[e] Unwinding of closed-circular PM2 DNA.
[f] Percentage of surviving Hep$_2$ cells in culture. Those marked * are significant.
[g] Sum of nonbonded and electrostatic interactions with dCpG, after global energy minimization.

ranking order of the calculated interaction energies (Table II) for these compounds is in good agreement with the various experimentally obtained measures of DNA interaction (apart from unwinding angles) and in overall qualitative agreement with their relative cell growth–inhibitory properties. It can be concluded that the modeling can identify the specific features responsible for optimal DNA binding, and that this in turn correlates with extent of cell kill for this series of derivatives. It will be of some interest to ascertain whether equivalent correlations can be made for the anthraquinone pyrazoles that have recently been reported to have high experimental anticancer activity (57); their molecular structures are suggestive of good yet sterically restricted intercalative ability.

VI. Acridine–DNA Interactions

Acridines have a long history as potential anticancer agents, and many such compounds have been prepared and tested. The 9-anilinoacridines have been especially studied by the New Zealand group (18), who have established activity for over 700 compounds in this class. One of them, *m*-AMSA (Fig. 1), which has promising clinical activity, has been the subject of numerous DNA-binding studies, since the overwhelming biological evidence points to DNA being the critical receptor for the drug.

An X-ray crystallographic analysis of *m*-AMSA has shown that there is a high degree of conformational flexibility about the two C—N bonds of the amine bridge linking acridine and methanesulphonanilide moieties, and that the severally observed crystallographic conformations are readily interconvertible with only modest energy cost. Molecular modeling of *m*-AMSA with the standard dinucleoside duplex model for DNA should take this factor into account. Inclusion of these two extra degrees of conformational freedom by means of a comprehensive, five-dimensional energy calculation (these two together with two translational and one rotational degrees of freedom in the intercalation plane) has not as yet been attempted. Instead, the low-energy forms of *m*-AMSA (as salt and "base" conformers) with dCpG and with dTpA dinucleosides have been determined (Z. H. L. Abraham and S. Neidle, unpublished observations). Several points emerge from these results:

1. The two conformers of *m*-AMSA have significantly different energies of interaction and indeed indicate different grooves for the most stable arrangements, for dCpG at least. This strongly suggests that drug-receptor modeling in general needs to take into explicit account the flexibility of drug conformation.

2. *m*-AMSA is most stable in the minor groove of a dCpG sequence (Fig. 6), although one would expect some major groove binding, depending on the relative ease of solvent displacement.

3. The flexibility of *m*-AMSA is markedly diminished on intercalation, and the nonintercalated region of the drug is not free to undergo molecular motion (Fig. 7). Intercalation from either groove results in the methane-sulphonanilide group protruding out from the complex. Since this group is both polar and has hydrogen-bonding acceptor potential, it could in prin-

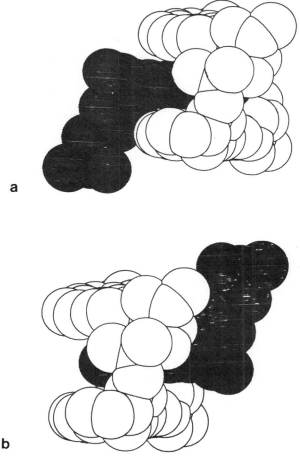

a

b

Fig. 6. Computer-drawn views of *m*-AMSA bound in (a) the major groove and (b) the minor groove of the dCpG model for DNA, shown in van der Waals representation with the drug molecule shaded.

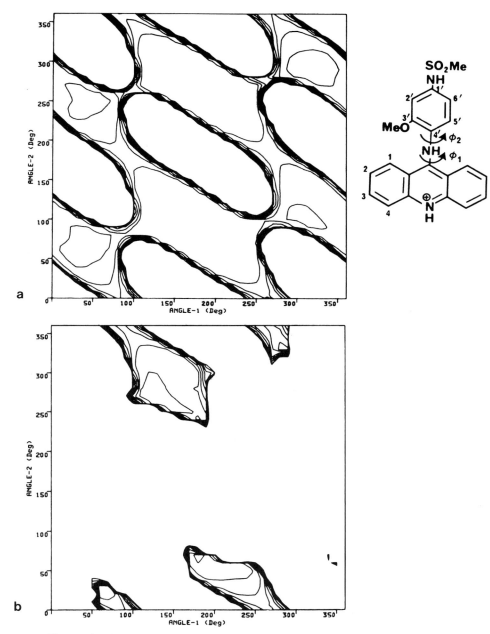

Fig. 7. Conformational maps of (a) *m*-AMSA, (b) the *m*-AMSA–dCpG minor groove complex, and (c) the *m*-AMSA–dCpG major groove complex. In each case, the torsion angles varied are as indicated in the insert. The contours have been drawn at 10-kcal·mole^{-1} intervals and enclose low-energy conformational regions.

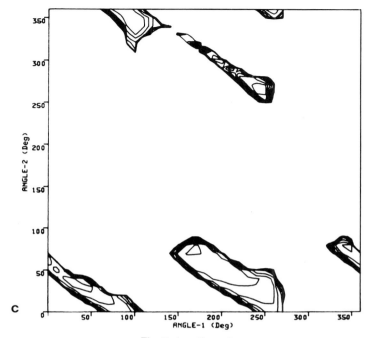

Fig. 7 *(continued)*

ciple interact with an appropriate protein to form a ternary complex, as has been suggested for DNA topoisomerase II.

4. The flexibility of the drug means that the two outer A and C rings of the acridine chromophore are equivalent in terms of the intercalative interaction, although at any one binding site, only one of these rings is at all stacked between base pairs (Fig. 8). The intercalation is a partial one in comparison with less sterically hindered drugs, since the substituents at the 5′ and 3′ positions on the phenyl ring (a hydrogen atom and a methoxy group) effectively prohibit deeper entry of the drug into the binding site.

5. The net atomic charges on the *m*-AMSA molecule (Table III) do not alter significantly on change of conformation.

These detailed models for *m*-AMSA interaction enable several conclusions to be readily made concerning the likely effect of various substituents:

1. Groups at the 1 position of the acridine ring could have the most profound effect by virtue of steric hindrance with the neighboring phenyl group. The 1-methyl derivative of *m*-AMSA has a severely buckled and

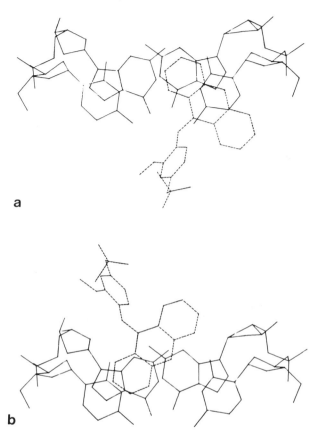

Fig. 8. Views of the *m*-AMSA–dCpG complexes projected onto the base-pair planes: (a) the major groove, and (b) the minor groove complex.

nonplanar acridine group for this reason (18a), and accordingly is a weaker DNA binder (and much less potent inhibitor of L1210 cells in culture).

2. The 2,3 and 4 positions on the acridine ring appear at first sight (Fig. 8) not to permit substituents, since they would not enable the intercalative stacking interactions to be retained. However, since these positions could equally be on the acridine C rather than A ring, they are fully allowed. Electron-withdrawing substituents at appropriate positions would enhance the electron deficiency of the chromophore and thus serve to increase the strength of intercalative binding. This effect has been noted (7). In general, very bulky substituents at positions 2,3 or 4 on both A and C

TABLE III

Net Atomic Charges Calculated for the Anilino Ring of *m*-AMSA and Derivatives, Using the CNDO/2 Method

	m-AMSA[a]	*m*-AMSA[b]	*o*-AMSA	AMSA	AMSA-3′-Cl[c]	AMSA-3′-NHCH$_3$[d]
C1′	0.138	0.168	0.101	0.116	0.120	0.140
C2′	0.096	−0.010	0.145	−0.027	−0.022	−0.093
C3′	0.158	0.176	0.070	−0.034	0.051	0.120
C4′	0.080	0.048	0.120	0.130	0.140	0.074
C5′	−0.066	0.004	−0.037	−0.035	−0.034	−0.013
C6′	−0.049	−0.062	−0.017	−0.021	−0.016	−0.056
H2′	0.020	0.038	—	0.009	0.026	0.018
H3′	—	—	0.032	0.009	—	—
H5′	−0.004	−0.013	−0.012	−0.010	0.017	0.008
H6′	0.005	0.042	0.042	0.024	0.029	0.103
N1′	−0.266	−0.201	−0.194	−0.214	−0.215	−0.214
N4′	−0.215	−0.205	−0.216	−0.276	−0.269	−0.271

[a] In conformation found for salt.
[b] In conformation found for base.
[c] Net charge on the chlorine atom in −0.167.
[d] Net charges on NHCH$_3$ substituents are N: −0.208; H: 0.104; C: 0.072; H(Me): 0.009, −0.007, −0.0016.

rings of the acridine would be expected to markedly reduce binding, as they would either interfere with the sugars of the DNA backbone or the anilino group of the drug (Fig. 7). The —CH(CH$_3$)$_2$ group at the 2 or 3 positions of *m*-AMSA reduces its DNA binding constant by between 25 and 30% (Fig. 7).

3. Substitution at the 3′ position in the anilino ring can critically alter the conformation of the drug, with a bulky substituent such as —N(Me)$_2$ having a deleterious effect, as well as itself hindering intercalation. Conversely, a hydrogen atom at the 3′ position will increase the flexibility of the drug. Table IV shows that this compound, AMSA, is calculated to bind almost as tightly as *m*-AMSA, whereas the 3′-chloro derivative interacts less effectively. The *o*-AMSA isomer interacts less effectively than *m*-AMSA or AMSA, as judged by the modeling. The experimentally found DNA-binding superiority of *o*-AMSA and AMSA over *m*-AMSA (Table V), in apparent conflict with these results, may well be a manifestation of the deficiencies of the intercalation model used, as discussed later; it is, however, notable that the calculated ranking order is more in agreement with the L1210 activities. Nevertheless we believe that this model, although it cannot provide information about interactions with nucleotide residues other than those immediately at the binding site, does enable

TABLE IV

Energies of Interaction Calculated between AMSA Derivatives and Double-Stranded DNA Dinucleoside Sequence[a]

	dCpG		dTpA	
Derivative	Major groove	Minor groove	Major groove	Minor groove
m-AMSA salt	−90.3	−85.5	−70.7	−79.7
m-AMSA base	−99.8	−113.3	−80.6	−96.3
1′Mesyl-*m*-AMSA	−88.1	−92.3	−71.4	−74.4
o-AMSA	−94.6	−106.0	−72.5	−89.5
AMSA	−104.3	−102.7		
AMSA-3′-Cl	−76.8	−86.6		

[a] Energies are as defined in the text and are given in kcal · mole^{-1}.

meaningful conclusions about the intercalative interactions themselves to be made. Table V indicates, for the limited range of 3′-substituents examined to date, that the net atomic charges in the anilino ring distant from the 3′ position do not change significantly. The 3′-NHMe analogue of *m*-AMSA has a DNA binding constant nearly 10 times higher than that of *m*-AMSA and is reported to bind more strongly than any other 3′ derivative. Its activity against the P388 tumor *in vivo* is also higher than that of *m*-AMSA (5). Preliminary molecular modeling studies on this compound

TABLE V

DNA Binding and Biological Data for Selected AMSA Derivatives

Derivative	K ($10^5 M^{-1}$)[a]	Unwinding (degrees)[b]	L1210 activity (ID$_{50}$)[c]
m-AMSA	3.7	20.5	35
o-AMSA	13.0	20.6	550
AMSA	15.9	20.9	35
m-AMSA-3′-Cl	2.8	—	1300
m-AMSA-3′-NHCH$_3$	26.3	—	71
m-AMSA-3′-N(Me)$_2$	2.2	—	520

[a] Wilson *et al.* (70); Atwell *et al.* (4); Ferguson *et al.* (22) for binding to poly (dA-dT).

[b] Waring (65).

[c] Nanomolar drug concentration for inhibition of L1210 cells in culture by 50%.

indicate that this enhanced binding is due to the possibility of drug–DNA intermolecular hydrogen bonding involving the 3' group. The minor groove orientation has a N(3')—H. . .N(3G) hydrogen bond, and the major groove has a N(3')—H. . .O(6G) (Fig. 9). These are bound to the same guanine residue in both cases and, for the major groove (which is energetically preferred), indicate a base preference for guanine at the binding site.

Molecular modeling of DNA interactions in the 9-anilinoacridine series is not yet at the stage at which reliable indications of binding properties can consistently be made, probably because a longer stretch of DNA than the dinucleoside duplex used may be involved, with the nearest-neighbor nucleotide residue to the intercalation site participating in largely electro-

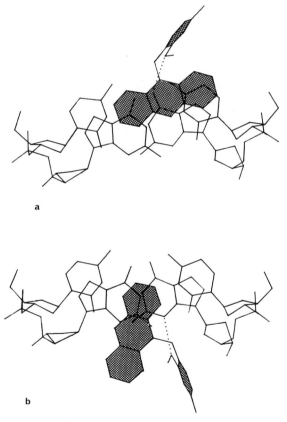

Fig. 9. Views of the 3'-NHMe-AMSA–dCpG complex (a) in the major groove and (b) in the minor groove. The dotted lines indicate hydrogen bonds.

static interactions with the methanesulphonyl group. Current studies are directed to this issue.

VII. Conclusions

Molecular modeling studies of drug intercalation are being used to understand the fundamental nature of the binding of particular drugs to their presumed major macromolecular target, especially when no crystallographic data are available. This information has predictive use in the rational design of new analogs and potentially in the design of radically new classes of intercalating molecules. To date, the available evidence suggests that the approach, when compared with experimental solutions-binding data, is a fruitful one. Since in many series of compounds, DNA binding is a necessary, though by itself insufficient, prerequisite for antitumor activity, the overall modeling process could be improved by incorporation of lipophilicity considerations. The fact that the extent of inhibition of nucleic acid synthesis *in vitro* may be rather better predicted at present by computer modeling (on a relative scale) than antitumor activity is a reflection of the inherent problems of extrapolating from *in vitro* to *in vivo* situations. The models used for intercalated DNA itself do have several defects, some of which can be expected to be overcome in the near future. Principally, the models contain insufficient nucleotide residues for "complex" and some classes of "simple" intercalators. Crystallographic data on relevant complexes will undoubtedly contribute to our understanding of this problem. The effects of solvent, especially of solvent displacement from tightly bound DNA coordination sites, have not yet been considered in any modeling study in this field. They are of considerable importance, especially in terms of estimating entropic changes. Charge and dipole polarization effects are not explicitly estimated by the molecular mechanics force fields commonly used for DNA molecular structures, not the least because of the lack of computationally accessible theory suitable for drug-design studies.

Acknowledgments

We are grateful to the Cancer Research Campaign for support, and to many colleagues and collaborators for advice and encouragement in various aspects of these studies, especially R. M. Acheson, H. M. Berman, J. R. Brown, W. A. Denny and J. Goodfellow. One of us (D.A.C.) thanks the S.E.R.C. and Glaxo Group Research Ltd. for a CASE research studentship.

References

1. Abraham, Z. H. L., Cutbush, S. D., Kuroda, R., Neidle, S., Acheson, R. M., and Taylor, G. N. (1985). Nucleic acid binding drugs. Part 12. X-ray crystallographic and conformational studies on the anti-cancer drug m-AMSA and its mesyl derivative. *J. Chem. Soc., Perkin Trans. 2*, pp. 461–645.

2. Aggarwal, A., and Neidle, S. (1985). Nucleic acid binding drug. Part 13. Molecular motion in a drug-nucleic acid model system: Thermal motion analysis of a proflavine-dinucleoside crystal structure. *Nucleic Acids Res.* **13**, 5671–5684.

3. Aggarwal, A., Islam, S. A., Kuroda, R., and Neidle, S. (1984). X-ray crystallographic analysis of a ternary intercalation complex between proflavine and the dinucleoside monophosphates CpA and UpG. *Biopolymers* **23**, 1025–1041.

4. Atwell, G. J., Cain, B. F., Baguley, B. C., Finlay, G. J., and Denny, W. A. (1984). Potential antitumour agents. 43. Synthesis and biological activity of dibasic 9-aminoacridine-4-carboxamides, a new class of antitumour agent. *J. Med. Chem.* **27**, 1481–1485.

5. Atwell, G. J., Rewcastle, G. W., Denny, W. A., Cain, B. F., and Baguley, B. C. (1984). Potential antitumour agents. 41. Analogues of amsacrine with electron-donor substituents in the anilino ring. *J. Med. Chem.* **27**, 367–372.

6. Baguley, B. C., and Nash, R. (1981). Antitumour activity of substituted 9-anilinoacridines—comparison of *in vivo* and *in vitro* testing systems. *Eur. J. Cancer* **17**, 671–679.

7. Baguley, B. C., Denny, W. A., Atwell, G. J., and Cain, B. F. (1981). Potential antitumour agents. 35. Quantitative relationships between antitumour (L1210) potency and DNA binding for 4'-(9-acridinylamino)methanesulfon-m-anisidine analogues. *J. Med. Chem.* **24**, 520–525.

8. Baguley, B. C., Denny, W. A., Atwell, G. J., and Cain, B. F. (1981). Potential antitumour agents. 34. Quantitative relationships between DNA binding and molecular structure for 9-anilinoacridines substituted in the anilino ring. *J. Med. Chem.* **24**, 170–177.

9. Berman, H. M., and Neidle, S. (1979). Modelling of drug-nucleic acid interactions. Intercalation geometry of oligonucleotides. *In* "Nucleic Acid Geometry and Dynamics" (R. H. Sarma, ed.), pp. 325–340. Pergamon, Oxford.

10. Berman, H. M., and Young, P. R. (1981). The interaction of intercalating drugs with nucleic acids. *Annu. Rev. Biophys. Bioeng.* **10**, 87–114.

11. Berman, H. M., Neidle, S., and Stodola, R. K. (1978). Drug-nucleic acid interactions: Conformational flexibility at the intercalation site. *Proc. Natl. Acad. Sci. U.S.A.* **75**, 828–832.

12. Berman, H. M., Stallings, W., Carrell, H. L., Glusker, J. P., Neidle, S., Taylor, G., and Achari, A. (1979). Molecular and crystal structure of an intercalation complex: proflavin cytidylyl-(3',5')-guanosine. *Biopolymers* **18**, 2405–2429.

13. Broyde, S., and Hingerty, B. (1979). Conformational origin of the pyrimidine (3', 5') purine base sequence preference for intercalation into RNAs. *Biopolymers* **18**, 2905–2910.

14. Cheng, C. C., and Zee-Cheng, R. K. Y. (1983). The design, synthesis and development of a new class of potent antineoplastic anthraquinones. *Prog. Med. Chem.* **20**, 83–118.

15. Dean, P. M., and Wakelin, L. P. G. (1979). The docking manoeuvre at the drug receptor: a quantum mechanical study of intercalative attack of ethidium and its carboxylated derivative on a DNA fragment. *Philos. Trans. R. Soc. London* **287**, 571–607.

16. Dearing, A., Weiner, P., and Kollman, P. A. (1981). Molecular mechanical studies of proflavine and acridine orange intercalation. *Nucleic Acids Res.* **9**, 1483–1497.

17. Denny, W. A., Cain, B. F., Atwell, G. J., Hansch, C., Panthanalickal, A., and Leo, A.

(1982). Potential antitumour agents. 36. Quantitative relationships between experimental antitumour activity, toxicity and structure for the general class of 9-anilinoacridine antitumour agents. *J. Med. Chem.* **25,** 276–315.

18. Denny, W. A., Baguley, B. C., Cain, B. F., and Waring, M. J. (1983). Antitumour acridines. *In* "Molecular Aspects of Anti-Cancer Drug Action" (S. Neidle and M. J. Waring, eds.), pp. 1–34. Macmillan, New York.

18a. Neidle, S., Webster, G. D., Baguley, B. C., and Denny, W. A. (1986). Nucleic Acid Binding Drugs. Part 14. The crystal structure of 1-methyl amsacrene hydrochloride; relationships to DNA-binding ability and anti-tumour activity. *Biochem. Pharmacol.* (in press).

19. Dickerson, R. E., Drew, H. R., Conner, B. N., Wing, R. M., Fratini, A. V., and Kopka, M. L. (1982). The anatomy of A-, B-, and Z-DNA. *Science* **216,** 475–485.

20. Durr, F. E., Wallace, R. E., and Citarella, R. V. (1983). Molecular and biochemical pharmacology of mitozanthrone. *Cancer Treat. Rev.* **10,** 3–11.

21. Feigon, J., Denny, W. A., Leupin, W., and Kearns, D. R. (1984). Interactions of antitumour drugs with natural DNA: 'H NMR study of binding mode and kinetics. *J. Med. Chem.* **27,** 450–465.

22. Ferguson, L. R., MacPhee, D. G., and Baguley, B. C. (1983). Comparative studies of mutagenic, DNA binding and antileukaemic properties of 9-anilino acridine derivatives and related compounds. *Chem.-Biol. Interact.* **44,** 53–62.

23. Gale, E. F., Cundliffe, E., Reynolds, P. E., Richmond, M. H., and Waring, M. J. (1981). "The Molecular Basis of Antibiotic Action", 2nd ed. Wiley, New York.

24. Gandecha, B. M., Brown, J. R., and Crompton, M. R. (1985). Dissociation kinetics of DNA-anthracycline and DNA-anthraquinone complexes determined by stopped-flow spectrophotometry. *Biochem. Pharmacol.* **34,** 733–736.

25. Islam, S. A., and Neidle, S. (1983). Nucleic acid binding drugs. VII. Molecular mechanics studies on the conformational properties of the anti-cancer drug daunomycin: Some observations on the use of differing potential-energy functions. *Acta Crystallogr. Sect. B* **B39,** 114–119.

26. Islam, S. A., and Neidle, S. (1984). Nucleic acid binding drugs. X. A theoretical study of proflavine intercalation into RNA and DNA fragments: Comparison with cyrstallographic results. *Acta Crystallogr., Sect. B* **B40,** 424–429.

27. Islam, S. A., Neidle, S., Gandecha, B. M., and Brown, J. R. (1983). Experimental and computer graphics simulation analyses of the DNA interaction of 1,8-bis-(2-diethylaminoethylamino)-athracene-9,10-dione, a compound modelled on doxorubicin. *Biochem. Pharmacol.* **32,** 2801–2808.

28. Islam, S. A., Neidle, S., Gandecha, B. M., Partridge, M., Patterson, L. H., and Brown, J. R. (1985). Comparative computer graphics and solution studies of the DNA interaction of substituted anthraquinones based on doxorubicin and mitoxanthrone. *J. Med. Chem.* **28,** 857–864.

29. Jain, S. C., Tsai, C. C., and Sobell, H. M. (1977). Visualisation of drug-nucleic acid interactions at atomic resolution. II. Structure of ethidium/dinucleoside monophosphate crystalline complex, ethidium: 5-iodocytidylyl(3′,5′)guanosine. *J. Mol. Biol.* **114,** 217–231.

30. Kollman, P. A. (1984). Drug-receptor binding forces. *In* "X-ray Crystallography and Drug Action" (A. S. Horn and C. J. De Ranter, eds), pp. 63–82. Oxford Univ. Press, London and New York.

31. Lerman, L. S. (1961). Structural considerations in the interaction of DNA and acridines. *J. Mol. Biol.* **3,** 18–30.

32. Low, C. M. L., Drew, H. R., and Waring, M. J. (1984). Sequence-specific binding of

echinomycin to DNA; evidence for conformational changes affecting flanking sequences. *Nucleic Acids Res.* **12**, 4865–4879.

33. Lown, J. W., and Hanstock, C. C. (1985). High field H¹-NMR analysis of the 1 : 1 intercalation complex of the antitumour agent mitoxanthrone and the DNA duplex [d(CpGpCpG)]. *J. Biomol. Struct. Dyn.* **2**, 1097–1106.

34. Malhotra, D., and Hopfinger, A. (1980). Conformational flexibility of dinucleoside dimers during unwinding from the B-form to an intercalation structure. *Nucleic Acids Res.* **8**, 5289–5305.

35. Marshall, B., Darkin, S., and Ralph, R. K. (1983). Evidence that m-AMSA induces topoisomerase action. *FEBS Lett.* **161**, 75–78.

36. Max, N. L., Mahotra, D., and Hopfinger, A. (1981). Computer graphics and the generation of DNA conformations for intercalation studies. *Comput. Chem.* **5**, 19–27.

37. Miller, K. J., and Newlin, D. D. (1982). Interactions of molecules with nucleic acids VI. Computer design of chromophoric intercalating agents. *Biopolymers* **21**, 633–652.

38. Miller, K. J., and Pycior, J. F. (1979). Interaction of molecules with nucleic acids II. Two pairs of families of intercalation sites, unwinding angles, and the neighbour-exclusion principle. *Biopolymers* **18**, 2683–2719.

39. Murdock, K. C., Child, R. G., Fabio, P. F., Angier, P. F., Wallace, R. E., Durr, F. E., and Citarella, R. V. (1979). Antitumour agents. 1. 1,4-bis[(aminoalkyl)amino]-9,10-anthracenediones. *J. Med. Chem.* **22**, 1024–1030.

40. Neidle, S. (1979). The molecular basis for the action of some DNA-binding drugs. *Prog. Med. Chem.* **16**, 151–221.

41. Neidle, S. (1984). Computer graphics in the study of drug-nucleic acid interactions. *Biochem. Soc. Trans.* **12**, 1008–1011.

42. Neidle, S. (1986). Computer-aided design of new DNA intercalators. *In* "Mechanisms of DNA Damage and Repair" (M. G. Simic, ed.), pp. 257–264. Plenum, New York.

43. Neidle, S., and Abraham, Z. (1984). Structural and sequence-dependent aspects of drug intercalation into nucleic acids. *CRC Crit. Rev. Biochem.* **17**, 73–121.

44. Neidle, S., and Berman, H. M. (1983). X-ray crystallographic studies of nucleic acids and nucleic acid- complexes. *Prog. Biophys. Mol. Biol.* **41**, 43–66.

45. Neidle, S., and Waring, M. J., eds. (1983). "Molecular Aspects of Anti-Cancer Drug Action." Macmillan, New York.

46. Neidle, S., Berman, H. M., and Shieh, H. S. (1980). Highly structured water network in crystals of a deoxynucleoside-drug complex. *Nature (London)* **288**, 129–133.

47. Nelson, E. M., Tewey, K. M., and Liu, L. F. (1984). Mechanism of antitumour drug action: poisoning of mammalian DNA topoisomerase II on DNA by 4′-(9-acridinylamino)-methanesulfon-*m*-anisidide. *Proc. Natl. Acad. Sci. U.S.A.* **81**, 1361–1365.

48. Nuss, M. E., and Kollman, P. A. (1979). Electrostatic potentials of deoxydinucleoside monophosphates. 1. Deoxydinucleoside monophosphate and actinomycin chromophore interactions. *J. Med. Chem.* **22**, 1517–1524.

49. Nuss, M. E., Marsh, F. J., and Kollman, P. A. (1979). Theoretical studies of drug-dinucleotide interactions. Empirical energy function calculations on the interaction of ethidium, 9-aminoacridine and proflavin cations with the base-paired dinucleotides GpC and CpG. *J. Am. Chem. Soc.* **101**, 825–833.

50. Pommier, Y., Zwelling, L., Kao-Shan, C.-S., Whang-Peng, J., and Bradley, M. O. (1985). Correlations between intercalator-induced DNA strand breaks and sister chromatid exchanges, limitations and cytotoxicity in Chinese hamster cells. *Cancer Res.* **45**, 3143–3149.

51. Quigley, G. J., Wang, A.H-J., Ughetto, G., van der Marel, G., van Boom, J. H., and

Rich, A. (1980). Molecular structure of an anticancer drug-DNA complex: daunomycin plus d(CpGpTpApCpG). *Proc. Natl. Acad. Sci. U.S.A.* **77**, 7204–7208.

52. Reddy, B. S., Seshadri, T. P., Sakore, T. D., and Sobell, H. M. (1979). Visualisation of drug-nucleic acid interactions at atomic resolution. V. Structure of two aminoacridine-dinucleoside monophosphate crystalline complexes, proflavin-5-iodocytidylyl-(3′,5′)guanosine and acridine orange-5-iodo-cytidylyl(3′,5′)guanosine. *J. Mol. Biol.* **135**, 787–812.

53. Ross, W. E., and Bradley, M. D. (1981). DNA double-strand breaks in mammalian cells after exposure to intercalating agents. *Biochim. Biophys. Acta* **654**, 129–134.

54. Ross, W. E., Glaubiger, D., and Kohn, K. W. (1979). Qualitative and quantitative aspects of intercalator-induced DNA strand breaks. *Biochim. Biophys. Acta* **562**, 41–50.

55. Schwartz, H. S. (1979). Biochemical action and selectivity of intercalating drugs. *Adv. Cancer Chemother.* **1**, 1–59.

56. Shieh, H-S., Berman, H. M., Dabrow, M., and Neidle, S. (1980). The structure of drug-deoxydinucleoside phosphate complex: generalised conformational behaviour of inter-calation complexes with DNA and RNA fragments. *Nucleic Acids Res.* **8**, 85–97.

57. Showalter, H. D. H., Johnson, J. L., Werbel, L. M., Leopolde, W. R., Jackson, R. C., and Elslager, E. F. (1984). 5[(aminoalkyl)amino]-substituted anthra[1,9-cd]-pyrazol-6(2H)-ones as novel anticancer agents. Synthesis and biological evaluation. *J. Med. Chem.* **27**, 253–255.

58. Stuart-Harris, R. C., Bozek, T., Pavlidis, N. A., and Smith, I. E. (1984). Mitoxan-throne: An active new agent in the treatment of advanced breast cancer. *Cancer Che-mother. Pharmacol.* **12**, 1–4.

59. Takusagawa, F., Dabrow, M., Neidle, S., and Berman, H. M. (1982). The structure of a pseudointercalated complex between actinomycin D and the DNA binding sequence d(GpC). *Nature (London)* **296**, 466–469.

60. Taylor, E. R., and Olson, W. K. (1983). Theoretical studies of nucleic acid interactions I. Estimates of conformational mobility in intercalated chains. *Biopolymers* **22**, 2667–2702.

61. Tewey, K. M., Chen, G. L., Nelson, E. M., and Liu, L. F. (1984). Intercalative antitu-mour drugs interfere with the breakage-reunion reaction of mammalian DNA topoiso-merase. II. *J. Biol. Chem.* **259**, 9182–9187.

62. Ughetto, G., Wang, A. H-J., Quigley, G. J., van der Marel, G. A., van Boom, J. H., and Rich, A. (1985). A comparison of the structure of echinomycin and triostin A complexed to a DNA fragment. *Nucleic Acids Res.* **13**, 2306–2323.

63. van Dyke, M. M., and Dervan, P. B. (1984). Echinomycin binding sites on DNA. *Science* **225**, 1122–1127.

64. Wang, A. H-J., Ughetto, G., Quigley, G. J., Hakoshima, T., van der Marel, G., van Boom, J. H., and Rich, A. (1984). The molecular structure of a DNA-triostin complex. *Science* **225**, 1115–1121.

65. Waring, M. J. (1976). DNA-binding characteristics of acridinylmethanesulphonanalide drugs: Comparison with antitumour properties. *Eur. J. Cancer* **12**, 995–1001.

66. Waring, M. J. (1981). DNA modification and cancer. *Annu. Rev. Biochem.* **50**, 159–192.

67. Weiner, P. K., Langridge, R., Blaney, J. M., Schaefer, R., and Kollman, P. A. (1982). Electrostatic potential molecular surfaces. *Proc. Natl. Acad. Sci. U.S.A.* **79**, 3754–3758.

68. Wells, R. D., and Larson, J. E. (1970). Studies on binding of actinomycin D to DNA and DNA model polymers. *J. Mol. Biol.* **49**, 319–342.

69. Wilman, D. E. V., and Connors, T. A. (1983). Molecular structure and antitumour

activity of alkylating agents. *In* "Molecular Aspects of Anti-Cancer Drug Action" (S. Neidle and M. J. Waring, eds.), pp. 223–282. Macmillan, New York.

70. Wilson, W. R., Baguley, B. C., Wakelin, L. P. G., and Waring, M. J. (1981). Interaction of the antitumour drug 4'-(9-acridinylamino)methanesulfon-*m*-anisidide and related acridines with nucleic acids. *Mol. Pharmacol.* **20,** 404–414.

71. Yang, L., Rowe, T. C., Nelson, E. M., and Liu, L. F. (1985). *In vivo* mapping of DNA topoisomerase II - specific cleavage sites on SV40 chromatin. *Cell (Cambridge, Mass.)* **41,** 127–132.

72. Zee-Cheng, R. K. Y., and Cheng, C. C. (1978). Antineoplastic agents. Structure-activity relationship study of bis(substituted-aminoalkylamino)anthraquinones. *J. Med. Chem.* **21,** 291–294.

PART II

Biochemical Modulation of Drug Activity

Biochemical Modulation: Perspectives and Objectives

DANIEL S. MARTIN

Department of Developmental Chemotherapy
Memorial Sloan-Kettering Cancer Institute
New York, New York
and Department of Cancer Research
Catholic Medical Center of Brooklyn and Queens
Woodhaven, New York

NEW AVENUES IN DEVELOPMENTAL
CANCER CHEMOTHERAPY

I. Introduction

Conceptual changes in cancer treatment take a relatively long time to reach clinical acceptance. Combination chemotherapy, the most important, and indeed, the only treatment shown capable of curing some *advanced* human cancers (32), was first advanced as a concept (108) and was demonstrated to be more effective therapy than single agents against experimental tumors in the 1950s, (59,98,105,108,155), but its clinical utility was not accepted until the 1970s (43,69). In contrast, although the concept of applying biochemical knowledge to improve combination chemotherapy was also documented in preclinical studies in the 1950s, most clinical advances in combination chemotherapy have been achieved empirically. Even the recent clinical trials seeking to reproduce preclinical findings of biochemical modulation are still largely disappointing. There are a number of probable reasons for these frustrations. The essential problem is the failure to translate properly the preclinical findings into the design of clinical protocols involving biochemical modulation. These errors, as will be discussed, if appropriately corrected, should permit therapeutic success with biochemical modulation in the clinic.

II. Biochemical Modulation, the Therapeutic Index, and Selectivity

Biochemical modulation refers to the pharmacologic manipulation of intracellular metabolic pathways by an agent (either a metabolite or an antimetabolite called the modulating agent) to produce either the selective enhancement of the antitumor effect or the selective protection of the host from an anticancer agent (called the effector agent). Potential advances in biochemical modulation are usually initially identified through *in vitro* studies. All too frequently these initial *in vitro* findings are taken directly (except for toxicity tests in normal animals) to cancer patients without further preclinical testing in *in vivo* tumor systems. In the clinic, however, effective treatment must be defined as a therapeutic index, that is, the relative effects of a chemotherapeutic regimen on a target tissue as compared to normal host tissues. *In vitro* systems simply cannot address this absolutely crucial question. Enhanced toxicity to tumor cells *in vitro* does not exclude similar enhancement of toxicity to bone marrow, intestine, and other normal tissues *in vivo*. The *in vivo* toxicity of the combination then leads to dose reductions, and the clinical investigator eventually ends up with a tolerable regimen with response rates no better than those seen with the maximally tolerated dose of the effector agent alone. A conclusion under these circumstances that the clinical trial of the *in vitro* biochemical modulation finding is disappointing is simply not warranted, for an appropriate preclinical *in vivo* test might well have demonstrated the futility of clinical trial. (Or, more importantly, preclinical studies of dosage ratios and schedules might have uncovered information that would have produced a successful clinical result with the particular modulated combination under study.) Selectivity is as important in biochemical modulation as it is in traditional combination chemotherapy. Biochemical modulation will be of advantage only if the therapeutic index is improved, i.e., if there is less toxicity with unchanged efficacy or more efficacy with unchanged toxicity.

III. The Significance of the Sequence and Scheduling Interval between Agents

A. 6-Methylmercaptopurine, 6-Mercaptopurine, and the Scheduling Interval

The design of an appropriate clinical trial of biochemical modulation should take into account all of the key details upon which the success of the preclinical findings were dependent. This is not always done. For example, although the sequence of modulating agent and effector agent is often critical to therapeutic success, a review of the clinical combination chemotherapy literature reveals that this important scheduling detail has been ignored in some clinical trials. To illustrate, a series of preclinical reports stressed that 6-methylmercaptopurine (MMPR) could enhance the anticancer effect of 6-MP only when administered in sequence with MMPR prior to 6-mercaptopurine (6-MP) (131,139,152). Nevertheless, when the clinical trial was done, the combination of MMPR and 6-MP was administered without sequence, and the simultaneous administration of the combination was reported as not offering better results than 6-MP alone (73). Also, in addition to proper sequence, the appropriate timing interval between the administration of the modulating agent and the effector agent may be critical. Scholar *et al.* (152) not only found the MMPR → 6-MP sequence to be necessary to yield augmented results but found that maximal enhancing effects required a 6- to 12-hr interval between the two agents. Thus, the design of this MMPR + 6-MP clinical trial ignored both sequence and timing interval. Saunders (148) has stated that "it has been a fact of scientific life in the United States that with respect to cancer, fundamental biomedical research and applied clinical research have not generally been carried out in a coordinated way."

B. PALA, 5-Fluorouracil, and the Scheduling Interval

The lowering of intracellular pyrimidine pools by N-(phosphonacetyl)-L-aspartic acid (PALA), an inhibitor of pyrimidine biosynthesis (36), can markedly augment the antitumor activity of 5-fluorouracil (FUra) (5,82,110,114), and this effect is both dose and time dependent. Thus, the *in vitro* potentiating therapeutic effect by a biochemically active dose of PALA on FUra was found to require PALA pretreatment for a period of 12–18 hr, and an interval period of 24 hr was reported best in *in vivo* preclinical studies (95,100,110,116). These preclinical findings indicate that the specific time sequence of administration of PALA and FUra is an important determinant in the outcome of biochemical modulation studies with these two drugs. However, some clinical trials (which were reported as negative) employed only a 3-hr period between PALA and FUra administration (8), which is likely too short a "modulating" interval on the basis of the preclinical findings.

C. Methotrexate, FUra, and the Scheduling Interval

The timing interval is also important for the enhanced FUra cytotoxicity seen when the folic acid antagonist, methotrexate (MTX), precedes FUra (15,25,109). 5-Phosphoribosyl-1-pyrophosphate (PRPP) is a common precursor for both purine and pyrimidine biosynthesis. MTX, as a consequence of its inhibition of *de novo* purine synthesis, causes an accumulation of the supplies of intracellular PRPP that is not utilized in the MTX-inhibited purine synthetic pathway. Since PRPP is a necessary substrate that is rate limiting in the enzymatic pathway for the activation of FUra to its antitumor nucleotides, the MTX-induced increase in levels of PRPP allows for greater production of the cytotoxic FUra-containing nucleotides. However, an appropriate time period after administration of MTX is required for optimal enlargement of the PRPP pools (25).

Initially, it had been shown that the interval between the sequential administration of MTX prior to FUra in preclinical studies may be as short as only 1 hr and may still produce enhanced cytotoxicity both *in vitro* (25) and *in vivo* (15,109). A number of clinical studies, therefore, were conducted with this interval (16,21–23,26,28,34,137). However, in the clinic, the optimal timing for the sequenced MTX–FUra combination apparently requires an interval greater than 1 hr between the two agents to yield enhanced tumor response rates in patients. Although as yet all reports are only preliminary clinical findings, the studies in Table I with the 1-hr interval between MTX and FUra (16,23,28,137) have been reported *not* to have an advantage over nonsequenced MTX + FUra, whereas clinical studies with intervals ranging from 4 to 24 hr

TABLE I

Results of Clinical Trials with Sequential Methotrexate (MTX) → 5-Fluorouracil (FUra)[a] with a 1-hr Scheduling

MTX → FUra Interval (hr)	% Responders	Reference
1[b]	N.S.[d]	21
1	N.S.[d]	22,36
1	6	34
1	0	35
1	0	36
1	6	40
1	N.S.[d]	38
4	42	25
7	50	24,39
7	32	41
12[c]	39	42
24	32	23
24	57	43

[a] High-dose MTX (except Refs. 23,42) → FUra followed by leucovorin.
[b] Cytoxan and prednisone in addition to MTX → FUra.
[c] Mitomycin C in addition to MTX → FUra.
[d] N.S., not significant.

(49,71,72,76,86,146,174) have been reported to show apparently success-fully enhanced tumor response rates. Although the latter results are also preliminary and await verification in appropriate phase III clinical trials, it is apparent that the initially observed preclinical 1-hr scheduling interval between MTX and FUra does not transpose like a recipe directly into successful clinical trial.

The lack of appreciation of the fact that in addition to the need for appropriate sequence, a sufficient time interval between modulating agent and effector agent is crucial to achieve a synergistic result is unfortunate, for a number of clinical trials with the MTX → FUra sequence have been conducted with an apparently inappropriate interval. More recently, pre-clinical studies have been reported, indicating that intervals in the range of 12–24 hr between MTX and FUra are optimal (13,70), and it is hoped that there will soon be reports of adequately controlled clinical trials of such time intervals (e.g., 24 hr).

IV. Quantitative Differences between Preclinical Tumor Models and Human Tumors

The "recipe" approach to clinical investigation, wherein a schedule found to be optimally effective in the preclinical model (e.g., the 1-hr MTX → FUra interval) is assumed to be directly transferable to clinical schedule, is rarely successful. Carrying over therapeutic results from one model cancer system to one human cancer requires corrections for quan-titative differences. For example, allowance must be made for the quanti-tative difference in tumor size when treatment is initiated (the animal tumor is usually small, whereas the human cancer is large) as well as for the quantitative difference in the criteria for tumor response (the criterion for an effectively treated animal tumor usually is growth inhibition, a relatively sensitive end point, whereas a very different and much more rigorous end point, tumor regression, is the criterion employed in the clinic) (113). Further, the quantitative difference in cell growth rates may have therapeutic significance (the usual animal tumor is fast-growing, whereas the human tumor is slow) (see Table II).

The following quantitative data may help explain why preclinical sched-uling observations, although qualitatively applicable, may simply not be quantitatively relevant to *in vivo* clinical circumstances: the L1210 murine leukemia has a doubling time of 10 hr (144), whereas the human leukemic cells have a doubling time *in vivo* of approximately 36 hr (93), and the average cell generation time for a variety of human solid tumors is 50–60 hr (10). Metabolic processes may proceed more slowly in the slower-

TABLE II

Some Quantitative Differences between Preclinical Model Tumor Systems and Clinical Human Cancer Studies

Model or study consideration	Tumor model	Human cancer
1. Type of study	Often *in vitro*	*In vivo*
2. Therapeutic index	Not obtainable *in vitro*	Inherent
3. *In vivo* tumor size when Rx begun	Small	Large
4. Minimal criterion for therapeutic response	Growth inhibition	Tumor regression
5. Tumor cell growth rate	Fast	Slow

growing human tumor cells, and, therefore, changes in intracellular metabolites may require longer pretreatment intervals. Whatever the exact explanation, one usually cannot transpose (i.e., not the "recipe" approach) the laboratory findings directly to clinical trial. Instead one has to "translate."

A. "Translation" of Preclinical Findings into Clinical Trial

"Translation" means the quantitative changes in regimen required to achieve a therapeutic response in a specific tumor system (e.g., cancer in humans) which will be similar to the therapeutic response produced by a particular treatment protocol in a different tumor system (e.g., an animal tumor model) (106,113). Translation can and, whenever possible, should be considered in "both directions," i.e., from clinic to laboratory and vice versa (116,119,156), as will be discussed further. Whenever possible, comparative cellular biochemical pharmacology (i.e., quantitative biochemical measurements at the cellular level in the preclinical animal tumor model and in patients undergoing treatment) should be the scientific basis for clinical treatment program design.

B. "Translation" of PALA → FUra in "Both Directions"

1. The Significance of the Appropriate Dosage Ratio between Agents

An example of "translation" and the utilization of biochemical pharmacology to select the doses and timing interval for a clinical modulation trial has been reported for the combination of PALA prior to FUra

(116,119). PALA, an inhibitor of *de novo* pyrimidine biosynthesis, can lower a murine tumor's intracellular level of uridine triphosphate (UTP) (Fig. 1) that competes with 5-fluorouridine triphosphate (5-FUTP) for incorporation into ribonucleic acid. PALA, administered 24 hr prior to FUra, can thereby increase 5-FUra incorporation into tumor cell RNA (Fig. 2), the result being a greater antitumor effect (116). In the laboratory, moderate to high doses of PALA alone display anticancer activity, and any ratio of such therapeutic doses of PALA and FUra in combination (e.g., high PALA to low FUra, or moderate PALA to high FUra) is able to display enhanced antitumor activity.

In the clinic, even high doses of PALA alone are devoid of demonstrable therapeutic activity. Unfortunately, only a high PALA dosage in combination with FUra was investigated in the clinical trials of this combination (8,52,123,134). The toxicity of this high PALA dosage permitted tolerable drug combination only with low FUra dosage, and the resulting antitumor activity of this combination in the clinic was found no better than the clinical maximal tolerated dose (MTD) of FUra alone.

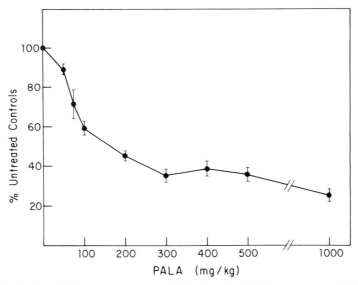

Fig. 1. Effect of 24-hr treatment with PALA on CD8F1 breast tumor UTP pools. Tumor-bearing CD8F1 mice received the indicated dose of PALA (intraperitoneally). After a 24-hr exposure, the animals were anesthetized with sodium pentobarbital, and the tumors were removed and immediately homogenized in ice-cold perchloric acid. The acid-soluble fraction was analyzed by high-pressure liquid chromatography for measurements of UTP. The levels of UTP were normalized to the amount of protein recovered in the acid-insoluble pellet. Bars, S.E.

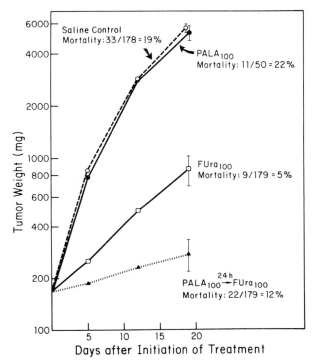

Fig. 2. Enhancement of antitumor activity of FUra by a nontherapeutic, but "modulating," dose of PALA. Pool of five experiments in male CD8F1 mice (10 mice per group) bearing advanced CD8F1 mammary tumor transplants. Subscripts = mg/kg. Bars, S.E.

The use of a dose of a modulating agent high enough to require a significant reduction of the dose of the effector agent (when the latter has a steep dose–response curve and is at its MTD in the historical controls) is likely to be self-defeating in comparison with the historical controls employing high-dose therapeutic activity of the effector agent. As Sartorelli and Creasey (147) have noted, the dosage ratio in drug combinations can be of major therapeutic significance on a biochemical basis. Dosage ratio can be a crucial detail in the design of clinical protocols.

Although the reported clinical studies of high PALA : low FUra were negative, they nevertheless provide evidence that PALA, a therapeutically inactive agent clinically, must be "modulating" pyrimidine activity in cancer patients, since it raises the therapeutic effect of the low FUra dose to the same degree of therapeutic activity found with the higher MTD of FUra alone. Moreover, these clinical findings further "translate" into the logic that a *low*-PALA "modulating" dose (i.e., a biochemically active dose, even if low) might permit a clinically tolerable combination with a high FUra dose at or close to its MTD and thereby might effect useful synergistic antitumor activity over that of the MTD of FUra alone. Since PALA's target enzyme, aspartate transcarbamylase, is in lower concentration in tumor than in normal cells, selectivity should be attained in the presence of a *low biochemically active* dose of PALA (116,126).

2. Specific Requirements for Appropriate Translation of the PALA–FUra Combination

On the basis of the preceding facts and reasoning, appropriate "translation" of PALA–FUra combination would require (1) finding a low dose of PALA in laboratory tumors *in vivo* that emulates the clinical findings in being nontherapeutic and having biochemical activity; (2) determining whether such a low PALA dose can usefully enhance the *in vivo* antitumor activity of a high dose of FUra; (3) if the laboratory answers are encouraging, identifying a similar, low, "modulating" dose of PALA in patients; and (4) clinically testing this low dose in combination with the highest tolerated dose of FUra, which, it is hoped, is the clinical MTD of FUra.

a. Required Preclinical Data. A study of the PALA–FUra combination in the laboratory on the basis of the aforementioned "translation" did indeed show that a low (100 mg/kg), *nontherapeutic* dose of PALA, chosen on the basis of demonstrated biochemical effects at that dose (i.e., the selected low dose of PALA lowered UTP pools *in vivo*), could selectively potentiate the antitumor effects of the MTD of FUra without undue toxicity despite its lack of therapeutic activity as a single agent at that low dose (116) (see Figs. 1–3).

b. Required Clinical Data. On the basis of these encouraging laboratory findings, a subsequent clinical biochemical pharmacology study determined that a low dose of PALA could effectively inhibit pyrimidine synthesis in patients, and a subsequent phase I clinical trial demonstrated that this clinically low, "modulating" dose of PALA (250 mg/m^2) could be administered weekly in sequenced combination with the weekly "historical" MTD of FUra (600 mg/m^2) without causing undue toxicity (30). This low PALA : high FUra dosage ratio has not yet undergone phase II clinical trial to evaluate its potential for therapeutic benefit. However, the combined laboratory and clinical studies clearly demonstrate the process of "translation" and that the use of biochemical pharmacology at the clinical level can usefully determine a "modulating" dose for a modulat-

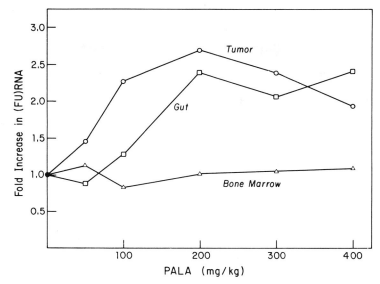

Fig. 3. Effect of PALA dose on the level of (FUra)RNA in CD8F1 breast tumor, intestinal epithelium, and bone marrow. CD8F1 mice bearing the advanced transplant mammary carcinoma were given the indicated dose of PALA 24 hr prior to receiving [³H]FUra (FUra = 50 mg/kg containing 80 mCi of tritiated FUra per kilogram). After a 2-hr labeling period, the animals were sacrificed by cervical dislocation, and the incorporation of FUra into RNA was determined. Animals which received only FUra served as controls to calculate the relative increase in (FUra)RNA.

ing agent and that a modulating agent need not necessarily have antitumor activity either as a single agent or at a "modulating" dose (116,119).

V. Heterogeneity: Quantitative as Well as Qualitative

The scientifically based rules of biochemical modulation in combination chemotherapy differ from the empirically derived rules of combination chemotherapy. The first rule of empirical combination chemotherapy is to combine only drugs with activity as single agents, and this view is based on the perception of the heterogeneity of neoplastic cell populations as qualitative in nature. However, in addition to the qualitative, there is also quantitative heterogeneity; namely, a subset of cancer cells can possess a gradient of responsiveness to a single agent. Under *in vivo* conditions the low chemotherapeutic indices of most agents (e.g., FUra) can make the eradication of even slightly resistant cells impossible at *in vivo* tolerated drug doses. Thus, the use of a modulating agent (e.g., PALA) to selectively manipulate intratumoral biochemical mechanisms to amplify the tumor cytotoxicity of an effector agent (e.g., FUra) can facilitate the chemotherapeutic attack, even though the modulating agent itself appears to have no antitumor activity. Simply adding more agents with single-agent clinical activity directed at qualitatively different subsets of cancer cells may worsen the quantitative aspects of drug resistance, if adding additional agents causes unacceptable toxicity that necessitates reducing the dose of the drugs in the combination. Indeed, quantitative differences in cells whose sensitivity is qualitatively similar necessitates the utilization of selective biochemical modulation to increase the therapeutic effectiveness of individual effector agents in a drug combination.

VI. The Different Needs of Classical and "Modulatory" Combination Chemotherapy

The inclusion of a certain agent(s) in a modulating combination is not for the ability of this modulating agent(s) to kill tumor cells per se but rather to obtain a desired intracellular biochemical alteration in the tumor cells which will permit greater differential toxicity in the tumor cells by the appropriate effector agent(s) in the combination. Therefore, parameters of dosage ratios of agents and the sequence and time interval between administration of agents are much more critical in this approach than in the classical approach, in which the independent activity of each agent is the desired effect. It has become apparent that the translation of preclinical results with biochemical modulation to the clinic requires careful attention to specific details.

In classical combination chemotherapy it was necessary simply to find the highest tolerable doses of the drugs in a combination. Therefore, in going from preclinical murine studies to clinical trials, the usual phase I dosage finding was an adequate preliminary for a definitive trial. In "modulating" chemotherapy, it may not be desirable to use the highest possible dose of some of the agents, and as mentioned before, sequence and timing may be critical. In this approach, therefore, comparative pharmacological and biochemical studies become essential if a drug combination that has been found to be valuable in a preclinical murine model is to be adequately tested in humans. The objective in clinical biochemical modulation studies is to find in humans the parameters of dosage and timing necessary to obtain the desired biochemical change(s) that was associated with successful modulation of the concerned antitumor effector agent in

the preclinical model. It is obvious that the translation of successful protocols of biochemical modulation to clinical fruition will be more difficult
than the translation of classical combination chemotherapy. Nevertheless, the exciting preclinical results obtained with biochemical modulation
indicate that the additional effort will be rewarded ultimately by significant advances in cancer treatment.

VII. More than One Modulating Agent May Be Necessary to Induce Unequivocally Improved Tumor Regression Rates by a "Modulated" Effector Agent in the Clinic

In the PALA → FUra example noted previously, an outstanding difference between the preclinical and clinical antitumor findings with PALA
emerges. Against experimental tumors, both moderate and high doses of
PALA are reported to exert antitumor activity, whereas in the clinic, even
high doses of PALA are considered therapeutically inactive. One major
reason for this apparent difference in therapeutic activity is that entirely
different end points are utilized for determining therapeutic activity in
animal tumor models and in the clinic (106,113). In the clinic, drugs are
defined as clinically active only if the drugs elicit tumor regression (≥50%
in at least 20% of evaluable patients). In marked contrast, inhibition of
tumor growth is the criterion of effectiveness employed to define the same
tumor agents as active in the laboratory tumor models.

The fact that different end points are being used to identify anticancer
activity in humans and animals merits consideration in the design of clinical trials involving biochemical modulation. In the laboratory tumor
model, various degrees of tumor growth inhibition can be discerned and
interpreted as evidence for therapeutic gain. For example, both PALA →
FUra and MTX → FUra can be clearly shown to be better than the MTD
of FUra alone on the basis of tumor growth inhibition measurements,
even though a very low and unimpressive percentage of chemotherapeu-
tically induced partial tumor regressions is evident (117). In the clinic,
however, the therapeutic incremental gains induced by each of these
single manipulations of FUra metabolism may not be sufficient (particularly in the usual small pilot study) to overcome the inherent extreme
tumor heterogeneity at the level of statistically significant improvement in
the number of tumor regressions.

Sequential modulation at several steps in the metabolic activation of
FUra has been demonstrated in experimental tumors to be more effective
than manipulation of a single step in the metabolism of FUra at the level

TABLE III

More than One Biochemical Modulator in Appropriate Sequence to 5-Fluorouracil (FUra) Is Necessary to Clearly Induce Unequivocally Improved Tumor Regression Rates[a]

Group	Treatment	% of PR[b]
1	FUra	0
2	PALA → FUra → LV + UR "rescue"	5
3	MTX → FUra → LV + UR "rescue"	3
4	PALA → MTX → FUra → LV + UR "rescue"	27–32

[a] Pooled data from four murine experiments with advanced CD8F1 breast cancer (Tables 5, 6, 7 of Ref. 45). Methotrexate (MTX) and PALA are administered in nontherapeutic but biochemically active regimens. LV, leucovorin; UR, uridine. FUra is at its MTD in group 1, as are each of the drug combinations in groups 2–4, but the UR "rescue" allows for the safe administration of FUra at higher doses than would be otherwise tolerated.

[b] PR, partial regressions of ≥50% of initial tumor size.

of tumor regressions (117); thus, whereas the very small number of partial regressions induced by PALA → FUra (3%) or MTX → FUra (5%) is not persuasive of therapeutic gain, the triple combination of (PALA + MTX) → FUra followed by appropriate rescue is clearly a therapeutic advance in producing 27–32% partial tumor regressions in advanced murine breast cancers (117) (see Table III). The message in these experimental studies is that the concurrent administration of several appropriate modulating agents in biochemically active regimens can enhance the opportunity for discerning clinical success with biochemical modulation of an effector agent.

VIII. Modulation of Pyrimidine Pools and Enhancement of ara-C Cytotoxicity

The anticancer nucleoside, cytosine arabinoside (ara-C), is therapeutically inactive and must be phosphorylated to the triphosphate, ara-CTP, to exert its cytoxic effect by inhibition of DNA polymerase and incorporation into DNA (97). The rate-limiting enzyme in this regard is CdR kinase, which is feedback-inhibited by high pool sizes of dCTP (31,78). A high level of dCTP has been shown to be a mechanism of resistance to ara-C in both murine (125) and human neoplasms (165). Therefore, reduction of dCTP pools might be expected to result in increased enzyme activity, with a consequent increase in the activation of ara-C. Furthermore, since ara-CTP competes with dCTP for DNA polymerase, a reduction of the dCTP pool would be expected to favor increased incorporation of ara-CTP into DNA, with consequently greater antitumor activity (31).

As noted in an earlier section, one way to lower intracellular pyrimidine pools is through the use of PALA, which inhibits the second enzyme of *de novo* pyrimidine synthesis (36,164). L-(αS,5S)-α-Amino-3-chloro-4,5-dihydro-5-isoxazoleacetic acid (acivicin) also is useful in this regard. Acivicin can inhibit several enzymes which catalyze the transfer of the amide group of L-glutamine (80), including two reactions in the *de novo* biosynthesis of pyrimidines: the first enzymatic step in the pyrimidine pathway, formation of carbamylphosphate by carbamylphosphate synthetase II (4); and the conversion of UTP to CTP by CTP synthetase (87). Synergistic effects have been reported on inhibition of pyrimidine biosynthesis when acivicin and PALA are used in combination, both in terms of biochemical and therapeutic end points (87,101).

It is particularly pertinent that the combination of acivicin and PALA has been reported (in *in vitro* studies on L1210 cells) to result in more than additive depletion of dCTP pools and has been recommended on this basis for combination therapy with ara-C (101). The effect of the combination of acivicin and PALA, administered prior to ara-C for therapeutic activity, with cytidine nucleotide and ara-CTP levels *in vivo* against very advanced, large murine breast tumors has been reported (161). Figure 4 records a significant and longer-lasting depletion of tumor cytidine nucleotides with a sequenced acivicin + PALA combination than that obtained with either drug alone. Cytidine nucleotide levels were essentially unchanged in bone marrow from mice treated with the same drug combination (161).

The depression of the cytidine nucleotide levels in the tumors is viewed as indicative of similar depression in dCTP pools, since reported results obtained with the acivicin–PALA combination have suggested that measurement of changes in CTP pools provides a good estimate of the changes in dCTP pools (101). Therefore, at a time when dCTP pools were apparently at low levels following acivicin + PALA (Fig. 4), ara-C was administered (Table IV).

Table IV records a representative experiment (of four), in which the triple combination of acivicin and PALA, administered prior to the MTD of ara-C as a single agent, is evaluated for therapeutic activity against very advanced (25 days of growth), and large (100 mg), murine CD8F1 breast tumor transplants.

The CD8F1 tumors are a member of the NCI tumor model panel (60), and, when advanced, are more difficult to treat than other experimental

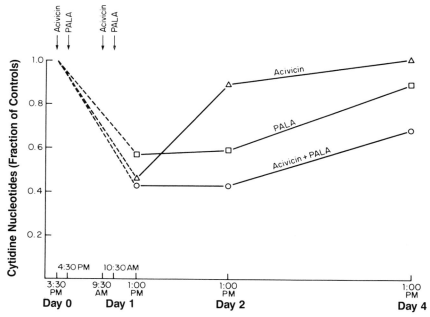

Fig. 4. Effect of acivicin and PALA on cytidine nucleotides in CD8F1 breast tumors. Tumor-bearing CD8F1 mice received either acivicin (10 mg/kg), PALA (100 mg/kg), or acivicin (10 mg/kg) followed 1 hr later by PALA (100 mg/kg) on two successive days with an 18-hr interval. At $2\frac{1}{2}$, $26\frac{1}{2}$, and $74\frac{1}{2}$ hr after the second PALA injection, the animals were sacrificed. Perchloric acid extracts were prepared from the tumors and were heated to convert cytidine nucleotides to CMP which was quantitated by high-pressure liquid chromatography.

tumor transplants, because in addition to the large tumor size of 100 mg when treatment is begun, they are first-generation transplants from spontaneous mammary tumors and, hence, carry a much higher degree of heterogeneity than the long-transplanted, common experimental tumors (112,160). It should also be noted that this is a solid tumor and ara-C is not considered active against solid tumors in the clinic. However, although ara-C is widely used in the treatment of leukemia and has recently been reported active against advanced human ovarian cancer (90,104), this agent has not been adequately evaluated in the treatment of most clinical solid tumors (173). It should be noted that deoxycytidine kinase, the enzyme that activates ara-C, is present in human solid tumor cells (7,104). Therefore human cancers have the capacity for cellular formation of ara-C nucleotides. If higher ara-C drug levels [e.g., as can be obtained clinically with therapeutically effective intraperitoneal chemotherapy against

TABLE IV

"Modulatory" Combination Chemotherapy: Enhancement of the Anticancer[a] Activity of the Maximum Tolerated Dose of Cytosine Arabinoside (ara-C) Alone by Prior Biochemical Modulation with a Sequenced Combination of Two Inhibitors of Pyrimidine Biosynthesis, Acivicin (ACIV) and PALA

Group	Weekly treatment[b]		Antitumor activity		Host toxicity	
	Day 1	Day 2	Tumor weight (mg)	Significance (vs. group)[c]	Weight change (%)	Dead/total
1		Saline	3077		+2	1/10
2	$ACIV_{10}$	$ACIV_{10}$	3368	NS (1)	+6	0/10
3	$PALA_{100}$	$PALA_{100}$	3140	NS (1)	+6	0/10
4	$ACIV_{10} \xrightarrow{1\ hr} PALA_{100}$	$ACIV_{10} \xrightarrow{1\ hr} PALA_{100}$	1377	S (1)	−5	0/10
5		$ara\text{-}C_{4000}$	1102	S (1)	−5	0/10
6	$ACIV_{10}$	$ACIV_{10} \xrightarrow{2\frac{1}{2}\ hr} ara\text{-}C_{4000}$	960	S (1); NS (5)	−5	0/10
7	$PALA_{100}$	$PALA_{100} \xrightarrow{1\frac{1}{2}\ hr} ara\text{-}C_{4000}$	926	S (1); NS (5)	−3	0/10
8	$ACIV_{10} \xrightarrow{1\ hr} PALA_{100}$	$ACIV_{10} \xrightarrow{1\ hr} PALA_{100} \xrightarrow{1\frac{1}{2}\ hr} ara\text{-}C_{4000}$	418	S (1–7)	−11	0/10

[a] Experiment 1421: Advanced (25-days-old), first-generation transplants of CD8F1 breast tumor transplants in male CD8F1 mice, averaging 100 mg when therapy began. Observations 5 days after third week's course.

[b] Three weekly courses at the indicated time intervals with an 18-hr interval between the 2 days of injections per week, and a 7-day interval between each of the three courses. Subscript = mg/kg intraperitoneally.

[c] Significance = statistical significance S to group indicated in parentheses; NS = not significant, Student's t test: $p \leq .05$.

ovarian cancer with ara-C (90,104)] than can be achieved with conventional chemotherapy are necessary for sufficient ara-C nucleotide synthesis, biochemical modulation as described here will facilitate such higher levels to be achieved selectively in tumor cells. The following enhanced antitumor effects with the acivicin–PALA–ara-C triple combination against a marginally sensitive ara-C solid experimental tumor, the CD8F1 breast cancer, and an ara-C refractory solid cancer, the Lewis lung tumor, are of decided interest against this background information.

In Table IV, note that neither the schedule of acivicin alone (group 2) nor that of PALA alone (group 3) exerts antitumor activity compared to the saline-treated, CD8F1 tumor–bearing animals (group 1). However, the combination of the two pyrimidine inhibitors, acivicin and PALA (group 4), exerts significant antitumor activity compared to the saline-treated controls (group 1). Ara-C as a single agent at its MTD (group 5) exerts modest tumor inhibitory activity as compared to the saline-treated controls (group 1). Neither the group receiving just acivicin prior to ara-C (group 6) nor the prior administration of just PALA to ara-C (group 7) show antitumor activity greater than that of ara-C alone (group 5). However, the administration of both pyrimidine antagonists prior to ara-C (group 3) resulted in a statistically significant increase in antitumor activity compared to that observed in mice treated with either the MTD of ara-C alone (group 5), or the double combination of acivicin + PALA (group 4).

Since neither acivicin alone (group 2) nor PALA as a single agent (group 3) evidenced antitumor activity but did so when given together (group 4 versus group 1), it is clear that these two agents are therapeutically synergistic in combination against this solid tumor, as they are against L1210 leukemia (101). The enhanced therapeutic effect obtained by administering the combination of acivicin and PALA prior to ara-C is a gratifying incremental gain against very advanced, large murine breast tumors. It may be possible to further "modulate" and improve this regimen's therapeutic results by the addition of excess thymidine (TdR) to cause an expansion of the intracellular dTTP pools. According to Kinahan *et al.* (89) an elevated level of dTTP can enhance the phosphorylation of ara-C by interfering with the inhibition of CdR kinase by dCTP. Also, high levels of dTTP feedback-inhibit the enzyme, ribonucleotide reductase, thereby lowering dCTP pools and activating ara-C (20,35,40,61,66,79, 142). Moreover, a high level of dTTP can inhibit an important ara-C degradative enzyme, dCMP deaminase (31). The balance between activating and degrading enzymes appears to be crucial in determining the quantity of ara-C converted to the active intermediate, ara-CTP, and this balance varies greatly among cell types (31). Further, the combination of TdR + PALA prior to ara-C has previously been shown to enhance ara-C antitumor activity against the CD8F1 breast tumor (114). Thus, the addition of TdR to the acivicin + PALA treatment prior to ara-C regimen may add further antitumor efficacy and result in synergistic therapeutic activity. Such exploration is under way in our laboratory.

Biochemical modulation with the acivicin + PALA combination prior to ara-C administration can convert an ara-C-refractory tumor to ara-C sensitivity. The Lewis lung tumor does not respond to ara-C as a single agent (143). Nor does pretreatment of ara-C with either PALA or acivicin convert the Lewis lung tumor to ara-C sensitivity. Table V demonstrates, however, that treatment of the ara-C-refractory Lewis lung tumor with the combination of acivicin and PALA prior to ara-C (group 4) results in antitumor activity that is statistically significantly greater than that effected by either the double combination of acivicin + PALA (group 3) or the MTD dose of ara-C alone (group 2). Based on calculation (94) of the growth inhibitory activity of the components of the three drug combination, 12% tumor growth by the triple combination (group 4) would be "expected" in comparison to the saline controls (group 1). In marked contrast, a 3% tumor growth is actually obtained in group 4 compared to group 1, suggesting therapeutic synergism. These are striking therapeutic findings with ara-C in an ara-C-refractory tumor.

Biochemical studies in the Lewis lung tumor are necessary to verify the biochemical rationale upon which this successful ara-C-containing therapeutic regimen was based. Previous studies of acivicin in the Lewis lung tumor have demonstrated that acivicin alone produces a 30% reduction in CTP pools (87), that PALA markedly lowers pyrimidine pools (88), and that the combination of acivicin with PALA effects synergistic therapeutic activity (87). The prospect for documenting biochemical evidence in the Lewis lung tumor, that appreciably lowered dCTP pools are effected by the two pyrimidine inhibitors acting in combination, which in turn is then responsible for allowing increased activation of ara-C by CdR kinase to therapeutic levels in this otherwise ara-C-refractory tumor, is promising. In another experimental tumor that is partially resistant to ara-C therapy, biochemical modulation has also been reported to result in therapeutic synergism (35). Since human tumor cells are markedly heterogeneous with populations of cells in which there is a wide spectrum of sensitivity to ara-C, the combination of acivicin and PALA prior to ara-C against presumed ara-C-sensitive tumors (e.g., leukemia) might be expected to yield better therapeutic results (both additive and synergistic at the cellular level) than could be obtained with ara-C alone.

TABLE V

Conversion of a Cytosine Arabinoside (ara-C)-Resistant Tumor to ara-C Sensitivity by Biochemical Modulation with Prior Administration of Acivicin (ACIV) and PALA[a]

Group	Weekly treatment[b]		Antitumor activity		Host toxicity	
	Day 1	Day 2	Tumor weight (mg)	Significance[c] (vs. group)	Weight change (%)	Dead/total
1		Saline	4804		−1	0/10
2		ara-C$_{4000}$	4035	NS (1)	−13	1/10
3	ACIV$_{10}$ $\xrightarrow{1\ hr}$ PALA$_{100}$	ACIV$_{10}$ $\xrightarrow{1\ hr}$ PALA$_{100}$	692	S (1)	+6	0/10
4	ACIV$_{10}$ $\xrightarrow{1\ hr}$ PALA$_{100}$	ACIV$_{10}$ $\xrightarrow{1\ hr}$ PALA$_{100}$ $\xrightarrow{1½\ hr}$ ara-C$_{4000}$	150	S (1–3)	+10	0/10

[a] Experiment L 11: Well-established (7-day-old) Lewis lung tumors in B6D2F1 male mice, averaging 130 mg when therapy began. Observations 5 days after the third week's course.

[b] Three weekly courses at the indicated time intervals with an 18-hr interval between the 2 days of injections per week, and a 7-day interval between each of the three courses. Subscript = mg/kg intraperitoneally.

[c] Significance = statistical significance S to group indicated in parentheses; NS = not significant, Student's t test: $p \leq .05$.

Moreover, these therapeutic findings on solid murine tumors augur well for similar results to be obtained in human solid tumors. As noted earlier, ara-C has antitumor cytotoxicity against advanced human ovarian cancer (90,104), and biochemical modulation therefore might be expected to enhance this activity. Advanced breast cancer would be another candidate solid tumor. Significant levels of CdR kinase, the enzyme that activates ara-C, along with low levels of the deaminase enzyme that inactivates ara-C, have been reported for human breast cancer (7). It should also be noted that the positive effects with the acivicin–PALA–ara-C triple combination against the CD8F1 mammary carcinoma may be considered as further supportive evidence warranting trial in human breast cancer, since the CD8F1 tumor has an excellent correlation in sensitivity to those agents shown clinically active against the human disease (112).

IX. Agents That "Rescue" FUra

A. Preclinical Studies with Uridine "Rescue" of High-Dose FUra

As indicated earlier in the discussion on Table III, Section VI, biochemical modulation by "rescue" techniques may also be employed to improve the therapeutic index of an effector agent. An appreciation of the relevance of the incorporation of FUra into tumor RNA to FUra's cytotoxic activity (48,53,56,68,74,95,96,103,120,121,129,149,158,172,175) provided the rationale (92,118) for the selection of uridine (UR) as a potential rescue agent. Appropriate studies have demonstrated that prolonged administration of UR following FUra can selectively protect or "rescue" normal host tissues from cytotoxicity (92,118), while antitumor efficacy is retained or even augmented by the UR-provided safe opportunity to increase the dose of the effector agent, FUra (91,92,118).

Enhanced therapeutic efficacy with the FUra–UR combination has been demonstrated in mice bearing colon tumor 26 (118), and a similar enhancement of the therapeutic index with this two-drug combination has been found in mice bearing the B16 melanoma (91). In these studies, protection of normal tissues with UR permitted the safe use of higher and more potent doses of FUra, resulting in greater antitumor effect without increased host toxicity.

Another way to administer what effectively amounts to a higher dose of

FUra is to modulate at several steps in the anabolism of FUra to its active nucleotides. The triple combination of PALA and MTX prior to FUra noted in Table III is one such example. PALA and MMPR prior to FUra is another. MMPR acts like MTX, but at a different metabolic point, in also being able to augment intracellular levels of PRPP, an obligatory substrate for the enzymatic conversion of FUra to its cytotoxic nucleotides. By virtue of its elevation of intracellular levels of PRPP, MMPR can, when given in combination with PALA (which, as explained earlier, favorably modulates FUra metabolism by lowering its competing pyrimidine pools), further enhance the antitumor activity of FUra (12, 24,96,114,115,149). Figure 5 records that in the presence of these two metabolic modulators MMPR and PALA, doubling the MTD of FUra in the triple combination causes 100% mortality, but the same lethal dose of FUra in the combination can be safely administered when a UR rescue schedule is administered following each course of the triple combination;

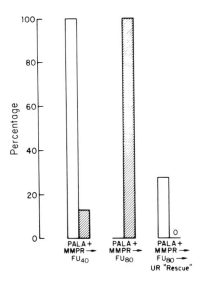

Fig. 5. Selective modulation by uridine (UR) "rescue" of a high-dose FUra combination. Advanced colon carcinoma #26 transplants in CO_2 male mice. □, Tumor Growth; ▨ Mortality.

and, most importantly, significantly greater antitumor activity is achieved in the UR rescue group without host toxicity (118).

The biochemical basis by which UR allows for selective rescue of host normal tissues from FUra with retention of FUra's antitumor activity is, however, not clear, since uridine administration also effects an enhanced clearance of FUra from tumor RNA, similar to that observed in bone marrow (118). In this regard, Sawyer et al. (150) have noted that tissues can have differing sensitivities to FUra in RNA, as Glazer and Lloyd (56) have reported. The latter investigators have demonstrated that in a human colon carcinoma cell line, cell survival correlated well with the absolute level of FUra in RNA rather than with inhibition of DNA synthesis. After reaching a threshold level of incorporation, cell viability decreased sharply with small increases in (FUra)RNA. Conversely, a small decrease in (FUra)RNA can produce a large increase in survival if the decrease reduces the (FUra)RNA level below the threshold level for that particular tissue. Thus, an equal percentage of reduction can produce a different result in different tissues if one tissue is reduced below its threshold level while the other remains above it. Perhaps this is the explanation for the selective retention of antitumor activity with host protection in the presence of a high-dose FUra/UR regimen despite the similar clearance of FUra from both tumor and bone marrow RNA.

At present, the biochemical basis for the selectivity between tumor and host tissues that can be attained by proper dose and scheduling of FUra and UR remains to be determined. If a tumor is sensitive to (FUra)RNA as the mechanism of cytotoxic action, then quantitative biochemical differences between cancer and normal host tissues may be responsible. For example, tissues differ in reparative activity, and these differences include the ability of cells to degrade FUra-altered molecules (9). Also, since the activity of uridine kinase and uridine phosphorylase can vary between different tumors (2,166) and between tumor and host tissues, quantitative differences in the utilization of UR in tumor as compared to normal host tissues might allow for a selective antitumor effect. An alternative possibility is that a tumor may contain a subset of cells that is sensitive to the DNA-directed action of an FdUMP block on thymidylate synthetase. The qualitative biochemical difference between these FdUMP-sensitive tumor cells and normal cells which are sensitive to the RNA-directed action of FUra may explain the ability of UR to selectively reverse the normal tissue toxic effects of FUra with retention of the antitumor effect.

B. Early Clinical Trials of UR and Its Potential to Rescue FUra Toxicity

Phase I clinical trials of high-dose UR have been initiated (99,168,169). Continuous infusions of UR were discontinued due to the rapid onset of fever. An intermittent infusion of UR, 3 hr on followed by 3 hr off for 72 hr, mostly at 2–3 g/m²/hr, was considered tolerable and safe (168). Only mild to moderate rises in temperature occurred during a number of courses. The only other problem noted was phlebitis, which could be circumvented by infusion into a central vein.

The pretreatment plasma level of uridine was 3–8 μM (99). At doses of 2 or 3 g/m²/hr, peak uridine levels of around 1 mM were achieved at the end of each 3-hr infusion period. During the 3-hr treatment-free intervals, UR concentration decreased rapidly but was still markedly elevated (0.1–0.4 mM) at the start of the next 3-hr infusion (168). It appears, therefore, that this intermittent UR schedule can provide prolonged clinical periods (72 hr) of relatively high UR exposure.

As yet, no definite conclusions can be drawn from this preliminary assessment of an intermittent UR infusion schedule for its potential to "rescue" patients from FUra toxicity. In one of two patients with FUra-induced toxicity there was evidence that the intended UR reversal of FUra toxicity was achieved.

C. Other Agents That Effect Selective "Rescue" of FUra Toxicity in Normal Host Tissues

1. Benzylacyclouridine

Uridine rescue may be limited due to the pyrogenic reactions (at least, with the aforementioned dose and schedule) with regard to the increase in the FUra dose that is tolerated. The pyrogenic toxicity is related to the large doses of UR that are required due to the efficiency with which UR is catabolized by uridine phosphorylase in normal tissues (55,85,128). The use of an inhibitor, benzylacyclouridine (BAU) (33,132,133), of this UR-catabolizing enzyme has been suggested to allow a lowering of the administered UR dose in UR "rescue" regimens in order to diminish or, one hopes, to prevent the UR-induced pyrogenic reactions (41,42). A combination of BAU and UR has been demonstrated to permit the administration of otherwise intolerably high doses of FUra, with the result of a significantly greater growth inhibition of murine colon tumor 38 than could be obtained with the maximally tolerated dose of FUra alone (42). Thus, the administration of BAU + UR in clinical UR "rescue" regimens may permit the safe administration of higher doses of FUra, with a corresponding increase in therapeutic effectiveness, and, due to the BAU, this improvement in FUra therapy may be accomplished with lower doses of UR.

2. Cytidine Rescue of FUra Toxicity in Normal Host Tissues

Uridine is nontoxic to humans, but high dosage causes fever that precludes the use of continuous infusion of high-dose UR (99,168,169). Although long-term exposure to moderately elevated UR levels has been achieved in patients by intermittent infusion, the low-grade fever that occurs may preclude the possibility of increasing the UR dose further, and therefore it may not be possible to increase FUra doses sufficiently to achieve therapeutic improvement (168).

Since the *Limulus* test for pyrogens is negative for clinically formulated UR, the UR-induced pyrogenic reaction is believed not to be related to bacterial pyrogens or to an accumulation of UR catabolites, but is likely inherent in the UR molecule (140,141). A FUra-protecting substitute for UR might, therefore, obviate the pyrogenic problem.

Cytidine (CR), which is deaminated *in vivo* to UR, has been compared to UR in rabbits because there is a positive correlation between drug-induced pyrogenic reactions in rabbits and humans (38,140,141). Unlike UR, CR does not produce hyperthermia in rabbits (38,140), and it therefore would not be expected to do so in humans. These findings have led, therefore, to the evaluation of CR as a rescue agent for FUra toxicity.

Table VI compares the ability of CR and UR to protect normal (tumor-

TABLE VI

Both Uridine (UR) and Cytidine (CR) Rescue 5-Fluorouracil (FUra)-Associated Toxicity[a]

Group	Treatment[b]	WBC/mm^3 [e] (Day 0)	WBC/mm^3 [e] (Day 21)	% Body weight change (day 26)	Dead/ total (day 30)
1	FUra	22,089 (±1823)	4,425 (±718)	−25	5/9
2	FUra $\xrightarrow{2\ hr}$ UR rescue[c]	21,711 (±1444)	17,889 (±1778)	−4	0/9
3	FUra $\xrightarrow{2\ hr}$ CR rescue[d]	22,022 (±1469)	17,167 (±1436)	−1	0/9

[a] Normal (tumor-free) CD8F1 female mice.
[b] FUra was administered in a known toxic regimen of 130 mg/kg on days 0, 7, 14, and 21.
[c] UR 1500 mg/kg $\xrightarrow{2\frac{1}{2}\ hr}$ UR 3500 mg/kg $\xrightarrow{17\ hr}$ UR 3500 mg/kg $\xrightarrow{7\ hr}$ UR 3500 mg/kg.
[d] CR 2000 mg/kg $\xrightarrow{2\frac{1}{2}\ hr}$ CR 5000 mg/kg $\xrightarrow{17\ hr}$ CR 5000 mg/kg $\xrightarrow{7\ hr}$ 5000 mg/kg.
[e] WBC, White blood cells.

free) mice (CD8F1) from a known toxic regimen of FUra (130 mg/kg)
administered once a week for four weekly injections). This toxic regimen
of FUra induces leukopenia, a 25% body weight loss, and a mortality rate
of 56%. The delayed administration of either a UR rescue regimen (group
2), or a CR rescue regimen, beginning 2 hr after FUra, resulted in complete prevention of FUra-induced leukopenia, weight loss, and mortality.
Accordingly, since CR appears equally as capable as UR in controlling
FUra toxicity, and since it appears, on the basis of the negative pyrogenic
rabbit tests with CR (38,140), that CR will not be pyrogenic in humans,
CR has been evaluated in tumor-bearing animals to determine whether,
like uridine (118), CR rescue can selectively protect the host from FUra
toxicity with retention of antitumor activity by FUra.

Table VII records one of three similar experiments demonstrating the
beneficial effects of delayed CR rescue on the therapeutic index of a
regimen of acivicin and PALA administered sequentially prior to the
MTD of FUra in CD8F1 mice bearing large breast tumors averaging 130
mg at initiation of therapy. The reasons for administering the sequential
acivicin $\rightarrow$ PALA combination (i.e., to lower intracellular pyrimidine
pools) prior to the administration of a pyrimidine antagonist) have
been previously discussed in Sections III,B,1 and VII and in published reports (87,88,101) documenting their synergistic effects on the inhibition of pyrimidine biosynthesis. In addition, the beneficial therapeutic
effect of low-dose PALA on the antitumor activity of the MTD (100
mg/kg) of FUra against the CD8F1 tumor has been presented (see Fig. 3)
(116). The fractionated acivicin–PALA weekly regimen (i.e., schedule,
dosage, and timing intervals) in Table VII is the same ($ACIV_{10} \xrightarrow{1\ hr}$
$PALA_{100} \xrightarrow{17\ hr} ACIV_{10} \xrightarrow{1\ hr} PALA_{100}$; subscripts = mg/kg) as that
previously presented in Section VII and Tables IV and V.

Without CR rescue, this acivicin–PALA regimen, administered
prior to the MTD of FUra, is a lethal combination, as is a fractionated
weekly schedule of just PALA prior to the MTD of FUra (i.e.,
$PALA_{100} \xrightarrow{18\ hr} PALA_{100} \xrightarrow{1\frac{1}{4}\ hr} FUra_{100}$), as well as a fractionated
weekly schedule of just acivicin prior to the MTD of FUra (i.e.,
$ACIV_{10} \xrightarrow{18\ hr} ACIV_{10} \xrightarrow{2\frac{1}{4}\ hr} FUra_{100}$). (These data are not presented in
Table VII, due to the virtually complete mortality.)

Note in Table VII in the "p (versus group)" column, that the MTD of
FUra alone (group 2) exerts its usual significant inhibitory antitumor activity compared to the saline-treated controls (group 1). The administra-
tion of $PALA_{100}$ $2\frac{1}{2}$ hr prior to $FUra_{100}$ (group 3) results in a greater antitumor effect than that produced by FUra alone (group 2), although in this
particular experiment the difference between these two groups is just
short of statistical significance. Neither FUra alone (group 2) nor the

TABLE VII

"Modulated" Combination Chemotherapy: Acivicin (ACIV) + PALA prior to 5-Fluorouracil (FUra) Followed by Cytidine (CR) Rescue

Group	Weekly treatment[a]		Antitumor activity		Host toxicity		
	Day 1	Day 2	Tumor weight (mg)	Significance (vs. group)	% of PR[c]	Weight change (%)	Dead/total
1		Saline	5814		0	−10	0/10
2		$FUra_{100}$	522	S (1)	0	−12	0/10
3	$PALA_{100} \xrightarrow{19\frac{1}{2}\ hr}$	$FUra_{100}$	267	NS (2)	0	−8	1/10
4	$ACIV_{10} \xrightarrow{1\ hr} PALA_{100}$	$ACIV_{10} \xrightarrow{1\ hr} PALA_{100} \xrightarrow{1\frac{1}{2}\ hr} FUra_{100} \xrightarrow{2\ hr} CR^{d}$	64	S (2,3)	80	−13	1/10

[a] Experiment 1537: Advanced (19-day-old), first-generation CD8F1 breast tumor transplants in female CD8F1 mice, averaging 130 mg at initiation of treatment. Three weekly courses at the indicated time intervals with a 17-hr interval between the 2 days of injections per week and a 7-day interval between each of the three courses. Subscripts = mg/kg intraperitoneally. Observations 5 days after the third week's course.

[b] Statistical significance S to group indicated in parentheses; Student's t test: $p \leq .05$, NS = not significant.

[c] PR = partial tumor regression (≥50% of initial tumor size).

[d] CR rescue = 2000 mg/kg 2 hr after receiving FUra, then 5000 mg/kg 2½ hr later, followed by 5000 mg/kg 17 hr later, and 5000 mg/kg again 7 hr later.

double combination of PALA and FUra (group 3) yields any partial tumor regressions. In marked contrast, group 4, the quadruple combination of sequenced acivicin, PALA, and FUra followed by CR rescue, exerts a *regressing* antitumor effect (i.e., a treatment-induced average tumor weight of 64 mg as compared to the initial tumor weight of 130 mg and, most importantly, an impressive 80% partial tumor regression rate. The group 4 average body weight loss is only 13%, and the mortality rate is virtually nil. These therapeutic results indicate that appropriate CR rescue can spare host toxicity with retention of the antitumor activity of FUra, at least in this experimental tumor and under these conditions. Whether CR modulation (i.e., rescue) will permit similar therapeutic gain with high-dose FUra in other tumors requires further evaluation.

It must be noted that the use of UR rescue does not improve the therapeutic effectiveness of FUra *alone* (i.e., in the absence of modulating agents) in either the L1210 murine leukemia (91) or in the CD8F1 murine mammary tumor (111,117). In contrast, however, in the same murine breast tumor model, UR rescue of high-dose FUra in a modulating combination of PALA plus high-dose MTX prior to high-dose FUra followed by both UR and leucovorin rescue allows for striking improvement in the therapeutic index (Table III) (117). Along with these findings, the marked therapeutic gain allowed by UR rescue of a PALA–MMPR–FUra combination against colon tumor 26 (Fig. 5) (118) further indicates that modulation at several steps in the metabolism of FUra is very much more effective than manipulation of a single metabolic stage of FUra activity (see discussion under Section VI).

3. Poly I: Poly C Can Modulate FUra Cytotoxicity in Normal Host Tissue

The cytotoxic activity of most anticancer agents is proliferation-dependent (167). Thus, since human tumor cells do not necessarily proliferate faster than normal cells do, normally proliferating host cells, such as those of hematopoietic tissue and intestinal epithelium, usually are cytotoxic targets, and toxic symptoms associated with cell loss in these normal tissues limits the dose of drug that can be administered with safety. Because of the general propensity of tumor cells to continue cycling under conditions which discourage normal cells from cycling, a therapeutic strategy has been developed in which selective differential cell cycle slowing of normal cells versus tumor cells results in differential protection of normal tissue from the toxicity of antitumor therapy which consequently can be administered at higher doses with a greater antitumor effect. Various substances that have been reported promising in this regard include cyclic adenosine 3′, 5′-monophosphate reduction of hydroxyurea-induced killing of normal versus SV-40-transformed baby hamster kidney cells (138); cyclohexamide protection of bone marrow damage induced by ara-C (11); asparaginase amelioration of myelosuppression by methotrexate (29); puromycin aminonucleoside selective protection against hydroxyurea-induced normal cell toxicity (18); selective protection by anguidine of normal versus transformed cells against ara-C and adriamycin (75); methylglyoxal *bis*-(guanylhydrazone)–selective protection of normal cells against hydroxyurea (145); difluoromethylornithine inhibition of proliferation of normal cells while potentiating killing of transformed cells (163); histidinol protection of marrow cells while augmenting the toxicities of ara-C and FUra for L1210 leukemia cells (171); interferon-selective protection of normal versus leukemic colony-forming units in culture against ara-C (62); and amelioration of the host toxicity of FUra by the interferon inducer, poly I: poly C (162), which allowed an increase in both the MTD of FUra and the antitumor effect of FUra in mice bearing L1210 leukemia (77) and colon tumor 26 (159).

The aforementioned inhibition of proliferation of normal cells as a means of reducing their susceptibility to chemotherapeutic drugs usually has been demonstrated only in cell culture systems (18,62,75,138,145, 163), with some of the agents ineffective or untested *in vivo* or, when assessed, possessing too great a toxicity for *in vivo* applicability (11). However, a few agents have demonstrated selective protection of the host animals from chemotherapeutic toxicity with retention of antitumor activity (29,77,159,171).

Table VIII records the results of three once-a-week intraperitoneal injections of combination therapy with high-dose FUra in conjuction with polyI: poly C in mice bearing advanced subcutaneous colon tumor 26 (averaging 340 mg when treatment was initiated). The 85-mg/kg dose of

TABLE VIII

Combination Therapy of Colon Tumor 26 with FUra and Poly I : Poly C[a]

Group	Treatment	Tumor weight (mg)[b]	Body weight change (%)	Dead/total
1	Saline	2284	−30	3/13
2	$FUra_{85}$	557	−21	2/13
3	$FUra_{100}$	Toxic	—	9/15
4	$FUra_{130}$ + poly I : poly C_4	309	−16	0/13

[a] Three courses of the indicated treatment were administered intraperitoneally with a 1-week interval between courses to mice bearing colon tumor 26 averaging 340 mg when treatment was initiated. Subscripts refer to doses in mg/kg.

[b] Group 2 versus group 4: $p = .017$.

FUra alone (group 2) resulted in a statistically significant inhibition of tumor growth, compared to the saline-treated controls of group 1 ($p = 6 \times 10^{-6}$), and a small mortality rate. A higher dose of FUra alone at 100 mg/kg (group 3) resulted in appreciable mortality (60%). Nevertheless, when combined with concomitantly administered poly I: poly C, a still higher weekly dose (130 mg/kg) of FUra (group 4) could be tolerated without mortality, and significantly greater tumor inhibition was obtained than with FUra alone at 85 mg/kg/week (group 2), $p = .017$. Doses of FUra higher than 130 mg/kg were not protected by the interferon inducer, poly I: poly C.

Both mouse interferon and hybrid human recombinant alpha A/D interferon (which has been demonstrated to cross species barriers in murine cells) can protect mice from weight loss, leukopenia, and mortality due to a known toxic regimen of FUra at 130 mg/kg/week for 3 courses (159). Since it has been demonstrated that poly I: poly C can produce inhibition of cell cycling in normal murine marrow for a period of approximately 48 hr after administration (162), it is presumably this decreased rate of proliferation in normal host tissues which accounts for the decreased toxicity of FUra to the murine host. Poly I: poly C does not evidence anticancer activity for colon tumor 26 (162). If tumor cells are not susceptible or are less susceptible than normal host cells to the anti-proliferative action of the interferon inducer, poly I: poly C, then the coadministration of the latter agent with FUra permits the use of higher doses of FUra than normally tolerable, with a resultant increase in therapeutic efficacy of FUra.

The preceding *in vivo* results indicate that differential cytokinetic modulation with poly I: poly C as an antiproliferative agent, and possibly other antiproliferative agents (64), may provide a new approach for improving clinical results in cancer therapy with available drugs.

X. Inhibition of Cellular Repair Mechanisms: A Potential Target for Biochemical Modulation

A. 6-Aminonicotinamide and Mitomycin C

It is now generally accepted that a combination of active chemotherapeutic drugs with different pathways of activation and different mechanisms of action will be required to overcome the very substantial biochemical heterogeneity in the neoplastic cell population of a single malignant tumor in order to achieve cure. Ideally, all of the chemotherapeutic agents should be administered *simultaneously,* so that cells that may be resistant to one of the agents would be killed by another, and therefore the greatest number of tumor cells, hopefully all, would be killed at the earliest possible time, thereby circumventing the problem of continued proliferation of residual cells with the possibility of further mutational development of drug resistance. Unfortunately, the toxicity of many active agents overlaps in normal tissues, and therefore a potentially totally effective combination of drugs may not be tolerable therapeutically. An alternative approach, suggested by the mathematical modeling of Goldie and Coldman (58) of judicious sequencing of either tolerable regimens of individual agents or tolerable regimens of drug combinations, may prove useful. In any event, the problem is formidable, and we believe that it will be necessary to maximize the therapeutic efficacy of each individual agent whenever possible in an ultimate curative therapeutic regimen. Quantitative heterogeneity—i.e. a subset of cancer cells possessing a gradient of responsiveness to a single agent—requires that the low *in vivo* therapeutic indices of most anticancer agents be increased to facilitate the eradication of slightly resistant cells at *in vivo* tolerated doses.

In view of the extensive clinical use of alkylating agents, it appears important to investigate whether an enhanced therapeutic index can be obtained with biochemical modulation of these clinically effective drugs. An alkylating agent's margin of tolerance between tumor response and systemic toxicity of the host is narrow. Steroids and pharmacologic depletion of glutathione to modulate the toxicity and antitumor activity of certain alkylating drugs have been used successfully in a few experimental tumor systems (65,122,153), but there appears to be a need for other approaches to widen the therapeutic index.

There are a number of biochemical methods that might be employed to augment the therapeutic activity of alkylating agents. Regardless of the specific methodology, if the toxicity of the "modulated" alkylating drug can be controlled adequately, the "modulating" agent should be administered simultaneously as part of a combination chemotherapy regimen. If not, the strategy would be to employ the "modulated" alkylating combination as a first line of attack to eradicate large numbers of tumor cells, which then would be expected to result in a shift of residual tumor cells out of the refractory G_0 compartment and into an actively proliferating stage which would be more vulnerable to a subsequently administered combination of modulated antimetabolite antitumor agents.

The alkylating agent, mitomycin C (Mito-C), is an antibiotic which selectively inhibits DNA synthesis as a result of DNA alkylation and cross-linking. The drug must be activated *in vivo* by enzymatic reduction of the quinone group. Mito-C has shown clinical activity against a variety of human neoplasms, including adenocarcinoma of the stomach (37), colon, pancreas, and breast and squamous-cell carcinomas of the head and neck (39). Alkylation and cross-linking in DNA resulting from the activity of Mito-C and other alkylating agents is subject to repair by intracellular enzymes, and the magnitude of cytotoxicity produced by an alkylating agent is dependent upon the level of activity of these repair mechanisms. Therefore, cellular repair mechanisms appear to provide an appropriate target for biochemical modulation in alkylating chemotherapy which has not yet been adequately exploited.

Polyadenosine diphosphoribose [poly(ADP-ribose)] is believed to be involved in the regulation of DNA replication and repair. Poly (ADP-ribose) polymerase, a chromatin-bound enzyme, responds to DNA damage by synthesizing poly(ADP-ribose) from nicotinamide adenine dinucleotide (NAD). NAD is utilized as an ADP-ribosyl donor with elimination of nicotinamide (67). NAD analogs can inhibit poly(ADP-ribose) polymerase, can interfere with the DNA repair process, and can enhance the cytotoxicity of DNA-damaging agents, such as N-methyl-N-nitrosourea and 1,3-*bis*-(2-chloroethyl)-1-nitrosourea (BCNU) (14,50,67,102,130,157). Documented inhibitors of poly(ADP-ribose) polymerase include such diverse compounds as pyridine analogs [for example, 6-aminonicotinamide (6-AN)] and purine analogs [for example, 6-mercaptopurine (6-MP)] (154).

6-AN is the most potent antagonist of nicotinamide (83). *In vivo* it may be incorporated into NAD in place of nicotinamide to give the corresponding NAD analog via an exchange reaction facilitated by the enzyme NAD glycohydrolase, which can remove nicotinamide from NAD (44,83). The 6-ANAD analog has been demonstrated to inhibit enzymatic reactions in which pyridine nucleotides play a part as coenzymes (44-46,135,136). The concentration of pyridine dinucleotide in neoplastic tissue has been shown to be low, as compared to normal tissue (57,81,107), and this suggests that an antagonist such as 6-AN may be much more active in tumor tissue than in normal tissue. In relation to poly(ADP-ribose) inhibition, 6-AN has demonstrated potentiation of the cytotoxic effects of DNA damage resulting from radio-therapy in L1210 cells and synergistic cytotoxicity in L1210 cells treated with BCNU (14).

All of the preceding information suggested the possibility that if 6-AN is indeed able to inhibit the cellular repair mechanism, poly(ADP-ribose), *in vivo,* it may be able to improve the antitumor effect of an alkylating agent such as Mito-C. Table IX records the results of one of three experiments with the combination of Mito-C + 6-AN in female mice (CD8F1) bearing spontaneous, autochthonous breast tumors. At the time of initiation of treatment, the tumors were very large, averaging close to 400 mg. Combination chemotherapy with Mito-C + 6-AN produced an augmentation in

TABLE IX

Therapy of Spontaneous, Autochthonous CD8F1 Breast Cancers with 6-Aminonicotinamide (6-AN) and Mitomycin C (Mito-C)

Group	Treatment[a]	Tumor weight (mg)		Significance (vs. group)[b]	% of PR[c]	Host toxicity	
		Initial	Final			Weight change (%)	Dead/total
1	Saline	403	1735		0	+6	0/13
2	Mito-C$_5$	379	436	S (1)	23	−5	0/13
3	Mito-C$_5$ + 6-AN$_{20}$	385	211	S (2)	54	−20	0/13

[a] Experiment R506: Three once-a-week courses of the indicated treatment with a 1-week interval between courses. Subscripts = mg/kg. Observations recorded 6 days after the third course of treatment.
[b] Student's t test. S = significant: $p \leq .05$ (versus group).
[c] PR = partial tumor regression of ≥50% of initial tumor size.

antitumor results, both in terms of inhibition of growth and partial regressions (PR) of tumors. The mean tumor weight in mice treated with Mito-C alone increased during the treatment period from 379 mg at the initiation of therapy to 436 mg, whereas the mean tumor weight in mice treated with Mito-C + 6-AN decreased from an initial size of 385 mg to 211 mg. The difference in posttreatment tumor weight between these two groups proved to be statistically significant, $p = .032$. The combination chemotherapy with Mito-C + 6-AN produced no mortality and a moderate body weight loss (20%). Body weight loss per se is not able to induce tumor regression. On an individual basis, 54% of the mice treated with the combination of Mito-C + 6-AN experienced tumor regressions of 50% or greater (i.e., partial regressions), compared to initial tumor size in these individual mice at the initiation of treatment. These results are particularly impressive in view of the fact that the therapeutic gain is in *regressions* of tumors in a very advanced stage of growth and the fact that these tumors are spontaneous. Owing to the limited number of spontaneous tumors that were available at the time, groups of tumor-bearing animals treated with 6-AN alone were omitted from this series of experiments. However, previous experience in two separate experiments in which 6-AN alone at the same dose (20 mg/kg) and weekly schedule was administered to mice bearing equisized CD8F1 spontaneous breast tumors demonstrated no mortality, an average body weight loss of 24%, and an average PR rate of only 11%.

These enhanced tumor-regressing therapeutic results are considered to be impressive and to augur well for ultimate integration of "modulated" alkylating chemotherapy with "modulated" combination antimetabolite chemotherapy. If the toxicity of an overall combination of "modulated" alkylating and antimetabolite agents can be controlled adequately, the two types of combination chemotherapy may be administered simultaneously; if not, it will be necessary to administer them sequentially. Selective "rescue" of host toxicity with nicotinamide may provide an opportunity for further improving the therapeutic index of the Mito-C + 6-AN combination. It is well documented that the toxic manifestations of 6-AN can be ameliorated by administration of the normal metabolite, nicotinamide, and amelioration of host toxicity from antimetabolite antitumor therapy with normal metabolites has proved useful with several antimetabolites.

One caveat should be noted. Neither the biochemical studies to explore the rationale for employing 6-AN to inhibit poly(ADP-ribose) in the CD8F1 tumor nor those to verify that this hypothesized mechanism is actually responsible for the augmented antitumor results obtained with the 6-AN–Mito-C combination have been completed. Poly(ADP-ribose) may not be involved at all. However, the biological results are stimulating: *in vivo* administration of 6-AN + Mito C produces a striking increase in regression rates of advanced, spontaneous, autochthonous solid tumors.

B. 6-AN, MMPR, and PALA

The purine antagonist, 6-methylmercaptopurine riboside (MMPR), also can by hypothesized to interfere with the formulation of poly(ADP-ribose). NAD, the substrate for poly(ADP-ribose) polymerase, is synthesized in the cell from nicotinamide mononucleotide (NMN) and ATP by an enzyme (NMN adenyltransferase) which catalyzes adenyl transfer to NMN. This enzyme can be competitively inhibited by a 6-MP metabolite, thioinosine triphosphate (thio-ITP), the result being inhibition of the biosynthesis of NAD. It is of further interest that thio-ITP is an analog of ATP, that it can be methylated *in vivo* (51), and that methylthio-IMP is also the active form of MMPR (27). It appears, therefore, not unreasonable to hypothesize that MMPR may act on tumors by facilitating the inhibition of a DNA repair mechanism involving poly(ADP-ribose), particularly in combination with a strong poly(ADP-ribose) polymerase inhibitor such as 6-AN.

There are certain factors favoring a differential effect by 6-AN on tumors as opposed to normal tissue. Metabolic antagonists, such as 6-AN, do not antagonize all systems dependent on the competing metabolite (i.e., nicotinamide) to the same degree (46,107); thus, an antagonist could be more selective in inhibiting the same enzyme in the tumor tissue than in normal tissue. Moreover, the concentration of the particular NAD-containing enzyme in tumor and normal tissues relative to that of the appropriate NAD antagonist is relevant to selectivity (46,107): "it should be possible to inhibit an enzyme present in cancer tissue in small amounts, while producing only inactivation of the enzyme in tissues containing larger amounts" (1). It therefore is pertinent that the concentration of pyridine dinucleotide in neoplastic tissue is low as compared to normal tissue (57,81,107,127). Also, the activity of the (NMN) adenyltransferase enzyme which is inhibited by thio-ITP (6) is considerably lower in a number of tumors than in comparable normal tissue (19). It seems reasonable that the low levels of pyridine nucleotides in tumors would make their neoplastic cells vulnerable to appropriate antagonist (i.e., 6-AN and thio-ITP via MMPR).

MMPR in high dosage can decrease pyrimidine ribonucleotide concentration (63,176). Since low-dose PALA can selectively inhibit pyrimidine synthesis in certain tumors (116), it seems reasonable to attempt to reinforce a high-dosage MMPR block on pyrimidine synthesis by adding PALA to MMPR.

On the basis of the aforementioned overall rationale, the triple combination of 6-AN + MMPR + PALA was evaluated in mice bearing advanced solid tumors, and striking tumor regression rates were demonstrated against large, well-established murine mammary carcinomas.

Table X records pooled data from three experiments with CD8F1 mice bearing CD8F1 mammary tumor first-generation transplants. The tumors were advanced, averaging 150 mg when treatment was initiated. The important therapeutic end point is in the percentage of PR of the treated tumors. The MTD of neither MMPR alone (group 2), 6-AN alone (group 3), nor the double combination of PALA + 6-AN (group 4) produced any partial regressions (although tumor growth was inhibited in each group compared to the saline-treated controls, group 1). The double combination of PALA and MMRP (group 5) and that of 6-AN and MMPR (group 6) produced relatively minor objective response rates, 7% and 17% PR rates, respectively. In marked contrast, the triple combination of 6-AN + MMPR + PALA effected an impressive 61% PR rate, without mortality and with only moderate body weight loss.

It is of interest that none of the single agents and none of the double combinations show a tumor regression rate that would be considered "active" in the clinic. By clinical criteria of activity (i.e., the need to demonstrate at least a 20% PR rate to be considered an "active" agent), these single agents would be dropped (tumor growth inhibition, even if complete, is not a clinical criterion of activity) and would not be put into

DANIEL S. MARTIN

TABLE X

**Combination Therapy with N-(Phosphonacetyl)-L-aspartate (PALA)
6-Aminonicotinamide (6-AN), and 6-Methylmercaptopurine Riboside (MMPR)[a]**

Group	Treatment[b]	% of PR[c]	Body weight change (%)	Dead/total
1	Saline	0/29	+17	4/29
2	$MMPR_{175}$	0/30	−3	0/30
3	$6\text{-}AN_{25}$	0/30	−25	5/30
4	$PALA_{100} \xrightarrow{18\ hr} 6\text{-}AN_{10}$	0/30	−3	10/30
5	$PALA_{100} \xrightarrow{18\ hr} MMPR_{150}$	2/28 (7%)	−14	2/28
6	$6\text{-}AN_{10} + MMPR_{150}$	5/29 (17%)	−11	0/29
7	$PALA_{100} \xrightarrow{18\ hr} 6\text{-}AN_{10} + MMPR_{150}$	17/28 (61%)	−22	0/28

For groups 6 and 7: $P = .01$

[a] Pooled data from three experiments (1164, 1170, 1171) in first-generation CD8F1 advanced breast tumors averaging 150 mg when therapy was initiated.

[b] Three courses of the indicated treatment were administered with a 1-week interval between courses. Subscripts = mg/kg. Observations 5 days after third course of treatment.

[c] PR = partial tumor regression ($\geq$50% of initial tumor size).

combination chemotherapy trial. Furthermore, in the unlikely event that two of the apparently "negative" compounds were put into a double combination trial, the minor objective response rates that resulted would likely preclude evaluation of the triple combination, at which the dramatic 61% PR rate broke through.

The biochemical mechanism postulated for the antitumor interactions between these three agents are in process of evaluation. It should be noted that the biochemical rationale for combining MMPR and 6-AN in order to interfere with poly(ADP-ribose) formation and the biochemical reason for adding PALA to this double combination are still only hypotheses. However, the biological result—striking regression rates of advanced, large murine solid carcinomas—is an impressive antitumor effect upon which to build further. Delayed "rescue" of host toxicity with nicotinamide (for 6-AN), guanosine (for MMPR), and pyrimidines (for PALA), may provide an opportunity for futher improving the therapeutic index of this triple combination. The addition of FUra to this combination may provide additional therapeutic gain, since both low-dose PALA and MMPR have been shown to be useful modulators of FUra.

XI. Inhibition of Spontaneous, Autochthonous Tumor Growth by Hydrocortisone and Therapeutic Implications

Many malignant tumors in animals and humans contain and secrete plasminogen activator (PA), the production of which is associated with tumor growth, cellular invasion, and metastases. Moreover, a correlation has been demonstrated between repression of PA production by hydrocortisone in the CD8F1 mammary tumor and inhibition of growth of this spontaneous, autochthonous tumor *in vivo* (124) (See Figure 6).

Although these antitumor effects are growth-inhibitory rather than tumor-regressing, these therapeutic findings nevertheless may be significant in general treatment, since glucocorticoid receptors and/or glucocorticoid sensitivity has been demonstrated in such a wide spectrum of human

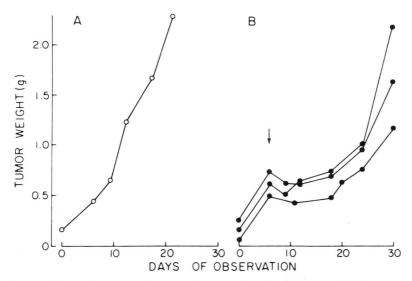

Fig. 6. Effect of hydrocortisone on the growth rate of primary CD8F1 mammary carcinomas. Twenty-five mice with palpable, progressively growing primary tumors were used for this experiment; 20 mice received implants of steroid pellets specified to release 0.5 mg hydrocortisone daily (for approximately 20 days), and 5 mice served as controls. (A) Growth rate of a representative tumor from a control mouse. (B) Three representative tumors from hydrocortisone-treated mice; (arrow) time of implantation of pellets. Growth inhibition was still evident at 18 days after pellet implantation; by 24 days, pellet hormone delivery had waned, and growth rates had returned to pretreatment levels.

tumors, including breast tumors (3), brain tumors (54), colon tumors (151), renal tumors (17), lung tumors (84), connective tissue tumors (170), and hepatomas (47). To elaborate further, it is recognized that between intermittent cycles of chemotherapy (the intermittency of which is necessary to allow for periods of recovery of host bone marrow and intestinal epithelium), residual tumor cells continue to proliferate; thus, at the next cycle of chemotherapy the tumor burden is larger and therefore more difficult to treat than it was at the end of the previous cycle. In addition, there is the potential problem that spontaneous mutation to drug resistance may occur, due to the opportunity for uninhibited tumor cells to proliferate during the untreated "off-period" from chemotherapy. Thus, treatment during the "off-period" (e.g., 2 weeks) between courses of chemotherapy with a tumor-inhibitory agent such as hydrocortisone may circumvent these problems and therefore may have considerable impact on the therapeutic outcome. At effective doses (124) hydrocortisone does not produce intestinal toxicity and does not adversely affect granulocytes. The immunosuppressive action of hydrocortisone is recognized as a potential problem in this strategy, but the treatment period would be short and the dose required may be low enough (124) so that meaningful immunosuppression does not occur.

XII. Summary and Conclusion: Clinical Potential for Biochemical Modulation in the Combination Chemotherapy of Cancer

In contrast to preclinical findings, in which many examples of successful biochemical modulation of anticancer drug activity have been reported in tumor models, clinical trials have not yet demonstrated a clear-cut improvement in the therapeutic indices of effector agents by modulating agents. This review has identified a number of probable reasons for these divergent results and suggested changes in the design of clinical trials involving biochemical modulation that should permit therapeutic success in the clinic.

The following quantitative differences between laboratory and clinical studies appear pertinent to attaining such success, and examples have been presented and discussed. Since *in vitro* drug studies cannot yield information concerning therapeutic indices, and since selectivity is as important in biochemical modulation as it is in traditional combination chemotherapy, *in vitro* preclinical findings of biochemical modulation studies must not be extrapolated directly to the clinic. Further, the appropriate sequence of administration of two drugs, the magnitude of the interval between their administration, and their dosage ratio all require careful incorporation into the design of the clinical biochemical modulation protocol. In contrast to the empirically based rules of combination chemotherapy, a modulating agent need not have therapeutic activity by itself in order to possess the ability to enhance the antitumor action of an effector agent. Indeed, employing a therapeutically ineffective modulating agent in high dosage to seek an antitumor effect may be counterproductive to a useful enhancement of the antitumor effect of the combination.

The only treatment proven capable of curing some *advanced* human cancers is combination chemotherapy. To pursue the lead of this important clinically demonstrated therapeutic advance, better single agents certainly should be sought, but it must be recognized that the finding of a "magic bullet" curative agent is not an expectation compatible with our current knowledge of the chemotherapeutic heterogeneity of neoplastic cell populations. The existence of chemotherapeutic heterogeneity implies that even for a very good new agent, it will be necessary to develop new drug combinations, with all of the problems of adding agents to seek cure without provoking undue toxicity. Although notable progress has been made with empirical combination chemotherapy, a more rational scientific approach, biochemical modulation, based on cellular biochemical pharmacology, should expedite therapeutic progress.

It must be recognized that in addition to qualitative heterogeneity, there is also quantitative heterogeneity; namely, a subset of cancer cells can possess a gradient of responsiveness to a single agent. Biochemical modulation can increase the antitumor effectiveness of individual agents in a drug combination to overcome the quantitative differences in cancer cells that are qualitatively similar in their sensitivity to an individual agent. Under *in vivo* conditions, the low chemotherapeutic indices of most antitumor drugs can make the eradication of even slightly resistant cells impossible at doses which are tolerated *in vivo*. Moreover, simply adding more agents in combination, each with single agent clinical antitumor activity directed at qualitatively different subsets of cancer cells, may worsen the quantitative aspects of drug resistance, because unless scientifically based on cellular biochemical pharmacology, adding additional agents can cause unacceptable host toxicity that necessitates reducing the dose of other drugs in the combination.

Biochemical modulation may be appropriately directed at a number of steps in the metabolism of a single effector antitumor agent. For example, each of the following—PALA, high-dose MTX-LV (LV, leucovorin), and UR—is an effective modulator for FUra, and the appropriate dose and sequenced combination of all of these agents is better tolerated while being more effective than the empirical combination of several effector agents. Nevertheless, although these are rationally based, more effective drug combinations, the preclinical results still fall short of cure and have evidenced a degree of toxicity which precludes the *simultaneous* addition of another rationally devised "modulatory" combination. However, there are potential strategies to overcome this problem. Alternating cycles of non-cross-resistant, optimally modulated chemotherapy regimens with "off-period" treatment by a relatively nontoxic agent that is inhibitory to tumor regrowth (e.g., glucocorticoids) awaits evaluation. Our successful "rescue" programs in preclinical studies have essentially only been evaluated with intermittent bolus administration of the rescue agents during the usual laboratory work day; continuous intraperitoneal administration day *and night* should permit further selective reduction in toxicity to a level at which the *simultaneous* administration of proven additional effective drug combinations would be possible. Programs to control host toxicity by agent-induced (e.g., poly I : poly C) differential modulation of proliferation in normal versus tumor tissue are promising and have only just begun evaluation.

Biochemical modulation can demonstrably enhance preclinical chemotherapeutic responses and thus has the potential to expedite the attainment of additional chemotherapeutic cure rates in the clinic. This potential can be realized if preclinical therapeutic studies, preclinical and clinical cellular biochemical pharmacology findings, and applied clinical research are carried out in a more coordinated way. Experience indicates that the initial design of the clinical protocol is all-important. Failure to obtain a positive result in the initial clinical trial usually leads to a loss of clinical interest sufficient to preclude additional and better-designed clinical investigations of a particular drug combination. It appears likely that a more coordinated "translation" from the laboratory of the *initial* design of drug sequence, schedule, timing, and dosage ratios of drugs in combination, scientifically based on cellular biochemical pharmacology, should lead to positive therapeutic results in clinical trials employing biochemical modulation.

References

1. Ackerman, W. W., and Potter, V. R. (1949). Enzyme inhibition in relation to chemotherapy. *Proc. Soc. Biol. Med.* **72**, 1–9.
2. Ahmed, N. K., Haggit, R. C., and Welch, A. D. (1982). Enzymes of salvage and *de novo* pathways of synthesis of pyrimidine nucleotides in human colorectal adenocarcinomas. *Biochem. Pharmacol.* **31**, 2485-2488.
3. Allegra, J. C., Lippman, M. E., Thompson, E. B., Simon, R., Barlock, A., Green, C.,

Huff, K. K., Do, H. M. T., and Aiken, S. C. (1979). Distribution, frequency, and quantitative analysis of estrogren, progesterone, and corticosteroid receptors on human breast cancer. *Cancer Res.* **39,** 1447-1454.

4. Aoki, T., Sebolt, J., and Weber, G. (1982). *In vivo* inactivation of carbamoylphosphate synthetase II in rat hepatoma by Acivicin. *Biochem. Pharmacol.* **31,** 927–932.

5. Ardalan, B., Glazer, R., Kensler, T., Jayarum, H., Cooney, D., and MacDonald, J. (1980). Biochemical mechanism for the synergism of 5-fluorouracil (5-FU) and phosphonacetyl-L-aspartate (PALA) in human mammary carcinoma cells. *Proc. Am. Assoc. Cancer Res.* **21,** 8.

6. Atkinson, M. R., Jackson, J. F., Morton, R. K., and Murray, A. W. (1962). Nicotinamide 6-metcaptopurine dinucleotide and related compounds: Potential sources of 6-mercaptopurine nucleotide in chemotherapy. *Nature (London)* **196,** 35–36.

7. Baxter, A., Currie, L. M., and Durham, J. P. (1978). *In vitro* metabolism of cytosine arabinoside in normal and tumor breast tissues. *Br. J. Cancer* **38**(1), 194.

8. Bedikian, A. Y., Stroehlein, J. R., Karlin, D. A., Bennets, R. W., Bodey, G. P., and Kaldivieso, M. (1981). Chemotherapy for colorectal cancer with a combination of PALA and 5-FU. *Cancer Treat. Rep.* **65,** 747–753.

9. Belousova, A. K., and Gerasimona, G. K. (1980). Search for the biochemical parameters of tumor cell sensitivity and resistance to antimetabolites. *Antibiot. Chemother. (Basel)* **28,** 48–52.

10. Belt, R. J., Haas, C. D., Kennedy, J., and Taylor, S. (1980). Studies of hydroxyurea administered by continuous infusion. Toxicity, pharmacokinetics, and cell synchronization. *Cancer (Philadelphia)* **46,** 455–462.

11. Ben-Ishay, Z., and Farber, E. (1975). Protective effects of an inhibitor of protein synthesis, cyclohexamide, on bone marrow damage induced by cytosine arabinoside or nitrogen mustard. *Lab. Invest.* **33,** 478–490.

12. Benz, C., and Cadman, E. (1981). Modulation of 5-fluorouracil metabolism and cytotoxicity by antimetabolite pretreatment in human colorectal adenocarcinoma HCT-8. *Cancer Res.* **41,** 994–999.

13. Benz, C., Tillis, T., Tattelman, E., and Cadman, E. (1982). Optimal scheduling of methotrexate and 5-fluorouracil in human breast cancer. *Cancer Res.* **42,** 2081–2086.

14. Berger, N. A., Catino, D. M., and Vietti, T. J. (1982). Synergistic antileukemic effect of 6-aminonicotinamide and 1,3-bis (2-chloroethyl)-l-nitrosourea on L1210 cells *in vitro* and *in vivo*. *Cancer Res.* **42,** 4382–4386.

15. Bertino, J., Sawicki, W. L., Lindquist, C. A., and Gupta, V. S. (1977). Schedule-dependent antitumor effects of methotrexate and 5-fluorouracil. *Cancer Res.* **37,** 327–328.

16. Blumenreich, M. S., Woodcock, T. M., Allegra, M., Richman, S. P., Kubota, T. T., and Allegra, J. C. (1982). Sequential therapy with methotrexate (MTX) and 5-fluorouracil (5-FU) for adenocarcinoma of the colon. *Proc. Am. Soc. Clin. Oncol.* **1,** 102.

17. Bojar, H., Maar, K., and Stalb, W. (1979). The endocrine background of human renal cell carcinoma IV glucocorticoid receptors as possible mediators of progestogen action. *Urol. Int.* **34,** 330-338.

18. Brady, M. O., Kohn, K. W., Sharkey, N. A., and Ewig, R. A. (1977). Differential cytotoxicity between transformed and normal human cells with combinations of aminonucleoside and hydroxyurea. *Cancer Res.* **37,** 2126–2131.

19. Branster, M. V. and Morton, R. K. (1956). Comparative rates of synthesis of diphosphopyridine nucleotide by normal and tumor tissue from mouse mammary gland, studies with isolated nuclei. *Biochem. J.* **63,** 640.

20. Breitman, J. R., and Keene, B. R. (1979). Synergistic cytotoxicity to melanoma and leukemias *in vitro* with thymidine (NSC-21548) and arabinofuranosylcytosine (NSC-63878). *Proc. Am. Assoc. Cancer Res.* **20,** 89.

21. Browman, G. P. (1984). Clinical application of the concept of methotrexate plus 5-FU sequence-dependent "synergy." How good is the evidence? *Cancer Treat. Rep.* **68,** 465–469.

22. Browman, G. P., Young, J. E. M., Archibald, S. C. Kiehl, K., Russell, R., and Levine, M. N. (1984). Prospective randomized trial of one hour sequential versus simultaneous methotrexate (MTX) + 5-Fluorouracil (5-FU) in squamous carcinoma of head and neck (SCHN). *Proc. Am. Soc. Clin. Oncol.* **2,** 158.

23. Burnet, R., Smith, F. P., Heerni, B., Lagarde, C., and Schein, P. (1981). Sequential methotrexate/5-fluorouracil in advanced measurable colorectal cancer: Lack of appreciable therapeutic synergism. *Proc. Am. Assoc. Cancer Res. ASCO* **22,** 370.

24. Cadman, E., Benz, C., Heimer, R., and O'Shaughnessy, J. (1981). Effects of *de novo* purine synthesis inhibitors on 5-fluorouracil metabolism and cytotoxicity. *Biochem. Pharmacol.* **30,** 2469–2472.

25. Cadman, E., Davis, L., and Heimer, R. (1979). Enhanced 5-fluorouracil nucleotide formation after methotrexate administration: explanation for drug synergism. *Science* **205,** 1135–1137.

26. Cadman, E., Glick, J., Cross, J., Horton, J., and Taylor, S. (1984). Sequential methotrexate and 5-FU in CMFP (cyclophosphamide, methotrexate, 5-FU, and prednisone) therapy for breast cancer. *Cancer Treat. Rep.* **68,** 877–879.

27. Caldwell, I. C., Henderson, J. F., and Paterson, A. R. P. (1966). The enzymatic formation of 6-(methylmercapto)purine ribonucleoside 5'-phosphate. *Can. J. Biochem.* **44,** 229.

28. Cantrell, J. E., Jr., Brunet, R., Lagarde, C., Schein, P. S., and Smith, F. P. (1982). Phase II study of sequential methotrexate-5-FU therapy in advanced measurable colorectal cancer. *Cancer Treat. Rep.* **66,** 1563–1565.

29. Capizzi, R. L. (1974). Biochemical interactions between asparaginase (A'ase) and methotrexate (MTX) in leukemia cells. *Proc. Am. Assoc. Cancer Res.* **15,** 77.

30. Casper, E. S., Vale, K., Williams, L. J., Martin, D. S., and Young, C. W. (1983). Phase I and clinical pharmacology evaluation of biochemical modulation of 5-fluorouracil with N-(phosphonacetyl)-L-aspartic acid (PALA). *Cancer Res.* **43,** 2324–2329.

31. Chabner, B. (1982). Cytosine arabinoside. *In* "Pharmacology of Anticancer Agents" (B. Chabner, ed.), pp. 387–396. Saunders, Philadelphia, Pennsylvania.

32. Chabner, B. A., Fine, R. L., Allegra, C. J., Yeh, G. W., and Curt, G. A. (1984). Cancer chemotherapy progress and expectations: *Cancer (Philadelphia)* **54,** 2529–2608.

33. Chu, M. Y. W., Naguib, R. N. M., Iltzsch, M. H., el Kouni, M. H., Chu, S. H., Cha, S., and Calabresi, P. (1984). Potentiation of 5-fluoro-2'-deoxyuridine antineoplastic activity by the uridine phosphorylase inhibitors benzylacyclouridine and benzyloxybenzylacyclouridine. *Cancer Res.* **44,** 1852–1856.

34. Coates, A. S., Tattersall, M. H. N., Swanson, C., Hedley, D., Fox, R. M., and Raghaven, D. (1984). Combination therapy with methotrexate and 5-fluorouracil: A prospective randomized clinical trial of order of administration. *J. Clin. Oncol.* **2,** 756–761.

35. Cohen, A., and Ullman, B. (1985). Analysis of the drug synergism between thymidine and arabinosyl cytosine using mouse S49 T lymphoma mutants. *Cancer Chemother. Pharmacol.* **14,** 70–73.

36. Collins, K. D., and Stark, G. R. (1971). Aspartate transcarbamylase, interaction with the transition state analogue N-(phosphonacetyl)-L-aspartate. *J. Biol. Chem.* **246**, 6599–6605.
37. Comis, R. L., and Carter, S. K. (1974). A review of chemotherapy in gastric cancer. *Cancer (Philadelphia)* **34**, 1576–1586.
38. Craddock, J. National Cancer Institute, National Institutes of Health (Personal communication: unpublished studies).
39. Crooke, S. T., and Bradner, W. T. (1976). Mitomycin C: A review. *Cancer Treat. Rev.* **3**, 121–139.
40. Danhauser, L. L., and Rustum, Y. M. (1985). Potential for selective enhancement of the *in vivo* metabolism of 1-B-D-arabinofuranosylcytosine in rats by thymidine pretreatment. *Cancer Res.* **45**, 2002–2007.
41. Darnowski, J. W., and Handschumacher, R. E. (1984). Pharmacokinetics of benzyluridine (BAU) and its utility as a potential rescuing agent from 5-fluorouracil (FUra) induced toxicity. *Proc. Am. Assoc. Cancer Res.* **25**, 358.
42. Darnowski, J. W., and Handschumacher, R. E. (1985). Tissue specific enhancement of uridine utilization and 5-fluorouracil therapy by benzylacyclouridine. *Cancer Res.* **45**, 5364–5368.
43. DeVita, V. T., and Schein, P. S. (1973). The use of drugs in combination for the treatment of cancer. *N. Engl. J. Med.* **288**, 998–1006.
44. Dietrich, L. S. (1975). Cytotoxic analogs of pyridine nucleotide coenzymes. *In* "Antineoplastic and Immunosuppressive Agents" pp. 539–542. (A. C. Sartorelli and D. G. Johns, eds.), Springer-Verlag, Berlin and New York.
45. Dietrich, L. S., Friedland, I. M., and Kaplan, L. (1958). Pyridine nucleotide metabolism: Mechanism of action of the niacin antagonist, 6-aminonicotinamide. *J. Biol. Chem.* **233**, 964–968.
46. Dietrich, L. S., Kaplan, L. A., Friedland, I. M., and Martin, D. S. (1958). Quantitative differences between tumor and host tissue. VI. 6-aminonicotinamide antagonism of DPN-dependent enzymatic systems. *Cancer Res.* **18**, 1272–1280.
47. Disurbo, D. M., Eisen, H. J., and Liwack, G. (1980). Characterization of the glucocorticoid receptors from a human primary liver cancer cell line. *Proc. Am. Assoc. Cancer Res.* **21**, 6.
48. Dolnick, B. J., and Pink, J. J. (1985). Effects of 5-fluorouracil on dihydrofolate reductase and dihyrofolate reductase in RNA from methotrexate-resistant K B cells. *J. Biol. Chem.* **260**, 3006–3014.
49. Drephin, R., McAloon, E., and Lyman, G. (1983). Sequential methotrexate (MTX) and 5-fluorouracil in advanced measurable colorectal cancer. *Proc. Am. Soc. Clin. Oncol.* **2**, 118.
50. Durkacz, B. W., Omidiji, O., Gray, D. A., and Shall, S. (1980). (ADP-ribose) participates in DNA excision repair. *Nature (London)* **283**, 593–596.
51. Elion, G. B. (1975). Interaction of anticancer drugs with enzymes. *In* "Pharmacological Basis of Cancer Chemotherapy" pp. 547–564. Williams & Wilkins, Baltimore, Maryland.
52. Erlichman, C., Donhower, R. C., Speyer, J. L., Klecker, R., and Chabner, B. (1982). Phase I-II trial of N-phosphonacetyl-L-aspartic acid given by intravenous infusion and 5-fluorouracil given by bolus injection. *JNCI, J. Natl. Cancer Inst.* **68**, 227–231.
53. Evans, R. M., Laskin, J. D., and Hakela, M. T. (1980). Assessment of growth limiting events caused by 5-fluorouracil in mouse cells and in human cells. *Cancer Res.* **40**, 4113–4122.

54. Freshney, R. I., Sherry, A., Hassanzadah, M., Freshney, M., Crilly, P., and Morgan, D. (1980). Control of cell proliferation in human glioma by glucocortocoids. *Br. J. Cancer* **41**, 857–866.

55. Gasser, T., Moyer, J. D., and Handschumacher, R. E. (1981). Novel single pass exchange of circulating uridine in rat liver. *Science* **213**, 777–778.

56. Glazer, R. I., and Lloyd, L. S. (1982). Association of cell lethality with incorporation of 5-fluorouracil and 5-fluorouridine into nuclear RNA in human colon carcinoma cells in culture. *Mol. Pharmacol.* **21**, 468–473.

57. Glock, G. E., and McLean, P. (1957). Levels of oxidized and reduced diphosphopyridine nucleotide and triphosphopyridine nucleotide in tumors. *Biochem. J.* **65**, 413–416.

58. Goldie, J. H., Goldman, A. J., and Gudauskas, G. A. (1982). Rationale for the use of alternating non-cross resistant chemotherapy. *Cancer Treat. Rep.* **66**, 439–449.

59. Goldin, A., Greenspan, E. M., and Schoenback, E. B. (1952). Studies on the mechanism of action of chemotherapeutic agents in cancer. VI. Synergistic (additive) action of drugs on a transplantable leukemia in mice. *Cancer (Philadelphia)* **5**, 153–160.

60. Goldin, A., Venditti, J. MacDonald, J., Muggia, F., Henney, J., and DeVita, V. T., Jr. (1981). Current results of the screening program at the Division of Cancer Treatment, National Cancer Institute. *Eur. J. Cancer Clin. Oncol.* **17**(3), 129–142.

61. Grant, S., Lehman, C., and Cadman, E. (1980). Enhancement of 1-B-D-arabinofuranosylcytosine accumulation within L1210 cells and increased cytotoxicity following thymidine exposure. *Cancer Res.* **40**, 1525–1531.

62. Greenberg, P. L., and Mosny, S. A. (1977). Cytotoxic effects of interferon *in vitro* on granulocytic progenitor cells. *Cancer Res.* **37**, 1794–1799.

63. Grindey, G. B., Lowe, J. K., Divekar, A. Y., and Hakala, M. T. (1976). Potentiation by guanine nucleosides of the growth inhibitory effects of adenosine analogs on L1210 and Sarcoma 180 cells in culture. *Cancer Res.* **36**, 379–383.

64. Guigon, M., Wdzieczak-Bakala, J., Mary, J. Y., and Lenfant, M. (1984). A convenient source of CFU-s inhibitors: the fetal calf liver. *Cell Tissue Kinet.* **7**, 49–55.

65. Hamilton, T. C., Winker, M. A., Louie, K. G., Batist, G., Fine, R. L., Behrens, B. C., Tsuruo, T., Grotzinger, K. R., McKoy, W. M., Young, R. C., and Ozols, R. E. (1985). Augmentation of adriamycin, melphalan, and cisplatin cytotoxicity by buthionine sulfoximine depletion of glutathionine in drug-resistant human overian cancer cell lines. *Proc. Am. Assoc. Cancer Res.* **26**, 345.

66. Harris, A. W., Reynolds, E. C., and Finch, L. R. (1979). Effect of thymidine on the sensitivity of cultured mouse tumor cells to 1-B-D-arabinofuranosylcytosine. *Cancer Res.* **39**, 538–541.

67. Hayaishi, O., and Ueda, K. (1982). Poly- and mono (ADP ribosyl)ation reactions: Their significance in molecular biology. *In:* ADP-Ribosylation Reactions Biology and Medicine'' pp. 3–16. (O. Hayaishi and K. Ueda, eds.), Academic Press, New York.

68. Heidelberger, C., Danenberg, P. V., and Moran, R. G. (1983). Fluorinated pyrimidines and their nucleosides. *Adv. Enzymol.* **54**, 58–119.

69. Henderson, E. H., and Samaha, R. J. (1969). Evidence that drugs in multiple combinations have materially advanced the treatment of human malignancies. *Cancer Res.* **29**, 2272–2280.

70. Herrmann, R., Kunz, W., Osswald, H., Ritter, M., and Port, R. (1985). The effect of methotrexate pretreatment on 5-fluorouracil kinetics in sarcoma 180 *in vivo*. *Eur. J. Cancer Clin. Oncol.* **21**, 753–758.

71. Herrmann, R., Manegold, C., Rithinghausen, R., Fritze, D., and Schettler, G. (1982). Sequential methotrexate (MTX) and 5-fluorouracil (FU) is effective in extensively pretreated breast cancer. *Proc. Am. Soc. Clin. Oncol.* **1**, 86.

72. Herrmann, R., Spehn, J., Beyer, J. H., von Franque, V., Schmieder, A., Holzman, K., and Abel, V. (1984). Sequential methotrexate and 5-fluorouracil: Improved response rate in metastatic colon cancer. *J. Clin. Oncol.* **2,** 591–594.

73. Hewlett, J. S. (1979). Combination 6-mercaptopurine and 6-methylmercaptopurine riboside in the treatment of adult acute leukemia: A Southwest Oncology Group Study. *Cancer Treat. Rep.* **63,** 156–157.

74. Houghton, J. A., Houghton, P. J., and Wooten, R. S. (1979). Mechanism of induction of gastrointestinal toxicity in the mouse by 5-fluorouracil, 5-fluorouridine, and 5-fluoro-2'-deoxyuridine. *Cancer Res.* **39,** 2406–2413.

75. Hromas, R., Barlogic, B., Swartzendruber, D., and Drewinko, B. (1983). Selective protection by anguidine of normal versus transformed cells against 1-B-D-arabino-furanosylcytosine and adriamycin. *Cancer Res.* **43,** 1135–1137.

76. Ignoffo, R. J., Friedman, M. A., Gribble, M., Hannigan, J., Reynolds, R., Yu, K. P., Schiff, S., and Congdon, J. E. (1984). Phase II study of sequential methotrexate and 5-FU plus mitomycin and leucovorin in patients with disseminated large bowel cancer. A Northern California Oncology Group study. *Cancer Treat. Rep.* **68,** 983–988.

77. Iigo, M., Chapekar, M. S., and Glazer, R. I. (1985). Synergistic antitumor effect of fluoropyrimidine and polyinosinic-polycytidylic acid against L1210 leukemia. *Cancer Res.* **45,** 4039–4042.

78. Ives, D. H., and Durham, I. P. (1970). Deoxycytidine kinase. III. Kinetic and allosteric regulation of the calf thymus enzyme. *J. Biol. Chem.* **245,** 2285–2294.

79. Jackson, R. C. (1978). The regulation of thymidylate biosynthesis in Novikoff hepatoma cells and the effects of amethopterin, 5-fluorodeoxyuridine, and 3-deazauridine. *J. Biol. Chem.* **253,** 7440–7446.

80. Jayaram, H. N., Cooney, D. A., Ryan, J. A., Neil, G., Dion, R. L., and Bono, V. H. (1975). L-(αS, 5S)-α-amino-3-chloro-4, 5-dihydro-5-isoxazoleacetic acid (NSC-163501). A new amino acid antibiotic with the properties of an antagonist of L-glutamine. *Cancer Treat. Rep.* **59,** 481–491.

81. Jediken, L. A. and Weinhouse, S. (1955). Metabolism of neoplastic tissue. VI. Assay of oxidized and reduced diphosphopyridine nucleotide in normal and neoplastic tissues. *J. Biol. Chem.* **213,** 271–280.

82. Johnson, R. K., Clement, J. J., and Howard, W. S. (1980). Treatment of murine tumors with 5-fluorouracil in combination with *de novo* pyrimidine synthesis inhibitors PALA or pyrazofurin. *Proc. Am. Assoc. Cancer Res.* **21,** 292.

83. Johnson, W. J., and McColl, J. D. (1955). 6-Aminonitotinamide—A potent nicotinamide antagonist. *Science,* **122,** 834.

84. Jones, K. L., Anderson, N. S., and Addiron, J. (1978). Glucocorticoid-induced growth inhibition of cells from human lung alveolar cell carcinoma. *Cancer Res.* **38,** 1688–1693.

85. Karle, J. M., Anderson, L. W., Dietrick, D. D., and Cysk, R. L. (1981). Effect of inhibitors of the *de novo* pyrimidine biosynthetic pathway on serum uridine levels in mice. *Cancer Res.* **41,** 4952–4955.

86. Kemeny, N., Ahmed, T., Michaelson, R., Harper, H., and Yip, L. (1984). Activity of sequential low-dose Methotrexate and Fluorouracil in advanced colorectal carcinoma: attempt at correlation with tissue and blood levels of phosphoribosylpyrophosphate. *J. Clin. Oncol.* **2,** 311–315.

87. Kensler, T. W., Jayaram, H. N., and Cooney, D. A. (1982). Effects of Acivicin and PALA, singly and in combination, on *de novo* pyrimidine biosynthesis. *Adv. Enzyme Regul.* **20,** 57–73.

88. Kensler, T. W., Mutter, G., Hankerson, J. G., Reck, L. J., Johnson, R. K., Jayaram,

H. N., and Cooney, D. A. (1981). Mechanism of resistance of variants of the Lewis lung carcinoma to N-(phosphonacetyl)-L-aspartic acid. *Cancer Res.* **41**, 894–904.

89. Kinahan, J. J., Kowal, E. P., and Grindey, G. B. (1981). Biochemical and antitumor effects of the combination of thymidine and 1-B-D-arabinosylcytosine against leukemia L1210. *Cancer Res.* **41**, 445–451.

90. King, M. E., Pfeifle, C. E., and Howell, S. B. (1984). Intraperitoneal cytosine arabinoside therapy in ovarian carcinoma. *J. Clin. Oncol.* **2**, 662–669.

91. Klubes, P., and Cerna, I. (1983). Use of uridine rescue to enhance the antitumor selectivity of 5-fluorouracil. *Cancer Res.* **43**, 3182–3186.

92. Klubes, P., Cerna, I., and Meldon, M. (1982). Uridine rescue from the lethal toxicity of 5-fluorouracil in mice. *Cancer Chemother. Pharmacol.* **8**, 17–21.

93. Koeffler, H. D., and Golde, D. W. (1980). Human myeloid leukemia cell lines: A review. *Blood* **56**, 344–350.

94. Kovach, J. S., and Svingen, P. A. (1985). Enhancement of the antiproliferative activity of human interferon by polyamine depletion. *Cancer Treat. Rep.* **69**, 97–103.

95. Kufe, D. (1980). Metabolic enhancement of 5-fluorouracil incorporation into human tumor cell RNA. *Proc. Am. Assoc. Cancer Res.* **21**, 265.

96. Kufe, D. W., and Egan, E. M. (1981). Enhancement of 5-fluorouracil incorporation into human lymphoblast ribonucleic acid. *Biochem. Pharmacol.* **30**, 129–133.

97. Kufe, D. W., Major, P. P., Egan, E. M., and Beardsley, G. P. (1980). Correlation of cytotoxicity with incorporation of ara-C into DNA. *J. Biol. Chem.* **255**, 8997–9000.

98. Law, L. W. (1952). Effects of combinations of anti-leukemic agents on an acute lymphocyte leukemia of mice. *Cancer Res.* **12**, 871–878.

99. Leyva, A., van Groeningen, C. J., Kraal, I., Gall, H., Peters, G., Lankelma, J., and Pinedo, H. M. (1984). Phase I and pharmacokinetic studies of high-dose uridine intended for rescue from 5-fluorouracil toxicity. *Cancer Res.* **44**, 5928–5933.

100. Liang, C. M., Donehower, R., and Chabner, B. (1982). Biochemical interactions between N-(phosphonacetyl)-L-aspartate and 5-fluorouracil. *Mol. Pharmacol.* **21**, 224–230.

101. Loh, E., and Kufe, D. W. (1981). Synergistic effects with inhibitors of *de novo* pyrimidine synthesis, Acivicin and N-(phosphonacetyl)-L-aspartic acid. *Cancer Res.* **41**, 3419–3423.

102. Lunec, J. (1948). Introductory review: Involvement of ADP-ribosylation and cellular recovery from some forms of DNA damage. *Br. J. Cancer* **24**, Suppl. VI, 13–18.

103. Mandel, H. G., Klubes, P., and Fernandes, D. J. (1978). Understanding the actions of carcinostatic drugs to improve chemotherapy: 5-fluorouracil. *Adv. Enzyme Regul.* **16**, 65–77.

104. Markman, M., Cleary, S., Lucas, W. E., and Howell, S. B. (1985). Intraperitoneal chemotherapy with high-dose cisplatin and cytosine arabinoside for refractory ovarian carcinoma and other malignancies principally involving the peritoneal cavity. *J. Clin. Oncol.* **3**, 925–931.

105. Martin, D. S. (1958). Discussion of experimental design in combination chemotherapy. *Ann N.Y. Acad. Sci.* **76**, 926–929.

106. Martin, D. S., Balis, M. E., Fisher, B., Frei, E., Freireich, E. J., Heppner, G. H., Holland, J. F., Houghton, J. A., Houghton, P. J., Johnson, R., Mittelman, A., Rustum, Y., Sawyer, R., Schmid, F., Stolfi, R. L., and Young, C. W. (1986). The role of murine tumor models in cancer treatment research. *Cancer Res.* **46**, 2189–2192.

107. Martin, D. S., Dietrich, L. S., and Shils, M. E. (1957). Quantitative biochemical differences between tumor and host as a basis for cancer chemotherapy. V. Niacin and 6-aminonicotinamide. *Cancer Res.* **17**, 600–604.

108. Martin, D. S., and Gelhorn, A. (1951). Combinations of chemical compounds in experimental cancer chemotherapy. *Cancer Res.* **11,** 35–41.
109. Martin, D. S., Hayworth, P., Davin, E., Stolfi, R., and Fugmann, R. (1976). Methotrexate's activity against human breast cancer correlates with positive activity against a spontaneous murine (CD8F1) mammary tumor, alone and with 5-fluorouracil. *Proc. Am. Assoc. Cancer Res.* **17,** 130.
110. Martin, D. S., Nayak, R., Sawyer, R., Stolfi, R., Young, C., Woodcock, T., and Spiegelman, S. (1979). Enhancement of 5-flurorouracil chemotherapy with emphasis on the use of excess thymidine. *Cancer Bull.* **30,** 219–224.
111. Martin, D. S., and Stolfi, R. L. Unpublished data.
112. Martin, D. S., Stolfi, R. L., Hayworth, P. E., and Fugmann, R. A. (1975). A solid tumor animal model therapeutically predictive for human breast cancer. *Cancer Chemother. Rep.* **5,** 89–109.
113. Martin, D. S., Stolfi, R. L., and Sawyer, R. C. (1984). Commentary of clinical predictivity of transplantable tumor system in the selection of new drugs for solid tumors: Rationale for a three-stage strategy. *Cancer Treat. Rep.* **68,** 1317–1318.
114. Martin, D. S., Stolfi, R. L., Sawyer, R. C., Nayak, R., Spiegelman, S., Schmid, F., Heimer, R., and Cadman, E. (1981). Biochemical modulation of 5-fluorouracil and cytosine arabinoside with emphasis on thymidine, PALA, and 6-methyl-mercaptopurine riboside. *In* "Nucleosides and Cancer Treatment" (M. H. N. Tattersal and R. M. Fox, eds.), pp. 339–392. Academic Press, Australia.
115. Martin, D. S., Stolfi, R. L., Sawyer, R. C., Nayak, R., Spiegelman, S., Young, C., and Woodcock, T. (1980). An overview of thymidine. *Cancer (Philadelphia)* **45,** 1117–1128.
116. Martin, D. S., Stolfi, R. L., Sawyer, R. C., Spiegelman, S., Casper, E. S., and Young, C. (1983). Therapeutic utility of utilizing low doses of N-(phosphonoacetyl)-L-aspartic acid in combination with 5-fluorouracil: A murine study with clinical relevance. *Cancer Res.* **43,** 2317–2321.
117. Martin, D. S., Stolfi, R. L., Sawyer, R. C., Spiegelman, S., and Young, C. W. (1983). Improved therapeutic index with sequential N-phosphonacetyl-L-aspartate plus high dose methotrexate plus high-dose 5-fluorouracil and appropriate rescue. *Cancer Res.* **43,** 4653–4661.
118. Martin, D. S., Stolfi, R. L., Sawyer, R. C., Spiegelman, S., and Young, C. W. (1982). High-dose 5-fluorouracil with delayed uridine "rescue" in mice. *Cancer Res.* **42,** 3964–3970.
119. Martin, D. S., Stolfi, R. L., Sawyer, R. C., and Young, C. W. (1985). The application of biochemical modulation with a therapeutically inactive modulating agent in clinical trials of cancer chemotherapy. *Cancer Treat. Rep.* **69,** 421–423.
120. Martin, D. S., Stolfi, R. L., and Spiegelman, S. (1978). Striking augmentation of the *in vivo* anticancer activity of 5-fluorouracil (5-FU) by combination with pyrimidine nucleosides: An RNA effect. *Proc. Am. Assoc. Cancer Res.* **19,** 221.
121. Maybaum, J., Ullman, B., Mandel, H. G., Day, J. L., and Sadee, W. (1980). Regulation of RNA- and DNA-directed actions of 5-fluoropyrimidines in mouse 5-lymphoma (S-49) cells. *Cancer Res.* **40,** 4209–4215.
122. Meister, A., and Anderson, M. E. (1983). Glutathione. *Annu. Rev. Biochem.* **52,** 711–760.
123. Meshad, M. W., Ervin, T. J., Kufe, D. W., Johnson, R. K., Blum, R. H., and Frei, E. (1981). Phase I trial of combination chemotherapy with PALA and 5-FU. *Cancer Treat. Rep.* **65,** 331–334.
124. Mira-y-Lopez, R., Reich, E., Stolfi, R. L., Martin, D. S. and Ossowski, L. (1985).

Coordinate inhibition of plasminogen activator and tumor growth by hydrocortisone in mouse mammary carcinoma. *Cancer Res.* **45**, 2270–2276.

125. Momparler, R. L., Chu, M. Y., and Fischer, G. A. (1968). Studies on a new mechanism of resistance of L51784 murine leukemia cells to cytosine arabinoside. *Biochim. Biophys. Acta* **161**, 481–493.

126. Moore, C. E., Friedman, J., Valdivieso, M., Plunkett, W., Marti, J. R., Rusa, J., and Loo, T. L. (1982). Aspartate carbamoyltransferase activity drug concentrations and pyrimidine nucleotides in tissue from patients treated with N-(phosphonacetyl)-L-aspartate. *Biochem. Pharmacol.* **31**, 3317–3321.

127. Morton, R. K. (1958). Enzymatic synthesis of coenzyme 1 in relation to chemical control of cell growth. *Nature (London)* **181**, 540–542.

128. Moyer, J. D., Oliver, J. T., and Handshumacher, R. E. (1981). Salvage of circulating pyrimidine nucleosides in the rat. *Cancer Res.* **41**, 3010–3017.

129. Myers, C. E. (1981). The pharmacology of the fluoropyrimidines. *Pharmacol. Rev.* **33**, 1–15.

130. Nduka, N., Skidmore, C. J., and Shall, S. (1980). The enhancement of cytotoxicity of N-methyl-N-nitrosourea and of r radiation by inhibitors of poly (ADP-ribose) polymerase. *Eur. J. Biochem.* **105**, 525–530.

131. Nelson, J. A., and Parks, R. E., Jr. (1972). Biochemical mechanisms for the synergism between 6-thioguanine and 6-(methylmercapto) purine ribonucleoside in sarcoma 180 cells. *Cancer Res.* **32**, 2034–2041.

132. Niedzwicki, J. G., Chu, S. H., el Kouni, M. H., Rowe, E. C., and Cha, S. (1982). 5-Benzylacyclouridine and 5-benzyloxybenzylacyclouridine, potent inhibitors of uridine phosphorylase. *Biochem Pharmacol.* **31**, 1857–1861.

133. Niedzwicki, J. G., el Kouni, M. H., Chu, S. H., and Cha, S. (1981). Pyrimidine acyclonucleosides, inhibitors of uridine phosphorylase. *Biochem. Pharmacol.* **30**, 2097–2101.

134. O'Connell, M. J., Powis, G., Rubin, J., and Moertel, C. G. (1982). Pilot study of PALA and 5-FU in patients with advanced cancer. *Cancer Treat. Rep.* **66**, 77–80.

135. Ofori-Nkansah, N., and Bruchhausen, F. V. (1972). Metabolic alterations in Yoshida ascites tumor cells caused by 6-aminonicotinamide and prevented by nicotinamide. *Naunyn-Schmiedeberg's Arch. Pharmacol.* **272**, 156–168.

136. Ofori-Nkansah, N., and Bruchhausen, F. V. (1972). Some metabolic and morphological alterations in Yoshida ascites tumor cells caused by 6-amino-nicotinamide. *Z. Krebsforsch,* **77**, 64–76.

137. Panasci, D., and Margolese, R. (1982). Sequential methotrexate (MTX) and 5-fluorouracil (FU) in breast and colorectal cancer. Results of increasing the dose of FU. *Proc. Am. Soc. Clin. Oncol.* **1**, 101.

138. Pardee, A. B., and James, L. J. (1975). Selective killing of transformed baby hamster (BHK) cells. *Proc. Natl. Acad. Sci. U.S.A.* **72**, 4994–4998.

139. Paterson, A. R. P., and Wang, M. C. (1970). Mechanism of the growth potentiation arising from the combination of 6-mercaptopurine with 6-(methylmercapto) purine ribonucleoside. *Cancer Res.* **30**, 2379–2387.

140. Peters, G. J. Free University Hospital, Amsterdam, The Netherlands (Personal communication, unpublished studies).

141. Peters, G. J., van Groeingen, C. J., Leyva, A., Laurensse, E., Lankelma, J., and Pinedo, H. M. (1985). Species dependent effect of high-dose uridine (HD-UR) on body temperature. *Proc. Am. Assoc. Cancer Res.* **26**, 370.

142. Plagemann, P. G., Mary, R., and Wohlhueter, R. M. (1978). Transport and metabolism of deoxycytidine and 1-B-D-arabinofuranosylcytosine into cultured Novikoff rat hepa-

toma cells. Relationship to phosphorylation and regulation of triphosphate synthesis. *Cancer Res.* **38**, 978–989.

143. Rahman, Y. E., Patel, K. R., Cernny, E. A., and Maccos, M. (1984). The treatment of intravenously implanted Lewis lung carcinoma with two sustained release forms of 1-B-D-arabinofuranosylcytosine. *Eur. J. Cancer Clin. Oncol.* **20**, 1105–1112.

144. Rauscher, F., III, and Cadman, E. (1983). Biochemical and cytokinetic modulation of L1210 and HL-60 cells by hydroxyurea and effect on 1-B-D-arabinofuranosylcytosine metabolism and cytotoxicity. *Cancer Res.* **43**, 2688–2693.

145. Rupniak, H. T., and Paul, D. (1980). Selective killing of transformed cells by exploitation of their defective cell cycle control by polyamines. *Cancer Res.* **40**, 293–297.

146. Saks, S., Sambol, N., Benz, C., and Cadman, E., (1985). Prolonged sequential infusions of methotrexate (MTX) and 5-fluorouracil (5-FU) in advanced malignancy. *Proc. Am. Soc. Clin. Oncol.* **4**, 43.

147. Sartorelli, A. C., and Creasey, W. A. (1982). Combination chemotherapy. *In* "Cancer Medicine" (J. F. Holland and E. Frei, III, eds.), 2nd ed., pp. 720–730. Lea & Febiger, Philadelphia, Pennsylvania.

148. Saunders, J. P. (1978). Editorial. *Hosp. Pract.*, October.

149. Sawyer, R. C., Stolfi, R. L., Nayak, R., and Martin, D. S. (1981). Mechanism of cytotoxicity in 5-fluorouracil chemotherapy of two murine solid tumors. *In* "Nucleosides and Cancer Treatment" (M. H. N. Tattersall and R. M. Fox, eds.), pp. 309–338. Academic Press, New York.

150. Sawyer, R. C., Stolfi, R. L., Spiegelman, S., and Martin, D. S. (1984). Effect of uridine on the metabolism of 5-fluorouracil in the CD8F1 murine mammary carcinoma system. *Pharm. Res.* **2**, 69–75.

151. Schiffey, L. M., and Beaunschweiger, P. G. (1983). Suppression of colon tumor cell proliferation by dexamethesone (DEX). *Proc. Am. Soc. Clin. Oncol.* **2**, 1.

152. Scholar, E. M., Brown, P. R., and Parks, R. E., Jr. (1972). Synergistic effect of 6-mercaptopurine and 6-methylmercaptopurine ribonucleoside on the levels of adenine nucleotides of sarcoma 180 cells. *Cancer Res.* **32**, 259–269.

153. Shepherd, R., and Harrap, K. R. (1982). Modulation of the toxicity and antitumor activity of alkylating drugs by steroids. *Br. J. Cancer* **45**, 413–420.

154. Sims, J. L., Sikorski, G. W., Catino, D. M., Berger, S. J., and Berger, N. A. (1982). Poly (ADP-ribose) polymerase inhibitors stimulate unscheduled DNA synthesis in normal human lymphocytes. *Biochemistry* **21**, 1813–1821.

155. Skipper, H. E., Chapman, J. B., and Bell, M. (1951). The anti-leukemic action of combinations of certain known antileukemic agents. *Cancer Res.* **11**, 109–112.

156. Skipper, H. E. and Schabel, R. M., Jr. (1982). Quantitative and cytokinetic studies in experimental tumor systems. *In* "Cancer Medicine." (J. F. Holland and E. Frei, III, eds.), 2nd ed., pp. 663–685. Lea & Febiger, Philadelphia, Pennsylvania.

157. Smulson, M. E., Schein, P., Mullins, D. W., Jr., and Sudhaker, S. (1977). A putative role for nicotinamide adenine dinucleotide-promoted nuclear protein modification in the antitumor activity of N-methyl-N-nitrosourea. *Cancer Res.* **37**, 3006–3012.

158. Spiegelman, S., Sawyer, R., Nayak, R., Stolfi, R., and Martin, D. (1980). Improving the antitumor activity of 5-fluorouracil by increasing its incorporation into RNA via metabolic modulation. *Proc. Natl. Acad. Sci. U.S.A.* **77**, 4966–4970.

159. Stolfi, R. L., and Martin, D. S. (1985). Modulation of chemotherapeutic drug activity with polyribonucleotides or with interferon. *J. Biol. Response Modif.* **4**, 634–639.

160. Stolfi, R. L., Martin, D. S., and Fugmann, R. A. (1971). Spontaneous murine mammary carcinoma: Model system for the evaluation of combined modalities of therapy. *Cancer Chemother. Rep.* **55**, 239–251.

161. Stolfi, R. L., Sawyer, R. C., and Martin, D. S. (1985). Combination chemotherapy with Acivicin, N-(phosphonacetyl)-L-aspartic acid (PALA) and Ara-C against CD8F1 breast tumors. *Proc. Am. Assoc. Cancer Res.* **26**, 241.

162. Stolfi, R. L., Martin, D. S., Sawyer, R. C., and Spiegelman, S. (1983). Modulation of 5-fluorouracil-induced toxicity in mice with interferon or with the interferon inducer, polyinosinic-polycytidylic acid. *Cancer Res.* **43**, 561–566.

163. Sunkara, P., Fowler, S., and Nishioka, K. (1982). Selective killing of transformed cells in combination with inhibitors of polyamine biosynthesis and S-phase specific drugs. *Cell Biol. Int. Rep.* **5**, 991–997.

164. Swyrd, E. A., Seaver, S. S., and Stark, G. R. (1974). N-(phosphonacetyl)-L-aspartate a potent transition state analog inhibitor of aspartate transcarbamylase, blocks proliferation of mammalian cells in culture. *J. Biol. Chem.* **249**, 6946–6950.

165. Tattersall, M. H. N., Ganeshaguru, K., and Hoffbrand, A. V. (1974). Mechanisms of resistance of human acute leukemia cells to cytosine arabinoside. *Br. J. Haematol.* **27**, 39–46.

166. Umeda, M., and Heidelberger, C. (1968). Fluorinated pyrimidines. XXX. Comparative studies of fluorinated pyrimidines with various cell lines. *Cancer Res.* **28**, 2529–2538.

167. Valeriote, F. A., and Van Putten, L. (1975). Proliferation-dependent cytotoxicity of anti-cancer agents: A review. *Cancer Res.* **35**, 2619–2630.

168. van Groeningen, C. J., Leyva, A., Kraal, I., Peters, G. J., and Pinedo, H. M. (1986). Clinical and pharmacokinetic studies of prolonged administration of high-dose uridine intended for rescue from 5-fluorouracil toxicity. *Cancer Treat. Rep.* **70**, 745–750.

169. van Groeningen, C. J., Leyva, A., Peters, G. J., Kraal, I., and Pinedo, H. M. (1984). Development of a uridine (UR) administration schedule for rescue from 5-fluorouracil (5-FU) toxicity. *Proc. Am. Assoc. Cancer Res.* **25**, 169.

170. Walker, M. J., Chardhuri, P. K., Beattie, C. W., and DasGupta, T. K. (1980). Steroid receptors in malignant skeletal tumors. *Cancer (Philadelphia)* **45**, 3004–3007.

171. Warrington, R. C., and Fang, W. D. (1985). Histidinol-mediated enhancement of the specificity of two anticancer drugs in mice bearing leukemic bone marrow disease. *J. Natl. Cancer Inst.* **74**, 1071–1077.

172. Washtien, W. L. (1980). Comparison of 5-fluorouracil metabolism in two human gastrointestinal tumor cell lines. *Cancer Res.* **44**, 909–914.

173. Wasserman, T. H., Comis, R. L., Goldsmith, M. *et al.* (1975). Tabular analysis of the clinical chemotherapy of solid tumors. *Cancer Chemother. Rep.* **6**, 399–419.

174. Weinerman, B., Schachter, B., Schipper, H., Bowman, D., and Levitt, M. (1982). Sequential methotrexate and 5-FU in the treatment of colorectal cancer. *Cancer Treat. Rep.* **66**, 1553–1555.

175. Wilkinson, D. S., and Pitot, H. C. (1973). Inhibition of ribosomal acid maturation in Novikoff hepatoma cells by 5-fluorouracil and 5-fluorouridine. *J. Biol. Chem.* **248**, 63–68.

176. Woods, R. A., Henderson, R. M., and Henderson, J. F. (1978). Consequences of inhibition of purine biosynthesis *de novo* by 6-methylmercaptopurine ribonucleoside in cultured lymphoma L5178 Y cells. *Eur. J. Cancer* **14**, 765–770.

Does Modulation of 5-Fluorouracil by Metabolites or Antimetabolites Work in the Clinic?

JOSEPH R. BERTINO AND ENRICO MINI

Departments of Pharmacology and Medicine
Yale University School of Medicine
New Haven, Connecticut

I. Introduction

The concept that the cytotoxicity of an antitumor drug may be manipulated to improve its therapeutic index is an attractive one. In recent years, increased knowledge of the mechanism of drug action has resulted in a concerted effort to maximize or "modulate" the antitumor effects of chemotherapeutic agents in the clinic. These efforts have almost exclusively employed antimetabolites and generally consist of the use of a metabolite or a second drug to enhance the activity of the primary drug.

In this chapter, we review the clinical data of trials attempting to modulate 5-fluorouracil (FUra) antitumor activity. Since FUra is the most effective single agent in the treatment of adenocarcinoma of the gastrointestinal tract, attempts to improve this limited activity are clearly worthwhile. FUra also has good single-agent activity in patients with cancer of the breast and as a 4- to 5-day infusion against cancer of the head and neck region (54). Also worth considering is the possibility that FUra [or 5-fluorodeoxyuridine (FdUrd)] may be converted to an active drug by appropriate modulation in circumstances in which it has little or no single-agent activity. For example, *in vitro* studies in this laboratory have shown marked potentiation of FUra and FdUrd cytotoxicity by leucovorin [5-formyltetrahydrofolate (LV)] against human lymphoblastic leukemia cells CCRF-CEM (72).

Figure 1 illustrates some of the ways in which FUra has been modulated to increase its cytotoxicity. Inhibition of its catabolism *in vivo* by thymidine (dThd) can increase its potency (65). Increased activation by increasing phosphoribosyl pyrophosphate (PRPP) pools via drugs that inhibit purine biosynthesis [e.g., methotrexate (MTX) or 6-methylmercaptopurine riboside (6MMPR)], by depleting competing pyrimidine pools

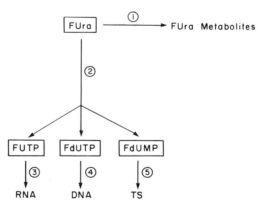

Fig. 1.   Metabolism and sites of actions of FUra. Circled numbers refer to the metabolic steps, that can be altered by a "modulator," resulting in increased drug cytotoxicity. (1) Degradation to the end products CO_2, ammonia, urea, and α-fluoro-β-alanine via pyrimidine-catabolizing enzymes. (2) Activation to fluorinated nucleotides via orotate phosphoribosyl transferase, uridine and thymidine phosphorylases, and kinases. (3) Incorporation into RNA via RNA polymerase. (4) Incorporation into DNA via DNA polymerase. (5) Inhibition of thymidylate synthase (TS).

[phosphonoacetyl-L-aspartic acid (PALA)], or by increasing levels of ri-bose-1-phosphate by guanosine administration have all been reported to enhance FUra cell kill (24,45,47,56). These drugs increase the intracellu-lar fluoronucleotide pools, resulting in increased levels of fluorouridine triphosphate (FUTP) and its incorporation into RNA. Increased levels of fluorodeoxyuridine monophosphate (FdUMP), a potent inhibitor of thy-midylate biosynthesis also occurs as well as increased incorporation of fluorodeoxyuridine triphosphate (FdUTP) into DNA. Enhanced and pro-longed inhibition of thymidylate synthase (TS) by FdUMP may also be achieved by increasing the levels of the coenzyme, 5,10-methylenetetra-hydrofolate (CH_2–FH_4) via LV administration (11,96). MTX pretreatment may also increase levels of dihydrofolate polyglutamates in cells, which also enhances FdUMP binding to TS (39). Decreasing the deoxyuridylate (dUMP) pool size, the substrate for TS, by inhibition of ribonucleotide reductase, e.g., by hydroxyurea, will also result in enhanced inhibition of TS by FdUMP (73).

II. Sequential Use of Methotrexate and 5-Fluorouracil in the Clinic

A large literature now exists that shows in experimental tumor models that the sequence MTX followed by FUra gives enhanced cell kill, while the opposite sequence gives less than additive cell kill (5,7,10,13,17,23,31,32,39,42,56,57,64,72,76). When murine tumor cells were used *in vitro* or *in vivo,* most studies showed that short intervals (1–2 hr) between MTX and FUra administration sufficed for synergy to be observed (5,13,23,31,42). However, synergistic cell kill of human tumor cells (breast, colon) was observed when the interval between MTX and FUra was 12–24 hr and was correlated with an increased level of PRPP and FUra nucleotide formation (7,10,38,64). In this regard, it is important to point out that little or no knowledge exists concerning the effects of increasing the treatment interval on normal sensitive tissues (i.e., bone marrow or gastrointestinal tract). From data available, it seems clear that in patients, treatments using short intervals between MTX and FUra administration may be less toxic to normal cells and may be administered weekly, while biweekly administration appears to be necessary when longer intervals are used between MTX and FUra administration. Thus, while the longer intervals using this sequence may be more effective in terms of tumor cell kill, it is not clear as to whether the therapeutic index is improved.

A. Head and Neck Cancer

Following encouraging reports of activity of this combination using a 1-hr interval in the treatment of patients with head and neck cancer (83,88), two randomized studies have examined the importance of the sequential use of these drugs (16,29). In the study by Browman *et al.* (16), a 1-hr interval (MTX → FUra) was compared to giving the drugs rapidly sequentially (MTX → FUra), referred to as "simultaneous" administration. The response rate was higher in patients given the drugs simultaneously as compared to the sequence (Table IA).

However, there was no difference in the response rates of stage IV patients; in contrast, 0 of 4 stage III patients responded to sequential MTX–FUra, while 8 of 9 patients with stage III disease responded to simultaneous MTX–FUra. Thus, the difference observed could be attributed to the small number of stage III patients in the sequential arm together with the very high response rate of stage III patients in the "simultaneous" group. There was no difference in survival between the groups. In the study by Coates *et al.* (29), the sequence MTX → FUra was compared to a FUra → MTX sequence; the interval in both arms was 1 hr (Table IB). In this investigation the MTX → FUra sequence produced a higher response rate than FUra → MTX, although the difference was not significant ($p = .18$, in previously untreated patients). Again, there were no differences in survival between the two groups.

These studies together with two of three other studies (48,83,88) report a high response rate in head and neck cancer to this combination. While the response rates reported are higher than those expected with single-agent treatment with MTX (ca. 30%), thus far this issue has not been addressed in a comparative trial. It also seems clear that the 1-hr sequence (MTX → FUra) seems not to have any advantage over simultaneous or the opposite sequence administration. In view of the *in vitro* data

TABLE I

Effect of Sequence of MTX and FUra on Response Rate in Patients with Head and Neck Cancer[a]

Sequence	Interval (hr)	No. patients	CR + PR (%)	Reference
A. MTX → FUra	1	37	38	(16)
MTX → FUra	"Simultaneous"[b]	42	62	
B. MTX → FUra	1	26	65	(19)
FUra → FUra	1	23	47	

[a] Not previously treated with chemotherapy.
[b] MTX was administered first, followed immediately by FUra.

using human breast carcinoma cells and colon carcinoma cells in culture, of great interest will be the result of a study in progress by Browman *et al.* employing a longer interval between MTX and FUra administration in patients with this malignancy.

The development of another effective combination for this disease (*cis*-platinum plus a 4- to 5-day FUra infusion) (53) and the preliminary results from our clinic indicating that patients failing MTX → FUra chemotherapy are still responsive to *cis*-platinum–FUra make it logical to attempt treatment of patients with these two combinations in an alternating fashion. Preliminary results from our clinic (unpublished observations) and from Ensley *et al.* (36) are encouraging in this regard.

B. Colorectal Cancer

A large number of studies have been reported, using sequential MTX and FUra in colorectal cancer (15,18,20,25,29,33,34,41,44,50,51,63,68,81, 87,91,94,99,100). What emerges from these studies, many with small numbers of patients, is that response rates when intervals of 4 hr or longer are used between MTX and FUra administration are higher than when shorter intervals (1–3 hr) were used (Table II).

The results of the studies using longer treatment intervals are encouraging. However, since the largest series reported consisted of 42 evaluable patients (44), there is an urgent need for controlled studies demonstrating that the interval of 4 hr or longer is better than the 1-hr interval and indeed that the combination MTX–FUra is more efficacious treatment than FUra alone. We are currently engaged in a randomized study testing a 1- versus 24-hr interval between treatment in patients with advanced or recurrent colorectal cancer. In addition, we are also examining the effectiveness of the sequential use of dichloromethotrexate and FUra via intraarterial administration (22-hr interval) to patients with isolated hepatic metastasis from colorectal cancer. This study, based on *in vitro* work using human

TABLE II

Responses to Sequential MTX–FUra in Patients with Colorectal Cancer

MTX–FUra interval (hr)	No. patients	No. CR + PR (%)
1–3	118	18 (15)
4–6	93	25 (27)[a]
7–24	153	48 (31)[b]

[a] Significantly increased over 1- to 3-hr interval, $p < .05$.
[b] Significantly increased over 1- to 3-hr interval, $p < .01$.

colorectal cancer cells (90), is encouraging in that 2 of the first 3 patients entered have had a response to treatment.

In a study conducted by the Northern California Oncology Group, sequential MTX–FUra (12-hr interval) was given with mitomycin C to patients with disseminated colon cancer (46). The response rate in 49 evaluable patients was 39%, and the median survival of patients responding was 13.6 months. The addition of mitomycin C to the sequential MTX–FUra regimen increased, however, the incidence of adverse effects, particularly myelodepression and renal toxicity. These results encourage further comparative studies of this three-drug combination in patients with colon cancer.

C. Gastric Cancer

While there have been few studies of gastric cancer reported using this sequence, one study is of particular interest. Klein *et al.* (55) employed high-dose MTX (1500 mg/m^2) followed 1 hr later with high-dose FUra (1500 mg/m^2), alternating biweekly with adriamycin, 30 mg/m^2. In a series of 65 patients, 68% have responded, and 4 patients achieved a complete response. Median survival of patients achieving a response was greater than 18 months.

D. Breast Cancer

As in colon cancer, several studies using this sequence have been reported (35,40,43,50,81,82,84,94), mainly in patients previously treated, some with CMF (cyclophosphamide, MTX, FUra). The response rate noted in these patients is usually higher than would be expected using either drug alone (40,43,84), although the value of the sequence and the importance of sequential use of these drugs has not been evaluated. In a pilot study of the Eastern Cooperative Oncology Group, the sequence MTX → FUra was used with a 1-hr interval in the CMFP regimen (cyclophosphamide, MTX, FUra, prednisone). The response rate obtained was not higher than that expected from conventional CMFP (22).

Since MTX and FUra are cycle-active drugs and might be expected to be more efficacious against experimentally growing tumor populations, this sequence has potential value in the adjuvant treatment of breast cancer (12), as well as in breast cancer cells synchronized by hormonal treatment. Following the initial favorable results of Allegra (1) utilizing sequential tamoxifen–premarin to synchronize breast cancer cells, Lippman *et al.* (58) have utilized a similar program with the addition of cyclophosphamide and adriamycin at the start of the cycle to treat patients with locally advanced disease. Very encouraging early results have been obtained with this program, in that an impressive 90% overall response rate has been observed in a series of 41 patients, with 46% complete responses.

The National Surgical Adjuvant Breast Program (NSABP) is utilizing this sequence as adjuvant therapy to treat patients with ER-negative, node-negative breast cancer. Since both MTX and FUra have not been reported to have carcinogenic effects, this combination is attractive both for theoretical as well as toxicological considerations. This large, randomized trial (versus no treatment) will be of great interest in regards to the effectiveness of this antimetabolite combination in the adjuvant setting.

III. 5-Fluorouracil and High-Dose Leucovorin in Advanced Adenocarcinoma of the Gastrointestinal Tract

Stimulated by the laboratory studies of Ullman et al. (96), Waxman and Bruckner (98), and Evans et al. (38) that demonstrated marked improvement in cytotoxic effects when FUra was used with high doses of LV, clinical trials with this combination were initiated. These studies have been, of necessity, phase I–II trials, since dose schedules and toxicities have had to be evaluated. When LV is administered either orally or parenterally, rapid conversion to 5-methyltetrahydrofolate (MeFH$_4$) occurs (69,77,93), and the blood level of this compound exceeds that of the physiological (l)-diastereoisomer of LV within 2 hr of drug administration (Fig. 2). Fortunately, MeFH$_4$ also gives synergistic effects when administered in high doses with FUra, and this rapid conversion of LV to MeFH$_4$ is not inhibitory (72). The relatively long half-life of the nonphysiologic (d)- diastereoisomer of LV and its persistence in relatively high concentration has not been explored fully in regards to this combination. Trave et al. (95) recently reported that high-dose LV may affect FUra pharmacokinetics, perhaps reflecting alterations in the cellular metabolism of this drug.

Based on these considerations, doses of LV used have ranged from 20 mg/m^2 to doses as high as 500 mg/m^2, administered as a bolus, short term or long term (daily × 4–5 days) infusions. These doses have been used with three different dosage schedules of FUra; a weekly bolus schedule (59,62), a daily bolus × 4 to 5-day schedule (14,19,21,61,86), or a 4- to 5-day infusion schedule (19,74). Table III summarizes the results of these studies. The largest study reported is by Machover et al. (61). These authors have now treated with FUra–LV over 84 patients with colorectal

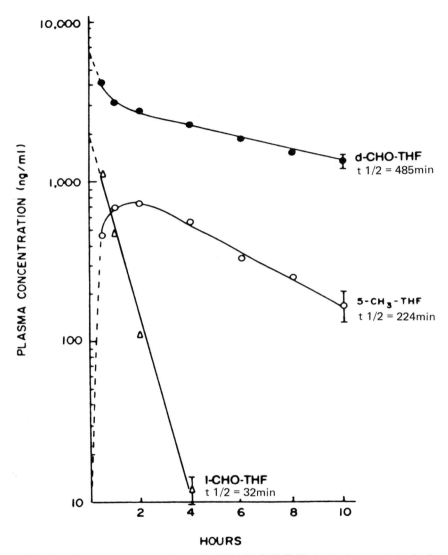

Fig. 2. Plasma concentrations of (d)-LV[d-CHO-THF (methylene tetrahydrofolate), ●], (l)-LV (l-CHO-THF, △), and MeFH₄ (5-CH₃-THF, ○) after a 5-min, intravenous infusion of 50 mg of (dl)-LV. [From Straw *et al.* (93), with permission.]

TABLE III

LV and FUra in Advanced Colorectal Cancer

LV dose[a] (mg/m²)	FUra dose[a] (mg/m²)	Schedule	No. patients	% (CR + PR)	Toxicity	Reference
200	370–400	Day 1–5, q. 3 weeks	84	33	++	(61)
200	350–400	Day 1–5, q. 4 weeks	43	12	+	(21)
75	330–550	Day 1–5, q. 4 weeks				(19)
60	600–1200	Day 1–4, q. 4 weeks	36	39	++	
(Continuous infusion)	(Continuous infusion)					
500	370	LV day 1–6, FUra day 2–6, q. 4 weeks	19	26	++	(14)
500 (Over 2 hr)	300–500	q. 1 week	23	39	+++	(62)
60 (q. 6 hr)	600–800 (Over 24 hr)	Day 1–4, q. 4 weeks	20	15	++	(74)
20–30	400–850	q. 1 week	7	57	++	(59)
200	370–400	Day 1–5, q. 3 weeks	8	0	NS	(86)

[a] Intravenous bolus, unless otherwise stated.

TABLE IV

Summary of LV–FUra Clinical Trials

Cancer	No. of trials	Tumor response		
		Previously FUra-treated patients	Previously FUra-untreated patients	Total patients
Colorectal	5	14/78 (18%)	47/127 (37%)	61/205 (30%)
Gastric	1	0/1 (0%)	13/26 (50%)	13/27 (48%)

cancer. Of interest is the activity of the combination, even in patients previously treated with FUra (Table IV), a response rate equal to FUra treatment alone in untreated patients. The results of five completed studies are summarized in Table IV (14,19,21,61,62). The response rate in previously untreated colon cancer is 37%, or about double that expected from FUra treatment alone. A large randomized study comparing FUra treatment to two different dosage regimens of FUra–LV is now in progress under the sponsorship of the Gastrointestinal Study Tumor Group.

Of interest also is the response rate of 50% in gastric cancer reported by Machover *et al.* (61) (Table IV). Use of this combination in gastric cancer is deserving further study.

IV. Combination Therapy with *N*-(Phosphonacetyl)-L-aspartic Acid, Thymidine, and 5-Fluorouracil

In both *in vitro* and *in vivo* experimental tumor models, *N*-(phosphonacetyl)-L-aspartic acid (PALA), an inhibitor of *de novo* pyrimidine biosynthesis (29a,75), enhances the antitumor activity of FUra (2,49,56,66) by depleting the intracellular pools of the normal pyrimidine nucleotides, deoxyuridine monophosphate (dUMP), and uridine triphosphate (UTP) that compete with FUra for its metabolic targets. Based on these positive results, phase I–II clinical trials with PALA and FUra were initiated in patients with various solid tumors, in particular with colorectal cancer. Most clinical trials have used relatively high doses of PALA by either continuous intravenous infusions (3,70,101,102), daily injections (6,37,79) for 5 days, or as single injection (6), prior to FUra administration, resulting in reduced tolerance to the fluoropyrimidine. In all studies, therapeutic results were disappointing in that response rates were not higher than those obtained by single-agent FUra, even in untreated patients (Table V).

TABLE V

Phase I–II Clinical Trials of PALA–FUra Combinations in Advanced Solid Tumors

PALA dose (mg/m²)[a]	Interval PALA–FUra (hr)	FUra dose (mg/m²)[a]	Schedule	No. responses/ no. evaluable patients	Dose-limiting toxicity	Reference
750 (Over 24 hr)	24	275	Day 1–5, q. 4 weeks	3/16	Mucositis	(70)
625 (Over 0.15 hr)	0	250–300	Day 1–5, q. 5 weeks	2/14	Mucositis	(79)
850 (Over 24 hr)	24	560 (Over 24 hr)	Day 1–5, q. 5 weeks	1/21	Mucositis	(102)
1000 (Over 0.25 hr)	0	200	Day 1–5, q. 3 weeks	1/30	Mucositis, GI tract toxicity[c]	(37)
850 (Over 24 hr)	24	300	Day 1–5, q. 4 weeks	6/43	Mucositis	(101)
940 (Over 24 hr)	0	250 (Over 24 hr)	q. 1 week	2/18	Mucositis	(3)
1600 (Over 1 hr)	4	360 (Over 0.5 hr)	q. 1 week	4/24[b]	Mucositis, GI tract toxicity,[c] skin rash	(6)
640 (Over 1 hr)	4	320 (Over 0.5 hr)	Day 1–5, q. 4 weeks	3/26[b]	Mucositis, GI tract toxicity,[c] skin rash	(6)
250 (Over 0.5 hr)	24	600	Day 1,8,15, q. 5 weeks	1/32	None	(27)

[a] Intravenous bolus, unless otherwise stated. Indicated doses of phase I trials are those suggested for phase II trials.
[b] Colorectal carcinoma patients.
[c] GI, gastrointestinal.

A more recent laboratory study has shown that low, nontherapeutic doses of PALA, capable, however, of inhibiting pyrimidine biosynthesis, could still enhance the therapeutic efficacy of FUra without undue toxicity (67). A phase I clinical trial based on these laboratory results has indicated that low-dose PALA (250 mg/m^2) can produce an effective inhibition of pyrimidine synthesis in humans and can be safely administered before FUra at standard doses (600–750 mg/m^2) once weekly (27). It would be of interest to assess the antitumor activity of this low-dose PALA/standard-dose-FUra combination further.

When given in large doses, dThd is able to block the degradation of FUra, since thymine generated by it competes for pyrimidine-catabolizing enzymes, resulting in prolonged FUra plasma half-life (4,52,103) and increased cellular exposure to the drug. Although dThd pretreatment would be expected to increase both the FUra antitumor activity and the host toxicity to levels comparable to those achievable with higher doses of FUra, increased therapeutic indices in several rodent tumor systems have been observed (65,89,91a). Therapeutic synergism was correlated with increased incorporation of FUra into RNA (65,91a).

Although preliminary clinical studies had suggested some antitumor activity of this combination in patients with advanced colorectal cancer, some of these patients being resistant to single-agent FUra (97,103), further clinical trials failed to demonstrate improved response rate of colorectal as well as other carcinomas to FUra by coadministration of dThd (60,85,92) (Table VI). On the contrary, dThd pretreatment appeared to increase the toxicity of FUra, in that dose-limiting myelosuppression occurred at FUra doses ranging from one-half to two-thirds of the standard tolerated dose of FUra alone (60,80,85,92,97), and relevant central nervous system toxicity at high dThd doses was observed (60).

Since improved therapeutic results with the three-drug regimen of PALA–dThd-FUra over those with the combinations of PALA–FUra or dThd-FUra have been more recently obtained in the CD8F1 murine mammary tumor (67), pilot clinical trials have been carried out to determine the antitumor activity and toxicity of this combination in patients with advanced solid tumors (26,28,78) (Table VII). O'Connell et al. (78) have reported a promising response rate of 27% in patients with colorectal cancer, with higher responses seen in patients with rapidly growing tumors. Two other studies, however, using a different dosage regimen have not documented any significant activity of this combination in a variety of advanced solid tumors, including colorectal cancer patients, most of them heavily pretreated with fluoropyrimidines (26,28). A high incidence of neurologic toxicity consisting of dizziness, lethargy, and confusion was observed in these two studies that used very high doses of dThd (30 and 45 gm/m^2), limiting possible clinical application of this combination.

TABLE VI

Phase I–II Clinical Trials of dThd–FUra Combinations in Advanced Solid Tumors

dThd dose (gm/m²)[a]	Interval dThd–FUra (hr)	FUra dose (mg/m²)[a]	Schedule	No. responding/ no. evaluated patients	Dose-limiting toxicity	Reference
8 (Over 24 hr)	2	200–400	Day 1–5, q. 4–5 weeks	NS/10	Myelotoxicity	(80)
8 (Over 2.5 hr)	0	400	q. 4–5 weeks	NS/10	Myelotoxicity	(80)
8 (Over 24 hr)	0	300 (Over 24 hr)	Day 1–5, q. 4 weeks	2/12[b]	Myelotoxicity	(97)
15[c]	1	300–400	q. 3–4 weeks	4/37	Myelotoxicity	(103)
9 (Over 0.25 hr)	1	225	q. 4 weeks	3/27	Myelotoxicity	(85)
16 (Over 0.5 hr)	2	1500 (Over 120 hr)	q. 4 weeks	1/22[b]	Myelotoxicity	(92)
18–32 (Over 0.5 hr), then 52 over 144 hr	0	100	q. 1 week	0/26[b]	Neurotoxicity, gastrointestinal tract toxicity	(60)
27 (Over 3 hr) (Over 1.5 hr)	0.5	175	q. 1 week	0/26[b]	Neurotoxicity	(60)

[a] Intravenous bolus, unless otherwise stated. Indicated doses of phase I trials are those suggested for phase II trials.
[b] Colorectal carcinoma patients.
[c] Total dose.

TABLE VII

Phase I–II Clinical Trials of PALA–dThd–FUra Combinations in Advanced Solid Tumors

PALA dose (mg/m²)[a]	Interval PALA–dThd (hr)	dThd dose (gm/m²)[a]	Interval dThd–FUra (hr)	FUra dose (mg/m²)[a]	Schedule	No. responding/ no. evaluated patients	Dose-limiting toxicity	Reference
4000 (Over 1 hr)	24	15 (Over 0.5 hr)	+1	200 (Over 3 hr)	q. 4 weeks	10/37[b]	Myelotoxicity, neurotoxicity	(78)
250–2000 (Over 0.5 hr)	24	45 (Over 1.5 hr)	−0.5	100–150	q. 3 weeks	0/15	Neurotoxicity, myelotoxicity	(26)
1000 (Over 1 hr)	24	30 (Over 3 hr)	0	150–300 (Over 3 hr)	q. 4 weeks	2/28	Gastrointestinal tract toxicity, neurotoxicity	(28)

[a] Intravenous bolus, unless otherwise stated.
[b] Colorectal carcinoma patients.

V. Conclusions

It is difficult to conclude from clinical studies published thus far that modulation chemotherapy of FUra with either MTX or LV has been successful in the clinic. Of necessity, problems of defining toxicity and optimum dosage scheduling have been addressed, and large randomized trials have been only recently initiated. Sufficiently encouraging response rates with both of these treatments have been reported in colorectal and gastric cancer, which should stimulate further study, especially in those tumors in which treatment options are limited. The problem exists in breast and head and neck cancer as not only how to define the activity of these regimens but how to integrate these treatments into combination programs with other effective drugs. Clinical studies of modulation of FUra with either LV or MTX in leukemia and lymphoma are also clearly warranted based upon experimental tumor results (71,72). Since levels of hypoxanthine and thymidine in the serum or bone marrow may affect the therapeutic outcome, measurement of these compounds in patients receiving this therapy may be of importance (9).

It may also be possible to modulate the FUra effect with both LV and MTX, and preliminary efforts in this direction have already been initiated (8,30). However, the complexity of a three-drug program in regards to dosing and scheduling is larger and should rely as much as possible on biochemical and pharmacologic guidance.

Biochemical modulation of FUra antitumor activity via PALA and/or dThd has led to poor therapeutic results in the clinic. Although further trials using different drug doses or schedules of administration are in progress, it appears that there are small margins to improve response rates over those of single-agent FUra, using this approach.

Acknowledgments

This work was supported by Grants CA08341 and CA08010 from the USPHS.

References

1. Allegra, J. C. (1983). Methotrexate and 5-fluorouracil following tamoxifen and premarin in advanced breast cancer. *Semin. Oncol.* **10,** Suppl. 2, 23–28.
2. Ardalan, B., Glazer, R. I., Kensler, T. W., Jayaram, H. N., Pham, T. V., MacDonald, J. S., and Cooney, D. A. (1981). Synergistic effects of 5-fluorouracil and N-(phosphonacetyl)-L-aspartate on cell growth and ribonucleic acid synthesis in a human mammary carcinoma. *Biochem. Pharmacol.* **30,** 2045–2049.

3. Ardalan, B., Jamin, D., Jayaram, H. N., and Presant, C. A. (1984). Phase I study of continuous-infusion PALA and 5-FU. *Cancer Treat. Rep.* **68,** 531–534.

4. Au, J. L-S., Rustum, Y. M., Ledesma, E. J., Mittelman, A., and Creaven, P. J. (1982). Clinical pharmacological studies of concurrent infusion of 5-fluorouracil and thymidine in treatment of colorectal carcinoma. *Cancer Res.* **42,** 2930–2937.

5. Bareham, C. R., Griswold, D. E., and Calabresi, P. (1974). Synergism of methotrexate with imuran and with 5-fluorouracil and their effects on hemolysis plaque-forming cell production in the mouse. *Cancer Res.* **34,** 571–575.

6. Bedikian, A. Y., Stroehlein, J. R., Karlin, D. A., Bennetts, R. W., Bodey, G. P., and Valdivieso, M. (1981). Chemotherapy for colorectal cancer with a combination of PALA and 5-FU. *Cancer Treat. Rep.* **65,** 747–753.

7. Benz, C., and Cadman, E. (1981). Modulation of 5-fluorouracil metabolism and cytotoxicity by antimetabolite in human colorectal adenocarcinoma, HCT-8. *Cancer Res.* **41,** 994–999.

8. Benz, C., DeGregorio, M., Saks, S., Sambol, N., Holleran, W., Ignoffo, R., Lewis, B., and Cadman, E. (1985). Sequential infusions of methotrexate and 5-fluorouracil in advanced cancer: Pharmacology, toxicity, and response. *Cancer Res.* **45,** 3354–3358.

9. Benz, C., Sambol, N., Yawitz, B., Wilbur, B., and DeGregorio, M. (1985). Serum purines and pyrimidines correlate with methotrexate (MTX) and 5-fluorouracil (5FU) response and toxicity. *Proc. Am. Soc. Clin. Oncol.* **4,** 43.

10. Benz, C., Tillis, T., Tattelman, E., and Cadman, E. (1982). Optimal scheduling to methotrexate and 5-fluorouracil in human breast cancer. *Cancer Res.* **42,** 2081–2086.

11. Berger, S., and Hakala, M. T. (1984). Relationship of dUMP and free FdUMP pools to inhibition of thymidylate synthase by 5-fluorouracil. *Mol. Pharmacol.* **25,** 303–309.

12. Bertino, J. R. (1982). Keynote address—Adjuvant chemotherapy and cancer cure. *Int. J. Radiat. Oncol. Biol. Phys.* **8,** 109–113.

13. Bertino, J. R., Sawicki, W. L., Lindquist, C. A., and Gupta, V. S. (1977). Schedule-dependent antitumor effects of methotrexate and 5-fluorouracil. *Cancer Res.* **37,** 327–328.

14. Bertrand, M., Doroshow, J. H., Multhauf, P., Newman, E., Blayney, D. W., Carr, B. I., and Goldberg, D. (1984). Combination chemotherapy with high-dose continuous infusion leucovorin and bolus 5-fluorouracil in patients with advanced colorectal cancer. *In* "Advances in Cancer Chemotherapy" (H. W. Bruckner and Y. M. Rustum, eds), pp. 73–76. Wiley, New York.

15. Blumenreich, M. S., Woodcock, T. M., Allegra, M., Richman, S. P., Kubota, T. T., and Allegra, J. C. (1982). Sequential therapy with methotrexate (MTX) and 5-fluorouracil (5-FU) for adenocarcinoma of the colon. *Proc. Am. Soc. Clin. Oncol.* **1,** 102.

16. Browman, G. P., Archibald, S. D., Young, J. E. M., Hryniuk, W. M., Russell, R., Kiehl, K., and Levine, M. N. (1983). Prospective randomized trial of one hour sequential versus simultaneous methotrexate plus 5-fluorouracil in advanced and recurrent squamous cell head and neck cancer. *J. Clin. Oncol.* **1,** 787–792.

17. Brown, I., and Ward, H. W. C. (1978). Therapeutic consequences of antitumor drug interactions: Methotrexate and 5-fluorouracil in the chemotherapy of C3H mice with transplanted mammary adenocarcinoma. *Cancer Lett.* **5,** 291–297.

18. Bruckner, H., and Cohen, J. (1983). MTX/5-FU trials in gastrointestinal and other cancers. *Semin. Oncol.* **10,** Suppl. 2, 32–39.

19. Bukowski, R. M., and Cunningham, J. (1984). Efficacy of 5-fluorouracil in combination with leucovorin in patients with colorectal carcinoma: continuous infusion of low

doses. *In* "Advances in Cancer Chemotherapy" (H. W. Bruckner and Y. M. Rustum, eds.), pp. 69–72. Wiley, New York.

20. Burnet, R., Smith, F. P., Hoerni, B., Lagarde, C., and Schein, P. (1981). Sequential methotrexate-5-fluorouracil in advanced measurable colorectal cancer: Lack of appreciable therapeutic synergism. *Proc. Am. Assoc. Cancer Res.* **22,** 370.

21. Byrne, P. J., Treat, J., McFadden, M., McVie, G., Huiniuk, T. B., Schein, P. S., and Wooley, P. V. (1971). Therapeutic efficacy of the combination of 5-fluorouracil and high-dose leucovorin in patients with advanced colorectal carcinoma: Single daily intravenous dose for five days. *In* "Advances in Cancer Chemotherapy" (H. W. Bruckner and Y. M. Rustum, eds.), pp. 65–67. Wiley, New York.

22. Cadman, E. C., Glick, J. H., Cross, J., Horton, J., and Taylor, S. G., IV (1984). Sequential methotrexate and 5-FU in CMFP (cyclophosphamide, methotrexate, 5-FU, and prednisone) therapy for breast cancer. *Cancer Treat. Rep.* **68,** 877–879.

23. Cadman, E., Heimer, R., and Benz, C. (1981). The influence of methotrexate pretreatment on 5-fluorouracil metabolism in L1210 cells. *J. Biol. Chem.* **256,** 1695–1704.

24. Cadman, E., Heimer, R., and Davis, L. (1979). Enhanced 5-fluorouracil nucleotide formation after methotrexate administration: Explanation for drug synergism. *Science* **205,** 1135–1137.

25. Cantrell, J. E., Jr., Burnet, R., Lagarde, C., Schein, P. S., and Smith, F. P. (1982). Phase II study of sequential methotrexate-5-FU therapy in advanced measurable colorectal cancer. *Cancer Treat. Rep.* **66,** 1563–1565.

26. Casper, E. S., Michaelson, R. A., Kemeny, N., Martin, D. S., and Young, C. W. (1984). Phase I evaluation of a biochemically designed combination: PALA, thymidine, and 5-FU. *Cancer Treat. Rep.* **68,** 539–541.

27. Casper, E. S., Vale, K., Williams, L. J., Martin, D. S., and Young, C. W. (1983). Phase I and clinical pharmacological evaluation of biochemical modulation of 5-fluorouracil with N-(phosphonacetyl)-L-aspartic acid. *Cancer Res.* **43,** 2324–2329.

28. Chiuten, D. F., Valdivieso, M., Bedikian, A., Bodey, G. P., and Freireich, E. J. (1985). Phase I-II clinical trial of thymidine, 5-FU and PALA given in combination. *Cancer Treat. Rep.* **69,** 611–613.

29. Coates, A. S., Tattersall, M. H. N., Swanson, C., Hedley, D., Fox, R. M., and Raghavan, D. (1984). Combination therapy with methotrexate and 5-fluorouracil: A prospective randomized clinical trial of order of administration. *J. Clin. Oncol.* **2,** 756–761.

29a. Collins, K. D., and Stark, G. R. (1971). Aspartate transcarbamylase, interaction with the transition state analogue N-(phosphonacetyl)-L-aspartate. *J. Biol. Chem.* **246,** 6599–6605.

30. Denny, A., Slavik, M., Chien, S. C., Taylor, S., Fabian, C., and Stephens, R. (1985). Initial clinical and pharmacokinetic study of oral (PO) methotrexate (MTX), intravenous (IV) 5-fluorouracil (5-FU) and high dose folinic acid (FA). *Proc. Am. Assoc. Cancer Res.* **26,** 167.

31. DiLorenzo, J. A., Griswold, D. E., Bareham, C. R., and Calabresi, P. (1974). Selective alteration of immunocompetence with methotrexate 5-fluorouracil. *Cancer Res.* **34,** 124–128.

32. Donehower, R. C., Allegra, J. C., Lippman, M. E., and Chabner, B. A. (1980). Combined effects of methotrexate and 5-fluoropyrimidine on human breast cancer cells in serum-free culture. *Eur. J. Cancer* **16,** 655–661.

33. Drapkin, R., Griffiths, E., McAloon, E., Paladine, W., Sokol, G., and Lyman, G. (1981). Sequential methotrexate (MTX) and 5-fluorouracil (5-FU) in adenocarcinoma of the colon and rectum. *Proc. Am. Assoc. Cancer Res.* **22,** 453.

34. Drapkin, R., McAloon, E., and Lyman, G. (1983). Sequential methotrexate (MTX) and 5-fluorouracil in advanced measurable colorectal cancer. *Proc. Am. Soc. Clin. Oncol.* **2,** 118.
35. Ellison, J., Bernath, A. M., Gallagher, J. G., Porter, P. A., Rine, K. T., and Lewis, G. O. (1985). Toxicity without benefit for sequential MTX/5FU. *Proc. Am. Soc. Clin. Oncol.* **4,** 26.
36. Ensley, J., Kish, J., Jacobs, J., Weaver, A., Kinzic, J., Crissman, J., and Al-Sarraf, M. (1985). The use of a five course, alternating regimen in advanced squamous cell carcinoma of the head and neck. *Proc. Am. Soc. Clin. Oncol.* **4,** 143.
37. Erlichman, C., Donehower, R. C., Speyer, J. L., Klecker, R., and Chabner, B. A. (1982). Phase I-phase II trial of N-phosphonacetyl-L-aspartic acid given by intravenous infusion and 5-fluorouracil given by bolus injection. *JNCI, J. Natl. Cancer Inst.* **68,** 227–231.
38. Evans, R. M., Laskin, J. D., and Hakala, M. T. (1981). Effects of excess folates and deoxyinosine and the activity and site of action of 5-fluorouracil. *Cancer Res.* **41,** 3288–3295.
39. Fernandes, D. J., and Bertino, J. R. (1980). 5-Fluorouracil-methotrexate synergy. Enhancement of 5-fluorodeoxyuridine binding to thymidilate synthetase by dihydropteroylpolyglutamates. *Proc. Natl. Acad. Sci. U.S.A.* **77,** 5663–5667.
40. Gewirtz, A. M., and Cadman, E. (1981). Preliminary report on the efficacy of sequential methotrexate and 5-fluorouracil in advanced breast cancer. *Cancer (Philadelphia)* **47,** 2552–2555.
41. Hansen, R., Ritch, P., and Anderson, T. (1983). Sequential methotrexate (MTX), 5-fluorouracil (5-FU) and leucovorin (LCV) in colorectal cancer. *Proc. Am. Soc. Clin. Oncol.* **2,** 117.
42. Heppner, G. H., and Calabresi, P. (1977). Effect of sequence of administration of methotrexate, leucovorin, and 5-fluorouracil on mammary tumor growth and survival in syngeneic C3H mice. *Cancer Res.* **37,** 4580–4583.
43. Herrmann, R., Manegold, C., Schroeder, M., Tigges, F. J., Bartsch, H., Jungi, F., and Fritze, D. (1984). Sequential methotrexate and 5-FU in breast cancer resistant to the conventional application of these drugs. *Cancer Treat. Rep.* **68,** 1279–1281.
44. Herrmann, R., Spehn, J., Beyer, J. H., von Franque, U., Schmieder, A., Holzmann, K., and Abel, U. (1984). Sequential methotrexate and 5-fluorouracil: Improved response rate in metastatic colorectal cancer. *J. Clin. Oncol.* **2,** 591–594.
45. Houghton, J. A., Tice, A. J., and Houghton, P. J. (1982). The selectivity of action of methotrexate in combination with 5-fluorouracil in xenografts of human colon adenocarcinomas. *Mol. Pharmacol.* **22,** 771–778.
46. Ignoffo, R. J., Friedman, M. A., Gribble, M., Hannigen, H., Reynolds, R., Yu, K.-P., Schiff, S., and Congdon, J. E. (1984). Phase II study of sequential methotrexate and 5-FU plus mitomycin and leucovorin in patients with disseminated large bowel cancer: A Northern California Oncology Group study. *Cancer Treat. Rep.* **68,** 983–988.
47. Iigo, M., and Hoshi, A. (1984). Effect of guanosine on antitumor activity of fluorinated pyrimidines against P 388 leukemia. *Cancer Chemother. Pharmacol.* **13,** 86–90.
48. Jacobs, C. (1982). Use of methotrexate and 5-FU for recurrent head and neck cancer. *Cancer Treat. Rep.* **66,** 1925.
49. Johnson, R. K., Clement, J. J., and Howard, W. S. (1980). Treatment of murine tumors with 5-fluorouracil in combination with *de novo* pyrimidine synthesis inhibitors PALA or pyrazofurin. *Proc. Am. Assoc. Cancer Res.* **21,** 292.
50. Kaye, S. B., Sangster, G., Hutcheon, A., Habeshaw, T., Crossling, F., Ferguson, C., McArdle, C., Smith, D., George, W. D., and Calman, K. C. (1984). Sequential metho-

trexate plus 5-FU in advanced breast and colorectal cancers: A phase II study. *Cancer Treat. Rep.* **68,** 547–548.

51. Kemeny, N. E., Ahmed, T., Michaelson, R. A., Harper, H. D., and Yip, J. L. C. (1984). Activity of sequential low-dose methotrexate and fluorouracil in advanced colorectal carcinoma: Attempts at correlation with tissue and blood levels of phosphoribosylpyrophosphate. *J. Clin. Oncol.* **2,** 311–315.

52. Kirkwood, J. M., Ensminger, W., Rosowsky, A., Papathanasopoulos, N., and Frei, E., III (1980). Comparison of pharmacokinetics of 5-fluorouracil and 5-fluorouracil with concurrent thymidine infusions in a phase I trial. *Cancer Res.* **40,** 107–113.

53. Kish, J., Drelichman, A., Jacobs, J., Hoshner, J., Kinzic, J., Loh J., Weaver, A., and Al Sarraf, M. (1982). Clinical trial of cisplatin and 5-FU infusion as initial treatment for advanced squamous cell carcinoma of the head and neck. *Cancer Treat. Rep.* **66,** 471–474.

54. Kish, J., Tapazoglou, J., Ensley, J., and Al Sarraf, M. (1985). Activity of 96 hour to 120 hour 5-fluorouracil (5-FU) infusion in advanced and recurrent head and neck cancer. *Proc. Am. Assoc. Cancer Res.* **26,** 168.

55. Klein, H. O., Wickramanayake, P. D., Schulz, V., Mohr, R., Oerkermann, H., and Farrokh, G. R. (1984). 5-Fluorouracil, adriamycin and methotrexate: A combination protocol (FAMETH) for the treatment of metastasized stomach cancer. *In* "Fluoropyrimidines in Cancer Therapy'' (K. Kimura, S. Fujii, G. P. Ogawa, G. P. Bodey, and P. Alberto, eds.), pp. 2280–2287. Elsevier, Amsterdam.

56. Kufe, D. W., and Egan, E. M. (1981). Enhancement of 5-fluorouracil incorporation into human lymphoblast ribonucleic acid. *Biochem. Pharmacol.* **30,** 129–133.

57. Lee, Y. N., and Khwaja, T. A. (1977). Adjuvant postoperative chemotherapy with 5-fluorouracil and methotrexate: Effect of schedule of administration on metastasis of 13762 mammary adenocarcinoma. *J. Surg. Oncol.* **9,** 469–479.

58. Lippmann, M., Sorace, R., Bagley, C., Lichter, A., Danforth, A., Wesley, M., and Young, R. (1985). Effective systemic management of locally advanced breast cancer. *Proc. Am. Soc. Clin. Oncol.* **4,** 65.

59. Lopez, A. R., Van Tilburg, A., Bradley, T., Jensen, B., Ziegler, J., Engelberg, C., and Deisseroth, A. (1984). Treatment of advanced malignancy with 5-fluorouracil (5-FU) combined with folinic acid (FA). *Proc. Am. Assoc. Cancer Res.* **25,** 178.

60. Lynch, G., Kemeny, N., Chun, H., Martin, D., and Young, C. (1985). Phase I evaluation and pharmacokinetic study of weekly iv thymidine and 5-FU in patients with advanced colorectal cancer. *Cancer Treat. Rep.* **69,** 179–184.

61. Machover, D., Goldschmidt, E., Chollet, P., Meztzger, G., Schwarzenberg, L., Misset, J. L., Timus, M., Vandenbulcke, J., Zittoun, J., Schneider, M., and Mathé, G. (1985). Treatment of advanced colorectal (CRC) and gastric adenocarcinomas (GC) with 5-FU and high dose folinic acid (FA). *Proc. Am. Assoc. Cancer Res.* **26,** 175.

62. Madajewicz, S., Petrelli, N., Rustum, Y. M., Campbell, J., Herrera, L., Mittelman, A., Perry, A., and Creaven, P. J. (1984). Phase I-II trial of high-dose calcium leucovorin and 5-fluorouracil in advanced colorectal cancer. *Cancer Res.* **44,** 4667–4669.

63. Mahajan, S. L., Ajani, J. A., Kanojia, M. H., Veilenkoop, L., and Bodey, G. P. (1983). Comparison of two schedules of sequential high-dose methotrexate (MTX) and 5-fluorouracil (5-FU) for metastatic colorectal carcinoma. *Proc. Am. Soc. Clion. Oncol.* **2,** 122.

64. Major, P. P., Egan, E. M., Sargent, L., and Kufe, D. W. (1982). Modulation of 5-fluorouracil metabolism in human MCFR-7 breast carcinoma cells. *Cancer Chemother. Pharmacol.* **8,** 87–91.

65. Martin, D. S., Nayak, K. R., Sawyer, R. L., Stolfi, R. L., Young, C. W., Woodcock, T., and Spiegelman, S. (1978). Enhancement of 5-fluorouracil chemotherapy with emphasis on the use of excess thymidine. *Cancer Bull.* **30,** 219–224.

66. Martin, D. S., Stolfi, R. C., Saywer, R. C., Nayak, R., Spiegelman, S., Schmid, F., Heimer, R., and Cadman, E. (1981). Biochemical modulation of 5-fluorouracil and cytosine arabinoside with emphasis on thymidine, PALA, and 6-methylmercaptopurine riboside. *In* "Nucleosides and Cancer Treatment" (M. H. N. Tattersall and R. M. Fox, eds.), pp. 339–382. Academic Press, Sydney, Australia.

67. Martin, D. S., Stolfi, R. L., Sawyer, R. C., Spiegelman, S., Casper, E. S., and Young, C. W. (1983). Therapeutic utility of utilizing low doses of N-(phosphonoacetyl)-L-aspartic acid in combination with 5-fluorouracil: A murine study with clinical relevance. *Cancer Res.* **43,** 2317–2321.

68. Mehrotra, S., Rosenthal, C. J., and Gardner, B. (1982). Biochemical modulation of antineoplastic response in colorectal carcinoma: 5-fluorouracil (F), high dose methotrexate (M) with calcium leucovorin (L) rescue (FML) in two sequences of administration. *Proc. Am. Soc. Clin. Oncol.* **1,** 100.

69. Mehta, B. M., Gisolfi, A. L., Hutchinson, D. J., Nirenberg, A., Kellick, M. G., and Rosen, G. (1978). Serum distribution of citrovorum factor and 5-methyltetrahydrofolate following oral and in administration of calcium leucovorin in normal adults. *Cancer Treat. Rep.* **62,** 345–350.

70. Meshad, M. W., Ervin, T. J., Kufe, D., Johnson, R. K., Blum, R. H., and Frei, E., III (1981). Phase I trial of combination therapy with PALA and 5-FU. *Cancer Treat. Rep.* **65,** 331–334.

71. Mini, E., and Bertino, J. R. (1982). Time and dose relationships for methotrexate (MTX), fluorouracil (FUra) and combinations of these drugs for maximum cell kill in human CCRF-CEF cells. *Proc. Am. Assoc. Cancer Res.* **23,** 181.

72. Mini, E., Moroson, B. A., and Bertino, J. R. (1985). Leucovorin (LV)-fluoropyrimidine synergy in the human leukemic lymphoblast cell line CCRF-CEM. *Proc. Am. Assoc. Cancer Res.* **26,** 324.

73. Moran, R. G., Danenberg, P. V., and Heidelberg, C. (1982). Therapeutic response of leukemic mice with fluorinated pyrimidines and inhibitors of deoxyuridylate synthesis. *Biochem. Pharmacol.* **31,** 2929–2935.

74. Mortimer, J., and Higano, C. (1985). Continuous infusion 5-fluorouracil (FU) and folinic acid (FA) in disseminated colorectal cancer: A phase I-II study. *Proc. Am. Assoc. Cancer Res.* **26,** 171.

75. Moyer, J. D., and Handschumacher, R. E. (1979). Selective inhibition of pyrimidine synthesis and depletion of nucleotide pools by N-(phosphonacetyl)-L-aspartate. *Cancer Res.* **39,** 3089–3094.

76. Mulder, J., Smink, T., and Van Putten, L. (1981). 5-Fluorouracil and methotrexate combination chemotherapy: The effect of drug scheduling. *Eur. J. Cancer Clin. Oncol.* **17,** 831–837.

77. Nixon, P. F., and Bertino, J. R. (1972). Effective absorption and utilization of oral formyltetrahydrofolate in man. *N. Engl. J. Med.* **286,** 175–179.

78. O'Connell, M. J., Moertel, C. G., Rubin, J., Hahn, R. G., Kvols, L. K., and Schutt, A. J. (1984). Clinical trial of sequential N-phosphonacetyl-L-aspartate, thymidine, and 5-fluorouracil in advanced colorectal carcinoma. *J. Clin. Oncol.* **10,** 1133–1138.

79. O'Connell, M. J., Powis, G., Rubin, J., and Moertel, C. G. (1982). Pilot study of PALA and 5-FU in patients with advanced cancer. *Cancer Treat. Rep.* **66,** 77–80.

80. Ohnuma, T., Roboz, J., Waxman, S., Mandel, E., Martin, S. D., and Holland, J. F.

Clinical pharmacological effects of thymidine plus 5-FU. *Cancer Treat. Rep.* **64,** 1169–1177.

81. Panasci, L., and Margolese, R. (1982). Sequential methotrexate (MTX) and 5-fluorouracil (FU) in breast and colorectal cancer. Results of increasing the dose of FU. *Proc. Am. Soc. Clin. Oncol.* **1,** 101.

82. Perrault, D. J., Erlichman, C., Hasselback, R., Tannock, I., and Boyd, N. (1983). Sequential methotrexate (MTX) and 5-fluorouracil (5FU) in refractory metastatic breast cancer. *Proc. Am. Soc. Clin. Oncol.* **2,** 100.

83. Pitman, S. W., Kowal, C. D., and Bertino, J. R. (1983). Methotrexate 5-fluorouracil in sequence on squamous head and neck cancer. *Semin. Oncol.* **10,** Suppl. 2, 15–19.

84. Plotkin, D., and Waugh, W. J. (1982). Sequential methotrexate 5-fluorouracil (M → F) in advanced breast carcinoma. *Proc. Am. Soc. Clin. Oncol.* **1,** 80.

85. Presant, C. A., Multhauf, P., Klein, L., Chan, C., Chang, F.-F., Hum, G., Opfell, J. R., Lemkin, S., Shiftan, T., and Plotkin, D. (1983). Thymidine and 5-FU: A phase II pilot study in colorectal and breast carcinomas. *Cancer Treat. Rep.* **67,** 735–736.

86. Price, F. (1984). The failure of 5-fluorouracil with high-dose folinic acid to induce meaningful responses in patients with advanced colon cancer and high performance status. *Proc. Am. Soc. Clin. Oncol.* **3,** 132.

87. Rangineni, R. R., Ajani, J. A., Bedikian, A. T., McKelvey, E. M., and Bodey, G. P. (1983). Sequential conventional dose methotrexate (MTX) and 5-fluorouracil (5-FU) in the primary therapy of metastatic colorectal carcinoma. *Proc. Am. Soc. Clin. Oncol.* **2,** 125.

88. Ringborg, U., Ewert, G., Kinnman, J., Lundquist, P. G., and Strander, N. (1983). Sequential methotrexate-5-fluorouracil treatment of squamous cell carcinoma of the head and neck. *Semin. Oncol.* **10,** Suppl. 2, 20–22.

89. Santelli, G., and Valeriote, F. (1978). *In vivo* enhancement of 5-fluorouracil cytotoxicity to AKR leukemia cells by thymidine in mice. *JNCI, J. Natl. Cancer Inst.* **61,** 843–847.

90. Sobrero, A. F., and Bertino, J. R. (1983). Sequence dependent synergism between dichloromethotrexate and 5-fluorouracil in a human colon carcinoma line. *Cancer Res.* **43,** 4011–4103.

91. Solan, A., Vogl, S. E., Kaplan, B. H., Berenzweig, M., Richard, J., and Lanham, R. (1982). Sequential chemotherapy of advanced colorectal cancer with standard or high-dose methotrexate followed by 5-fluorouracil *Med. Pediatr. Oncol.* **10,** 145–149.

91a. Spiegelman, S., Sawyer, R., Nayak, R., Ritzi, E., Stolfi, R., and Martin, D. (1980). Improving the anti-tumor activity of 5-fluorouracil by increasing its incorporation into RNA via metabolic modulation. *Proc. Natl. Acad. U.S.A.* **77,** 4966–4970.

92. Sternberg, A., Petrelli, N. J., Au, J., Rustum, Y., Mittelman, A., and Creaven, P. (1984). A combination of 5-fluorouracil and thymidine in advanced colorectal cancer. *Cancer Chemother. Pharmacol.* **13,** 218–222.

93. Straw, J. A., Szapary, D., and Wynn, W. T. (1984). Pharmacokinetics of diastereoisomers of leucovorin after intravenous and oral administration to normal subjects. *Cancer Res.* **44,** 3114–3119.

94. Tisman, G., and Wu, S. J. G. (1980). Effectiveness of intermediate dose methotrexate and high dose 5-fluorouracil as sequential combination chemotherapy in refractory breast cancer and as primary therapy in metastatic adenocarcinoma of the colon. *Cancer Treat. Rep.* **64,** 829–835.

95. Trave, F., Rustum, Y. M., Mazzoni, A., Petrelli, N., Madajewicz, S., Mittleman, A., and Creaven, P. (1985). Possible effects of high dose 5-formyltetrahydrofolate (dlCF)

on the pharmacokinetics of 5-fluorouracil (FUra) in patients with colorectal carcinoma. *Proc. Am. Soc. Clin. Oncol.* **4,** 30.

96. Ullman, B., Lee, M., Martin, D. W., and Santi, D. V. (1978). Cytotoxicity of 5-fluoro-2'-deoxyuridine: Requirement for reduced folate cofactors and antagonism by methotrexate. *Proc. Natl. Acad. Sci. U.S.A.* **75,** 980–983.

97. Vogel, S. J., Presant, C. A., Ratkin, G. A., and Klahr, C. (1979). Phase I study of thymidine plus 5-fluorouracil infusions in advanced colorectal carcinoma. *Cancer Treat. Rep.* **63,** 1–5.

98. Waxman, S., and Bruckner, H. (1982). Enhancement of 5-fluorouracil antimetabolic activity by leucovorin, menadione and -tocopherol. *Eur. J. Cancer Clin. Oncol.* **18,** 685–692.

99. Weinerman, B., Maroun, J., Stewart, D. J., Bowman, D., Levitt, M., and Schacter, B. (1984). Phase II trial of methotrexate (M) and 5-fluorouracil (F) (M-F) in metastatic colorectal cancer (CRC) II. *Proc. Am. Soc. Clin. Oncol.* **3,** 133.

100. Weinerman, B., Schacter, B., Schipper, H., Bowman, D., and Levitt, M. (1982). Sequential methotrexate and 5-FU in the treatment of colorectal cancer. *Cancer Treat. Rep.* **66,** 1553–1555.

101. Weiss, G. R., Ervin, T. J., Meshad, M. W., and Kufe, D. W. (1982). Phase II trial of combination therapy with continuous-infusion PALA and bolus-injection 5-FU. *Cancer Treat. Rep.* **66,** 299–303.

102. Weiss, G. R., Ervin, T. J., Meshad, M. W., Schade, D., Branfman, A. R., Bruni, R. J., Chadwick, M., and Kufe, D. W. (1982). A phase I trial of combination therapy with continuous-infusion PALA and continuous-infusion 5-FU. *Cancer Chemother. Pharmacol.* **8,** 301–304.

103. Woodcock, T. M., Martin, D. S., Damin, L. A. M., Kemeny, N. E., and Young, C. W. (1980). Combination clinical trials with thymidine and fluorouracil: A phase I and clinical pharmacologic evaluation. *Cancer (Philadelphia)* **43,** 1135–1143.

PART III

Initiation of Cell Differentiation

7

Induction of Cell Differentiation and Bypassing of Genetic Defects in Cancer Therapy

LEO SACHS

Department of Genetics
Weizmann Institute of Science
Rehovot, Israel

I. Introduction

The multiplication and differentiation of normal cells is controlled by different regulatory molecules. These regulators have to interact to achieve the correct balance between cell multiplication and differentiation during embryogenesis and during the normal functioning of the adult individual. The origin and further progression of malignancy results from genetic changes that uncouple the normal balance between multiplication

NEW AVENUES IN DEVELOPMENTAL
CANCER CHEMOTHERAPY

and differentiation so that there are too many growing cells. This uncoupling can occur in various ways (52,54,56,56a). What changes uncouple normal controls so as to produce malignant cells? When cells have become malignant, can malignancy again be suppressed so as to revert malignant back to nonmalignant cells? Malignant cells can have different abnormalities in the controls for multiplication and differentiation. Do all the abnormalities have to be corrected, or can they be bypassed in order to reverse malignancy? These questions can now be answered.

II. Normal Growth Factors and Differentiation Factors

An understanding of the mechanisms that control multiplication (growth) and differentiation in normal cells would seem to be an essential requirement to elucidate the origin and reversibility of malignancy. The development of appropriate cell culture systems has made it possible to identify the normal regulators of growth (growth factors) for various types of cells and also in some cell types the normal regulators of differentiation (differentiation factors). This approach has been particularly fruitful in identifying the normal growth factors for all the different types of hematopoietic cells, first for myeloid cells (36,49,50,52,54,56a) and then for other cell types, including T lymphocytes (38) and B lymphocytes (39). The growth and differentiation factors for hematopoietic cells are different proteins that can be secreted by the cells that produce them. The normal differentiation factors but not the growth factors for myeloid cells are DNA binding proteins (65). It will be interesting to determine how far this applies to normal differentiation factors for other cell types.

In cells of the myeloid series four different growth-inducing proteins have been identified. These are now called macrophage and granulocyte inducers, type 1 (MGI-1), or colony-stimulating factors (CSF) (36,52,54, 57). Of the four growth factors, one protein (M) induces the development of clones with macrophages, another (G) clones with granulocytes, the third (GM) clones with both macrophages and granulocytes, and the fourth (also called interleukin-3, IL-3), clones with macrophages, granulocytes, eosinophils, mast cells, erythroid cells, or megakaryocytes. Cloning of the genes for the IL-3 (16,68) and GM (17) growth factors has shown that these two genes are completely unrelated in their nucleotide sequence. This multigene family represents a hierarchy of growth factors for different stages of hematopoietic cell development as the precursor cells become more restricted in their developmental program. It can be assumed that in the normal developmental program IL-3 functions as a growth factor at an early stage when the precursors have the potential to develop into six cell types, GM functions at a later stage when the precursors have a more limited potential and can develop into two cell types, and that G and M are growth factors when the developmental potential is still more restricted to produce only one cell type. There is presumably also such a hierarchy of growth factors in the developmental program of other types of cells.

How do normal myeloid precursor cells induced to multiply by these growth factors develop into clones that contain mature differentiated cells that stop multiplying when they terminally differentiate? It appears unlikely that a growth factor which induces cell multiplication is also a differentiation factor whose action includes the stopping of cell multiplication in mature cells. Proteins that act as myeloid cell differentiation factors have been identified, and these have been called MGI-2, or differentiation factors (DF) (44,52,54,57,62). Experiments with normal myeloid cell precursors have shown that in these cells the growth factors induce growth (cell viability and multiplication) and also production of differentiation factors (30,31,52,54). The myeloid differentiation factors induce differentiation directly, whereas the growth factors induce differentiation indirectly by inducing the production of differentiation factors (Table I). This induction of differentiation factor by growth factor thus ensures the normal coupling of growth and differentiation, a coupling mechanism that may also apply to other cell types. Differences in the time of the switch-on of the differentiation factor would produce differences in the amount of

TABLE I

Growth Factors and Differentiation Factors in the Development of Myeloid Hematopoietic Cells

Types of factors	Nomenclature	Differentiated cell type	Induction of differentiation	
			Direct	Indirect[a]
Growth factors	MGI-1M = M-CSF	Macrophages	−	+
	MGI-1G = G-CSF	Granulocytes	−	+
	MGI-1GM = GM-CSF	Macrophages and granulocytes	−	+
	IL-3	Macrophages, granulocytes and others	−	+
Differentiation factors	MGI-2 = DF	Myeloid	+	−

[a] Growth factor induces production of differentiation factor.

cell multiplication before differentiation. There is more than one type of differentiation factor (56). Different growth factors may switch on different differentiation factors, which may determine the differentiated cell type. The results thus show that there are different proteins that participate in the developmental program of myeloid cells, growth factors, and differentiation factors, and that growth factors can induce the synthesis of differentiation factors in normal myeloid precursors. In addition to their production by normal myeloid precursors, the differentiation factors can also be produced by some other cell types and can induce differentiation when supplied externally to the target cells (44,52,54,56,57).

III. The Uncoupling of Normal Controls

Identification of these normal growth and differentiation factors and the cells that produce them has made it possible to identify the different types of changes in the production of, or response to, these normal regulators that occur in malignancy. The normal myeloid growth factors can be produced by various cell types. However, these growth factors are not made by the normal myeloid precursors (30,31), so that the normal precursors require an external source of growth factor for cell viability and growth. Cells that become malignant have escaped some normal control, and in myeloid leukemic cells different clones of malignant cells have been identified which have shown the various possible changes that can occur in the normal response to growth and differentiation factors (50,52,54,56,56a). There are different leukemic clones that (1) are independent of the normal growth factor for growth, (2) constitutively produce their own growth factor, (3) are blocked in the ability of the growth factor to induce production of the differentiation factor, (4) are changed in their requirement for the normal growth factor but can still respond normally to the normal differentiation factor, or (5) are defective in their ability to respond to the normal differentiation factor. The cells blocked in the ability of growth factor to induce production of differentiation factor include some cell lines in culture which require an external source of growth factor for growth (30,31). There are thus different ways to uncouple the normal controls of growth and differentiation and different ways for the cells to become malignant. The uncoupling of normal controls and these different ways for the cells to become malignant were associated with changes from an induced to a constitutive expression of certain genes (25,52). The various types of changes that have been found in myeloid leukemic cells can serve as a model system to identify the different changes that can give rise to malignant cells.

Growth factors induce cell viability and cell multiplication. Independence from normal growth factor or constitutive production of their own growth factor can also explain the survival and growth of metastasizing malignant cells in places in the body where the growth factor required for the survival of normal cells is not present. In cells that are malignant and may still need some growth factor, the organ preference of metastasis could be due to production of the required growth factor in the organ in which the metastasis occurs.

The transformation of normal into malignant cells requires a number of genetic changes, and the genes involved in the expression of malignancy are now called "oncogenes" (4,9,24). The changes of normal genes to oncogenes are always associated with changes in the structure or regulation of the normal genes. As in the case of normal genes not all oncogenes have the same function. The *sis* oncogene is derived from the normal genes for platelet-derived growth factor (11,63), the *erb B* oncogene from the gene for the receptor for epidermal growth factor (12), and the *erb A* oncogene from the gene for carbonic anhydrase that is involved in erythroid differentiation (10). The origin and progression of malignancy can involve different genetic changes including changes in gene dosage (49), gene mutations, deletions, and gene rearrangements (24). The different genetic changes in the structure or regulation of the normal genes that control growth and differentiation can thus produce in different ways the uncoupling of normal controls that is required for the origin and further progression of malignancy.

IV. Induction of Differentiation in Malignant Cells by Normal Differentiation Factors

The different types of myeloid leukemic cells include clones that have changed their normal requirement for growth factor and in which growth factor no longer switches on production of differentiation factor but which can still be induced to differentiate to mature nondividing cells by a normal differentiation factor. These clones, which are called D^+ clones (D for differentiation) can be induced to differentiate normally to mature macrophages and granulocytes via the normal sequence of gene expression that occurs during differentiation by incubating the cells with normal differentiation factor (49,50,52,54). The mature cells, which can be formed from all the cells of a leukemic clone, then stop multiplying like normal mature cells and are no longer malignant. The differentiation factor can thus act on these leukemic cells when supplied externally. Experiments carried out in animals have shown that normal differentiation of these myeloid leukemic cells to mature nondividing cells can be induced not only in culture but also in the body (16a,27,29,32,32a,64). These leukemias, therefore, grow progressively when there are too many leukemic cells for the normal amount of differentiation factor in the body. The development of leukemia can be inhibited in mice having these leukemic cells by increasing the normal amount of differentiation factor either by injecting it or by injecting a compound that increases production of differentiation factor by cells in the body (29,32).

The culture of different clones of myeloid leukemic cells in the presence of differentiation factor has shown that in addition to D^+ clones there are also differentiation-defective clones (called D^- clones). Some of these clones were induced to an intermediate stage of differentiation which then slows down the growth of the cells, and others could not be induced to differentiate even to this intermediate stage (49,50,54) (Fig. 1). Since normal differentiation factor can induce differentiation to mature, nondividing cells in the D^+ clones, it can be suggested the D^+ clones are the early stages of leukemia and that the formation of the different types of D^- clones may be later stages in the further progression of malignancy. Does this further progression include complete loss of the genes for differentiation in D^- clones? To answer this, experiments were carried out to determine whether compounds other than normal differentiation factor can induce differentiation in myeloid leukemic cells.

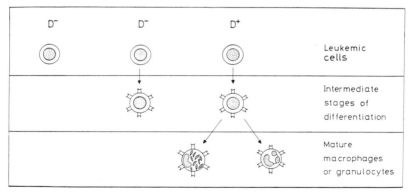

Fig. 1. Classification of different types of clones of myeloid leukemic cells according to their ability to be induced to differentiate by normal differentiation factor. Some differentiation-defective (D^-) clones can be induced by normal differentiation factor to intermediate stages of differentiation, whereas other D^- clones were not induced to differentiate by this factor even to an intermediate stage.

V. Induction of Differentiation in Malignant Cells by Other Compounds

Studies with a variety of chemicals other than normal differentiation-inducing protein have shown that many compounds can induce differentiation in D^+ clones of myeloid leukemic cells. These include certain steroid hormones; chemicals such as cytosine arabinoside, adriamycin, methotrexate; and other chemicals that are used today in cancer chemotherapy. X-Irradiation also induces differentiation (Table II). At high doses both these compounds used in cancer therapy and X-irradiation kill cells, whereas at low doses they can induce differentiation. Not all these compounds are equally active on the same leukemic clone. A variety of chemicals can also induce differentiation in clones that are not induced to differentiate by normal differentiation factor, and in some clones induction of differentiation requires combined treatment with different compounds (50,54,56). The results show that although the response for induction of differentiation by differentiation factor has been altered, the D^- clones have not lost all the genes for differentiation. In addition to certain steroids and chemicals used today in chemotherapy and irradiation, other compounds that can induce differentiation in myeloid leukemic cells include insulin, bacterial lipopolysaccharide, certain plant lectins, and phorbol esters, together with or without differentiation factor (50,56). It is probable that all myeloid leukemic cells no longer susceptible to the normal differentiation factor by itself can be induced to differentiate by the choice of the appropriate combination of compounds.

The ability of a variety of compounds to induce differentiation in malignant cells is not restricted to myeloid leukemic cells. Erythroleukemic cells can be induced to differentiate by various chemicals (15,35). Erythropoietin, a normal protein that induces the production of hemoglobin in normal erythrocytes, did not induce hemoglobin in these erythroleuke-

TABLE II

Compounds Used Today in Cancer Therapy That Can Induce Differentiation in Clones of Myeloid Leukemic Cells at Low Doses

Adriamycin	Methotrexate
Cytosine arabinoside	Mitomycin C
Daunomycin	Prednisolone
Hydroxyurea	X-Irradiation

mias. These erythroleukemias are thus like D^- myeloid leukemias that are not induced to differentiate by the normal myeloid differentiation factor. It has also been shown that some of the compounds that induce differentiation in leukemic cells can induce differentiation in tumors derived from other types of cells (35).

VI. Different Pathways for Inducing Differentiation

Studies on how different compounds act in myeloid leukemic cells have shown that there are different pathways for inducing differentiation. Some compounds induce differentiation by inducing the production of differentiation-inducing protein in the D^+ leukemic cells, whereas others such as the steroid hormones induce differentiation without inducing this protein. Various compounds can also induce differentiation in D^- clones that are not induced to differentiate by normal differentiation factor. Not all clones respond to the same compound, and in some clones differentiation requires combined treatment with more than one compound. Not all compounds act in the same way, and in cases of combined treatment each compound induces changes not induced by the other. The combined treatment then produces, by complementation, the appropriate gene expression that is required for differentiation (50,54,56).

Further evidence that there are different pathways of inducing differentiation in leukemic cells was obtained from studies on changes in the synthesis of cellular proteins in normal myeloid precursors and different types of myeloid leukemic cells (8,25,52). These experiments have shown that there are protein changes that have to be induced in normal cells and are constitutive in leukemic cells. The leukemic cells were found to be constitutive for changes in the synthesis of a group of proteins that were only induced in the normal cells after the addition of growth factor. These protein changes, which include the appearance of some proteins and the disappearance of others, were constitutive in all the leukemic clones studied that were derived from different leukemias. They have been called C_{leuk}, constitutive in leukemia. D^+ leukemic cells can be induced to differentiate to mature cells by normal differentiation factor. This showed that the differentiation program induced by differentiation factor can proceed normally, even when the protein changes induced in normal cells by growth factor have become constitutive. There were other protein changes that were induced by differentiation factor in normal and D^+ leukemic clones but were constitutive in the differentiation-defective D^- leukemic clones. With this group of proteins, the most differentiation-defective clones showed the highest number of constitutive protein changes. These protein changes have been called C_{def}, constitutive in differentiation defective (Fig. 2).

The protein changes during differentiation of normal myeloid precursors are induced as a series of parallel multiple pathways of gene expression. It can be assumed that normal differentiation requires synchronous initiation and progression of these multiple parallel pathways. The presence of constitutive instead of induced gene expression for some pathways can be expected to produce asynchrony in the coordination required for differentiation. Depending on the pathways involved, this asynchrony can then produce blocks in the induction and termination of the differentiation program (8,25,52). D^- leukemic cells can be treated to induce the reversion of C_{def} proteins from the constitutive to the induced state. This reversion was associated with restoration of inducibility for differentiation by the normal differentiation factor. Reversion from constitutive to the induced state in these cells thus restored the synchrony of gene expression that is required for differentiation (60).

The study of different mutants of myeloid leukemic cells has shown that in addition to the existence of constitutive protein changes that inhibit differentiation of myeloid leukemic cells by normal differentiation factor, there are also constitutive protein changes that inhibit differentiation by

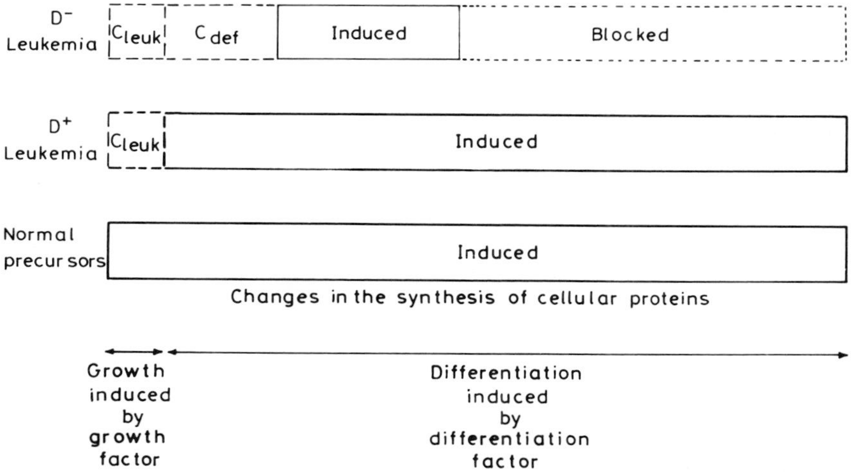

Fig. 2. Schematic summary of changes in the synthesis of cellular proteins associated with growth and differentiation. C_{leuk}, constitutive expression of changes in all the clones of myeloid leukemic cells compared to normal myeloblasts. C_{def}, constitutive expression of changes in differentiation-defective (D^-) clones of leukemic cells compared to differentiation-competent (D^+) leukemic clones and normal myeloblasts. The most differentiation-defective D^- clones (Fig. 1) showed the highest number of C_{def} constitutive protein changes (25).

the steroid hormone dexamethasone. The constitutive changes that inhibit differentiation by dexamethasone are different from those that inhibit differentiation by normal differentiation factor (8). These experiments have thus identified different pathways of gene expression for inducing differentiation and have also shown that genetic changes which block differentiation by one compound need not affect differentiation by another compound that uses alternative pathways. Since the normal differentiation factor for myeloid cells has been identified and leukemic clones have been found that respond to this normal differentiation factor, it was possible to compare the ability of clones of myeloid leukemic cells to be induced to differentiate by the normal inducer and by other compounds. Even though the normal differentiation factors for many other cell types have not yet been identified, it seems likely that the conclusions on the different pathways of inducing differentiation derived from studies with myeloid leukemic cells will also apply to other types of tumors.

VII. Oncogene Suppressors and Bypassing of Genetic Defects in the Reversibility of Malignancy

The change of normal into malignant cells involves a sequence of genetic changes. Evidence has, however, been obtained with various types of tumors including sarcomas (49), myeloid leukemias (49,50), and teratocarcinomas (59), that malignant cells have not lost the genes that control normal growth and differentiation. This was first shown in sarcomas by the finding that it was possible to reverse the malignant to a nonmalignant phenotype with a high frequency in cloned sarcoma cells whose malignancy had been induced by chemical carcinogens, X-irradiation, or by a tumor-inducing virus (45,46,49). In sarcomas induced by chemical carcinogens or X-irradiation, this reversibility of malignancy included reversion to the limited life-span found with normal fibroblasts (47).

Chromosome studies on normal fibroblasts, sarcomas, revertants from sarcomas which had regained a nonmalignant phenotype, and re-revertants showed that the difference between these malignant and nonmalignant cells is controlled by the balance between genes for expression (E) and suppression (S) of malignancy (5,6,18,46,49,67). When there is enough S to neutralize E, malignancy is suppressed, and when the amount of S is not sufficient to neutralize, E malignancy is expressed. These early experiments, (5,6,18,46,49,67) have shown that in addition to genes for expression of malignancy (E) (oncogenes), there are other genes, S genes [that have now been called soncogenes (55) or anti-oncogenes (9a)] that can suppress the action of oncogenes. Suppression of the action of the *Ki-ras* oncogene in revertants (9a, 43) is presumably due to such suppressor genes. The balance between oncogenes and their suppressors also seems to determine malignancy in other tumors, including human retinoblastomas (42).

In the mechanism found with sarcomas (see 49,55) reversion was obtained by chromosome segregation, resulting in a change in gene dosage due to a change in the balance of specific chromosomes. This reversion of malignancy by chromosome segregation, with a return to the gene balance required for expression of the nonmalignant phenotype, occurred without hybridization between different types of cells. The nonmalignant cells were thus derived from the malignant ones by genetic segregation. Reversion of the malignant phenotype associated with chromosome changes has also been found after hybridization between different types of cells (3,13,22,23,48,58). These studies on cell hybrids have led to similar conclusions to those obtained from the reversal of malignancy in sarcomas without hybridisation between different cell types.

In addition to this reversion of malignancy by chromosome segregation, another mechanism of reversion was found in myeloid leukemia. These leukemic cells also have an abnormal chromosome composition (1). In this second mechanism, reversion to a nonmalignant phenotype was also obtained with a higher frequency in certain clones, but this reversion was not associated with chromosome segregation. Phenotypic reversion of malignancy in these leukemic cells was obtained by induction of the normal sequence of cell differentiation by the normal differentiation factor (49,50,52,54). In this reversion of the malignant phenotype, the stopping of cell multiplication by inducing differentiation to mature cells bypasses genetic changes in the requirement for the normal growth factor, and the block in the ability of growth factor to induce differentiation factor, that produced the malignant phenotype. Genetic changes which make cells defective in their ability to be induced to differentiate by the normal differentiation factor occur in the evolution of myeloid leukemia. But even these cells can be induced to differentiate by other compounds, either singly or in combination, that can induce the differentiation program by other pathways (50,52,56). Also in these cases the stopping of cell multiplication by inducing differentiation by these alternative pathways bypasses the genetic changes that block response to the normal differentiation factor. This bypassing of genetic defects if presumably also the mechanism for the reversion of malignancy by inducing differentiation in other types of tumors such as erythroleukemias and neuroblastomas. There is also the possibility that all the oncogenes are lost (14) or that changes of normal genes into oncogenes are actually reversed. Chromo-

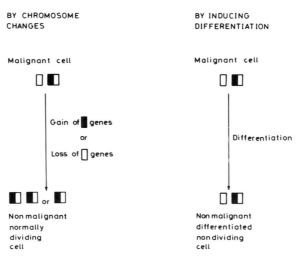

DIFFERENT WAYS OF REVERTING MALIGNANCY

Fig. 3. Malignancy can be suppressed in different ways. (Left) By chromosome changes that change the balance between (□) genes for the expression of malignancy (oncogenes), and (■) genes for the suppression of malignancy (soncogenes or anti-oncogenes). (Right) The stopping of cell multiplication by inducing differentiation to mature cells can bypass genetic changes that produce the malignant phenotype. Chromosome changes can also change malignant cells from D^- to D^+ so that the cells can then be induced to differentiate when exposed to normal differentiation factors.

some changes can also change malignant cells from D^- to D^+ (1) so that the cells can then be induced to differentiate when exposed to normal differentiation factors.

It can therefore be concluded that the change of normal genes into oncogenes that result in the expression of malignancy does not mean that this expression of malignancy cannot again be suppressed. The results on the reversibility of malignancy have shown that there are different ways of reverting malignancy (Fig. 3), that reversion does not have to restore all the normal controls, and that the stopping of cell multiplication by inducing differentiation to mature cells can bypass genetic abnormalities that give rise to malignancy.

VIII. Differentiation Therapy

It has been suggested from these results that the reversibility of malignancy provides new possibilities for therapy (49–51). This is an alternative approach to therapy based on the use of cytotoxic agents which, with the agents used so far, kill many normal cells as well as tumor cells. The reversion of malignancy by correcting genetic abnormalities may be of therapeutic value in the future. However, the therapeutic possibilities of reverting malignancy by inducing differentiation and thus bypassing the genetic abnormalities are already now testable. Results showing that the development of myeloid leukemia can be inhibited in mice with D^+ leukemic cells by injecting the normal differentiation factor or injecting a compound that increases the production of this differentiation factor in the body (29,32) indicate a therapeutic potential for normal differentiation factors. The induction of growth of normal myeloid precursors by myeloid growth factors and their differentiation to macrophages and granulocytes by the differentiation factors also suggest that injection of these factors and the use of compounds that increase their production in the body could be of value in restoring the normal macrophage and granulocyte population after cytotoxic therapy. The use of these factors may also be of value for treating nonmalignant macrophage and granulocyte defects (50,51).

Chemicals and irradiation used today in cancer therapy at high doses to kill cells can induce differentiation in leukemic cells at low doses. Not all these compounds are equally active on the same clone. The existence of differences in the ability of clones to be induced to differentiate may help to explain differences in response to therapy in different patients. The induction of differentiation factors by these compounds may also play a role in the therapeutic effects that can be obtained. As a result of these experiments it has been suggested (50,51) that there could be a form of therapy based on induction of differentiation by using in addition to the normal differentiation factors some of these other compounds, which can also affect mutant malignant cells that are no longer susceptible to the normal differentiation factor. Therapy should include prescreening of the leukemic cells from each patient to select the most effective compounds (28,33), either singly or in combination, and using these compounds at low doses to induce differentiation. Differentiation therapy could also in some cases be combined with cytotoxic therapy to reduce the number of malignant cells. Based on these suggestions some encouraging clinical results with myeloid leukemia have been obtained with low doses of cytosine arabinoside (2,7,19–21,34,37,40,41,61,66), which is one of the compounds that can induce differentiation in myeloid leukemic cells (26,50). Differentiation therapy should also be applicable to tumors derived from other types of cells whose growth and differentiation are controlled by other normal factors.

IX. Summary

Identification of normal growth and differentiation factors and how they interact in normal development has made it possible to identify the mechanisms that uncouple growth and differentiation so as to produce malignant cells. When cells become malignant the malignant phenotype can again be suppressed. Results on the reversibility of malignancy in different types of tumors have shown that in addition to genes for the expression of malignancy (oncogenes), there are other genes (called soncogenes or anti-oncogenes) that can suppress the action of oncogenes; that reversion does not have to restore all the normal controls; and that stopping cell multiplication by inducing differentiation to mature cells can bypass genetic abnormalities that give rise to malignancy. These results have provided new possibilities for cancer therapy.

Acknowledgments

This research is now supported by the National Foundation for Cancer Research, Bethesda, the Julian Wallerstein Foundation, and the Farleigh S. Dickinson, Jr., Foundation.

References

1. Azumi, J., and Sachs, L. (1977). Chromosome mapping of the genes that control differentiation and malignancy in myeloid leukemic cells. *Proc. Natl. Acad. Sci. U.S.A.* **74**, 253–257.
2. Baccarani, M., and Tura, S. (1979). Correspondence. Differentiation of myeloid leukemic cells; new possibilities for therapy. *Br. J. Haematol.* **42**, 485–487.
3. Benedict, W. F., Weissman, B. E., Mark, C., and Stanbridge, E. J. (1984). Tumorigenicity of human HT1080 fibrosarcoma × normal fibroblast hybrids: Chromosome dosage dependency. *Cancer Res.* **44**, 3471–3479.
4. Bishop, J. M. (1983). Cellular oncogenes and retroviruses. *Annu. Rev. Biochem.* **52**, 301–354.
5. Bloch-Shtacher, N., and Sachs, L. (1976). Chromosome balance and the control of malignancy. *J. Cell. Physiol.* **87**, 89–100.
6. Bloch-Shtacher, N., and Sachs, L. (1977). Identification of a chromosome that controls malignancy in Chinese hamster cells. *J. Cell. Physiol.* **93**, 205–212.
7. Castaigne, S., Daniel, M. T., Tilly, H., Herait, P., and Degos, L. (1983). Does treatment with ara-C in low dosage cause differentiation of myeloid leukemic cells? *Blood* **62**, 85–86.
8. Cohen, L., and Sachs, L. (1981). Constitutive gene expression in myeloid leukemia and cell competence for induction of differentiation by the steroid dexamethasone. *Proc. Natl. Acad. Sci. U.S.A.* **78**, 353–357.

9. Cooper, G. M. (1982). Cellular transforming genes. *Science* **218**, 801–806.

9a. Craig, R. W., and Sager, R. (1985). Suppression of tumorogenicity in hybrids of normal and oncogene transformed CHEF cells. *Proc. Natl. Acad Sci. U.S.A.* **82**, 2062–2066.

10. Debuire, B., Henry, C., Benaissa, M., Biserte, G., Claverie, J. M., Saule, S., Martin, P., and Stehelin, D. (1984). Sequencing the *erb* A gene of avian erythroblastosis virus reveals a new type of oncogene. *Science* **224**, 1456–1459.

11. Doolittle, R. F., Hunkapiller, M. W., Hood, L. E., Devare, S. G., Robbins, K. C., Aaronson, S. A., and Antoniades, H. N. (1983). Simian sarcoma virus onc gene, v-sis, is derived from the gene (or genes) encoding a platelet-derived growth factor. *Science* **221**, 275–277.

12. Downward, J., Yarden, Y., Mayers, E., Scrace, G., Totty, N., Stockwell, P., Ulrich, A., Schlessinger, J., and Waterfield, M. D. (1984). Close similarity of epidermal growth factor receptor and v-*erb-B* oncogene protein sequences. *Nature (London)* **307**, 521–527.

13. Evans, E. P., Burtenshaw, M. D., Brown, B. B., Hennion, R., and Harris, H. (1982). The analysis of malignancy by cell fusion. IX. Re-examination and clarification of the cytogenetic problem. *J. Cell. Sci.* **56**, 113–130.

14. Frankel, A. E., Haapala, D. K., Newbouer, R. L., and Fischinger, P. J. (1976). Elimination of the sarcoma genome from murine sarcoma virus transformed cat cells. *Science* **191**, 1264–1266.

15. Friend, C. (1978). The phenomenon of differentiation in murine erythroleukemic cells. *Harvey Lect.* **72**, 253–281.

16. Fung, M. C., Hapel, S. J., Ymer, S., Cohen, D. R., Johnson, R. M., Campbell, H. D., and Young, I. G. (1984). Molecular cloning of cDNA for murine interleukin-3. *Nature (London)* **307**, 233–237.

16a. Gootwine, E., Webb, C. G., and Sachs, L. (1982). Participation of myeloid leukemic cells injected into embryos in haematopoietic differentiation in adult mice. *Nature (London)* **299**, 63–65.

17. Gough, N. M., Gough, J., Metcalf, D., Kelso, A., Grail, D., Nicola, N. A., Burgess, A. W., and Dunn, A. R. (1984). Molecular cloning of cDNA encoding a murine haematopoietic growth regulator, granulocyte-macrophage colony stimulating factor. *Nature (London)* **309**, 763–767.

18. Hitotsumachi, S., Rabinowitz, Z., and Sachs, L. (1971). Chromosomal control of reversion in transformed cells. *Nature (London)* **231**, 511–514.

19. Housset, M., Daniel, M. T., and Degos, L. (1982). Small doses of Ara-C in the treatment of acute myeloid leukemia: Differentiation of myeloid leukemia cells? *Br. J. Haematol.* **51**, 125–129.

20. Ishikura, H., Sawada, H., Okazaki, T., Mochizuki, T., Izumi, Y., Yamagishi, M., and Uchino, H. (1984). The effect of low dose Ara-C in acute non-lymphoblastic leukaemias and atypical leukaemia. *Br. J. Haematol.* **58**, 9–18.

21. Jensen, M. K., and Ahlbom, G. (1985). Low dose cytosine arabinoside in the treatment of acute non-lymphocytic leukaemia. *Scand. J. Haematol.* **34**, 261–263.

22. Kitchin, R. M., Gadi, I. K., Smith, B. L., and Sager, R. (1982). Genetic analysis of tumorogenesis. X. Chromosome studies of transformed mutants and tumor-derived CHEF/18 cells. *Somatic Cell Genet.* **8**, 677–689.

23. Klein, G. (1981). The role of gene dosage and genetic transposition in carcinogenesis. *Nature (London)* **194**, 313–318.

24. Land, H., Parada, L. F., and Weinberg, R. A. (1983). Cellular oncogenes and multistep carcinogenesis. *Science* **222**, 771–778.

25. Liebermann, D., Hoffman-Liebermann, B., and Sachs, L. (1980). Molecular dissection

of differentiation in normal and leukemic myeloblasts: Separately programmed pathways of gene expression. *Dev. Biol.* **79**, 46–63.

26. Lotem, J., and Sachs, L. (1974). Different blocks in the differentiation of myeloid leukemic cells. *Proc. Natl. Acad. Sci. U.S.A.* **71**, 3507–3511.

27. Lotem, J., and Sachs, L. (1978). *In vivo* induction of normal differentiation in myeloid leukemic cells. *Proc. Natl. Acad. Sci. U.S.A.* **75**, 3781–3785.

28. Lotem, J., and Sachs, L. (1980). Potential pre-screening for therapeutic agents that induce differentiation in human myeloid leukemic cells. *Int. J. Cancer* **25**, 561–564.

29. Lotem, J., and Sachs, L. (1981). *In vivo* inhibition of the development of myeloid leukemia by injection of macrophage and granulocyte inducing protein. *Int. J. Cancer* **28**, 375–386.

30. Lotem, J., and Sachs, L. (1982). Mechanisms that uncouple growth and differentiation in myeloid leukemia cells. Restoration of requirement for normal growth-inducing protein without restoring induction of differentiation-inducing protein. *Proc. Natl. Acad. Sci. U.S.A.* **79**, 4347–4351.

31. Lotem, J., and Sachs, L. (1983). Coupling of growth and differentiation in normal myeloid precursors and the breakdown of this coupling in leukemia. *Int. J. Cancer* **32**, 127–134.

32. Lotem, J., and Sachs, L. (1984). Control of *in vivo* differentiation of myeloid leukemic cells. IV. Inhibition of leukemia development by myeloid differentiation-inducing protein. *Int. J. Cancer* **33**, 147–154.

32a. Lotem, J., and Sachs, L. (1985). Control of *in vivo* differentiation of myeloid leukemic cells. V. Regulation by response to antigen. *Leukemia Res.* **9**, 1479–1486.

33. Lotem, J., Berrebi, A., and Sachs, L. (1985). Screening for induction of differentiation and toxicity to blast cells by chemotherapeutic compounds in human myeloid leukemia. *Leuk. Res.* **9**, 249–258.

34. Manoharan, A. (1983). Low dose cytarabine therapy in hypoplastic acute leukemia. *N. Engl. J. Med.* **309**, 1652–1653.

35. Marks, P., and Rifkind, R. A. (1978). Erythroleukemia differentiation. *Annu. Rev. Biochem.* **47**, 419–448.

36. Metcalf, D. (1985). The granulocyte-macrophage colony-stimulating factors. *Science* **299**, 16–22.

37. Michalewicz, R., Lotem, J., and Sachs, L. (1984). Cell differentiation and therapeutic effect of low doses of cytosine arabinoside in human myeloid leukemia. *Leuk. Res.* **8**, 783–790.

38. Mier, J. W., and Gallo, R. C. (1980). Purification and some characteristics of human T-cell growth factor from phytohemagglutinin-stimulated lymphocyte-conditioned media. *Proc. Natl. Acad. Sci. U.S.A.* **77**, 6134–6138.

39. Möller, G., ed. (1984). B cell growth and differentiation factors. *Immunol. Rev.* **78**, 1.

40. Moloney, W. C., and Rosenthal, D. S. (1981). Treatment of early acute nonlymphocytic leukemia with low dose cytosine arabinoside. *Haematol. Bluttransfus.* **26**, 59–62.

41. Mufti, G. J., Oscier, D. G., Hamblin, T. J., and Bell, A. J. (1983). Low doses of cytarabine in the treatment of myelodysplastic syndrome and acute myeloid leukemia. *N. Engl. J. Med.* **309**, 1653–1654.

42. Murphree, A. L., and Benedict, W. F. (1984). Retinoblastoma: Clues to human oncogenesis. *Science* **223**, 1028–1033.

43. Noda, M., Selinger, Z., Scolnick, E. M., and Bassin, R. H. (1983). Flat revertants isolated from Kirsten sarcoma virus-transformed cells are resistant to the action of specific oncogenes. *Proc. Natl. Acad. Sci. U.S.A.* **80**, 5602–5606.

44. Olsson, I., Sarngadharan, M. G., Breitman, T. R., and Gallo, R. C. (1984). Isolation and

characterisation of a T lymphocyte-derived differentiation inducing factor for the myeloid leukemic cell line HL-60. *Blood* **63**, 510–517.

45. Rabinowitz, Z., and Sachs, L. (1968). Reversion of properties in cells transformed by polyoma virus. *Nature (London)* **220**, 1203–1206.

46. Rabinowitz, Z., and Sachs, L. (1970). Control of the reversion of properties in transformed cells. *Nature (London)* **225**, 136–139.

47. Rabinowitz, Z., and Sachs, L. (1970). The formation of variants with a reversion of properties of transformed cells. V. Reversion to a limited life span. *Int. J. Cancer* **6**, 388–398.

48. Ringertz, N. R., and Savage, R. E. (1976). "Cell Hybrids." Academic Press, New York.

49. Sachs, L. (1974). Regulation of membrane changes, differentiation and malignancy in carcinogenesis. *Harvey Lect.* **68**, 1–35, Academic Press, New York.

50. Sachs, L. (1978). Control of normal cell differentiation and the phenotypic reversion of malignancy in myeloid leukemia. *Nature (London)* **274**, 535–539.

51. Sachs, L. (1978). The differentiation of myeloid leukemia cells. New possibilities for therapy. *Br. J. Haematol.* **40**, 509–517.

52. Sachs, L. (1980). Constitutive uncoupling of pathways of gene expression that control growth and differentiation in myeloid leukemia: A model for the origin and progression of malignancy. *Proc. Natl. Acad. Sci. U.S.A.* **77**, 6153–6156.

53. Sachs, L. (1981). Induction of normal differentiation in malignant cells as an approach to cancer therapy. *In* "Molecular Actions and Targets for Cancer Chemotherapeutic Agents" (A. C. Sartorelli, J. S. Lazo, and J. R. Bertino, eds.), pp. 579–589. Academic Press, New York.

54. Sachs, L. (1982). Normal developmental programmes in myeloid leukaemia: Regulatory proteins in the control of growth and differentiation. *Cancer Surv.* **1**, 321–342.

55. Sachs, L. (1984). Normal regulators, oncogenes and the reversibility of malignancy. *Cancer Surv.* **3**, 219–228.

56. Sachs, L. (1985). Regulators of growth, differentiation and the reversion of malignancy. Normal hematopoiesis and leukemia. *In* "Molecular Biology of Tumor Cells," Nobel Conf., (B. Wahren, G. Holm, S. Hammarström, and P. Perlmann, eds.), pp. 257–280. Raven Press, New York.

56a. Sachs, L. (1986). Growth differentiation and the reversal of malignancy. *Scientific American* **254**, 40–47.

57. Sachs, L., and Lotem, J. (1984). Haematopoietic growth factors. *Nature (London)* **312**, 407.

58. Stanbridge, E. J., Der, C. J., Doersen, C.-J., Nishimi, R. Y., Peehl, D. M., Weissman, B. E., and Wilkinson, J. E. (1982). Human Cell Hybrids: Analysis of transformation and tumorigenicity. *Science* **215**, 252–259.

59. Stewart, T. A., and Mintz, B. (1981). Successive generations of mice produced from an established culture line of euploid teratocarcinoma cells. *Proc. Natl. Acad. Sci. U.S.A.* **78**, 6314–6318.

60. Symonds, G., and Sachs, L. (1983). Synchrony of gene expression and the differentiation of myeloid leukemic cells: Reversion from constitutive to inducible protein synthesis. *EMBO J.* **2**, 663–667.

61. Tilly, H., Castaigne, S., Bordessoule, D., Sigaux, F., Daniel, M.-T., Monconduit, M., and Degos, L. (1985). Low-dose cytosine arabinoside treatment for acute nonlymphocytic leukemia in elderly patients. *Cancer* **55**, 1633–1636.

62. Tomida, M., Yamamoto-Kamaguchi, Y., and Hozumi, M. (1984). Purification of a factor inducing differentiation of mouse myeloid leukemic M1 cells from conditioned medium from mouse fibroblast L929 cells. *J. Biol. Chem.* **259**, 10978–10982.

63. Waterfield, M. D., Scrace, G. T., Whittle, N., Stroobant, P., Johnsson, A., Wasteson, A., Westermark, B., Heldin, C. H., Huang, J. S., and Deuel, T. F. (1983). Platelet-derived growth factor is structurally related to the putative transforming protein p28^{sis} of simian sarcoma virus. *Nature (London)* **304,** 35–39.

64. Webb, C. G., Gootwine, E., and Sachs, L. (1984). Developmental potential of myeloid leukemia cells injected into mid-gestation embryos. *Develop. Biol.* **101,** 221–224.

65. Weisinger, G., and Sachs, L. (1983). DNA-binding protein that induces cell differentiation. *EMBO J.* **2,** 2103–2107.

66. Wischz, J. S., Griffin, J. D., and Kuffe, D. W. (1983). Response of preleukemic syndromes to continuous infusion of low-dose cytarabine. *N. Engl. J. Med.* **309,** 1599–1602.

67. Yamamoto, T., Rabinowitz, Z., and Sachs, L. (1973). Identification of the chromosomes that control malignancy. *Nature (London),* New Biol. **243,** 247–250.

68. Yokota, T., Lee, F., Rennick, D., Hall, C., Arai, N., Mosmann, T., Nabel, G., Cantor, H., and Arai, K-I. (1984). Isolation and characterization of a mouse cDNA clone that expresses mast-cell growth-factor activity in monkey cells. *Proc. Natl. Acad. Sci. U.S.A.* **81,** 1070–1074.

The Regulatory Role of Commitment in Gene Expression during Induction of Leukemic Cell Differentiation

ASTERIOS S. TSIFTSOGLOU, JACK HENSOLD,
STEPHEN H. ROBINSON, AND WILLIE WONG

Charles A. Dana Research Institute
Harvard-Thorndike Laboratory
Department of Medicine
Beth Israel Hospital
Harvard Medical School
Boston, Massachusetts

I. Introduction

Acute leukemias are hemopoietic malignancies characterized by clonal expansion of aberrant hemopoietic progenitor cells which self-renew themselves and are unable to differentiate (42,55). These malignant cells,

NEW AVENUES IN DEVELOPMENTAL
CANCER CHEMOTHERAPY

which in many other respects resemble their normal counterparts, have undergone alterations in their developmental program (38) such that they fail to mature and continue to proliferate. The mechanisms by which leukemic cells are maintained at the level of early hemopoietic progenitors are as yet not well understood. Detailed analysis of the events which control hemopoiesis at the cellular and molecular level would lead to a better understanding of the leukemias and may lead to more effective treatment of these disorders.

During the last several years a number of permanent cell lines have been established from murine cells (MEL, ML-1) (16,37) and human leukemic cells (HL-60, K-562, HEL-1, U937, KG-1) (8,29,39,41,64). These have served as models for studying various aspects of hemopoietic malignancies. With some of these cell lines, it has been possible to convert the leukemic cells into cells resembling normal mature hemopoietic cells by treatment with various chemical inducers of differentiation (8,16,48,53) (Fig. 1). The observation that some cultured leukemic cells can differentiate into more than one cell type may allow delineation of how early multipotential hemopoietic progenitors are able to express different phenotypes and how this capacity is impaired in leukemia. The initiation of leukemic cell differentiation by chemical and/or pharmacological agents has supported the view that leukemic development might be a reversible lesion of hemopoietic cell differentiation (54,56) and raises the possibility that such agents may offer a new, noncytotoxic approach to the selective eradication of leukemic cells. *In vivo* studies to test the clinical effective-

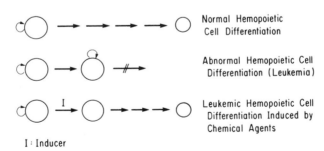

I : Inducer

Fig. 1.   Normal, leukemic, and induced leukemic hemopoietic cell differentiation. Normal early hemopoietic progenitor cells react to known and unknown regulators of growth and differentiation and give rise to mature blood cells. Unlike normal hemopoiesis, in leukemias, transformed early hemopoietic cells remain anaplastic and highly proliferative and fail to differentiate into blood cells. Leukemic cells, however, can be converted into cells resembling normal mature blood cells after treatment with chemical inducers *in vitro*.

ness of chemical inducers such as retinoic acid and hexamethylene-bis-acetamide (HMBA) have already begun.

This chapter will describe cellular and molecular aspects of leukemic cell differentiation and will focus on the regulatory role of commitment in maturation of hemopoietic cells as elucidated by studying the differentiation of murine erythroleukemia (MEL) and human promyelocytic leukemia (HL-60) cells. In addition, the chapter will present similarities and differences concerning the patterns of gene expression on committed proerythroid and myeloid leukemia cells and will explore the potential role of alterations in chromatin structure in leukemic cell differentiation. This information may provide insights regarding the central role of commitment in hemopoietic cell development and leukemic cell growth.

II. Induction of Leukemic Cell Differentiation

A. Differentiation of Murine Erythroleukemia Cells

MEL cells were originally isolated from virus-infected spleen cells (16). These cells are grown in culture and induced to differentiate along the erythrocytic pathway by treatment with various structurally unrelated agents which include polar solvents [dimethyl sulfoxide (DMSO), dimethylformanide (DMF)], butyric acid, antitumor agents (actinomycin D, anthracyclines), purine derivatives, urea and thiourea analogs, bis-acetamides, pyridine derivatives, metabolic inhibitors and antimetabolites, and several other agents including hemin and proteases, as reviewed elsewhere (40,57,70). MEL cells induced to differentiate undergo a series of morphological and biochemical alterations which resemble those occurring during the differentiation of normal proerythroid cells into orthochromatophilic normoblasts; these alterations include, among others, a decrease in cell volume, cell surface alterations, activation of iron-transport and heme biosynthesis, accumulation of globin mRNA, hemoglobin production, expression of erythrocytic antigens and spectrin (10), alterations in nucleoprotein composition, nuclear condensation, and programmed limitation of proliferative capacity (see, for review, 40,57,70). Terminally differentiated cells can extrude their nuclei and give birth to physically unstable reticulocyte-like cells in culture (71,79). Due to a lack of evidence showing differentiation of the MEL cell to a lineage other than erythroid, these cells provide a model system for the analysis of differentiation of unipotent proerythroid cells (22). MEL cell differentiation in response to inducers occurs stochastically (19) (Fig. 2).

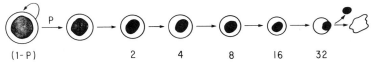

Fig. 2. Differentiation of unipotent murine erythroleukemia cells. MEL cells treated with an inducer commit to terminal maturation stochastically with a given probability *P*. In contrast to uncommitted cells that form large (>32 cells), undifferentiated colonies without hemoglobin when plated in semisolid media, committed cells divide a few times and form colonies of <32 differentiated cells full of hemoglobin (19). Under certain culture conditions, terminally differentiated MEL cells can extrude the nucleus and can produce physically unstable reticulocyte-like cells (72,79).

B. Differentiation of Human Promyelocytic HL-60 Leukemia Cells

The HL-60 cells were originally isolated from the peripheral blood of a patient with acute promyelocytic leukemia (8). These cells are myeloid in nature and can be induced to differentiate into either mature granulocytes (polymorphonuclear leukocytes) by treatment with a variety of chemical agents (i.e., DMSO, retinoic acid, 6-thioguanine, 5-azacytidine, tunicamycin, anthracyclines) (4, 7, 8, 45, 49, 58) or monocyte/macrophage-like cells by incubation with the phorbol ester phorbol-12-myristate-13-acetate (TPA) (26,51), 1a,25-dihydroxyvitamin D_3 (65), or cytosine arabinoside (18). More recent evidence indicates that cultured HL-60 cells can also be converted into eosinophil-like cells by culture and under alkaline conditions (13). In contrast to the unipotent MEL cells, these cells provide a model system with which to study the differentiation of multipotent

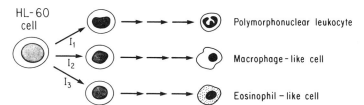

Fig. 3. Differentiation of multipotent HL-60 leukemia cells. HL-60 cells differentiate into either granulocytes (polymorphonuclear leukocytes) when induced with DMSO or retinoic acid (I_1); monocyte- or macrophage-like cells when induced with TPA or 1a,25-dihydroxyvitamin D_3 (I_2), or eosinophilic-like cells when cultured under alkaline conditions (I_3) (see text). Committed cells form colonies of fewer than 32 cells, with differentiated cells widely dispersed due to acquired motility (77). HL-60 cells serve as a model for differentiation of multipotent myeloid cells (14,69).

myeloid progenitor cells (Fig. 3). HL-60 cells undergoing induced differentiation exhibit biochemical and morphological changes similar to those seen during normal granulocyte, macrophage, and/or eosinophil development. The events associated with HL-60 cell differentiation are specific for each phenotype and include irreversible cessation of DNA replication, induction of phagocytic properties, acquisition of migratory capacity, decrease in cell size, condensation of nuclear material, attachment to substratum, changes in cell surface glycoproteins, decrease in transferrin receptor number, decrease in myeloperoxidase activity, expression of nitroblue tetrazolium-(NBT-)reducing activity, increase in O_2^- production, appearance of fibronectin receptors, expression of myeloid antigens, induction of hexose-monophosphate shunt activity, induction of α-naphylacetate esterase activity, secretion of complement, and others as described elsewhere (46,69). As in the case of MEL cells, the differentiating HL-60 cells undergo a programmed loss of proliferative capacity. Terminally differentiated cells fail to renew themselves and to form colonies (12,77) and exhibit a diminished DNA (52) and RNA synthetic activity (77). The gradual loss of proliferative activity and the expression of NBT-reducing activity during HL-60 cell maturation are shown in Fig. 4.

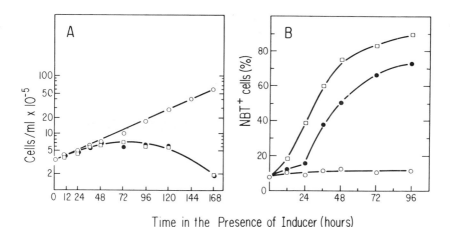

Time in the Presence of Inducer (hours)

Fig. 4. Alterations in cell growth and kinetics of accumulation of NBT$^+$-positive cells in HL-60 cell cultures treated with DMSO or retinoic acid. HL-60 cells were incubated in liquid culture with no drug, DMSO (1.5% v/v) or retinoic acid (RA) (2 μM). At various times, duplicate samples (0.1 ml) of the cell suspension were removed, counted in a Coulter counter, and examined for the ability to reduce NBT dye. (A) Cell growth of control (O———O), DMSO-treated (●———●), and retinoic acid–treated (□———□) cells. (B) Accumulation of NBT-positive cells in control (O———O), DMSO-treated (●———●), and retinoic acid–treated (□----□) cells. [From Tsiftsoglou et al. (77).]

III. Commitment to Maturation: Clonal and Biochemical Assessment

Time-course studies have indicated that exposure of MEL cells to an inducer is followed by biochemical and cellular events, some of which occur immediately, and others at a later time (70). Both the onset and maintenance of the early events depend on the continuous presence of the inducer in the culture medium. Upon removal of the inducer, the early events revert rapidly. Longer exposure of cells to the inducer leads to permanent changes which proceed to completion of the differentiation program in the absence of the inducer. These observations indicate that MEL cell differentiation is characterized by unstable early and stable late processes separated from each other by a critical event which occurs concurrently with an irreversible decision to mature.

A detailed analysis of these early and late events requires precise determination of the kinetics of differentiation at the level of individual cells. Clonal analysis in which cells are removed from culture and plated in secondary, inducer-free cultures has allowed determination of the proportion of cells entering the differentiation pathway well before these cells express the differentiated phenotype (11,19), which is characterized by a limitation of proliferative capacity, nuclear condensation, and synthesis of hemoglobin, as shown in Fig. 5.

Committed MEL and HL-60 cells exposed to the inducer DMSO and subsequently plated in drug-free plasma clots form small colonies (<32 cells) of differentiated cells expressing erythroid and myeloid markers, respectively. In contrast to MEL cells which form compact colonies composed of hemoglobinized differentiated cells (19), the colonies derived from differentiating HL-60 cells are composed of mature NBT-positive cells which are widely dispersed due to the acquisition of migratory capacity and loss of intercellular attachment (77).

Biochemical characterization has indicated that the majority of the early reversible events occurring in MEL cell differentiation appear to be membrane-mediated processes (i.e., ion transport changes, alterations in cell surface architecture) (63,70) whose function is necessary but not sufficient to promote commitment. In contrast, most if not all of the irreversible changes appear to be metabolic events (cessation of DNA replication and transcription, changes in nucleoprotein composition) that contribute to gradual nuclear condensation and accumulation or disappearance of specific proteins. How the early unstable processes are linked to commitment and how commitment leads to an irreversible, terminally differentiated state is unknown. Experiments which used metabolic inhibitors and membrane-active agents of known function (24,25) have sug-

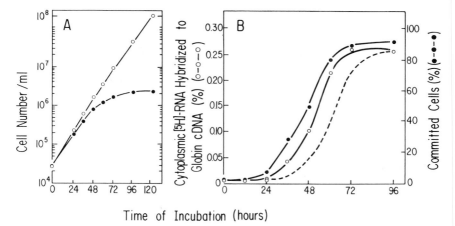

Fig. 5. Kinetics of cell growth, commitment, and rate of globin mRNA accumulation in MEL cells exposed continuously to DMSO. MEL cells were incubated in the presence of DMSO (1.5% v/v) at a concentration of 3×10^4 to 3×10^5 cells/ml. At various times during incubation, cell number was determined and clonal analysis of committed cells was performed. In parallel, cells were labeled with 50 μCi/mmol [³H]uridine (specific activity, 21 Ci/mmole) for 2 hr. Labeled RNA was prepared at each time point and was hybridized to an excess of globin cDNA-oligo(dT)-cellulose. Plasma clot clonal analysis of commitment, preparation of [³H]RNA, and hybridization with globin cDNA were carried out as described elsewhere (72). (A) Cell growth of control (O——O) and DMSO-treated (●——●) cells. (B) Proportion of committed cells (●——●); proportion of cytoplasmic [³H]RNA hybridized to mouse globin cDNA (O——O). The dashed line (- - -) indicates an accumulation of hemoglobin in differentiating MEL cells, as determined spectrophotometrically (72). [From Tsiftsoglou *et al.* (72); Tsiftsoglou and Wong (70).]

gested that a number of distinguishable processes operate at various levels during differentiation. The patterns by which these several processes are coordinated appear to be complex. The finding that an inhibitor such as dexamethasone erases "memory response" and blocks initiation of commitment without abrogating all of the early events (e.g., cell size alterations) of MEL cell differentiation (75) argues against a sequential pattern of coordination. Furthermore, analysis of MEL cells exposed to both DMSO and cycloheximide [CH, an inhibitor of protein synthesis (32)] and/or cordycepin [CD, 3'deoxyadenosine, an inhibitor of mRNA synthesis and RNA methylation (30,35) indicated that at least two discrete processes acting in parallel rather than sequentially occur just prior to, or at the time of, commitment (25). One appears to be a protein synthesis–dependent function that acts in a rate-limiting manner (32) and slowly builds up as a quite stable component. The other process(es) that is sensitive to CD acts rapidly at the time of commitment and can synchronize the commitment event in an MEL cell population undergoing maturation (25,35). Inhibition of the CD-sensitive event does not inhibit the CH-sensitive process. This information is consistent with a model of parallel processes described elsewhere (70). It may be possible, however, that the developmental program of MEL cells comprises initial parallel processes which are linked to a series of sequential rapidly acting events undetectable by current methodology. The information presented thus far refers to commitment of MEL cells. It remains to be seen whether commitment in HL-60 cells follows a similar pattern.

Discontinuous exposure of MEL cells to DMSO has shown that inducer-treated cells subsequently deprived of, and then rechallenged with, inducer several hours later commit immediately. This suggests that inducer-treated cells acquire a "memory response" during the first exposure to inducer, which allows them to initiate differentiation without a significant lag (33). "Memory response" that has been initiated by one inducer can be continued by other inducers, independent of the structural features of the second inducer (A. S. Tsiftsoglou, unpublished observations). Expression of memory response may play an important role in initiation of both commitment and cytoplasmic accumulation of mRNA and for maintenance of globin mRNA levels in differentiating cells. In a typical "memory experiment" presented elsewhere (24), both commitment and accumulation of globin mRNA were interrupted when the inducer was removed from culture and began to increase simultaneously again when cells were re-exposed to the inducer. Erasure of "memory response" by inhibitors of commitment such as CH, CD (34), and dexamethasone (75), a steroid hormone with repressing action on initiation of transcription of globin genes (43), suggests that "memory response" may be carried by a macromolecule whose synthesis and stability is a pivotal part of the differentiation program.

In both the differentiation systems studied, MEL and HL-60 cells, it has been shown that commitment to terminal maturation is closely associated with expression of differentiation markers such as enzymatic activities, cell surface antigens, and a variety of other types of molecules characteristic of the differentiated phenotype. In most of these studies, it has been difficult to delineate whether the expression of the differentiation markers is an integral part of the commitment process or if commitment and expression of differentiation markers are independent from each other. The finding that hemin, an agent that activates globin mRNA synthesis, does not cause commitment as determined by clonal analysis in both mouse and human erythroleukemia K-562 cells (20,53) first suggested that expression of erythroid markers may not necessarily be linked to commitment to terminal maturation. Further experiments with imidazole, which is a potent inhibitor of hemoglobin accumulation but does not block commitment and cessation of proliferation in MEL cells (21), suggested that hemoglobin synthesis is regulated independently of commitment; that is, there are at least two distinguishable subprograms in erythroid cell maturation (70). One is responsible for activating iron uptake, heme biosynthesis, and hemoglobin synthesis, and the other for commitment (76). The former program may be related to the polarization of the mitochondrial membranes whose function appears to play an important role in heme synthesis (81).

IV. Gene Expression Patterns in Committed MEL and HL-60 Cells

Studies with MEL and HL-60 cells indicate that commitment is a central process in hemopoietic cell differentiation. It may perhaps occur independently of the expression of erythroid (e.g., hemoglobin) and presumably myeloid markers (e.g., NBT-reducing activity, cell surface myeloid antigens) and controls the programmed proliferative limitation of leukemic cells as they mature. Characterization of specific events that occur at or shortly after commitment would represent an important step toward understanding the molecular basis of the commitment process. During differentiation of MEL and HL60 cells into orthochromatophilic normoblasts and granulocytes, respectively, a number of gene products (i.e., proteins) accumulate selectively (e.g., IP-25 or H1 nucleoprotein, spectrin, and hemoglobin in MEL cells; myeloid antigens and 60K nucleoprotein in HL-60 cells), whereas others disappear (69,70). These include several membrane proteins, enzymes, nucleoproteins, and proteins of unknown function. Meanwhile, the nucleus becomes progressively pyknotic, and in the case of polymorphonuclear maturation of the HL-60 cells, segmented. The appearance of new proteins and the disappearance of others which are associated with commitment (e.g., IP-25) indicate that the transcriptional activity of both MEL and HL-60 leukemic cells is altered during differentiation. It is reasonable, then, to propose that some of the alterations in protein makeup reflect changes in the transcription of genes during commitment and that commitment may be responsible for "switching on" or "turning off" gene activity during hemopoietic development. It is also possible that some of the changes in protein composition seen in committed cells may result from altered RNA processing and mRNA stability (78).

A fruitful approach in analyzing which genes are selectively controlled in committed cells is to expose cells to an inducer and to analyze the cellular RNA for transcripts levels by RNA blotting hybridization with ^{32}P-labeled, cloned DNA fragments coding for proteins with a demonstrable role in the regulation of cell proliferation. By carrying out such an analysis, we observed that commitment of MEL cells along the erythroid lineage is temporally correlated with globin mRNA accumulation and transcriptional inactivation of ribosomal DNA sequences coding for rRNAs (74). By following a similar approach, the pattern of expression of the *c-myc* and *p53* genes, which have a potential role in cell proliferation (68) and possibly in differentiation as well (2,61), was studied in committed MEL cells (23). As shown in Fig. 6, *c-myc* transcripts were detected in MEL cells unexposed to DMSO. Following exposure to DMSO for about 2 hr, the level of *c-myc* transcripts declined markedly and then increased again to a level comparable to that of control cells after 18–24 hr, a time that roughly corresponds with the onset of commitment in these cells. A progressive decrease in *c-myc* mRNA level occurred at a later time as the proportion of committed cells increased toward a maximum value. A similar biphasic pattern of expression was observed for *p53* gene transcripts (Fig. 6). DMSO-noninducible cells did not demonstrate the biphasic decrease in the level of either *c-myc* or *p53* transcripts that was seen in inducible cells (data not shown). These noninducible cells exhibited only

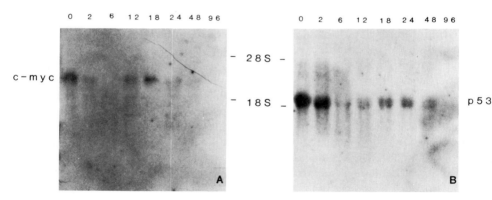

Fig. 6. Kinetics of cytoplasmic accumulation of *c-myc* and *p53* RNA transcripts in DMSO-inducible MEL Cells. MEL cells were incubated with or without DMSO (1.5 v/v). At time intervals indicated above each figure (in hours), total cytoplasmic RNA was prepared, separated electrophoretically on an agarose gel, transferred onto a nitrocellulose filter, and hybridized with either ^{32}P-labeled 1.7-kilobase (kb) *Eco*RI-Cla DNA fragment containing cloned human 3′ end *c-myc* DNA sequences (9) or ^{32}P-labeled 560-kb cDNA of mouse *p53* DNA sequences (1). The resulting autoradiograms of *c-myc* (B) and *p53* (A) RNA transcripts are shown. The positions of 28S and 18S rRNA are also indicated. [From Hensold *et al.* (23).

the initial but not the later, permanent decline in the accumulation of the *c-myc* transcripts. The *p53* mRNA levels did not decline at all following DMSO exposure of these cells. These results are consistent with those of Lachman and Skoultchi (31), who observed a biphasic pattern of repression of *c-myc* in inducer-treated MEL cells, and the results of others (2,61), who observed a decrease in *p53* protein in differentiating MEL cells. The observation that the expression of *c-myc* and *p53* genes is related to commitment to terminal maturation was further supported by analysis of *c-myc* and *p53* mRNA levels in hemin-treated MEL cells which fail to commit to maturation despite their capacity to accumulate large quantities of globin mRNA (23). To demonstrate whether the changes observed in *c-myc* and *p53* transcript levels were closely associated with changes in the proliferative status of the cells, DMSO-inducible and DMSO-uninducible MEL cells were exposed to DMSO, and the cell cycle distribution was recorded cytofluorographically using a fluorescent DNA-binding dye, propidium iodide. Exposure of inducible cells to DMSO led to a progressive arrest of cells in the G_1 (or G_0) phase of the cell cycle. However, no early changes in cell cycle distribution were recorded concomitant with the early declines in *c-myc* and *p53* transcript levels. DMSO treatment of the noninducible cells did not alter cell cycle distribution or did not result in the late decrease in *p53* transcripts (23), further demonstrating the relationship between the terminally differentiated state and the decrease in activity of these two growth-regulatory genes.

To determine whether initiation of commitment plays a regulatory role in gene expression in HL-60 cells that undergo a similar cell cycle arrest upon differentiation and to define differences and similarities between the patterns of gene expression in these two cell lines, we performed the following experiment. HL-60 cells were exposed to retinoic acid, DMSO, and/or TPA, and the level of expression of ribosomal DNA sequences, *c-myc*, and *β-actin* genes was determined. The former two genes appear to have a demonstrable role in control of cell growth, whereas the *β-actin* gene is involved in cytoskeleton functions which are induced during HL-60 cell differentiation (3). Our hypothesis was that the activity of these genes might change transcriptionally during commitment of HL-60 cells when the ability of cells to divide and migrate is dramatically changed. These studies have shown that commitment of HL-60 cells toward the granulocytic pathway induced by DMSO is accompanied by a gradual decline in the transcription of the ribosomal genes (77) and a marked suppression of the accumulation of *c-myc* mRNA, as shown in Fig. 7. A substantial decline of the amplified *c-myc* gene was also observed during TPA-induced macrophage maturation of HL-60 cells (Figs. 7,8). The repression of *c-myc* in TPA-treated cells exhibits a pattern different from

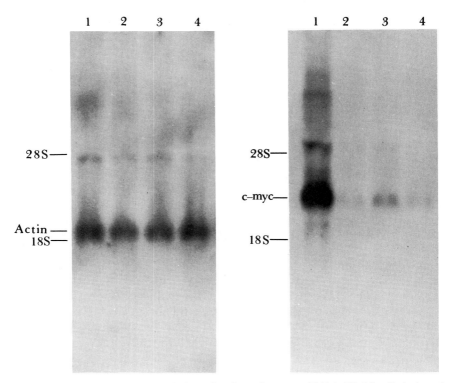

Fig. 7. Cytoplasmic accumulation of actin and *c-myc* mRNA in HL-60 cells induced to differentiate with DMSO, retinoic acid (RA), or TPA. Samples of 20 μg of total RNA prepared from untreated (lane 1), RA- (2 μM) (lane 2), DMSO- (1.5% v/v) (lane 3), or TPA-treated (0.1 μM) (lane 4) HL-60 cells for 96 hr were used for RNA blotting hybridization analysis (67). Hybridization probes were ^{32}P-labeled DNA fragments as follows: (Right) The *Eco*RI-Cla 1.7-kb DNA fragment derived from a human *c-myc* gene containing recombinant plasmid (9). (Left): The *Pst*I-*Hind*III 2.15-kb DNA fragment derived from chicken α-actin gene containing recombinant plasmid that hybridizes to human β-actin gene under certain conditions (59°C). The resulting autoradiograms and the migration pattern of both 28S and 18S rRNA are shown.

that observed in differentiating MEL cells (see Fig. 6). This decline in *c-myc* mRNA accumulation appears to follow that of rRNA synthesis, and we have most recently observed the pattern of repression of the transferrin receptor gene in HL-60 cells undergoing granulocytic and macrophage maturation (A. S. Tsiftsoglou, S. H. Robinson, J. Hensold, A. McClelland, F. Ruddle, and W. Wong, unpublished observations). Exposure of HL-60 cells to any inducer (DMSO, retinoic acid, or TPA) leads to no substantial alterations in the level of expression of β-actin genes during granulocytic and/or macrophage maturation of HL-60 cells (Figs. 7, 9).

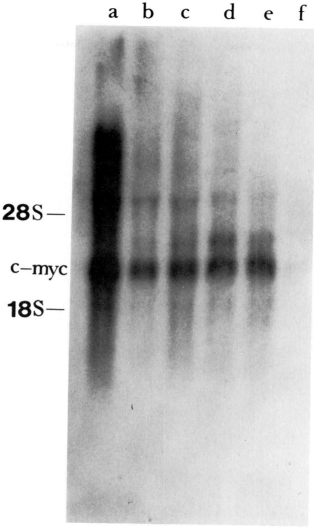

Fig. 8. Time-dependent *c-myc* mRNA accumulation in TPA-treated HL-60 cells. Samples of total RNA (20 μg) prepared from control (unexposed) (lane a: 0 hr) and cells exposed to TPA (1×10^{-7} *M*) for 4 (lane b), 10 (lane c), 20 (lane d), 36 (lane e), and 78 hr (lane f) of incubation were electrophoretically separated in an agarose/formaldehyde denaturing gel, transferred onto nitrocellulose filter, and hybridized with ^{32}P-labeled *Eco*RI-Cla 1.7-kb 3' end fragment of human *c-myc* DNA sequences, as described previously (9). The positions of the 28S and 18S rRNAs are indicated in the resulting autoradiograms.

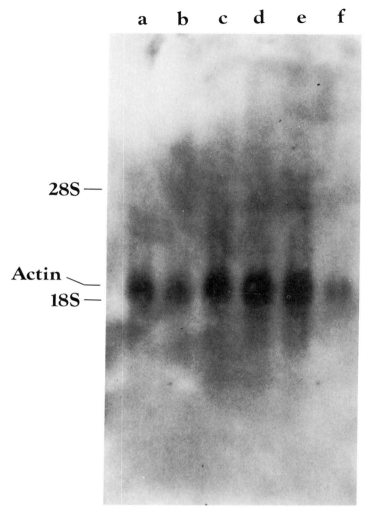

Fig. 9. Time-dependent accumulation of actin mRNA in TPA-treated HL-60 cells. Samples (20 μg) of total RNA extracted from TPA-treated cells, separated on an agarose gel, and transferred on a nitrocellulose filter, were hybridized with a ³²P-labeled *Pst*I-*Hind*III 2.15-kb DNA fragment derived from a chicken α-actin gene containing recombinant plasmid. This cloned fragment shares a significant degree of homology with human β-actin gene. The resulting autoradiograms are shown. The letter above each lane indicates the time point at which RNA was extracted from HL-60 cells. Lanes a, b, c, d, e, and f correspond to 0, 4, 10, 20, 36, and 78 hr of incubation.

These data indicate that commitment of HL-60 cells is associated with a similar pattern of repression of the ribosomal DNA sequences but a quite different pattern of repression of *c-myc* genes as compared to that of MEL cells. The lack of substantial alterations in the expression of actin genes in committed HL-60 cells indicates that the regulation of actin genes may not be an integral part of the commitment program.

V. Initiation of Commitment and Chromatin Structure

Despite the plethora of information concerning the kinetics of commitment in the MEL and HL-60 differentiation systems, the molecular basis of commitment remains elusive. Studies with various inhibitors of commitment (cycloheximide, dexamethasone, amiloride, procaine, cordycepin) (6,25) suggest that initiation of commitment is a very complex process which is regulated at several levels. Initiation of commitment and its relationship to cell cycle may differ among the hemopoietic progenitor cells; for example, evidence exists to indicate that commitment in HL-60 cells may be initiated at the S or S/G_2 interphase of the cell cycle (82), despite available evidence suggesting that HL-60 cell differentiation may not be linked to DNA replication and cellular division (52,66). In MEL cells, commitment occurs later and appears to be initiated within the first cell cycle, presumably at the G_1 or G_1/S interphase (17), although lengthening of G_1 during MEL cell differentiation does not strictly correlate with differentiation of these cells (15). It is possible that these differences in initiation, maintenance, and progression of commitment to maturation may be related to the developmental history of MEL and HL-60 cells, that is, to the unipotent and multipotent nature of these cells. Experiments in MEL cells have suggested that initiation of commitment depends on membrane-mediated events (such as Ca^{2+} uptake) (5,36,63,73) which may result in signals inside the nuclear compartment for activation and repression of gene activity. This may occur by trans-acting factors which recognize altered chromatin structure in committed cells and lead to sequential nuclear events such as transcription, nuclear condensation, and other events leading to maturation.

The structure–activity relationships of the chemical inducers used in cell differentiation of MEL cells have not defined unique structural features required for initiation of commitment. This lack of information makes the search for possible mechanisms of initiation of commitment quite difficult. Recent information on the structure of chromatin in committed cells has begun to shed some light into how commitment is related to transcription of several genes involved in hemoglobin synthesis and terminal maturation.

Progressive nuclear condensation and subsequent irreversible cessation of DNA replication together with other nuclear events (i.e., RNA synthesis, alterations in nucleoproteins) (57) are the most prominent events occurring in terminally differentiated cells. Digestion of nuclei isolated from both control (unexposed) and DMSO-induced MEL cells with DNAse I (44) and electrophoretic examination of the DNA pattern did not reveal substantial alterations in gross chromatin structure during initiation, progression, and completion of MEL cell maturation. A more effective approach which allows identification of alterations occurring at specific sites within chromatin indicated that changes in chromatin structure do occur during commitment. MEL cells exposed to inducers like HMBA exhibited an altered pattern in DNAse I–hypersensitive (59,62) and micrococcal nuclease- (MNase-)hypersensitive sites of globin DNA sequences (83). In particular, HMBA treatment increases DNAse I hypersensitivity of sequences located 5′ upstream from the cap sites of both α and β^{maj} globin genes and within the second intron (IVS_2) of the β^{maj} globin DNA sequences (59,60). Since such changes have not been observed in HBMA-noninducible cells (60), and since these changes in DNAse I–hypersensitive sites are blocked by the commitment inhibitor dexamethasone (27,62) and not by imidazole (83), potent abrogator, of hemoglobin synthesis, they are considered to be part of the commitment processes. According to Yu and Smith (83) an increase in DNAse I hypersensitivity precedes aquisition of MNase hypersensitivity in committed cells. These sequential alterations indicate that upon commitment, chromatin undergoes sequential changes which may be essential for terminal maturation and β-globin gene activation. How acquisition of increased DNAse I hypersensitivity is related to initiation of commitment and gene activation and/or repression is not clear. It is reasonable to assume that structural changes of chromatin might be recognized by diffusible trans-acting molecules which are induced during commitment and exert a regulatory role on gene expression by interaction with the genome.

The detection of DNA fragments in differentiating MEL cells by several investigators has attracted considerable interest in recent years (see review by Scher *et al.* (57). Although the precise role of this DNA strand scission remains obscure and its role as an important event in differentiation has been reconsidered (50), somatic cell hybrid studies (47) suggest that DNA fragmentation might be one of the major events of MEL cell maturation. These studies with fused, ultraviolet-irradiated BHK and nonirradiated BHK cells and DMSO-treated MEL cells suggested that two crucial events cooperate in the initiation of differentiation. One of these appears to be an ultraviolet-inducible, trans-acting (a) factor and the other a cis-element induced at the level of the chromatin of DMSO-treated cells.

VI. Concluding Remarks

Studies over the last several years have shown that leukemic cells of erythroid and myeloid origin can be induced to differentiate into cells resembling mature blood cells. Inducer-treated cells commit to maturation irreversibly within the first cell cycle. Commitment, the process by which an irreversible decision for maturation is made, appears to be a complex process regulated at several levels. Commitment is closely coordinated with the expression of differentiation markers and leads to a programmed loss of proliferative capacity and nuclear maturation, which are characterized by cessation of DNA replication, selective transcription of DNA sequences, and alterations in chromatin structure. Inhibition of initiation of commitment by agents with known mechanism(s) of action, such as dexamethasone, cycloheximide, cordycepin, procaine, and amiloride, indicates that several distinguishable processes occur prior to or at the time of commitment. One of these appears to be dependent on new protein synthesis and is an event required for the expression of "memory response" (the ability of inducer-treated cells to remember previous exposure to inducer). Another acts rapidly at commitment and is sensitive to cordycepin (3'-deoxyadenosine), an inhibitor of RNA synthesis and methylation. Initiation of commitment is causally related to alterations in the expression of the ribosomal DNA sequences, the protooncogene c-myc, the p53 gene, and the transferrin-receptor gene. Comparison of the patterns of gene expression in committed mouse proerythroid MEL and human myeloid HL-60 cells suggests that initiation of commitment leads to different patterns of expression of c-myc in these two types of hemopoietic cells. Commitment in HL-60 cells does not result in substantial alterations in the expression of the actin gene, despite the aquisition of migratory ability and altered cytoskelton functions in differentiating cells. This finding is consistent with the view that commitment can be dissociated from the expression of specific differentiative events such as hemoglobin synthesis in the case of MEL cells. The time point in the cell cycle when commitment is initiated in MEL and HL-60 cells is not precisely known. Experiments with synchronized MEL and HL-60 cells indicate that commitment may not be initiated at the same time in both cell systems. Commitment to maturation has been found to be causally related to sequential alterations in chromatin structure. These are characterized by acquisition of hypersensitive regions, as elucidated by micrococcal nuclease and/or DNAse I digestion of the nuclei and subsequent DNA blotting hybridization analysis. The possible mechanisms by which commitment is initiated are discussed.

Acknowledgments

This work was supported by USPHS grants AM17148 and CA 37727 and a grant by the American Cancer Society, Massachusetts Division. Dr. Hensold is the recipient of USPHS Physician-Scientist Award AM01392. Dr. Tsiftsoglou is a recipient of an American Cancer Society Junior Faculty Research Award.

Note Added in Proof

Most recently, it has been reported (Nomura, S., Yamagoe, S., Kamiya, T., and Oishu, M. (1986). *Cell* **44**, 663–669) that MEL cells contain an intracellular factor which when injected into cells shortly treated with DMSO promotes substantial degree of erythroid maturation.

References

1. Benchimol, S., Jenkins, J. R., Crawford, L. V., Leppard, K., Lamp, P., Williamson, N. M., Pim, D. C., and Harlow, E. (1984). Molecular analysis of the gene for the p53 cellular tumor antigen. *Cancer Cells* **2**, 383–391.
2. Ben-Dori, R., Resnitzki, D., and Kimchi, A. (1983). Reduction in p53 synthesis during differentiation of Friend erythroleukemia cells: Correlation with the commitment to terminal cell division. *FEBS Lett.* **162**, 384–389.
3. Bernal, S. D., and Chen, L. D. (1982). Induction of cytoskeleton-associated proteins during differentiation of human myeloid leukemia cell lines. *Cancer Res.* **42**, 5106–5116.
4. Breitman, J. R., Selonick, S. E., and Collins, S. J. (1980). Induction of differentiation of the human promyelocytic cell line HL-60 by retinoic acid. *Proc. Natl. Acad. Sci. U.S.A.* **77**, 2936–2940.
5. Bridges, K., Levenson, R., Housman, D., and Cantley, L. (1981). Calcium regulates the commitment of murine erythroleukemia cells to terminal erythroid differentiation. *J. Cell Biol.* **90**, 542–544.
6. Chen, Z. X., Banks, J., Rifkind, R. A., and Marks, P. A. (1982). Inducer-mediated commitment of murine erythroleukemia cells to differentiation: A multistep process. *Proc. Natl. Acad. Sci. U.S.A.* **79**, 471–475.
7. Christman, J. K., Menselsohn, N., Hersog, D., and Schneiderman, N. (1983). Effect of 5-aza-cytidine on differentiation and DNA metabolism in human promyelocytic leukemia (HL-60) cells. *Cancer Res.* **43**, 763–769.
8. Collins, S. J., Ruscetti, F. W., Gallanger, R. E., and Gallo, R. C. (1978). Terminal differentiation of human promyelocytic leukemia cells induced to dimethylsulfoxide and other polar compounds. *Proc. Natl. Acad. Sci. U.S.A.* **75**, 2458–2462.

9. Dalla-Favera, R., Gelman, E. P., Marinotti, S., Franchini, G., Papas, T. S., Gallo, R. C., and Wong-Staal, F. (1982). Cloning and characterization of different human sequences related to the *onc* gene (v-myc) of avian myelocytomatosis virus (MC29). *Proc. Natl. Acad. U.S.A.* **79,** 6497–6501.

10. Eisen, H., Bach, R., and Emery, R. (1977). Induction of spectrin in erythroleukemia cells transformed by Friend virus. *Proc. Natl. Acad. Sci. U.S.A.* **74,** 3898–3902.

11. Fibach, E., Reuben, R., Rifkind, R. A., and Marks, P. A. (1977). Effect of hexamethylene-bis-acetamide on the commitment to differentiation of murine erythroleukemia cells. *Cancer Res.* **37,** 440–444.

12. Fibach, E., Leled, T., and Rachmilewitz, E. A. (1982). Self-renewal and commitment to differentiation of human leukemic promyelocytic cells (HL-60). *J. Cell. Physiol.* **113,** 152–158.

13. Fischkoff, S. A., Pollack, A., Gleich, G. J., Testa, J. R., Misawa, S., and Reber, T. J. (1984). Eosinophilic differentiation of the human promyelocytic leukemic cell line HL-60 cells. *J. Exp. Med.* **160,** 179–196.

14. Fontana, J. A., Colbert, D. A., and Deisseroth, A. B. (1981). Identification of a population of bipotent stem cells in the HL-60 human promyelocytic leukemia cell line. *Proc. Natl. Acad. Sci. U.S.A.* **78,** 3863–3866.

15. Friedman, E. A., and Schildkraut, C. L. (1978). Lengthening of the G_1 phase is not strictly correlated with differentiation in Friend erythroleukemia cells. *Proc. Natl. Acad. Sci. U.S.A.* **75,** 3813–3817.

16. Friend, C., Scher, W., Holland, J., and Sato, T. (1971). Hemoglobin synthesis in murine erythroleukemia cells *in vitro:* Stimulation of erythroid differentiation by dimethysulfoxide. *Proc. Natl. Acad. Sci. U.S.A.* **68,** 378–382.

17. Geller, R., Levenson, R., and Housman, D. (1978). Significance of the cell cycle in commitment of murine erythroleukemia cells to erythroid differentiation. *J. Cell. Physiol.* **95,** 213–222.

18. Griffin, J., Munroe, D., Major, P., and Kufe, D. (1982). Induction of differentiation of human myeloid leukemia cells by inhibition of DNA synthesis. *Exp. Hematol.* **10,** 774–781.

19. Gusella, J. F., Geller, R., Clarke, B., Weeks, V., and Housman, D. (1976). Commitment to erythroid differentiation by Friend erythroleukemia cells: A stochastic analysis. *Cell (Cambridge, Mass.)* **9,** 221–229.

20. Gusella, J. F., Weil, S., Tsiftsoglou, A. S., Volloch, V., Newman, J. R., Keys, C., and Housman, D. (1980). Hemin does not cause commitment of murine erythroleukemia cells to terminal differentiation. *Blood* **56,** 481–487.

21. Gusella, J. F., Tsiftsoglou, A. S., Volloch, V., Weil, S., Neuman, J., and Housman, D. (1982). Dissociation of hemoglobin accumulation and commitment during erythroleukemia cell differentiation by treatment with imidazole. *J. Cell. Physiol.* **113,** 179–185.

22. Harrison, P. R. (1976). Analysis of erythropoiesis at the molecular level. *Nature (London)* **262,** 353–356.

23. Hensold, J., Robinson, S. H., and Tsiftsoglou, A. S. (1985). Biphasic repression of p53 gene activity during commitment of murine erythroleukemia cells to terminal maturation. (Submitted for publication.)

24. Housman, D., Volloch, V., Tsiftsoglou, A. S., Levenson, R., Gusella, J. F., Kernen, J., and Mitrani, A. (1979). Analysis of the molecular basis of commitment in murine erythroleukemia (MEL) cells. *In "In Vivo* and *In Vitro* Erythropoiesis: The Friend Cell System" (G. B. Rossi, ed.), pp. 273–282. Elsevier/North-Holland Biomedical Press, Amsterdam.

25. Housman, D., Levenson, R., Volloch, V., Tsiftsoglou, A. S., Gusella, J. F., Parker, D., Kernen, J., Mitrani, A., Weeks, V., Witte, O., and Besmer, P. (1980). Control of proliferation and differentiation in cells transformed by Friend virus. *Cold Spring Harbor Symp. Quant. Biol.* **44,** 1177–1185.

26. Huberman, E., and Callaham, M. F. (1979). Induction of terminal differentiation in human promyelocytic leukemia cells by tumor promoting agents. *Proc. Natl. Acad. Sci. U.S.A.* **76,** 1293–1297.

27. Kaneda, T., Murate, T., Sheffery, M., Brown, K., Rifkind, R. A., and Marks, P. A. (1985). Gene expression during terminal differentiation: Dexamethasone suppression of inducer-mediated a_1 and β^{maj}-globin gene expression. *Proc. Natl. Acad. Sci. U.S.A.* **82,** 5020–5024.

28. Keppel, F., Allet, B., and Eisen, H. (1977). Appearance of a chromatin protein during the erythroid differentiation of Friend virus-transformed cells. *Proc. Natl. Acad. Sci. U.S.A.* **74,** 653–656.

29. Koeffler, H. P., and Golde, D. W. (1980). Human leukemia cell lines: A review. *Blood* **56,** 344–350.

30. Kredich, N. M. (1980). Inhibition of nucleic acid methylation by cordycepin. *J. Biol. Chem.* **255,** 7380–7385.

31. Lachman, R., and Skoultchi, A. I. (1985). Expression of c-myc changes during differentiation of mouse erythroleukemia cells. *Nature (London)* **310,** 592–594.

32. Levenson, R., and Housman, D. (1979). Developmental program of murine erythroleukemia cells: Effect of inhibition of protein synthesis. *J. Cell Biol.* **82,** 715–725.

33. Levenson, R., and Housman, D. (1979). Memory of MEL cells to a previous exposure to inducer. *Cell (Cambridge, Mass.)* **17,** 485–490.

34. Levenson, R. and Housman, D. (1981). Erasure of the memory response in MEL cells. *Dev. Biol.* **86,** 81–86.

35. Levenson, R., Kernen, J., and Housman, D. (1979). Synchronization of MEL cell commitment with cordycepin. *Cell (Cambridge, Mass.)* **18,** 1073–1076.

36. Levenson, R., Housman, D., and Cantley, L. (1980). Amiloride inhibits murine erythroleukemia cell differentiation: Evidence for a Ca^{++} requirement for commitment. *Proc. Natl. Acad. Sci. U.S.A.* **77,** 5948–5952.

37. Lotem, J., and Sachs, L. (1974). Different blocks in the differentiation of myeloid leukemic cells. *Proc. Natl. Acad. Sci. U.S.A.* **71,** 3507–3511.

38. Lotem, J., and Sachs, L. (1983). Coupling of growth and differentiation in normal myeloid precursors and the breakdown of this coupling in leukemia. *Int. J. Cancer* **32,** 127–134.

39. Lozzio, C. B., and Lozzio, B. B. (1975). Human chronic myelogenous leukemia cell line with positive Philadelphia chromosome. *Blood* **45,** 321–334.

40. Marks, P. A., and Rifkind, R. A. (1978). Erythroleukemic differentiation. *Annu. Rev. Biochem.* **47,** 419–448.

41. Martin, P., and Papayanopoulou, T. (1982). HEL-cells: A new human erythroleukemia cell line with spontaneous and induced globin expression. *Science* **216,** 1233–1235.

42. McCulloch, E. A. (1982). Stem cells in normal and leukemic hemopoiesis (Henry Stratton Lecture, 1982). *Blood* **62,** 1–13.

43. Mierendorf, R. C., and Muller, G. C. (1982). The effect of dexamethasone on the initiation of β-globin gene transcription in differentiating Friend cells. *J. Biol. Chem.* **256,** 4496–4500.

44. Miller, D. M., Turner, P., Nienhuis, A. W., Axelrod, D. E., and Gopalakrishan, T. V. (1978). Active conformation of the globin genes in uninduced and induced mouse erythroleukemia cells. *Cell (Cambridge, Mass.)* **14,** 511–521.

45. Nakayasu, M., Terada, M., Tamura, G., Sugimura, T. (1980). Induction of the human and murine myeloid leukemia cells in culture by tunicamycin. *Proc. Natl. Acad. Sci. U.S.A.* **77**, 409–413.

46. Newburger, P., Chovaniec, M. E., Greenberger, J. S., and Cohen, H. (1979). Functional changes in human leukemia cell line HL-60. *J. Cell Biol.* **82**, 315–322.

47. Nomura, S., and Oishi, M. (1983). Indirect induction of erythroid differentiation in mouse Friend cells: Evidence for two intracellular reactions involved in the differentiation. *Proc. Natl. Acad. Sci. U.S.A.* **80**, 210–214.

48. Olsson, I., and Breitman, T. R. (1982). Induction of differentiation of the human histiocytic lymphoma cell line U-937 by retinoic acid and cAMP-inducing agents. *Cancer Res.* **42**, 3924–3927.

49. Papac, R. J., Brown, A. E., Schwartz, E. L., and Sartorelli, A. C. (1980). Differentiation of human promyelocytic leukemia cells *in vitro* by 6-thioguanine. *Cancer Lett.* **10**, 33–38.

50. Pulito, V. L., Miller, D. L., Sassa, S., and Yamane, T. (1983). DNA fragments in Friend erythroleukemia cells induced by dimethylsulfoxide. *Proc. Natl. Acad. Sci. U.S.A.* **80**, 5912–5915.

51. Rovera, G., Santolli, D., and Damsky, G. (1979). Human promyelocytic leukemia cells in culture differentiate into macrophage-like cells treated with phorbol diesters. *Proc. Natl. Acad. Sci.* **76**, 2729–2734.

52. Rovera, G., Olashaw, M., and Meo, P. (1980). Terminal differentiation in human promyelocytic leukemic cells in the absence of DNA synthesis. *Nature (London)* **284**, 69–70.

53. Rutherford, T., Clegg, J. B., Higgs, D. R., Jones, R. W., Thompson, J., and Weatherall, D. J. (1981). K-562 human leukemia cells: A model system for the study of hemoglobin switching? *In* "Hemoglobins in Development and Differentiation" (G. Stamatoyannopoulos, and A. W. Nienhuis, eds.), pp. 487–506. Liss, New York.

54. Sachs, L. (1978). Control of normal cell differentiation in the phenotypic reversion of malignancy in myeloid leukemia. *Nature (London)* **274**, 535–539.

55. Sachs, L. (1980). Constitutive uncoupling of pathways of gene expression that control growth and differentiation in myeloid leukemia: A model for the origin and progression of malignancy. *Proc. Natl. Acad. Sci. U.S.A.* **77**, 6152–6156.

56. Sachs, L. (1984). Reversibility of neoplastic transformation: Regulation of clonal growth in differentiation in hemopoiesis and the normalization of myeloid leukemia cells. *Adv. Viral Oncol.* **4**, 307–329.

57. Scher, W., Scher, B. M., and Waxman, S. (1983). Nuclear events during differentiation of erythroleukemia cells. *In* "Current Concepts of Erythropoiesis" (C. D. R. Dunn, ed.), pp. 301–338. Wiley, New York.

58. Schwartz, E. L., and Sartorelli, A. C. (1981). Structure activity relationships for induction of differentiation of human HL-60 acute promyelocytic cells by anthracyclines. *Cancer Res.* **42**, 2651–2655.

59. Sheffery, M., Rifkind, R. A., and Marks, P. A. (1982). Murine erythroleukemia cell differentiation: DNAse I hypersensitivity and DNA methylation near the globin genes. *Proc. Natl. Acad. Sci. U.S.A.* **79**, 1180–1184.

60. Sheffery, M., Rifkind, R. A., and Marks, P. A. (1983). Hexamethylene bisacetamide-resistant murine erythroleukemia cells have altered patterns of inducer-mediated chromatin changes. *Proc. Natl. Acad. Sci. U.S.A.* **80**, 5912–5915.

61. Shen, O. W., Real, F. X., DeLeo, A. B., Old, L. J., Marks, P. A., and Rifkind, R. A. (1983). Protein p53 and inducer-mediated erythroleukemia cell commitment to terminal cell division. *Proc. Natl. Acad. Sci. U.S.A.* **80**, 5919–5922.

62. Smith, R. D., and Yu, J. (1984). Alterations in globin gene chromatin conformation during murine erythroleukemia cells. *J. Biol. Chem.* **259**, 4609–4615.

63. Smith, R. L., Macara, I. G., Levenson, R., Housman, D., and Cantley, L. (1982). Evidence that a Na^+/Ca^{++} antiport system regulates murine erythroleukemia cell differentiation. *J. Biol. Chem.* **257**, 773–780.

64. Sundstrom, C., and Nillson, K. (1976). Establishment and characterization of human histiocytic lymphoma cell line (U-937). *Int. J. Cancer* **7**, 565–577.

65. Tanaka, H., Abe, E., Miyaura, C., Shiina, Y., and Suda, T. (1983). la,25-dehydroxyvitamin D_3 induces differentiation of human promyelocytic leukemia cells (HL-60) in monocyte/macrophages, but not into granulocytes. *Biochem. Biophys. Res. Commun.* **117**, 86–92.

66. Tarella, C., Ferrero, D., Gallo, E., Pagliad, L. G., and Ruscetti, F. W. (1982). Induction of differentiation of HL-60 cells by dimethylsulfoxide: Evidence for a stochastic model not linked to cell division. *Cancer Res.* **42**, 445–449.

67. Thomas, P. S. (1980). Hybridization of denatured RNA and small DNA fragments transferred to nitrocellulose. *Proc. Natl. Acad. Sci. U.S.A.* **77**, 5201–5205.

68. Thompson, C. B., Challoner, P. B., Neiman, P. E., and Groudine, M. (1985). Levels of c-myc oncogene mRNA are invariant throughout of the cell cycle. *Nature (London)* **314**, 363–366.

69. Tsiftsoglou, A. S., and Robinson, S. H. (1985). Differentiation of leukemic cell lines: A review focusing on murine erythroleukemia and human HL-60 cells. *Int. J. Cell Cloning* **3**, 349–366.

70. Tsiftsoglou, A. S. and Wong, W. (1985). Molecular and cellular mechanisms of leukemic cell differentiation: An analysis of the Friend system. *Anticancer Res.* **5**, 81–100.

71. Tsiftsoglou, A. S., Barrnett, R. J., and Sartorelli, A. C. (1979). Enucleation of differentiated murine erythroleukemia cells in culture. *Proc. Natl. Acad. Sci. U.S.A.* **76**, 6381–6385.

72. Tsiftsoglou, A. S., Gusella, J. F., Volloch, V., and Housman, D. (1979). Inhibition by dexamethasone of commitment to erythroid differentiation in murine erythroleukemia cells. *Cancer Res.* **39**, 3849–3865.

73. Tsiftsoglou, A. S., Mitrani, A., and Housman, D. (1981). Procaine inhibits the erythroid differentiation of MEL cells by blocking commitment: Possible involvement of calcium metabolism. *J. Cell. Physiol.* **108**, 327–335.

74. Tsiftsoglou, A. S., Wong, W., Volloch, V., Gusella, J. F., and Housman, D. (1982). Commitment of murine erythroleukemia (MEL) cells to terminal differentiation is association with coordinated expression of globin and ribosomal genes. *Prog. Clin. Biol. Res.* **102**, 69–79.

75. Tsiftsoglou, A. S., Wong, W., and Housman, D. (1983). Dexamethasone-sensitive and insensitive responses during *in vitro* differentiation of Friend erythroleukemia cells. *Biochim. Biophys. Acta* **759**, 160–169.

76. Tsiftsoglou, A. S., Nunez, M. T., Wong, W., and Robinson, S. H. (1983). Dissociation of iron transport and heme biosynthesis from commitment to terminal maturation of murine eythroleukemia cells. *Proc. Natl. Acad. Sci. U.S.A.* **80**, 7528–7532.

77. Tsiftsoglou, A. S., Wong, W., Hyman, R., Minden, M., and Robinson, S. H. (1985). Analysis of commitment of human leukemia HL-60 cells to terminal granulocytic maturation. *Cancer Res.* **45**, 2334–2339.

78. Volloch, V., and Housman, D. (1981). Stability of globin mRNA in terminally differentiating murine erythroleukemia cells. *Cell (Cambridge, Mass.).* **23**, 509–514.

79. Volloch, V., and Housman, D. (1982). Terminal differentiation of murine erythroleukemia cells: Physical stabilization of end-stage cells. *J. Cell. Biol.* **93,** 390–394.
80. Westin, E. H., Wong-Stadl, F., Gelman, E. P., Dalla-Favera, R., Paps, T. S., Lautenberger, J. A., Eva, A., Reddy, P., Tronick, S. R., Aaronson, S. A., and Gallo, R. C.
(1982). Expression of cellular homologues or retroviral *onc* genes in human hematopoietic cells. *Proc. Natl. Acad. Sci. U.S.A.* **79,** 2490–2494.
81. Wong, W., Robinson, S. H., and Tsiftsoglou, A. S. (1985). Relationship of mitochondrial membrane potential to hemoglobin synthesis during Friend cell maturation. *Blood*
66, 999–1001.
82. Yen, A., and Albright, K. L. (1984). Evidence for cell cycle phase-specific initiation of a
program of HL-60 cell myeloid differentiation mediated by inducer. *Cancer Res.* **44,**
2511–2515.
83. Yu, J., and Smith, R. D. (1985). Sequential alterations in globin gene structure during
erythroleukemia cell differentiation. *J. Biol. Chem.* **260,** 3035–3040.

Cancer Chemotherapeutic Agents as Inducers of Leukemia Cell Differentiation

ALAN C. SARTORELLI, MICHAEL J. MORIN,
AND KIMIKO ISHIGURO

Department of Pharmacology and Developmental Therapeutics Program
Comprehensive Cancer Center
Yale University School of Medicine
New Haven, Connecticut

I. Introduction

Cancer may be considered a disease of altered maturation in which the rate of proliferation of the cell population is increased relative to that of its maturation, resulting in an increase in tissue mass. There is considerable evidence, however, that many neoplastic cells retain the capacity to mature to adult, end-stage cells with a finite life-span. Differentiation to a nonmalignant state can be produced in a variety of malignant neoplasms, including teratocarcinoma, neuroblastoma, and leukemia (4,7,13,17,30, 31), by placing the neoplastic cells in an appropriate embryonic environment; such transformation demonstrates the reversibility of the malignant state. In addition, neoplastic cells can be induced to differentiate *in vitro* and *in vivo* by a wide variety of structurally diverse chemical agents. These include solvents (11,33), hormones (23), vitamins (1,3,36,41), tu-

NEW AVENUES IN DEVELOPMENTAL
CANCER CHEMOTHERAPY

mor promoters (16,24), and a number of cancer chemotherapeutic agents. The latter group consists of drugs such as aclacinomycin A and marcellomycin (27,35,37), bleomycin (34,40), mitomycin C (9,15,25,40), methotrexate (2), cytosine arabinoside (2,9,15,22,25), 6-mercaptopurine (14,25), 6-thioguanine (12,14,18,19,25,29,38), and actinomycin D (5,22,25,43). The differentiation-inducing activities of such a wide range of cancer chemotherapeutic agents suggest that their antineoplastic effects may be the result of a combination of both cytotoxic and maturative actions that lead to cellular forms in both instances with no capacity to proliferate. Since both cytotoxicity and terminal differentiation result in a cessation of replicative potential, it is difficult to distinguish between these two phenomena. It is conceivable that maturation and cytodestruction caused by cancer chemotherapeutic agents are linked processes caused by the same drug-induced biochemical events. Our laboratory has conducted studies, employing the anthracycline antibiotics and 6-thiopurine antimetabolites, that have permitted a distinction to be made between the termination of proliferation by differentiation from that caused by cytotoxicity; included in these investigations is a delineation of a portion of the programmed events involved in the termination of the replicative capability of the leukemia cells that results from the maturation process.

II. Anthracyclines as Inducers of HL-60 Leukemia Cell Differentiation

The polysaccharide-containing anthracycline antibiotics are effective inducers of the differentiation of HL-60 promyelocytic leukemia cells, both *in vitro* (27,35) and *in vivo* (37). The most active drugs of this class as initiators of the maturation of these leukemic cells were in the pyrromycinone group of anthracyclines; the structural formulas of these agents are shown in Fig. 1. The trisaccharide-containing antibiotics, marcellomycin and aclacinomycin A, were the most efficacious members of this class, while the disaccharides, musettamycin and 10-decarbomethoxymarcellomycin, were slightly less active; the monosaccharide pyrromycin had minimal activity, and other monosaccharide-containing anthracyclines, such as adriamycin and carminomycin, were inactive as inducers of the differentiation of HL-60 leukemia cells (35). These studies of the relationship between structure and activity demonstrated that the oligosaccharide side chain of the pyrromycinone class of anthracyclines was the predominant determinant of differentiation inducing-activity.

The anthracycline antibiotics were employed to obtain information on

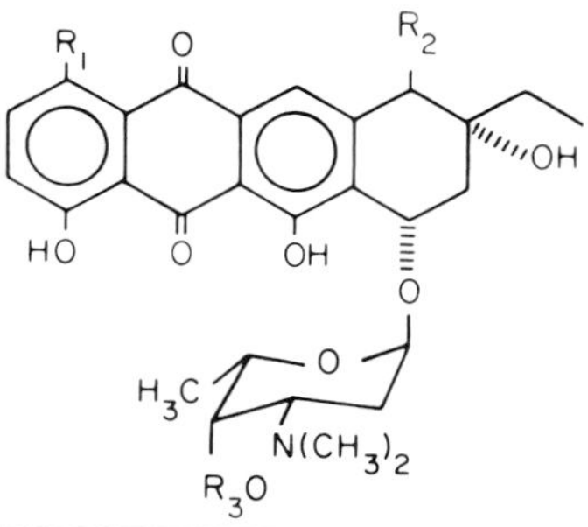

Compound	R_1	R_2	R_3
Pyrromycin	OH	$COOCH_3$	H
Musettamycin	OH	$COOCH_3$	2-Deoxyfucose
Marcellomycin	OH	$COOCH_3$	2-Deoxyfucose-2-deoxyfucose
Aclacinomycin A	H	$COOCH_3$	2-Deoxyfucose-2-cinerulose
10-Descarbomethoxy-marcellomycin	OH	H	2-Deoxyfucose-2-deoxyfucose

Fig. 1. Structures of anthracycline antibiotics active as inducers of the differentiation of HL-60 cells.

the biochemical events involved in the termination of cellular proliferation through the formation of end-stage, mature cellular forms produced by differentiation by comparison of some of the metabolic effects produced by aclacinomycin A and the related inactive compound adriamycin. The comparative effectiveness of these two anthracyclines on the replication and differentiation of HL-60 leukemia cells is shown in Fig. 2. A significant degree of differentiation of the leukemic cell population was produced by concentrations of aclacinomycin A from 30 to 50 nM, whereas adriamycin at identical levels caused similar degrees of inhibition of cellular replication but did not induce any differentiation as determined by the capacity of cells to reduce nitroblue tetrazolium, a functional measure of oxidative metabolism that accompanies phagocytosis.

Investigation of the biochemical basis for the differentiation-inducing activity of the trisaccharide-containing anthracyclines has provided infor-

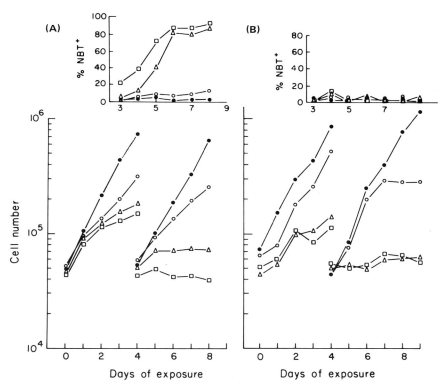

Fig. 2. Growth inhibition and induction of differentiation of HL-60 leukemia cells by aclacinomycin A (A) or adriamycin (B). HL-60 cells were seeded at an initial concentration of 5×10^4 cells/ml. On day 4, the cells in each group were washed and resuspended at 5×10^4 cells/ml in fresh medium containing anthracycline. Cell numbers were determined with a Model ZBI Coulter particle counter, and differentiation was assessed by nitroblue tetrazolium dye reduction. Cultures were treated as follows: (A) ●, no addition; ○, 10 nM aclacinomycin A; △, 30 nM aclacinomycin A; □, 50 nM aclacinomycin A. (B) ●, no addition; ○, 10 nM adriamycin; △, 30 nM adriamycin; □, 50 nM adriamycin. [From Morin and Sartorelli (27).]

mation on the mechanism by which HL-60 cells terminate their replicative potential. All of the anthracyclines tested intercalate into DNA and inhibit the biosynthesis of both DNA and RNA (46). Significant differences exist, however, between aclacinomycin and marcellomycin on the one hand and adriamycin and pyrromycin on the other, with respect to their potencies as inhibitors of nucleolar RNA synthesis, with the trisaccharide-containing antibiotics being markedly more potent (6). Thus, it is possible that the exceedingly great inhibition of the formation of nucleolar RNA by aclacinomycin A and marcellomycin may be involved in the initiation of the maturation of HL-60 leukemia cells.

A biochemical lesion unique to the trisaccharide-containing anthracyclines is the inhibition of the synthesis of glycoproteins containing asparagine-linked oligosaccharides (27). This alteration was initially demonstrated by the selective decrease produced by aclacinomycin and marcellomycin of the incorporation of radioactive mannose into lipid-insoluble, acid-precipitable glycoproteins of HL-60 cells relative to tritiated leucine incorporation into proteins (Fig. 3). In contrast, adriamycin and pyrromycin did not produce a differential blockage of the synthesis of lipid-linked oligosaccharides. The preferential interference with the biosynthesis of asparagine-linked oligosaccharides by aclacinomycin A and marcellomycin corresponded to an inhibitory effect by these agents on the

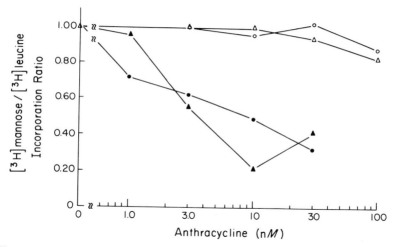

Fig. 3. Inhibition of [³H]mannose and [³H]leucine incorporation into intact HL-60 leukemia cells exposed to anthracyclines. Cells were suspended at an initial concentration of 2.5 × 10⁵ cells/ml in adriamycin, pyrromycin, aclacinomycin A, or marcellomycin at the concentrations indicated on the abscissa (logarithmic scale). Cells were incubated in the presence of anthracyclines (○, adriamycin; △, pyrromycin; ●, marcellomycin; ▲, aclacinomycin A) for 42 hr and then washed and resuspended at a concentration of 2.5 × 10⁵ cells/ml in media containing the same concentration of anthracycline plus L-[3,4,5-³H]leucine (0.50 Ci/ml) or D-[2-³H]mannose (2.25 Ci/ml). The incorporation of each precursor was determined after a 6-hr incubation period, at which time the cell pellets were washed, acid-precipitated, extracted, solubilized, and assessed for radioactivity. Data from three similar experiments were calculated as [³H]mannose : [³H]leucine incorporation ratios (counts per minute per milligram of protein for each precursor) and were expressed as a fraction of the value of the incorporation ratios of control groups. [From Morin and Sartorelli (27).]

TABLE I

Effects of Anthracyclines on HL-60 Leukemia Cell Transferrin Receptor Activity[a]

Treatment	Transferrin binding (counts per minute/2 × 10⁶ cells)			
	Total	Nonspecific	Specific	% of control
None	13,460 ± 540	1,230	12,230 ± 490	100 ± 4
Aclacinomycin A	6,950 ± 940	710	6,240 ± 860	51 ± 7
Marcellomycin	5,150 ± 1,480	630	4,520 ± 1,350	37 ± 11
Pyrromycin	13,780 ± 1,340	1,190	12,590 ± 1,220	103 ± 10
Adriamycin	13,530 ± 670	1,170	12,360 ± 610	101 ± 5

[a] HL-60 leukemia cells were untreated or grown in the presence of a 30 nM concentration of the indicated anthracyclines for 24 hr. At that time, cells were washed extensively, resuspended at a level of 10⁷ cells/ml, and assayed at 4°C for cell-surface transferrin receptor activity. Data represent three or more experiments for each treatment group, with four or more determinations of specific binding measured in each experiment (mean ± S.D.). [From Morin and Sartorelli (27).]

incorporation of tritiated mannose into lipid-linked oligosaccharides (27); adriamycin and pyrromycin, at equivalent growth-inhibitory concentrations, did not interfere with the formation of dolichol-linked oligosaccharides. It is also of particular interest that the anthracyclines, aclacinomycin A and marcellomycin, were markedly more potent than the classical inhibitor of this pathway, tunicamycin, in depressing the formation of dolichol-linked oligosaccharides.

As a consequence of the interference with glycoprotein biosynthesis by the active anthracycline inducers of maturation, the levels of cell-surface transferrin receptor, an N-glycosidically linked glycoprotein, decreased significantly (Table I). The ineffective anthracycline inducers of differentiation, pyrromycin and adriamycin, as expected, did not alter the levels of transferrin receptor. That the down-regulation of the transferrin receptor is a general phenomenon that constitutes an important event in the maturation of leukemia cells is shown by the decrease in transferrin receptor levels in a number of leukemia cell systems, including the M-1, K-562, and HL-60 myeloid cell lines, after exposure to a variety of inducers of differentiation (10,42,45). The importance of iron for the activity of ribonucleoside diphosphate reductase, a critical enzyme for the synthesis of the deoxyribonucleoside triphosphate building blocks of DNA, and the cytochromes, essential for the maintenance of ATP levels, mark the down-regulation of the transferrin receptor as one of the critical events in the programmed termination of replication through maturation. Thus, the comparative effects of the anthracycline antibiotics on the activity of the transferrin receptor have permitted a distinction between the termination of cellular proliferative capacity which results from maturation from that caused by the cytotoxic actions of these antibiotics. The findings imply that distinct biochemical events are involved in the cessation of replication by these two mechanisms.

III. 6-Thioguanine as an Inducer of Leukemia Cell Differentiation

Studies on the action of the purine antimetabolite 6-thioguanine as an initiator of a program of HL-60 leukemia cell differentiation have provided further evidence that the biochemical events responsible for the cytotoxicity of anticancer agents is distinct from the actions that produce maturation. The approach taken was to develop a series of mutants of the HL-60 leukemia deficient in enzymes involved in the anabolic metabolism of 6-thioguanine (19). The objective was to define the metabolic forms of the 6-thiopurine responsible for cytotoxicity and the induction of differentiation. Gusella and Housman (14) had reported that the 6-thiopurines induced erythroid differentiation in Friend leukemia cells that lacked hypoxanthine-guanine phosphoribosyltransferase (HGPRT) activity but were inactive in parental cells possessing this enzymatic activity. Based upon these findings these investigators postulated that the formation of 6-thioguanosine 5'-monophosphate (TGMP) and the incorporation of 6-thioguanine into DNA were not required for the induction of differentiation.

6-Thioguanine caused inhibition of cellular proliferation in parental HL-60 cells, with the 50% inhibitory concentration being 8 μM; no nitroblue tetrazolium–positive cells were produced in wild-type cells exposed to 6-thioguanine. In an HGPRT-negative subline of HL-60, however, the concentrations of 6-thioguanine that produced half-maximal induction of differentiation and inhibition of growth were 0.37 and 0.74 mM, respectively. The degree of differentiation as measured by the production of nitroblue tetrazolium–positive cells caused by 6-thioguanine in HGPRT-negative cells is shown in Fig. 4; greater than 95% of the cells acquired a mature phenotype. 6-Thioguanosine caused significantly less differentiation, which reached a maximum at 0.4 mM; increased levels of this nucleoside produced progressively greater inhibition of cellular differentiation. β-2'-Deoxythioguanosine was inactive as an initiator of maturation in this HGPRT-negative subline. The intracellular metabolites of 6-thioguanine formed by HGPRT-negative cells exposed to 6-thioguanine and its nucleosides are shown in Tables II–IV. Following the exposure of HL-60/

TABLE II

**Intracellular Metabolites of 6-Thioguanine
Formed by HL-60/HGPRT-Negative Cells Exposed
to 6-Thioguanine (TGua), 6-Thioguanosine (TGuo),
or β-2′-Deoxythioguanosine (dTGuo)**[a]

Treatment	Distribution (%)			
	TGua	TGuo	dTGuo	TGua nucleotides
TGua	98.4	1.6	0	0
TGuo	86.9	11.9	0	1.3
dTGuo	79.5	0	17.1	3.4

[a] HL-60/HGPRT-negative cells were exposed to 0.5 m*M* of either TGua, TGuo, or dTGuo for 24 hr. Cells were collected, and the intracellular distribution of metabolites was measured. [From Ishiguro and Sartorelli (19).]

HGPRT-negative cells to 6-thioguanine, the majority (>98%) of the material remained as the free base, with a small amount of 6-thioguanosine being formed (Table II). Cells exposed to 6-thioguanosine converted most (>86%) of the ribonucleoside analog to the free base, with a small percentage (1.3%) being anabolized to 6-thioguanine nucleotides (Table III). These findings imply that the free base, 6-thioguanine, was the form that induced the mature state. Although β-2′-deoxythioguanosine was also predominantly converted to the free base (>79%), a significant amount of thioguanine nucleotides was formed; the formation of these cytotoxic metabolites produced significant growth inhibition and prevented the formation of differentiated cells. The use of the potent inhibitor of purine

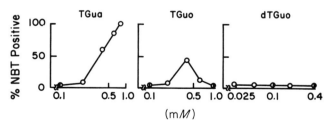

Fig. 4. Induction of differentiation of HL-60/HGPRT-negative cells by 6-thioguanine (TGua), 6-thioguanosine (TGuo), and β-2′-deoxythioguanosine (dTGua). HL-60/HGPRT-negative cells were exposed to various concentrations of each analog, and the extent of cellular differentiation was measured on day 8. [From Ishiguro and Sartorelli (19).]

TABLE III

Intracellular Metabolites of 6-Thioguanine Formed by HL-60/HGPRT-Negative Cells Exposed to 6-Thioguanine (TGua), 6-Thioguanosine (TGuo), or β-2′-Deoxythioguanosine (dTGuo) in the Presence of 8-Aminoguanosine[a]

Treatment	Distribution (%)			
	TGua	TGuo	dTGuo	TGua nucleotides
TGua	94.5	5.5	0	0
TGuo	31.6	56.6	0	12.9
dTGuo	11.9	0	76.2	11.9

[a] HL-60/HGPRT-negative cells were exposed to 0.5 mM of either TGua, TGuo, or dTGuo in the presence of 0.2 mM 8-aminoguanosine for 24 hr. Cells were collected, and the intracellular distribution of metabolites was measured. [From Ishiguro and Sartorelli (19).]

TABLE IV

Intracellular Metabolites of 6-Thioguanine Formed by Cells Deficient in HGPRT and Deoxycytidine Kinase Following Exposure to β-2′-Deoxythioguanosine (dTGuo) in the Absence or Presence of 8-Aminoguanosine (AGuo)[a]

Treatment	Distribution (%)	
	TGua	dTGuo
dTGuo	41.2	58.6
dTGuo + 0.1 mM AGuo	37.6	62.5
dTGuo + 0.3 mM AGuo	25.4	74.6

[a] HL-60 cells deficient in HGPRT and deoxycytidine kinase were exposed to β-2′-deoxythioguanosine in the absence or presence of 0.1 or 0.3 mM 8-aminoguanosine for 24 hr. Cells were collected, and the intracellular distribution of metabolites was measured. [From Ishiguro and Sartorelli (19).]

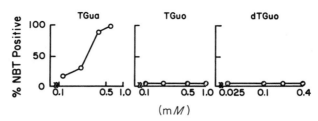

Fig. 5. Induction of the differentiation of HL-60/HGPRT-negative cells by 6-thioguanine (TGua), 6-thioguanosine (TGuo), and β-2′-deoxythioguanosine (dTGua) in the presence of 0.2 mM 8-aminoguanosine. Conditions were as described in Fig. 4. [From Ishiguro and Sartorelli (19).]

nucleoside phosphorylase, 8-aminoguanosine (20,39), to minimize the degradation of 6-thioguanosine and β-2′-deoxythioguanosine increased the intracellular concentration of 6-thioguanine nucleotides by four- to tenfold (Table III) and completely inhibited the differentiation produced by 6-thioguanosine (Fig. 5), supporting the idea that thioguanine nucleotides interfere with the maturation process.

A double-mutant deficient in both HGPRT and deoxycytidine kinase, an enzyme shown to be responsible for the phosphorylation of deoxyguanosine and deoxythioguanosine (8,28), was employed to demonstrate that β-2′-deoxythioguanosine had the capacity to induce maturation (Fig. 6). Since no 6-thioguanine nucleotides were formed in this cell line following exposure to the deoxyribonucleoside analog (Table IV), the results added further support to the concept that 6-thiopurine nucleotides are antagonistic to the attainment of a differentiated state. The use of 8-aminoguanosine to suppress the degradation of β-2′-deoxythioguanosine to 6-thioguanine (Table IV) did not completely prevent the formation of

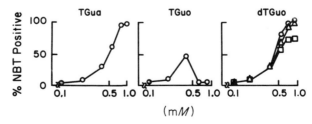

Fig. 6. Induction of the differentiation of HL-60 cells deficient in HGPRT and deoxycytidine kinase activities by 6-thioguanine (TGua), 6-thioguanosine (TGuo), and β-2′-deoxythioguanosine (dTGua) in the absence (○) and presence of 0.1 (△) or 0.3 (□) mM 8-aminoguanosine. Conditions were as described in Fig. 4. [From Ishiguro and Sartorelli (19).]

differentiated cells (Fig. 6), suggesting that β-2'-deoxythioguanosine may be a metabolic form that is capable of initiating maturation in this system; however, the decrease in the percentage of nitroblue tetrazolium–positive cells caused by the presence of 0.3-mM 8-aminoguanosine, which corresponded to a decrease in the intracellular levels of 6-thioguanine, makes it questionable as to whether β-2'-deoxythioguanosine is a form that induces differentiation.

The conclusion that 6-thioguanine nucleotides interfere with the maturation process was supported by the finding that the simultaneous administration of hypoxanthine or its nucleosides to parental HL-60 cells markedly lowered the accumulation of 6-thioguanine nucleotides in the acid-soluble fraction of parental HL-60 cells treated with the 6-thiopurine (Fig. 7) and caused a corresponding decrease in the cytotoxicity of 6-thioguanine for these leukemia cells (18). The prevention of the cytotoxic action of 6-thioguanine by the simultaneous administration of hypoxanthine or its nucleosides resulted in the expression of the differentiation inducing properties of the 6-thiopurine in parental HL-60 cells (Fig. 8).

Differences also occurred in the stage of the cell cycle at which parental HL-60 cells were arrested as a result of cytotoxicity compared to that of HL-60/HGPRT-negative cells, in which cellular replication was apparently terminated by conversion of cells to end-stage forms with a mature phenotype (38). Thus, about 85% of wild-type HL-60 cells treated with the 6-thiopurine accumulated in the S and G_2/M phases of the cell cycle, a finding in agreement with previous work with the L1210 leukemia (21,44)

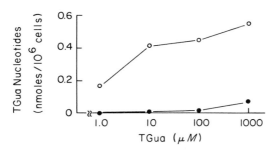

Fig. 7. Accumulation of 6-thioguanine (TGua) nucleotides in the acid-soluble fraction of parental HL-60 cells treated with TGua in the presence or absence of inosine. Parental HL-60 cells (1 × 10^6 cells/ml) were treated with TGua at various concentrations in the absence (○) or presence (●) of 1 mM inosine for 6 hr. The cells were washed extensively with medium and phosphate-buffered saline to remove nonphosphorylated metabolites of TGua and were extracted with cold perchloric acid. TGua nucleotides in the acid-soluble extracts were quantitated by fluorometry. [From Ishiguro and Sartorelli (18).]

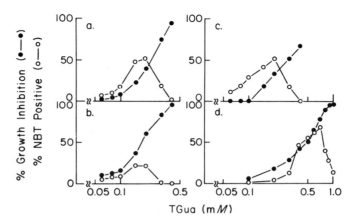

Fig. 8. Growth inhibition and induction of differentiation of parental and HL-60/HGPRT-negative cells treated with 6-thioguanine (TGua). Parental HL-60 cells (8 × 10⁴ cells/ml) were exposed to various concentrations of TGua in the presence of 2 m*M* inosine (a), deoxyinosine (b), or hypoxanthine (c). HL-60/HGPRT-negative cells were treated with TGua alone (d). On day 6, cell numbers were determined, and the cultures were diluted 50% with fresh medium containing TGua and the various protecting agents. On day 8, the extent of differentiation was measured by nitroblue tetrazolium reduction. Growth inhibition (●); differentiation (○). [From Ishiguro and Sartorelli (18).]

and Chinese hamster ovary (26) cells. In contrast, HL-60/HGPRT-negative cells treated with 6-thioguanine accumulated in G_1, the phase of the cell cycle in which many cell types reside in the mature state (32).

That differences existed in the mechanism involved in the termination of proliferation by differentiation and cytotoxicity was also demonstrated by measuring the concentration of transferrin receptors in parental HL-60 cells and in their HGPRT-negative counterparts treated with 6-thioguanine (Fig. 9). In wild-type cells, extensive cytotoxicity was produced as the concentration of 6-thioguanine was increased; these results were not accompanied by a marked change in cell-surface transferrin receptor activity. In contrast, a rapid and pronounced down-regulation of the transferrin receptor occurred in HL-60/HGPRT-negative leukemia cells, even under conditions in which little growth inhibition was produced, a finding consistent with a program of cell maturation being induced in this drug-sensitive subline by the 6-thiopurine. The collective findings suggest that the maturation produced by cancer chemotherapeutic agents is not simply related to their capacity to inhibit the replication of DNA. Furthermore, the results imply that molecular modifications of antineoplastic agents with differentiation-inducing properties are possible

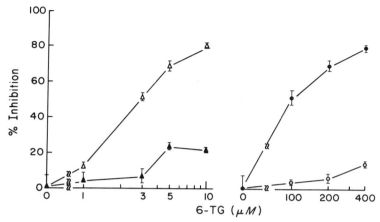

Fig. 9. The effects of various concentrations of 6-thioguanine (6-TG) on the growth and transferrin receptor activity of HL-60 and HL-60/HGPRT-negative cells. Cell growth was measured on day 5; HL-60 (△), HL-60/HGPRT-negative (○). Transferrin receptor activity was measured at 24 hr by ascertaining the extent of binding of [³H]transferrin at 4°C; HL-60 (▲), HL-60/HGPRT-negative (●).

to minimize their cytotoxic activities and to optimize their capacities to initiate the maturation process.

Acknowledgments

The research described in this report was supported in part by U.S. Public Health Service Grants CA-02817 and CA-28852 from the National Cancer Institute.

References

1. Abe, E., Miyaura, C., Sakagami, H., Takeda, M., Konno, K., Yamazaki, T., Yoshika, S., and Suda, T. (1981). Differentiation of mouse myeloid leukemia cells induced by 1,25-dihydroxyvitamin D₃. *Proc. Natl. Acad. Sci. U.S.A.* **78,** 4990–4994.
2. Bodner, A. J., Ting, R. C., and Gallo, R. C. (1981). Induction of differentiation of human promyelocytic leukemia cells (HL-60) by nucleosides and methotrexate. *JNCI, J. Natl. Cancer Inst.* **67,** 1025–1030.
3. Breitman, T. R., Selonick, S. E., and Collins, S. J. (1980). Induction of differentiation of the human promyelocytic leukemia cell line (HL-60) by retinoic acid. *Proc. Natl. Acad. Sci. U.S.A.* **77,** 2936–2940.
4. Brinster, R. L. (1974). The effects of cells transferred into the mouse blastocyst on subsequent development. *J. Exp. Med.* **140,** 1049–1056.

5. Collins, S. J., Bodner, A., Ting, R., and Gallo, R. C. (1980). Induction of morphological and functional differentiation of human promyelocytic leukemia cells (HL-60) by compounds which induce differentiation of murine leukemia cells. *Int. J. Cancer* **25,** 213–218.

6. Crooke, S. T., DuVernay, V. H., Golvan, L., and Prestayko, A. W. (1978). Structure-activity relationships of anthracyclines relative to effects on macromolecular synthesis. *Mol. Pharmacol.* **14,** 290–298.

7. DeCosse, J. J., Gossens, C. L., and Kuzma, J. F. (1973). Breast cancer: Induction of differentiation by embryonic tissue. *Science* **181,** 1057–1058.

8. Durham, J. P., and Ives, D. H. (1969). Deoxycytidine kinase. I. Distribution in normal and neoplastic tissues and interrelationships of deoxycytidine and 1-β-D-arabinofuranosylcytosine phosphorylation. *Mol. Pharmacol.* **5,** 358–375.

9. Ebert, P. S., Wars, I., and Buell, D. N. (1976). Erythroid differentiation in cultured Friend leukemia cells treated with metabolic inhibitors. *Cancer Res.* **36,** 1809–1813.

10. Felsted, R. L., Gupta, S. K., Glover, C. J., Fischkoff, S. A., and Gallagher, R. E. (1983). Cell surface membrane protein changes during the differentiation of cultured human promyelocytic leukemia HL-60 cells. *Cancer Res.* **43,** 2754–2761.

11. Friend, C., Scher, W., Holland, J. G., and Sato, T. (1971). Hemoglobin synthesis in murine virus-induced leukemia cells *in vitro:* Stimulation of erythroid differentiation by dimethyl sulfoxide. *Proc. Natl. Acad. Sci. U.S.A.* **68,** 378–382.

12. Gallagher, R. E., Ferrai, A. C., Zulich, A. W., Yen, R-W.-C., and Testa, J. R. (1984). Cytotoxic and cytodifferentiative components of 6-thioguanine resistance in HL-60 cells containing acquired double minute chromosomes. *Cancer Res.* **44,** 2642–2653.

13. Gootwine, E., Webb, C., and Sachs, L. (1982). Participation of myeloid leukemia cells injected into embryos in hematopoietic differentiation in adult mice. *Nature (London)* **299,** 63–67.

14. Gusella, J. F., and Housman, D. (1976). Induction of erythroid differentiation *in vitro* by purines and purine analogs. *Cell (Cambridge, Mass.)* **8,** 263–269.

15. Hayashi, M., Okabe, J., and Hozumi, M. (1979). Sensitization of resistant myeloid leukemia clone cells by anticancer drugs to factor-stimulating differentiation. *Gann* **70,** 235–238.

16. Huberman, E., and Callaham, M. F. (1979). Induction of terminal differentiation in human promyelocytic leukemia cells by tumor-promoting agents. *Proc. Natl. Acad. Sci. U.S.A.* **76,** 1293–1297.

17. Illmensee, K., and Mintz, B. (1976). Totipotency and normal differentiation of single teratocarcinoma cells cloned by injection into blastocysts. *Proc. Natl. Acad. Sci. U.S.A.* **73,** 549–553.

18. Ishiguro, K., and Sartorelli, A. C. (1985). Enhancement of the differentiation-inducing properties of 6-thioguanine by hypoxanthine and its nucleosides in HL-60 promyelocytic leukemia cells. *Cancer Res.* **45,** 91–95.

19. Ishiguro, K., Schwartz, E. L., and Sartorelli, A. C. (1984). Characterization of the metabolic forms of 6-thioguanine responsible for cytotoxicity and induction of differentiation of HL-60 acute promyelocytic leukemia cells. *J. Cell. Physiol.* **121,** 383–390.

20. Kazmers, I. S., Mitchell, B. S., Dadonna, P. E., Wotring, L. L., Townsend, L. B., and Kelley, W. N. (1981). Inhibition of purine nucleoside phosphorylase by 8-aminoguanosine: selective toxicity for T lymphoblasts. *Science* **214,** 1137–1139.

21. Lee, S. H., and Sartorelli, A. C. (1981). The effects of inhibitors of DNA biosynthesis on the cytotoxicity of 6-thioguanine. *Cancer Biochem. Biophys.* **5,** 189–194.

22. Lotem, J., and Sachs, L. (1974). Different blocks in the differentiation of myeloid leukemia cells. *Proc. Natl. Acad. Sci. U.S.A.* **71,** 3507–3511.

23. Lotem, J., and Sachs, L. (1975). Induction of specific changes in the surface membrane of myeloid leukemic cells by steroid hormones. *Int. J. Cancer* **15**, 731–740.

24. Lotem, J., and Sachs, L. (1979). Regulation of normal differentiation in mouse and human myeloid leukemia cells by phorbol esters and the mechanism of tumor promotion. *Proc. Natl. Acad. Sci. U.S.A.* **76**, 5158–5162.

25. Lotem, J., and Sachs, L. (1980). Potential pre-screening for therapeutic agents that induce differentiation in human myeloid leukemia cells. *Int. J. Cancer* **25**, 561–564.

26. Maybaum, J., and Mandel, H. G. (1983). Unilateral chromatid damage: A new basis for 6-thioguanine cytotoxicity. *Cancer Res.* **43**, 3852–3856.

27. Morin, M. J., and Sartorelli, A. C. (1984). Inhibition of glycoprotein biosynthesis by the inducers of HL-60 cell differentiation, aclacinomycin A and marcellomycin. *Cancer Res.* **44**, 2807–2812.

28. Nakai, Y., and LePage, G. A. (1972). Characterization of the kinase(s) involved in the phosphorylation of α- and β-2′-deoxythioguanosine. *Cancer Res.* **32**, 2445–2451.

29. Papac, R. J., Brown, A. E., Schwartz, E. L., and Sartorelli, A. C. (1980). Differentiation of human promyelocytic leukemia cells *in vitro* by 6-thioguanine. *Cancer Lett.* **10**, 33–38.

30. Pierce, G. B., and Wallace, C. (1971). Differentiation of malignant to benign cells. *Cancer Res.* **31**, 127–134.

31. Pierce, G. B., Pantazis, C. G., Caldwell, J. E., and Wells, R. S. (1982). Specificity of the control of tumor formation by the blastocyst. *Cancer Res.* **42**, 1082–1087.

32. Prescott, D. M. (1976). Cell cycle and control of cellular reproduction. *Adv. Genet.* **18**, 99–177.

33. Reuben, R. C., Rifkin, R. A., and Marks, P. A. (1980). Chemically induced murine erythroleukemia differentiation. *Biochim. Biophys. Acta* **605**, 325–346.

34. Scher, W., and Friend, C. (1978). Breakage of DNA and alterations in folded genomes by inducers of differentiation in Friend erythroleukemic cells. *Cancer Res.* **38**, 841–849.

35. Schwartz, E. L., and Sartorelli, A. C. (1982). Structure-activity relationships for the induction of differentiation of HL-60 human acute promyelocytic leukemia cells by anthracyclines. *Cancer Res.* **42**, 2651–2655.

36. Schwartz, E. L., Snoddy, J. R., Kreutter, D., Rasmussen, H., and Sartorelli, A. C. (1983). Synergistic induction of HL-60 differentiation by 1,25-dihydroxyvitamin D_3 and dimethyl sulfoxide (DMSO). *Proc. Am. Assoc. Cancer Res.* **24**, 18.

37. Schwartz, E. L., Brown, B. J., Nierenberg, M., Marsh, J. C., and Sartorelli, A. C. (1983). Evaluation of some anthracycline antibiotics in an *in vivo* model for studying drug-induced human leukemia cell differentiation. *Cancer Res.* **43**, 2725–2730.

38. Schwartz, E. L., Blair, O. C., and Sartorelli, A. C. (1984). Cell cycle events associated with the termination of proliferation by cytotoxic and differentiation-inducing actions of 6-thioguanine on HL-60 cells. *Cancer Res.* **44**, 3907–3910.

39. Stoeckler, J. D., Cambor, C., Kuhns, V., Chu, S.-H., and Parks, R. E., Jr. (1982). Inhibitors of purine nucleoside phosphorylase. C(8) and C(5′) substitutions. *Biochem. Pharmacol.* **31**, 163–171.

40. Sugano, H., Furusawa, M., Kawaguchi, T., and Ikawa, Y. (1973). Enhancement of erythrocyte maturation of Friend virus-induced leukemia cells *in vitro*. *Bibl. Haematol.* **39**, 943–954.

41. Takenaga, K., Hozumi, M., and Sakagami, Y. (1980). Effects of retinoids on induction of differentiation of cultured mouse myeloid leukemia cells. *Cancer Res.* **40**, 914–919.

42. Tei, D., Makino, Y., Sakagami, H., Kanamura, I., and Kanno, K. (1982). Decrease of transferrin receptor during mouse myeloid leukemia (M1) cell differentiation. *Biochem. Biophys. Res. Commun.* **107**, 1419–1424.

43. Terada, M., Epner, E., Nudel, U., Salmon, J., Fibach, E., Rifkind, R. A., and Marks, P. A. (1978). Induction of murine erytholeukemia differentiation by actinomycin D. *Proc. Natl. Acad. Sci. U.S.A.* **75,** 2795–2799.
44. Wotring, L. L., and Roti Roti, J. L. (1980). Thioguanine-induced S and G_2 blocks and their significance to the mechanism of cytotoxicity. *Cancer Res.* **40,** 1458–1462.
45. Yeh, C.-J. G., Papamichael, M., and Foulk, W. P. (1982). Loss of transferrin receptors following induced differentiation of HL-60 promyelocytic leukemia cells. *Exp. Cell Res.* **138,** 429–433.
46. Young, R. C., Ozols, R. F., and Myers, C. E. (1981). The anthracycline antineoplastic drugs. *N. Engl. J. Med.* **305,** 139–153.

10

The Role of Natural Differentiation Factors in Leukemic Cell Maturation Induced by Antineoplastic Agents

ALEXANDER BLOCH

Department of Experimental Therapeutics
Grace Cancer Drug Center
Roswell Park Memorial Institute
Buffalo, New York

I. Introduction

DNA-specific antineoplastic agents have been shown to be capable of inducing the *in vitro* differentiation of various human leukemia cell lines in culture (1–5,7,10–12,14,15). The mechanism by which this induction occurs has been obscure, and the studies reported in this chapter were designed to gain information on the nature of the induction process. ML-1 human myeloblastic leukemia cells were employed, since they differentiate readily to monocyte- and macrophage-like cells upon treatment with DNA-directed agents (14).

We had previously observed that in the absence of fetal bovine serum from the culture medium, DNA-specific agents fail to induce differentiation. That observation implicated serum as a component essential for

NEW AVENUES IN DEVELOPMENTAL
CANCER CHEMOTHERAPY

maturation. We had also demonstrated that fetal bovine serum (13) as well as pokeweed mitogen-stimulated, human leukocyte–conditioned medium (conditioned medium) (16) contain specific factors that induce ML cell differentiation, and we showed that partially purified preparations of such factors can take the place of serum or conditioned medium in the maturation-induction process. The study reported here was directed at establishing the role such differentiation factors play in bringing about drug-stimulated leukemic cell maturation.

II. Methods

ML-1 cells were maintained in RPMI 1640 medium containing penicillin, streptomycin, and 7.5% heat-inactivated fetal bovine serum (14). Assays for growth inhibition, viability, and differentiation were carried out with cultures inoculated with 3×10^5 cells/ml of RPMI 1640 medium to which drug and serum or conditioned medium were added at the specified concentrations. Cell numbers were determined by Coulter counter, viability by trypan blue exclusion, and differentiation by EA rosetting and morphological change (14).

III. Results and Discussion

As demonstrated by the representative experiments shown in Fig. 1, increasing the concentration of daunomycin in the presence of a low concentration (0.07%) of serum leads to an approximately 10% increase in the percentage of differentiated cells that emerges. As the drug concentration is increased, both growth and viability decrease. At the point at which the curves representing these two parameters intersect, inhibition of growth with retention of viability is optimized. Exactly at this point, the maximal number of differentiated cells is obtained, and the drug concentration that provides this effect is, therefore, designated as the optimal differentiation-sensitizing concentration (ODSC). At drug concentrations above and below the ODSC, a smaller percentage of differentiated cells emerges.

As the concentration of serum is increased to 0.5, 1, and 10%, the fraction of differentiated cells that is obtained increases in a concentration-dependent manner (Fig. 1). However, the concentration of drug at which maximal differentiation occurs remains the same, demonstrating that the increase in percentage of differentiated cells is a function of the serum concentration. When serum is replaced with conditioned medium

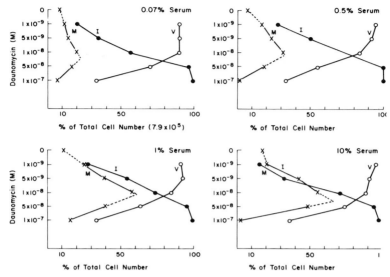

Fig. 1. Effect of varying concentrations of daunomycin and fetal bovine serum on the maturation (M, x-x); growth inhibition (I, ●——●); and viability (V, ○——○) of ML-1 human myeloblastic leukemia cells. Dotted lines represent extrapolations from experimental points.

containing a fixed level of serum (0.1%) (Fig. 2), the fraction of differentiated cells is increased as a function of conditioned medium. When the differentiation-inducing activity partially purified from conditioned medium is used in this assay system, the same result as provided by conditioned medium is obtained (data not shown). Actinomycin D and cytosine arabinoside exert a similar effect on maturation (M), growth inhibition (I), and viability (V) as does daunomycin (data not shown), but the ODSC of actinomycin D and cytosine arabinoside is 5×10^{-10} and 6×10^{-8} M, respectively, as compared to the ODSC of daunomycin, which is 3×10^{-8} M. Maturation is not induced effectively when agents that inhibit protein (Fig. 3) or RNA synthesis (not shown) are used as the differentiation-stimulating components, no matter what concentration of serum or conditioned medium is employed.

These results are generalized in Fig. 4, which summarizes the relationship between DNA-specific agents and natural differentiation factors in affecting the differentiation response. Segment A is a measure of the percentage of differentiated cells that is present in the cell culture free of drug. This fraction is rather small, and its size depends upon the amount of differentiation-inducing factors present in the culture, as well as on the

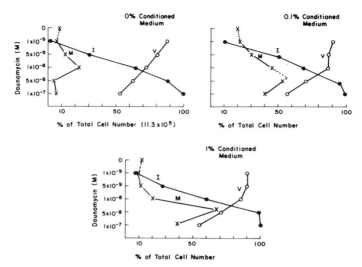

Fig. 2. Effect of varying concentrations of daunomycin and human leukocyte-conditioned medium on the maturation (M, x-x); growth inhibition (I, ●——●); and viability (V, O——O) of ML-1 human myeloblastic leukemia cells. Dotted lines represent extrapolations from experimental points.

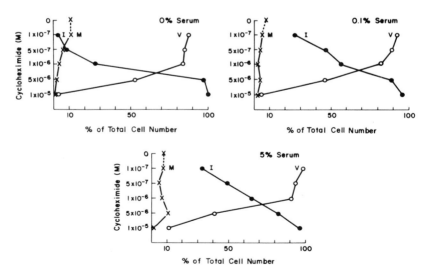

Fig. 3. Effect of varying concentrations of cycloheximide and fetal bovine serum on the maturation (M, x-x); growth inhibition (I, ●——●); and viability (V, O——O) of ML-1 human myeloblastic leukemia cells. Dotted lines represent extrapolations from experimental points.

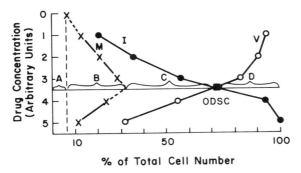

Fig. 4. Interrelationships between DNA-specific agents, natural differentiation factors, and differentiation response. See text for discussion.

relative sensitivity of the leukemic cells to the signal emitted by the factors.

The increase in the fraction of mature cells that occurs by virtue of the presence of the drug is given by segment B. The size of this segment also depends on the concentration of differentiation factors present in the medium. But no matter what this concentration, the maximal stimulatory effect of the drug occurs only at the ODSC. At lower concentrations, the maximal effect of the drug is not reached, and at concentrations above the ODSC, cytotoxicity becomes the determinant of decreased cell differentiation. This deduction is derived from the apparent parallelism that exists at adequate serum concentrations (10%) (Fig. 1), between the increase in differentiated cell fraction and the decrease in cell proliferation that occurs up to the ODSC and, above that level, between the decline in differentiated cell fraction alongside viability.

As visualized by Fig. 4, the total number of differentiated cells is the sum of segments A and B, and the magnitude of this sum is a function of the differentiation factor concentration. In the absence of such factors, the drug alone displays no differentiation-inducing activity. In their presence, the drug stimulates the differentiation of a greater number of cells than mature in the presence of differentiation factors alone.

At the ODSC, the growth of all viable cells is arrested, and segment C is a measure of the fraction of cells that is growth arrested but not recognizably due to maturation. Since the maturation of a cell population is a time-dependent event, the magnitude of this segment decreases with time, and its ultimate size depends on the level of differentiation factors.

Some loss of viability occurs among the drug-exposed cell population, but this loss may represent already damaged cells, whose death may have been accelerated by the presence of the drug. This low fraction of nonviable cells emphasizes the fact that the differentiation-stimulating activity of the drugs occurs at concentrations that are largely noncytocidal (8). Otherwise, maturation could not proceed.

This recognition is of fundamental importance to a differentiation-centered approach to therapy. Since the ODSC of a drug occurs at a specific drug concentration above and below which drug-stimulated differentiation is less effective, the administration of doses of a DNA-specific drug at or near the ODSC would appear essential for effective therapy. Since that critical concentration is difficult to establish *in vivo,* doses that produce a limited degree of toxicity are more likely to be effective than doses that are nontoxic or that produce overwhelming toxicity. Since conversion of the leukemic cells to stably mature forms depends, however, on the level of differentiation factors present in the environment, a maximal therapeutic result can be obtained only when adequate levels of such factors are produced by the host. When factor production is very low or signal recognition markedly impaired, significant remissions cannot be expected to occur with DNA-specific agents administered at their ODSC. In such a case, the parenteral administration of differentiation factors constitutes an essential auxiliary modality. By re-establishing some factor-centered control, it is likely that the cytoreductive regimens employed today are capable of effecting long-term remissions. The level of differentiation factors normally produced does not suffice for controlling a large tumor cell population which, by itself, elaborates factors that signal inhibition of stem cell renewal and precursor cell maturation (6). As a result, mature cells that generate many of the differentiation factors are not formed, leading to the perpetuation of the neoplastic state. In fact, the inability to produce adequate levels of differentiation factors can constitute the oncogenic event, and the application of highly cytotoxic regimens is likely to exacerbate the neoplastic state so generated. Thus, optimal therapeutic regimens based on a differentiation-centered approach need to include cytoreduction by the least toxic means, followed by the combined use of maturation factors and DNA-specific agents at their ODSC.

The molecular events responsible for the selective ability of DNA-specific agents to sensitize leukemic cells to respond to differentiation factors derives from their capacity to interfere with the transcription of the cells' proliferation program, including the expression of oncogenes (9). This interference results in the amplification of the maturation signals emitted by the differentiation factors, initiating the differentiation program unhindered by the DNA-specific inhibitors when these are present at their ODSC. At higher drug concentrations, the differentiation program is also interfered with, and loss of viability results. Because inhibitors of RNA and protein synthesis interfere with metabolic reactions required for the expression of both the proliferation and differentiation program, they lack the selectivity of action that attaches to DNA-specific drugs. It is likely because of this difference that only the DNA- but not the RNA- or protein-specific inhibitors are clinically effective antitumor agents.

References

1. Bloch, A. (1981). Purine and pyrimidine analogs in cancer chemotherapy. *In* "New Leads in Cancer Therapeutics" (E. Mihich, ed.), pp. 65–72. G. K. Hall and Co., Boston, Massachusetts.
2. Bloch, A. (1984). Antitumor agents and the molecular basis of cancer. *Prog. Clin. Biol. Res.* **172B**, 207–214.
3. Bloch, A. (1984). Induced cell differentiation in cancer therapy. *Cancer Treat. Rep.* **68**(1), 199–205.
4. Bloch, A. (1985). Chemotherapeutic agents as differentiation inducers. *In* "Biology and Therapy of Acute Leukemia" (L. Baker, F. Valeriote, and V. Ratanatharathain, eds.), pp. 97–105. Martinus Nijhoff, Boston, Massachusetts.
5. Bodner, A. J., Ting, R. C., and Gallo, R. C. (1981). Induction of differentiation of human promyelocytic leukemia cells (HL-60) by nucleosides and methotrexate. *JNCI, J. Natl. Cancer Inst.* **67**, 1025–1030.
6. Broxmeyer, H. E., Jacobsen, N., Kurland, J., Mendelsohn, N., and Moore, M. A. S. (1978). *In vitro* suppression of normal granulocytic stem cells by inhibitory activity derived from human leukemia cells. *J. Natl. Cancer Inst.* (*U.S.*) **60**, 497–510.
7. Collins, S. J., Bodner, A., Ting, R., and Gallo, R. C. (1980). Induction of morphological and functional differentiation of human promyelocytic leukemia cells (HL-60) by compounds which induce differentiation of murine leukemia cells. *Int. J. Cancer* **25**, 213–218.
8. Craig, R. W., Frankfurt, O. S., Sakagami, H., Takeda, K., and Bloch, A. (1984). Macromolecular and cell cycle effects of different classes of agents inducing the maturation of human myeloblastic leukemia (ML-1) cells. *Cancer Res.* **44**, 2421–2429.
9. Craig, R. W., and Bloch, A. (1984). Early decline in *c-myb* oncogene expression in the differentiation of human myeloblastic leukemia (ML-1) cells induced with 12-*O*-tetradecanoylphorbol-13-acetate. *Cancer Res.* **44**, 442–446.
10. Hozumi, M., Honma, V., Tomida, M., Okabe, J., Kasukabe, T., Sugiyama, K., Hayashi, M., Takenaga, K., and Yamamoto, V. (1979). Induction of differentiation of myeloid leukemia cells with various chemicals. *Acta Haematol. Jpn.* **42**, 941–952.
11. Lotem, J., and Sachs, L. (1980). Potential pre-screening for therapeutic agents that induce differentiation in human myeloid leukemia cells. *Int. J. Cancer* **25**, 561–564.
12. Papac, R. J., Brown, A. E., Schwartz, E. L., and Sartorelli, A. C. (1980). Differentiation of human promyelocytic leukemia cells *in vitro* by 6-thioguanine. *Cancer Lett.* **10**, 33–38.
13. Sakagami, H., Hromchak, R., and Bloch, A. (1984). Prevention of phorbol ester receptor down-modulation in human leukemia ML-1 cells by differentiation-stimulating serum components. *Cancer Res.* **44**, 3330–3335.
14. Takeda, K., Minowada, J., and Bloch, A. (1982). Kinetics of appearance of differentiation associated characteristics in a line of human myeloblastic leukemia cells (ML-1) treated with tetradecanoyl phorbol acetate, dimethylsulfoxide or with arabinofuranosyl cytosine. *Cancer Res.* **42**, 5153–5158.

15. Takeda, K., Minowada, J., and Bloch, A. (1983). The role of drug-induced differentiation in the control of tumor growth. *In* "Biological Characterization of Human Tumours" (W. Davis, C. Maltoni, and S. Tanneberger, eds.), pp. 275–281. Akademie Verlag, Berlin.
16. Takeda, K., Minowada, J., and Bloch, A. (1983). Differential ability of mitogen-stimulated human leukocyte-conditioned media to induce F_c receptors in human leukemia cells. *Cell. Immunol.* **79,** 288–297.

PART IV

Targeting with Monoclonal Antibodies

11

Treatment of Lymphoma with Antibody Preparations Which Rely on Recruiting Natural Effectors

G. T. STEVENSON

Lymphoma Research Unit
Tenovus Laboratory
General Hospital
Southampton, United Kingdom

I. Introduction

Monoclonal technology has yielded many antibodies of greater or lesser specificity for a variety of tumors (24). We remain, however, quite uncertain about the therapeutic possibilities presented by this development. The experience presented in this chapter derives from anti-idiotype antibodies (anti-Id) directed against B-lymphocytic tumors (10,22), a well-characterized system which could provide lessons of much wider applicability.

Antibody by itself alighting on a mammalian cell can trigger various

NEW AVENUES IN DEVELOPMENTAL
CANCER CHEMOTHERAPY

physiological changes, and some of these in the anti-Id system have been described by Glennie *et al.* (4). Rarely, if ever, will antibody in isolation threaten viability. To kill the target cell one must invoke one of two further strategies. The first, to be discussed here, is reliance on the natural effectors which antibody recruits. As far as present knowledge extends, the relevant effectors consist of complement, K cells, and mononuclear phagocytes. The second strategy, dealt with in other chapters in this volume, entails the use of antibodies as vectors to deliver to the cell an exogenous lethal agent such as a toxin, drug, or radioactive isotope. (A third strategy possibly available to anti-Id, the suppression of some physiologically responsive tumors by idiotypic regulation, will not be discussed.)

Treatment of B lymphoma and other tumors with unmodified antibody has proved relatively innocuous. One possible problem, the formation of immune complexes in extracellular fluid, is readily monitored. Another problem, damage to normal cells to which antibody attaches because of immunological cross-reaction or receptors for the Fc region of antibody, is minimized because the natural effectors succeed in destroying a target cell only if the invoking antibody is displayed at the surface in a sufficient density and is properly oriented.

Unfortunately this lack of toxicity has not been matched by therapeutic success. Among the cases of human B lymphoma known to us to have been treated with unmodified anti-Id there has been 1 prolonged complete remission (16), 11 partial remissions, and 6 cases showing no significant response (7,9,14,18). Given these results we are led to consider first the factors thwarting antibody and, second, one of those antibody derivatives which might prove therapeutically more effective while still relying on natural effectors.

II. Factors Thwarting Antibody

A. Inadequate Access to Tumor Cell Surfaces

The cells in nodal masses of lymphoma are reached by antibody given in adequate dosage (14), but a question remains about any tumors which find their way into "immunologically privileged" sites such as the central nervous system or the testis. Problems of accessibility here might prove similar to those encountered in chemotherapy of leukemia and lymphoma.

Even with the cells in accessible sites, antibody can be prevented from reaching the surfaces in adequate amounts by an extracellular barrier of either antigen or anti-antibody. Both of these do more than impede access of therapeutic antibody: the immune complexes they form will consume effector capacity and are an important source of toxicity.

The majority of B-lymphocytic tumors, whether presenting as chronic lymphocytic leukemia or non-Hodgkin's lymphoma, export small amounts of idiotypic immunoglobulin (Ig) (21). In most of our cases idiotypic IgM, in the exported pentameric form, can be found in plasma at 5–200 μg/ml. Although it can be lowered somewhat by plasmapheresis, the upper part of this range represents a serious barrier to anti-Id therapy (7,14). It is important to note that it arises from an export (secretory) pathway, not from turnover at the cell surface: thus there is no apparent correlation between the density of a cell's surface Ig and the rate it delivers antigenically detectable Ig to extracellular fluid.

Perhaps half the cancer patients treated with mouse monoclonal antibody have eventually exhibited a troublesome immune response to the mouse Ig. Such a response appears less common in patients with B-lymphocytic neoplasms, presumably reflecting the severe immunosuppression they so often exhibit. However, it was detected by Meeker et al. (14) in 5 of their 11 cases and at levels requiring termination of antibody therapy.

B. Inadequate or Maldistributed Surface Antigen

It has long been appreciated that insufficient antigen density on a target cell can lead to a failure of antibody plus complement to lyse it, and this has been demonstrated for surface Ig (6). Other effector mechanisms might not be so susceptible to a lowered antigen density (8,13). The surface antigen might be sparse because this is an inherent property of the particular tumor; the surface Ig of chronic lymphocytic leukemia is a good example. Alternatively a low density on a proportion of cells might represent the low end of a distribution reflecting random variation in this particular property; thus, we have often observed on flow cytometry what appears to be a lognormal distribution of surface Ig density on a population of neoplastic lymphocytes.

Recently there have been reports of emergence of idiotypic variants in human lymphoma (15,17). The frequency of such an event remains to be assessed. Monoclonal anti-Id antibodies, each having a specificity limited to one determinant, are clearly more susceptible than polyclonal anti-Id to a loss of reactivity when the target protein is altered by a point mutation.

Antigenic modulation, defined originally as antibody-induced resistance to the cytotoxic action of antibody plus complement, is associated with the redistribution of antigen–antibody complexes on the cell surface

(20). It does not require complete clearance of complexes from the surface, and in the case of surface Ig it can occur with a rapidity sufficient to provide some protection for cells confronted simultaneously by antibody and complement (5). It is likely that antigenic modulation inhibits the therapeutic activity of anti-Id, and it could well cause problems for many other monoclonal antibodies of therapeutic promise in cancer (19).

C. Failure to Recruit Appropriate Effectors

Failure of antibody in this category could result either from its being the wrong isotype (i.e., class) for recruitment of the effector or from exhaustion of the effector mechanism in dealing with cells and immune complexes. The difficulty we face here is that neither clinical nor experimental observations have yielded clear information as to which effector mechanisms are of prime importance in the antibody attack on tumor cells. This is well illustrated by experiments attempting to elucidate the role of complement.

In two systems employing antigens other than idiotype, the addition of exogenous complement appeared to enhance the destruction of neoplastic cells by antibody *in vivo* (1,11). However Lanier *et al.* (12), in investigating the therapeutic effect of anti-Id in a murine lymphoma, noted that

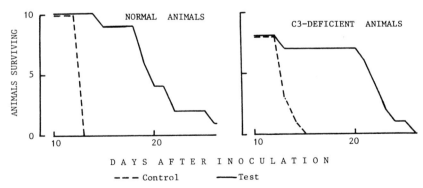

Fig. 1. Treatment of the L$_2$C leukemia in strain 2 guinea pigs with anti-Id. On day 0 each animal is inoculated intraperitoneally with 5 × 10^5 leukemic cells. Twenty-four hours later it receives a single intraperitoneal injection of 10 mg of IgG from either rabbit normal serum (control) or rabbit anti-Id serum (test). The leukemia has a doubling time *in vivo* of about 20 hr, so that therapeutic destruction of 90% of the cells will, by simple kinetic calculation, prolong life by 3 days. The complement-deficient variant of strain 2 animals has C3 at only 6% of the normal level, apparently due to hypercatabolism of a mutant molecule (2); this is similar to the C3 depletion achievable with cobra venom factor.

equally good responses to therapy were shown by C5-deficient or cobra venom factor–treated mice as by normal mice. Our recent experience with anti-Id treatment of the guinea pig L$_2$C leukemia adds weight to the proposition that complement is not playing a major role. A murine monoclonal IgG1 antibody, which could not mediate complement lysis *in vitro*, was broadly as effective as two polyclonal, complement-activating, anti-Id preparations (rabbit and sheep) in retarding the tumor. Furthermore, the rabbit antibody was no more therapeutically effective in normal guinea pigs than in a C3-deficient strain (Fig. 1).

It remains to be determined which, if any, of the other known candidate mechanisms (antibody-dependent cellular cytotoxicity, antibody-dependent cytostasis, phagocytosis) is useful in this context. The demonstration that F(ab')$_2$ fragments of anti-Id were therapeutically ineffective against a murine lymphoma (12) suggests that *some* effector mechanism is required.

III. Treatment of B Lymphoma with an FabIgG Derivative of Anti-Id

In order that a cell receive protection from antigenic modulation the surface antigens must be linked by bi- or multivalent antibody. Univalent antibody will avoid modulation, and *univalent antibody with an intact Fc region* will at the same time retain an ability to recruit effector mechanisms. Such a univalent antibody, Fab/c from rabbit anti-Id, was shown to be more effective than the bivalent parent in killing guinea pig lymphoma cells both *in vitro* and *in vivo* (3). As an extension of this approach we have prepared the *chimeric univalent antibody*, FabIgG. Here Fab'γ, derived from peptic digestion of antibody, is linked to normal IgG of the recipient species (Fig. 2). The linkage is via thioether bonds involving cysteine residues in the hinge region of both partners, an arrangement which permits only a limited number of orientations of the Fab'γ in relation to the IgG (23). In addition to avoiding antigenic modulation and retaining the ability to recruit effectors, it is designed to be minimally immunogenic and to have good metabolic survival. The yield (about 40% in terms of starting Fab'γ) is better than that obtainable with Fab/c, and it is available from a wider range of antibodies.

At the time of treatment B.R. was a 52-year-old woman with widespread B-cell lymphoma of the nodular, centrocytic/centroblastic type. The spleen was 4 cm below the costal margin, there was extensive lymphadenopathy and marrow infiltration, and neoplastic cells were present in the blood at about 7×10^9/liter. The cells exhibited surface IgM at a

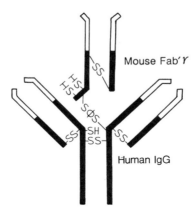

Fig. 2. The chimeric univalent antibody FabIgG (23). F(ab'γ)₂ from peptic digestion of mouse monoclonal antibody is lightly reduced and allowed to react with a large molar surplus of the cross-linker *o*-phenylenedimaleimide (25). The resultant Fab'γ with free maleimide groups then reacts with lightly reduced human normal IgG to give FabIgG linked via thioether bonds. It is separated by recycling chromatography on Sephacryl S300 (Pharmacia, Uppsala, Sweden).

density sparse compared with normal B cells. Plasma idiotypic Ig was at less than 2 μg/ml. She had not received any chemotherapy. An infusion of 200 mg of mouse monoclonal IgG1 anti-Id transiently reduced the circulating neoplastic cells to 3×10^9/liter. No other effects were noted from this infusion. Beginning 2 weeks later she was given a course of four infusions of 380–580 mg of FabIgG over a period of 11 weeks. Each infusion was followed by a fall in the number of circulating neoplastic cells, reaching a minimum of 5–50% of the preinfusion level after about 24 hr. The reductions were rather slower than those occurring in this and other patients after infusions of IgG antibody. For 3 days after infusion there was a raised level of the complement breakdown product C3c in the plasma. Four days after completion of each FabIgG infusion lymph nodes in all areas had swollen to about twice their previous size and were tender. They remained enlarged for 5–8 days and then subsided. There was no corresponding enlargement of the spleen. Four weeks after completing the course of infusions the number of circulating neoplastic cells was at about 50% of pretreatment level, the nodal masses had shrunk, and the spleen was palpable only on deep inspiration.

After each infusion of FabIgG the antibody disappeared from the plasma, with a half-life of less than 24 hr. This rapid consumption was thought to reflect uptake by the very large tumor mass. However it was thought important to confirm that the FabIgG was not merely being scavenged by the mononuclear phagocyte system or was not suffering some other unexpected metabolic demise. The patient therefore consented to a control infusion of FabIgG in which the Fab moiety had anti-idiotype activity against guinea pig L$_2$C cells and no activity against her tumor cells or against human normal lymphocytes; the IgG moiety was again normal human. Plasma levels of mouse Fab'γ were estimated only for 1 week after the infusion, but it became apparent that the half-life was >10 days and probably close to the approximate value of 20 days expected for human normal IgG. In contrast to this survival is a metabolic half-life of only 5 days observed for sheep IgG during the treatment of a patient with sheep polyclonal anti-idiotype (9). At no time during or after treatment could any antibody response to mouse Ig be detected.

We consider this a modest therapeutic result achieved at the cost of no significant toxicity. Surprise was occasioned by our failure to exceed the binding capacity of the tumor and its extracellular product even after a cumulative dose of 1.9 g of reagent. We feel that the patient will now be best served by reducing her tumor mass by chemotherapy and again treating her with FabIgG.

IV. Conclusion

Antibody treatment of neoplasm appears to be at the stage chemotherapy was in the 1940s, after the introduction of nitrogen mustard and methotrexate. Partial and only partially predictable therapeutic responses indicate the need for a long developmental period. Many mechanisms and variables need to be elucidated, quite apart from the strategic issue of whether it will be more rewarding to rely on antibody to recruit natural effectors or to deliver exogenous toxins. It will be surprising if we do not learn in some way to make good therapeutic use of these highly specific reagents now available in plentiful amounts.

Acknowledgments

This work has been supported by Tenovus, the Cancer Research Campaign, and the Leukaemia Research Fund.

References

1. Bernstein, I. D., Tam, M. R., and Nowinski, R. C. (1980). Mouse leukemia: Therapy with monoclonal antibodies against a thymus differentiation antigen. *Science* **207**, 68–71.

2. Burger, R., Gordon, J., Stevenson, G., Ramadori, G., Zanker, B., Hadding, U., and Bitter-Suermann, D. (1985). An inherited deficiency of the third component of complement, C3, in guinea pigs. *Eur. J. Immunol.* (in press).

3. Glennie, M. J., and Stevenson, G. T. (1982). Univalent antibodies kill tumour cells *in vitro* and *in vivo*. *Nature (London)* **295**, 712–714.

4. Glennie, M. J., Stevenson, F. K., Stevenson, G. T., and Virji, M. (1979). Cross-linking of lymphocytic surface immunoglobulin inhibits its production via a cyclic nucleotide mechanism. *Nature (London)* **281**, 305–307.

5. Gordon, J., and Stevenson, G. T. (1981). Antigenic modulation of lymphocytic surface immunoglobulin yielding resistance to complement-mediated lysis. II. Relationship to redistribution of the antigen. *Immunology* **42**, 13–17.

6. Gordon, J., Anderson, V. A., Robinson, D. S. F., and Stevenson, G. T. (1982). The influence of antigen density and a comparison of IgG and IgM antibodies in the anti-complementary modulation of lymphocytic surface immunoglobulin. *Scand. J. Immunol.* **15**, 169–177.

7. Gordon, J., Abdul-Ahad, A. K., Hamblin, T. J., Stevenson, F. K., and Stevenson, G. T. (1984). Mechanisms of tumour cell escape encountered in treating lymphocytic leukaemia with anti-idiotypic antibody. *Br. J. Cancer* **49**, 547–557.

8. Halloran, P. F., and Stylianos, S. K. (1980). Augmentation of antibody-dependent cell-mediated cytotoxicity by anti-immunoglobulin. *Clin. Exp. Immunol.* **42**, 127–135.

9. Hamblin, T. J., Abdul-Ahad, A. K., Gordon, J., Stevenson, F. K., and Stevenson, G. T. (1980). Preliminary experience in treating lymphocytic leukaemia with antibody to immunoglobulin idiotypes on the cell surfaces. *Br. J. Cancer* **42**, 495–502.

10. Hatzubai, A., Maloney, D. G., and Levy, R. (1981). The use of a monoclonal anti-idiotype antibody to study the biology of a human B cell lymphoma. *J. Immunol.* **126**, 2397–2402.

11. Kassel, R. L., Old., L. J., Carswell, E., Fiore, N., and Hardy, W. D. (1973). Serum-mediated leukemia cell destruction in AKR mice. Role of complement in the phenomenon. *J. Exp. Med.* **138**, 925–938.

12. Lanier, L. L., Babcock, G. F., Raybourne, R. B., Arnold, L. W., Warner, N. L., and Haughton, G. (1980). Mechanism of B-cell lymphoma immunotherapy with passive xenogeneic anti-idiotype serum. *J. Immunol.* **125**, 1730–1736.

13. Lawson, A. D. G., and Stevenson, G. T. (1983). Macrophages induce antibody-dependent cytostasis but not lysis in guinea-pig leukaemic cells. *Br. J. Cancer* **48**, 227–237.

14. Meeker, T. C., Lowder, J., Maloney, D. G., Miller, R. A., Thielemans, K., Warnke, R., and Levy, R. (1985). A clinical trial of anti-idiotype therapy for B cell malignancy. *Blood* **65**, 1349–1363.

15. Meeker, T. C., Lowder, J., Cleary, M. L., Stewart, S., Warnke, R., Sklar, J., and Levy, R. (1985). Emergence of idiotype variants during treatment of B-cell lymphoma with anti-idiotype antibodies. *N. Engl. J. Med.* **312**, 1658–1665.

16. Miller, R. A., Maloney, D. G., Warnke, R., and Levy, R. (1982). Treatment of B-cell lymphoma with monoclonal anti-idiotype antibody. *N. Engl. J. Med.* **306**, 517–522.

17. Raffeld, M., Neckers, L., Longo, D. L., and Cossman, J. (1985). Spontaneous alteration of idiotype in a monoclonal B-cell lymphoma. *N. Engl. J. Med.* **312**, 1653–1658.

18. Rankin, E. M., Hekman, A., Hardeman, M. R., and Hocfragel, C. A. (1984). Dynamic studies of lymphocytes labelled with indium-111 during and after treatment with monoclonal anti-idiotype antibody in advanced B cell lymphoma. *Br. Med. J.* **289**, 1097–1100.

19. Ritz, J., and Schlossman, S. F. (1982). Utilization of monoclonal antibodies in the treatment of leukemia and lymphoma. *Blood* **59**, 1–11.

20. Stackpole, C. W., Jacobson, J. B., and Lardis, M. P. (1974). Antigenic modulation *in*

vitro. I. Fate of thymus-leukemia (TL) antigen-antibody complexes following modulation of TL antigenicity from the surfaces of mouse leukemia cells and thymocytes. *J. Exp. Med.* **140,** 939–953.

21. Stevenson, F. K., Hamblin, T. J., Stevenson, G. T., and Tutt, A. L. (1980). Extracellular idiotypic immunoglobulin arising from human leukemic B lymphocytes. *J. Exp. Med.* **152,** 1484–1496.

22. Stevenson, G. T., and Stevenson, F. K. (1975). Antibody to a molecularly-defined antigen confined to a tumour cell surface. *Nature (London)* **254,** 714–716.

23. Stevenson, G. T., Glennie, M. J., Paul, F. E., Stevenson, F. K., Watts, H. F., and Wyeth, P. (1985). Preparation and properties of FabIgG, a chimeric univalent antibody designed to attack tumour cells. *Biosci. Rep.* **5,** 991–998.

24. Wright, G. L., ed. (1984). "Monoclonal Antibodies and Cancer." Dekker, New York.

25. Yoshitake, S., Hamaguchi, Y., and Ishikawa, E. (1979). Efficient conjugation of rabbit Fab' with β-D-galactosidase from Escherichia coli. *Scand. J. Immunol.* **10,** 81–86.

12

Immunotoxins

ELLEN S. VITETTA

Department of Microbiology
University of Texas Health Science Center at Dallas
Dallas, Texas

PHILIP E. THORPE

Drug Targeting Laboratory
Imperial Cancer Research Fund Laboratories
London, United Kingdom

I. Introduction

Many types of tumor cells express high levels of tissue-specific differentiation antigens, receptors for growth factors, or viral antigens on their surface. Antibodies against these antigens have been coupled to potent toxins to produce reagents (called "immunotoxins") which are power-

NEW AVENUES IN DEVELOPMENTAL
CANCER CHEMOTHERAPY

fully and selectively toxic to cells that express the appropriate target antigen (3,8,13,17,27,28,43). These antigens are often expressed in lower densities on normal tissue or at the same density on minor subpopulations of normal cells. However, if the normal tissues are not life-sustaining, these immunotoxins may be useful as tumor-specific reagents.

Several toxins produced by bacteria and plants have been used to arm antibody molecules. These toxins are proteins which, in their active forms, consist of a cell-binding B chain and a toxin A chain joined by a disulfide bond (22). The most widely used of these toxins is ricin from the seeds of the plant *Ricinus communis*. The B chain of ricin binds to galactose-containing glycoproteins and glycolipids that are expressed on the surface of most cell types (24,29). Following internalization of the toxin, the A chain penetrates the membrane of an endocytic vesicle (23) and kills the cell by catalytically inactivating its ribosomes.

II. Cytotoxic Activity of Immunotoxins

Two general strategies have been adopted for conferring selectivity of binding upon toxins. The first is to link the intact toxin directly to the antibody molecule. Immunotoxins of this type always exert potent cytotoxic effects on cells that express the appropriate antigens. However, immunotoxins prepared with holotoxins must be used in the presence of high concentrations of free galactose or lactose *in vitro* to antagonize their nonspecific binding to galactose-containing molecules on nontarget cells (21,35).

The second strategy is to link the antibody by a disulfide bond to the isolated toxin A chain or, alternatively, to one of the single-chain ribosome-inactivating proteins (RIP) (e.g., gelonin) that are widely distributed in the plant kingdom and whose action upon eukaryotic ribosomes is presently indistinguishable from that of the A chains of holotoxins (1). These immunotoxins, although lacking the problem of nonspecific binding, show great variability in their cytotoxic potency. Thus, some immunotoxins are as effective as native toxin (11,35), and others are only weakly toxic or nontoxic (35). Even when A-chain immunotoxins are highly effective, the kinetics of inhibition of protein synthesis are slower than when ricin immunotoxins are used (21,44). The major variables that determine the potency of immunotoxins include the density of cell-surface antigen to which the antibody is directed (25), the rate of endocytosis of the antigen–immunotoxin complex (which in turn depends upon the nature of the antigen on the target cell), the binding affinity and isotype of the antibody (4,18), and the stability of the linkage between the A chain and the antibody (11,18).

III. Potentiation of Toxicity of A-Chain Immunotoxins

The variability in target cell toxicity of A-chain immunotoxins and the finding that A-chain immunotoxins kill cells more slowly than ricin immunotoxins *in vitro* has made it desirable to develop methods to increase their potency. One approach for increasing specific toxicity is to use lysosomotropic agents such as ammonium chloride or chloroquine (4,26). These agents raise the pH of endosomal and lysosomal compartments of the cell and may also perturb membranes in other ways. These agents may enhance toxicity by decreasing the proteolysis of the ingested immunotoxin and thus increase the efficiency of A-chain translocation.

Another way to enhance the potency of A-chain immunotoxins is to use free ricin B chain. The addition of B chains to cells coated with the A-chain immunotoxins often gives a much improved and accelerated cytotoxic effect (19,44). Thus, the B chain of the toxin, in addition to its cell-binding property, also appears to facilitate the entry of the A-chain portion of the immunotoxin into cytoplasm. The mechasnism by which the B chain assists A-chain entry is unknown. The B chain could protect the A chain from proteolysis or could insert into the membrane of the endosome or lysosome and, either alone or in conjunction with its cell surface receptor, form a channel through which the A chain can enter the cytoplasm.

Vitetta *et al.* (41) have recently described the use of B-chain immunotoxins to potentiate killing by A-chain immunotoxins. The rationale was that if both immunotoxins were bound to the same cell, a portion of each would be endocytosed within the same vesicle. The A and B chains might be cleaved from their respective antibodies and thereby allow the B chain to potentiate translocation of the A chain. *In vitro* experiments in which A and B-chain immunotoxins of the same specificity were used showed a marked and specific potentiation of the toxicity of A-chain immunotoxins. B-chain immunotoxins, by themselves, were essentially nontoxic. Furthermore, the attachment of B chain to antibody resulted in significant attenuation of the galactose-binding site. Thus, synergy depended on specificity of the antibody portion of each immunotoxin for the target cell.

A variation of this approach is to generate B-chain immunotoxins in which the antibody is specific for the antibody component of the A-chain immunotoxin, i.e., a "piggyback" approach. This approach was highly effective (42). It also allowed the use of the F(ab') A-chain immunotoxin to coat the target cells. This has a potential advantage for *in vivo* use. Thus, the F(ab') A-chain immunotoxin should be removed relatively rapidly from the circulation (33) but should be retained on the target cell surface for prolonged periods of time because of its univalency. Thus, it might be possible to inject the B-chain immunotoxin after much of the F(ab') A-chain has been cleared from the circulation. This maneuver might minimize nonspecific toxicity and yet allow the potentiation of specific target cell toxicity.

IV. Modification of the Galactose Binding Sites of Ricin

The problem with using free ricin B chain or B-chain immunotoxins to enhance the cytotoxic activity of A-chain immunotoxins *in vivo* is that the B chain retains some or all of its ability to bind to galactose. Much of the free B chain or B-chain immunotoxin would, therefore, be absorbed by galactose-bearing cells and serum glycoproteins *in vivo,* thereby reducing the potentiation of the toxic effect upon the target cells. For this reason, we sought ways to modify the galactose-binding capacity of the B chain in intact ricin immunotoxins and in B-chain immunotoxins.

One way to attenuate galactose-binding activity is to utilize "blocked" ricin immunotoxins. Thorpe *et al.* (36) used a short thioether bond to link ricin to antibody and found that a proportion of the immunotoxin molecules then passed through an asialofetuin–Sepharose column, indicating that they had markedly diminished galactose-binding activity. The blockade of galactose binding sites appears to be a steric effect, i.e., the lectin sites on the B chain are "hidden" by the attached antibody. The result is the generation of a subset of immunotoxin molecules that retains the high potency of ricin-containing immunotoxins but that does not kill cells nonspecifically in the absence of galactose. Such immunotoxins are highly effective both *in vitro* and *in vivo*. However, they still retain significant nonspecific toxicity when used *in vivo,* possibly because cells of the reticuloendothelial system (RES) remove such molecules from the circulation (5,6,32,34,37), degrade them, and then release toxic fragments into the bloodstream.

A more permanent method of blocking the galactose binding sites of ricin was recently devised by E. S. Vitetta (39). Studies performed several years ago by Sandvig *et al.* (30) suggested that iodination of intact ricin by the chloramine T method resulted in loss of toxicity. It was unclear whether this loss of toxicity was related to iodination of the A and/or the B chains and to what extent each retained its normal function. A series of experiments was therefore aimed at investigating the effect of chloramine T–mediated iodination or of chloramine T treatment alone of the B chain on its galactose-binding ability. It was found that B chains treated with sodium iodide and chloramine T or chloramine T alone (under conditions in which the recovery of B chains was approximately 20–40%) had lost their ability to bind to asialofetuin. Nevertheless, when such treated B chains were covalently coupled to the appropriate antibody and evaluated in the "piggyback" killing of Daudi cells, they could still potentiate killing, albeit to a lesser extent than immunotoxins formed with native B chains. Moreover, the failure to couple modified B chains to antibody as effectively as native B-chains could account for the decreased toxicity.

These studies have implications beyond their obvious practical use since they indicate that the galactose-binding capacity of the B chain is not required for the potentiation of the toxicity induced by A-chain immunotoxin. This suggests that different domains of the B chain are responsible for lectin activity and A-chain translocation. Hence, modification of B chains by genetic engineering may be the strategy of choice for the future.

V. Antitumor Effects in Experimental Animals

Krolick and his colleagues (14) induced prolonged remissions in mice with advanced BCL_1 leukemia by a sequence of total lymphoid irradiation, splenectomy, and intravenous administration of an immunotoxin; the immunotoxin was constructed by linking ricin A chain to antibodies against immunoglobulin δ chain which is expressed on the leukemic cells. Mice that received cytoreductive therapy and "irrelevant" immunotoxin suffered early leukemic relapse and death. Less dramatic, but nevertheless convincing, antitumor effects have been obtained in mice by several other groups by administering ricin A-chain immunotoxins intraperitoneally or intratumorally.

Two reports of good antitumor effects of immunotoxins in guinea pigs have been described by Bernhard et al. (2) and Hwang et al. (10). These investigators demonstrated that the intravenous administration of anti-JJO hepatoma immunotoxins, prepared with diphtheria toxin A chain or abrin A chain, delayed or abolished the growth of established intradermal

JJO tumors. Abrin A-chain immunotoxin was also able to delay or inhibit tumor metastses to the lymph nodes: 20–40% of the treated animals had long-term remissions.

Recently, Thorpe and co-workers (38) linked saporin (an RIP from *Saponaria officinalis*) to monoclonal anti-Thy 1.1 antibody. A single intravenous injection of the immunotoxin into mice bearing a Thy 1.1-expressing lymphoma allograft prolonged survival time to an extent corresponding to that expected if 99.999% of the tumor cells had been eradicated. Interestingly, ricin A chain coupled to the same antibody was 100–1000 times less effective than the saporin immunotoxin as an antitumor agent *in vivo*, even though the two immunotoxins were equally cytotoxic to the lymphoma cells in tissue culture. This difference suggests that the saporin immunotoxins are either more stable *in vivo* than those prepared with ricin A chain or that they do not interact as extensively with cellular or noncellular components of the host (e.g., in a manner that would promote their clearance or would inhibit their diffusion throughout the tissues of the animal). Another unexpected finding to emerge from studies utilizing saporin immunotoxin was that it caused gross necrosis in the liver of the recipients, an effect that was not observed with the ricin A-chain immunotoxin. Clearly, a better understanding of the interactions of immunotoxins with host tissues is needed before their activity *in vivo* can be optimized and before they can be regarded as safe for administration to patients.

VI. Problems Confronting Immunotoxins for Therapy *in Vivo*

A. Linkage Instability

A disulfide bond between antibody and A chain gives the greatest cytotoxic effect. Unfortunately, when some antibodies are used, the disulfide bond introduced by reagents such as SPDP or 2-iminothiolane is unstable in animals. This could be due to the splitting of the immunotoxin by thiol-containing molecules in the bloodstream and peripheral tissues. In one study, blood samples removed from mice up to 48 hr after injecting radiolabeled abrin A-chain immunotoxins prepared with these reagents were analyzed by sodium dodecyl sulfate polyacrylamide gel electrophoresis (SDS-PAGE) and autoradiography (P. E. Thorpe *et al.*, unpublished results). The pattern of radiolabeled protein bands showed a gradual disappearance of SPDP- and 2-iminothiolane-linked immunotoxins, with a half-life in both cases of about 8 hr. During this time, free antibody appeared in the circulation; free A chain was not observed, since it was probably cleared very rapidly. We recently developed a new linking agent called "SMBT" to overcome this problem. This reagent generates a disulphide linkage that is shielded from thiol attack by a methyl group and benzene ring adjacent to the disulfide bond. Immunotoxins prepared with the SMBT reagent show no detectable breakdown after injection into mice and give superior antitumor effects as compared to immunotoxins prepared with the SPDP and 2-iminothiolane reagents (P. E. Thorpe *et al.*, unpublished results).

A second bond suspected of instability is the aliphatic carboxamide bond by which many of the cross-linkers currently available (e.g., SPDP) are attached to the antibody. The degradation of this linkage appears to be a property of certain types of tumor cells (e.g., AKR-A mouse lymphoma cells) rather than to host factors. A subpopulation (about 1%) of AKR-A cells survive exposure to SPDP-linked anti-Thy-1.1-abrin-A immunotoxins both *in vitro* and *in vivo*. This same subpopulation of cells can be killed by immunotoxins prepared with cross-linking agents (e.g., 2-iminothiolane and SMBT) that introduce other types of bonds. It is possible that the resistant cells have elevated levels of an enzyme capable of splitting aliphatic carboxamide bonds (P. E. Thorpe *et al.*, unpublished results).

B. Recognition by the Reticuloendothelial System

The cells of the reticuloendothelial system (RES) have receptors that bind the mannose-terminating oligosaccharides present on ricin and other toxins (32,37). As a result, they clear the immunotoxins rapidly from the bloodstream and are damaged (5). This problem has been overcome by chemically (37) or enzymatically (7) deglycosylating the toxins before their linkage to the antibody. In this regard, we have recently demonstrated (40) that immunotoxins prepared with deglycosylated ricin A or B chains are effective in the "piggyback" killing of Daudi cells *in vitro*. Futhermore, anti-Thy-1.1 antibodies coupled to deglycosylated A chains have a longer serum half-life and do not cause liver damage (D. Blakey and P. Thorpe, unpublished observations). Thus, the use of immunotoxins containing deglycosylated A chain, B chain, or holotoxin may improve antitumor effects *in vivo* and may decrease nonspecific uptake and damage to the RES.

C. Tumor Cell Heterogeneity

Antigen-negative tumor variants are likely to emerge unless cocktails of tumor-reactive immunotoxins are used. Similarly, toxin-resistant tumor variants may emerge unless cocktails of immunotoxins are prepared from toxins whose mode of entry and toxicity are different.

D. Immunogenicity

Neutralizing antibodies are certain to be produced by patients who are not severely immunosuppressed, making it imperative to alter the toxin and antibody components to ones antigenically dissimilar to those initially injected into the patient.

E. Failure to Permeate Solid Tumor Masses

The most promising results of *in vivo* administration of immunotoxins into experimental animals have utilized leukemia models in which the cells are freely available to systemically administered immunotoxin. The problems related to the penetration of solid tumors with immunotoxins are formidable. Solutions to this problem will probably involve utilizing fragments of antibody to prepare immunotoxins, and agents to facilitate escape of the immunotoxin from the vascular system supplying the solid tumor. The most promising strategy for treating advanced solid tumors in patients will probably be to use cytoreductive therapy or surgery to eliminate the vast majority of tumor cells nonspecifically and immunotoxin to kill residual cells.

VII. Genetically Engineered Immunotoxins

Over the past few years, numerous advances in molecular biology suggest that it will soon be feasible to tailor-make toxins for drug-targeting purposes. The structural genes encoding diphtheria toxin fragments (9,16) and the ricin precursor, preproricin (15), have been cloned in *Escherichia coli*. In the case of diphtheria toxin, the toxin fragments are synthesized and secreted into the periplasmic space of the bacterium and are enzymically active (16). Several groups are in the process of modifying toxin genes in order to delete the nonspecific, cell-binding property of the B chain. It is hoped that such mutagenized, recombinant ricin, once attached to a specific antibody, will retain its ability to insert into the membrane of the target cell and that the modified B chain will assist the entry of the A chain into the cytoplasm. Obviously, as we learn more about the mechanisms of A-chain translocation, new possibilities will arise for altering the A chain to make it more effective and for altering the B chain to improve its ability to affect translocation. It may also be possible to modify those regions of the gene that encode the antigenic domains of the toxin and to thereby avoid an antitoxin response.

Another goal is to produce immunotoxins entirely by recombinant DNA technology. Transfection of myeloma cells or bacteria with immunoglobulin genes ligated to toxin genes could facilitate the production of large quantities of immunotoxins provided that variants of the (myeloma) cells that are insensitive to the toxic effects of the A chain can be selected. The feasibility of this approach has been elegantly demonstrated by Neuberger and his colleagues who have ligated heavy-chain genes of monoclonal anti-hapten antibodies to the staphylococcal nuclease gene (20). Once transfected into myeloma cells producing the appropriate light chain, intact antibodies ligated to the enzyme are secreted by the hybridoma cells. The linkage of the A chain to an antibody *via* conventional DNA-splicing methods might prove problematic, since the A chain and the antibody must be cleaved in the endosome of the target cell. However, it is conceivable that these genes could be ligated with an intervening sequence encoding a polypeptide that can be split by proteolytic enzymes in the endosome but not in the serum.

Acknowledgments

This work was partially supported by NIH grant CA-28149. We thank Ms. A. Pereira and Ms. G. A. Cheek for secretarial assistance.

References

1. Barbieri, J., and Stirpe, F. (1982). Ribosome-inactivating proteins from plants: Properties and possible uses. *Cancer Surv.* **1**, 489–520.
2. Bernhard, M. J., Foon, K. A., Oeltmann, T. N., Key, M. F., Hwang, K. M., Clarke, G. C., Christensen, W. J., Hoyer, J. C., Hanna, M. G., and Oldham, R. K. (1983). Guinea pig line 10 hepatocarcinoma model: Characterization of monoclonal antibody and *in vivo* effect of unconjugated antibody and antibody conjugated to diphtheria toxin A chain. *Cancer Res.* **43**, 4420–4428.
3. Blythman, H. E., Casellas, P., Gros, O., Gros, P., Jansen, F. K., Paolucci, F., Pau, R., and Vidal, H. (1981). Immunotoxins: Hybrid molecules of monoclonal antibodies and a toxin subunit specifically kill tumor cells. *Nature (London)* **290**, 145–146.
4. Casellas, P., Bourrie, B. J. P., Gros, P., and Jansen, F. (1984). Kinetics of cytotoxicity induced by immunotoxins: Enhancement by lysosomotropic amines and carboxylic ionophores. *J. Biol. Chem.* **259**, 9359–9368.
5. Derenzini, M., Bonetti, E., Marinozzi, V., and Stirpe, F. (1976). Toxin effect of ricin. Studies on the pathogenesis of liver lesions. *Virchows. Arch. B* **20**, 15–17.

6. Fodstad, O., Olsnes, S., and Pihl, A. (1976). Toxicity, distribution and elimination of the cancerostatic lectins abrin and ricin after parenteral injection into mice. *Br. J. Cancer* **34**, 418–425.

7. Foxwell, R. M. J., Donovan, T. A., Thorpe, P. E., and Wilson, G. (1985). The removal of carbohydrates from ricin with endoglycosidases H, F and D and α-mannosidase. *Biochim. Biophys. Acta* **840**, 193–203.

8. Gilliland, D. G., Steplewski, Z., Collier, R. J., Mitchell, K. F., and Chang, T. H. (1980). Antibody-directed cytotoxic agents: Use of monoclonal antibody to direct the action of toxin A-chains to colorectal carcinoma cells. *Proc. Natl. Acad. Sci. U.S.A.* **77**, 4539–4553.

9. Greenfield, L., Bjorn, M. J., Horn, G., Fong, D., Buck, G. A., Collier, R. J., and Kaplan, D. A. (1983). Nucleotide sequence of the structural gene for diphtheria toxin carried by corynebacteriophage β. *Proc. Natl. Acad. Sci. U.S.A.* **80**, 6853–6857.

10. Hwang, K. M., Foon, K. A., Cheung, P., Pearson, J. W., and Oldham, R. K. (1984). Selective anti-tumor effect of L10 hepatocarcinoma cells of a potent immunoconjugate composed of the A-chain of abrin and a monoclonal antibody to a hepatoma-associated antigen. *Cancer Res.* **44**, 4578–4586.

11. Jansen, F. K., Blythman, H. E., Carriere, D., Casellas, P., and Gros, O. (1982). Immunotoxins: Hybrid molecules combining high specificity and potent cytotoxicity. *Immunol. Rev.* **62**, 185–216.

12. Kishida, K., Masuho, Y., Saito, M., Hara, T., and Fuji, H. (1983). Ricin A-chain conjugated with monoclonal anti-L1210 antibody. *In vitro* and *in vivo* anti-tumor activity. *Cancer Immunol. Immunother.* **16**, 93–97.

13. Krolick, K. A., Villemez, C., Isakson, P., Uhr, J. W., and Vitetta, E. S. (1980). Selective killing of normal or neoplastic B cells by antibody coupled to the A-chain of ricin. *Proc. Natl. Acad. Sci. U.S.A.* **77**, 5419–5423.

14. Krolick, K. A., Uhr, J. W., Slavin, S., and Vitetta, E. S. (1982). *In vivo* therapy of a murine B cell tumor (BCL$_1$) using antibody-ricin A-chain immunotoxins. *J. Exp. Med.* **155**, 1797–1809.

15. Lamb, F. I., Roberts, L. M., and Lord, J. M. (1985). Nucleotide sequence of cloned cDNA coding for preproricin. *Eur. J. Biochem.* **148**, 265–270.

16. Leong, D., Coleman, K. D., and Murphy, J. R. (1983). Cloned fragment A of diphtheria toxin is expressed and secreted into the periplasmic space of *Escherichia coli* K12. *Science,* **220**, 515–517.

17. Masuho, Y., and Harra, T. (1980). Target-cell cytotoxicity of a hybrid of Fab' of immunoglobulin and A-chain of ricin. *Gann* **71**, 75–79.

18. Masuho, Y., Kishida, K., Saito, M., Umemoto, N., and Hara, T. (1982). Importance of the antigen-binding valency and the nature of the crosslinked bond in ricin A-chain conjugates with antibody. *J. Biochem. (Tokyo)* **91**, 1583.

19. McIntosh, D. P., Edwards, D. C., Cumber, A. J., Parnell, G. D., Dean, C. J., Ross, W. C. J., and Forrester, J. A. (1983). Ricin B-chain converts a non-cytotoxic antibody-ricin A-chain conjugate into a potent and specific cytotoxic agent. *FEBS Lett.* **164**, 17–20.

20. Neuberger, M. S., Williams, G. T., and Fox, R. O. (1984). Recombinant antibodies possessing novel effector functions. *Nature (London)* **312**, 604–608.

21. Neville, D. M., Jr., and Youle, R. J. (1982). Monoclonal antibody-ricin or ricin A-chain hybrids: Kinetic analysis of cell killing for tumor therapy. *Immunol. Rev.* **62**, 75–92.

22. Olsnes, S., and Pihl, A. (1982). Toxic lectins and related proteins. *In* "Molecular Action of Toxins and Viruses" (P. Cohen and S. van Heyningen, eds.) pp. 503–513. Am. Elsevier, New York.

23. Olsnes, S., and Sandvig, K. (1983). Entry of polypeptide toxins into animal cells. *In*

"Receptor-Mediated Endocytosis" (I. Pastan and M. Willingham, eds.), pp. 189–236. Plenum, New York.

24. Olsnes, S., Saltvedt, E., and Pihl, A. (1974). Isolation and comparison of galactose-binding lectins from *Abrus precatorius* and *Ricinus communis. J. Biol. Chem.* **249**, 803–810.

25. Poncelet, P., Canat, X., Carayon, P., Casselles, P., and Laurent, G. (1983). Elimination of leukemic cells from autologous grafts with immunotoxins: Therapeutic implications of antigen density and heterogeneity on tumor cells. "International Symposium on Detection and Treatment and Minimal Residual Disease in Acute Leukemia." Rotterdam, The Netherlands.

26. Ramakrishnan, S., and Houston, L. L. (1984). Inhibition of human acute lymphoblastic leukemia cells by immunotoxins: Potentiation by chloroquin. *Science* **223**, 58.

27. Raso, V., and Griffin, T. (1982). Specific cytotoxicity of a human immunoglobulin-directed Fab'-ricin A-chain conjugate. *J. Immunol.* **125**, 2610–2616.

28. Ross, W. C. J., Thorpe, P. E., Cumber, A. J., Edwards, D. C., and Hinson, C. A. (1980). Increased toxicity of diphtheria toxin for human lymphoblastoid cells following covalent linkage to anti-(human lymphocyte) globulin or its F(ab')$_2$ fragment. *Eur. J. Biochem.* **104**, 381–390.

29. Sandvig, K., Olsnes, S., and Pihl, A. (1976). Kinetics of binding of the toxic lectins abrin and ricin to surface receptors of human cells. *J. Biol. Chem.* **251**, 3977–3984.

30. Sandvig, K., Olsnes, S., and Pihl, A. (1978). Chemical modifications of the toxic lectins abrin and ricin. *Eur. J. Biochem.* **84**, 323.

31. Seto, M., Umemoto, N., Saito, M., Masuho, Y., Hara, T., and Takahashi, T. (1982). Monoclonal anti-MM46 antibody: ricin A chain conjugate: *In vitro* and *in vivo* anti-tumor activity. *Cancer Res.* **42**, 5209–5215.

32. Skilleter, D. N., Paine, A. J., and Stirpe, F. (1981). A comparison of the accumulation of ricin by hepatic parenchymal and non-parenchymal cells and its inhibition of protein synthesis. *Biochim. Biophy. Acta* **677**, 495–500.

33. Spiegelberg, H. L., and Weigle, W. O. (1965). The catabolism of homologous and heterologous 7S gamma globulin fragments. *J. Exp. Med.* **121**, 323–338.

34. Stahl, P. D., Rodman, J. S., Miller, M. J., and Schlesinger, P. H. (1978). Evidence for receptor-mediated binding of glycoproteins, glycoconjugates, and lysosomal glycosidases by alveolar macrophages. *Proc. Natl. Acad. Sci. U.S.A.* **75**, 1399–1403.

35. Thorpe, P. E., and Ross, W. C. J. (1982). The preparative and cytotoxic properties of antibody-toxin conjugates. *Immunol. Rev.* **62**, 119–158.

36. Thorpe, P. E., Ross, W. C. J., Brown, A. N. F., Myers, C. D., Cumber, A. J., Foxwell, R. M. J., and Forrester, J. A. (1984). Blockade of the galactose-binding sites of ricin by its linkage to antibody: Specific cytotoxic effects of the conjugates. *Eur. J. Biochem.* **140**, 63–71.

37. Thorpe, P. E., Detre, S. J., Foxwell, R. M. J., Brown, A. N. F., Skilleter, D. N., Wilson, G., Forrester, J. A., and Stirpe, F. (1985). Modification of the carbohydrate in ricin with metaperiodate-cyanoborohydride mixtures. Effects on toxicity and *in vivo* distribution. *Eur. J. Biochem.* **147**, 197–206.

38. Thorpe, P. E., Brown, A. N. F., Bremner, J. A. G., Foxwell, B. M. J., and Stirpe, F. (1985). An immunotoxin composed of monoclonal anti-Thy 1.1 antibody and a ribosome-inactivating protein from *Saponaria officinalis:* potent anti-tumor effects *in vitro* and *in vivo. J. Natl. Cancer Inst.* **75**, 151–159.

39. Vitetta, E. S. (1986). Synergy between immunotoxins prepared with native ricin A chains and chemically modified ricin B chains. *J. Immunol.* **136**, 1880–1887.

40. Vitetta, E. S., and Thorpe, P. H. (1985). Immunotoxins containing ricin A or B chains

with modified carbohydrate residues act synergistically in killing neoplastic B cells *in vitro*. *Cancer Drug Delivery* **2,** 191–198.

41. Vitetta, E. S., Cushley, W., and Uhr, J. W. (1983). Synergy of ricin A-chain-containing immunotoxins and ricin B-chain-containing immunotoxins in the *in vitro* killing of neoplastic human B cells. *Proc. Natl. Acad. Sci. U.S.A.* **80,** 6332–6335.

42. Vitetta, E. S., Fulton, R. J., and Uhr, J. W. (1984). The cytotoxicity of cell-reactive immunotoxin containing ricin A-chain is potentiated with an anti-immunotoxin containing ricin B-chain. *J. Exp. Med.* **160,** 341–346.

43. Youle, R. J., and Neville, D. M., Jr. (1980). Anti-Thy 1.2 monoclonal antibody linked to ricin is a potent cell-type-specific toxin. *Proc. Natl. Acad. Sci. U.S.A.* **77,** 5483–5486.

44. Youle, R. J., and Neville, D. M., Jr. (1982). Kinetics of protein synthesis inactivation by ricin-anti-Thy 1.1 monoclonal antibody hybrids. *J. Biol. Chem.* **257,** 1598–1601.

13

Monoclonal Antibody 791T/36: Drug Conjugates for Cancer Therapy

R. W. BALDWIN

Cancer Research Campaign Laboratories
University of Nottingham
Nottingham, United Kingdom

I. Introduction

Monoclonal antibodies which react with antigens associated with malignant cells offer new approaches for targeting cytotoxic drugs (4,5,8). This may increase their therapeutic effectiveness by improving localization and retention in tumors. Antibody targeting may also provide a more effective approach for depositing anticancer agents in metastatic deposits. Additionally if normal tissues lack the antigens associated with malignant

NEW AVENUES IN DEVELOPMENTAL
CANCER CHEMOTHERAPY

cells, it should be possible to minimize drug toxicity, this being a major limitation in conventional cancer chemotherapy.

The design and evaluation of drug–antibody conjugates will be reviewed principally with respect to investigations with an anti-human tumor monoclonal antibody designated 791T/36, although the general concepts are relevant to other anti-tumor monoclonal antibodies (5). Monoclonal antibody 791T/36 is produced by a hybridoma obtained by fusion of splenocytes from a mouse immunized against cells of a human osteogenic sarcoma cell line 791T and murine myeloma P3NS1 (14). The antibody reacts with osteogenic sarcoma cells derived from long-term cultured cell lines (14) and also with primary and metastatic osteogenic sarcomas (25). Reactivity is not confined to sarcomas, however, and it has been found to bind to cells derived from primary and metastatic colorectal carcinomas (7,12) and to ovarian tumors (26). This is illustrated by the flow cytometry analysis of the binding of 791T/36 antibody to malignant cells derived from primary colorectal cancers as well as a range of metastases including lymph node, hepatic, and omental deposits (12). Tumor cells obtained by collagenase disaggregation of tumor tissue were reacted with 791T/36 antibody and bound antibody detected by reaction of tumor cells with fluorescein isothiocyanate (FITC) conjugated rabbit anti-mouse Ig. The mean linear fluorescence (MLF) of cells in the size range of malignant populations was then determined by flow cytometry (12). A typical analysis of binding of 791T/36 antibody to malignant cells derived from a primary colon carcinoma and lymph node and liver metastases derived from the same patient is illustrated in Fig. 1. This shows that

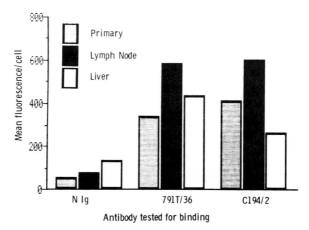

Fig. 1. Binding of monoclonal antibodies to primary and metastatic colon carcinoma cells as determined by flow cytometry (24).

monoclonal antibody 791T/36 binds to tumor cells derived from both the primary colon carcinoma and from lymph node and liver metastases, in this particular analysis the binding of 791T/36 being comparable to that observed with antibody recognizing CEA (194/2). Similar trials have been carried out on 50 primary colorectal carcinomas, of which 67% stained to varying degrees with 791T/36 (12). Also, tumor cells derived from lymph node metastases (13 patients) and distant metastases (9 patients) reacted with 791T/36 antibody (9).

II. Tumor Localization of Monoclonal Antibody 791T/36

Targeting of cytotoxic drugs requires that the antibody localizes in the tumor and ideally penetrates regions of the tumor which contributes to its progressive growth. This has been established with 791T/36 in a series of investigations showing that iodine-131- and 125-labeled ([131]I- and ^{125}I-labeled) antibody localizes in osteogenic sarcoma xenografts in immunodeprived mice (20,21). Localization of 791T/36 labeled with indium-111 (^{111}In) has also been demonstrated by gamma camera imaging and organ distribution of radioactivity in mice bearing xenografts of several different types of human tumor including osteogenic sarcomas (19) and colorectal carcinomas. The kinetics of tumor localization of ^{111}In-labeled 791T/36 is illustrated in Fig. 2, which shows the organ distribution of radioactivity between 1 and 8 days following injection of 0.1 MBq of ^{111}In-labeled antibody into immunodeprived mice bearing osteogenic sarcoma 788T xenografts (19). This clearly shows the good discrimination between tumor uptake of radioactivity and that in normal mouse tissues. Comparing the organ distribution of ^{111}In-labeled antibody with that of ^{131}I-labeled antibody (20) the absolute level of ^{111}In deposition in tumor (up to 60% of the whole body count per gram of tissue) is similar to that seen with ^{131}I-labeled preparations. Although the peak level of tumor localization was achieved more rapidly with ^{111}In-labeled 791T/36 (2 days compared with 4 days using ^{131}I-labeled antibody), both trials showed that radiolabeled antibody persisted in the tumor for 8 days. This is particularly important, since it indicates that prolonged tumor retention of targeted drug can be achieved, providing the drug–antibody linkage is not biodegradable.

A. Clinical Trials

Clinical imaging trials with ^{131}I-labeled 791T/36 antibody in colorectal cancer have shown consistent localization of antibody in primary tumors

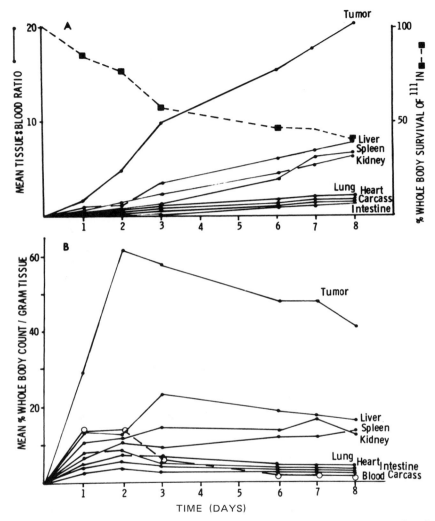

Fig. 2. Kinetics of ^{111}In-labeled 791T/36 monoclonal antibody distribution in mice with sarcoma 788T xenografts.

as well as local and distant metastases (1,16). With primary colon carcinomas 8/11 imaged positively, whereas imaging was negative in 4 patients with benign lesions. Rectal carcinomas also imaged, but excreted ^{131}I in the bladder obscured the tumor in 8/15 cases (1). Of particular importance to the application of 791T/36 for drug targeting was the finding that ^{131}I-labeled antibody localized in metastatic deposits. Of the 15 patients with metastatic (or recurrent tumors) all but 2 showed positive imaging for all sites. Monoclonal antibody labeled with ^{111}In has proved far superior to ^{131}I-labeled preparations for imaging, and positive images of primary and metastatic sites were recorded in 13/14 patients (2). Prospectively in the detection of recurrent colorectal cancer (25 patients) [131]I- and ^{111}In-labeled antibody detected 30/37 separate sites, including recurrences in liver (11/14), pelvis (10/12), abdomen (5/6), and other (5/6) sites (K. C. Ballantyne, A. C. Perkins, N. C. Armitage, M. V. Pimm, R. W. Baldwin, and J. D. Hardcastle, unpublished findings).

III. Monoclonal Antibody–Drug Conjugates

Conjugation of drugs to monoclonal antibodies aims to introduce the maximum number of drug residues using conditions which ensure optimal retention of both drug and antibody reactivities. In this respect, only a limited number of drug residues can be introduced by direct linkage to antibody without producing loss of antibody reactivity. This will be dependent upon the characteristics of the antibody and physical and chemical properties of the conjugated compound, but in general substitution ratios of greater that $10:1$ with respect to IgG antibodies produce a marked loss of antibody reactivity, and in many cases substitution of as few as four drug residues per antibody molecule produces unacceptable antibody damage (4).

In order to increase the amount of drug coupled to antibody, "drug-carrier" systems are being designed. In this case, the drug moiety is first linked to carrier molecules such as dextran (3) and human serum albumin (18), and then the complex is conjugated to antibody. Conjugates constructed in this manner can be produced with a "drug loading" at least 10 times as great as that produced by direct drug–antibody conjugation. But products using polymeric carriers such as polysaccharides and proteins, because of the considerable increase in molecular size, will have altered biodistribution patterns which may influence drug deposition in tumors.

A. Methotrexate–791T/36 Monoclonal Antibody Conjugates

Conjugates of methotrexate (MTX) with monoclonal antibody 791T/36 have been constructed, since MTX is highly cytotoxic for sarcoma 791T cells, 50% inhibition of growth in culture (IC_{50}) being produced at a concentration of $1 \times 10^{-8}M$ (18).

Conjugates containing MTX directly linked to antibody were prepared by incubating equimolar quantities of MTX, N-hydroxysuccinimide, and dicyclohexyl carbodiimide for several hours. Substituted 791T/36 antibody was then prepared by reacting the MTX ester with antibody in aqueous medium to yield products with an average molar substitution ratio in the range of 2–3.

Conjugates have also been synthesized using human serum albumin (HSA) as a carrier for MTX (18). Briefly, MTX–HSA conjugate was prepared by reacting an excess of MTX and ethyl carbodiimide with HSA, and unwanted polymeric products were removed by size-exclusion chromatography. Iodoacetyl-substituted 791T/36 was produced by reacting it with a three- to four-fold molar excess of N-hydroxysuccinimidyl iodoacetate. The MTX-HSA conjugate was treated with dithiothreitol to reduce free sulphydryl groups and was reacted with the iodoacetyl substituted antibody. Reaction products were separated by size-exclusion chromatography to yield conjugates (MTX–HSA–791T/36) in the molecular weight range of 200,000–400,000, with MTX : antibody ratios of the order of 30–40 : 1 (17,18).

IV. Characterization of Antibody Conjugates

A. Antibody Reactivity

Antibody binding properties of conjugates with tumor cells have been assessed using a flow cytometry technique (24). In this procedure conjugate is mixed with FITC-labeled 791T/36 antibody (FITC-791T/36), and the mixture is reacted with tumor cells under conditions of antibody excess. At equilibrium the relative amounts of FITC-labeled antibody bound to tumor cells is estimated by quantitative fluorescence measurements. The degree of competitive binding of antibody conjugate will reflect both qualitative and quantitative changes in antibody binding activity produced by MTX conjugation.

For these assays, binding of FITC-791T/36 to sarcoma 791T cells was measured by FACS IV flow cytometry. Titration of FITC-791T/36 established that saturation of antibody binding sites on 791T cells was obtained using 1 μg of FITC conjugate/2×10^5 cells. It was also found that with this level of FITC-791T/36, the tumor cell/antibody mixture could be analyzed without washing tumor cells to remove nonbound antibody, thereby allowing analysis of competition directly at equilibrium. When evaluating MTX–791T/36 conjugates, a comparison is made between the conjugate and unlabeled antibody. This then provides an assessment of antibody reactivity in conjugates relative to that of unconjugated antibody. Using

TABLE I

Characteristics of Methotrexate–791T/36 Monoclonal Antibody Conjugates

Preparation	MTX substitution MTX : 791T/36	Antibody reactivity (%)
MTX–791T/36		
MDC26	2.5 : 1	36
MDC29	1.9 : 1	68
MDC31	2.7 : 1	75
MTX–HSA–791T/36		
MT1	32 : 1	28
MT7	27 : 1	36
MT11	23 : 1	32
MT17	38 : 1	32

this procedure, it was shown that conjugates containing 2–3 moles of MTX directly linked to 791T/36 retained adequate levels of antibody reactivity (Table I). But when more than four MTX residues are linked to 791T/36 there was marked loss of antibody reactivity. Conjugates prepared using HSA as MTX carrier and containing 23–38 moles of MTX per mole of antibody retained 28–36% of the reactivity of unsubstituted antibody (Table I).

B. *In Vitro* Cytotoxicity of Methotrexate–791T/36 Antibody Conjugates

The *in vitro* cytotoxicity of MTX–791T/36 antibody conjugates was measured by incubating tumor cells with a range of concentrations of conjugate in microtiter plates for 24–48 hr and determining tumor cell survival by postincubation labeling with [^{75}Se]selenomethionine (15). The reactivity of conjugates was then assessed from the dose–response curve and was expressed as an IC_{50} dose, this being the amount of MTX in the conjugate producing 50% inhibition of tumor cell survival. Directly linked conjugates (MTX–791T/36) were tested against both sarcoma 791T cells, expressing approximately 6×10^5 791T/36 antibody binding sites per cell, and bladder carcinoma T24 cells, which express of the order of 10^4 antibody binding sites per cell. These conjugates were cytotoxic for both of these MTX-sensitive tumor cells but with reduced activity when compared to free MTX (Table II). Directly linked MTX conjugates were also tested against colon tumor cell lines developed from primary tumor speci-

TABLE II

Cytotoxicity of Methotrexate–791T/36 Antibody Conjugates

Reagent	Cytotoxicity (IC_{50} ng/ml) against	
	Osteogenic sarcoma (791T)	Bladder carcinoma (T24)
Direct conjugate		
MTX–791T/36 (MDC27)	204.0	112.0
MTX	6.6	2.5
MTX–791T/36 (MDC30)	178.0	178.0
MTX	6.0	5.0
MTX–791T/36 (MDC31)	70.8	ND[a]
MTX	12.6	ND
HSA carrier conjugate		
MTX–HSA–791T/36 (MT5)	18.6	251.0
MTX	6.2	6.3
MTX–HSA–791T/36 (MT17)	2.4	316.0
MTX	4.8	6.0
MTX–HSA–791T/36 (MT18)	50.0	ND
MTX	10.0	

[a] ND, no data.

mens and were shown to bind 791T/36 antibody (13). These colon tumor cells were resistant to free MTX, with IC_{50}'s in the range of 1000–8000 ng/ml of medium (Table III). In comparison MTX–791T/36 conjugates demonstrated enhanced cytotoxicity (IC_{50} of 63–170 ng/ml of medium).

Conjugates in which the level of MTX substitution was increased through the use of an HSA carrier were more cytotoxic for sarcoma 791T cells, and one of the three preparations summarized in Table I was more reactive than free MTX. Furthermore, with these conjugates it was possible to discriminate between the cytotoxicity for target cells expressing "high," e.g., sarcoma 791T, and "low," e.g., bladder carcinoma T24, levels of 791T/36 antibody binding.

The cytotoxicity of MTX–antibody conjugates has also been demonstrated using a clonogenic assay in which the influence of MTX or conjugates is assessed on tumor colony formation following coincubation for 5 days (Fig. 3). These assays showed that MTX–HSA–791T/36 conjugates completely suppressed colony formation by sarcoma 791T cells in some cases at concentrations (in terms of MTX) lower than that of free drug. For example, the IC_{50} with conjugate MT5 was 0.5 ng/ml in terms of free drug compared with an IC_{50} of 3 ng/ml for MTX.

TABLE III

Cytotoxicity of Methotrexate–791T/36 Conjugates against Tumor Cells

Target cell	Cytotoxicity (IC_{50} ng/ml)	
	MTX	MTX–791T/36
Osteogenic sarcoma		
791T	12	90
Colon tumor		
C146	1000	63
C168	8000	400
C170	1800	170

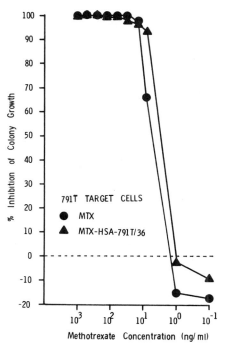

Fig. 3. Cytotoxicity of MTX–HSA–791T/36 conjugate against 791T osteogenic sarcoma cells, as measured by colony inhibition assay.

C. Therapeutic Activity of Methotrexate–HSA–791T/36 Antibody Conjugate

The therapeutic efficacy of MTX–HSA–791T/36 antibody conjugates has been assessed using the MTX-sensitive sarcoma 791T developing in immunodeprived mice. In these trials, therapy was intraperitoneal injection of free or conjugated MTX twice weekly. This dosing schedule was selected on the basis of tumor localization studies with 791T/36 antibody to maintain saturation of the developing tumor with antibody agents (20). When expressed as a ratio of tumor weights in treated (T) compared with control (C) mice (T/C ratio) 2 weeks after the final treatment, free MTX exerted a significant effect at a dose of 20 mg/kg body weight, and overall the data indicate a T/C ratio of 0.5 at 24 mg/kg body weight. The therapeutic response to MTX–HSA–791T/36 was more pronounced than that obtained with free MTX with a T/C of 0.5 at a dose (in terms of MTX) of 14 mg/kg body weight. In one test, virtually complete tumor suppression was achieved with MTX–HSA–791T/36 (18 mg MTX/kg body weight), whereas the maximum dose of free MTX tested (60 mg/kg) produced a T/C ratio of 0.30.

V. Discussion

Monoclonal antibody 791T/36 localizes in several types of human tumors, including colorectal carcinoma (1,16) and ovarian tumors (26). In the colorectal cancer series, localization of 791T/36 antibody has been demonstrated by gamma camera imaging of patients injected with [131]I- and ^{111}In-labeled preparations (1,2). Analysis of levels of radioactivity in surgically resected tissue specimens from patients injected with radioisotope-labeled 791T/36 antibody also demonstrated that the levels in colon tumor were at least two- to threefold greater than in adjacent normal colonic tissue (1,2). This reflected specific binding of antibody since ^{123}I-labeled normal mouse IgG2b did not localize in colorectal cancer and the colon carcinoma–associated antigen binding ^{131}I-labeled 791T/36 is a 72K glycoprotein with characteristics comparable to those of the product isolated from sarcoma 791T cells (23). Consistent with these findings, ^{131}I-labeled MTX–791T/36 conjugates have been shown to localize in primary colon carcinomas, with tumor/nontumor tissue ratios comparable to those of unconjugated antibody (K. C. Ballantyne, A. C. Perkins, M. V. Pimm, M. C. Garnett, N. C. Armitage, R. W. Baldwin, and J. D. Hardcastle, unpublished findings). This establishes that the antibody moiety of MTX-conjugates localizes in colonic tumors and allows trials to be developed to evaluate methotrexate deposition.

Antibody targeting of cytotoxic agents requires that the antibody local-izes in tumors and reacts with cells which contribute to its progressive growth. In this respect, tumor cells derived by collagenase treatment from primary colorectal carcinomas have been shown by flow cytometry to bind 791T/36 antibody (Fig. 1), and this was confirmed by immunohisto-logy (12). Furthermore, a similar pattern of reactivity with 791T/36 was observed with lymph node and distant (hepatic/omental) metastases. This is particularly important in view of the finding that 20–30% of colorectal cancer patients have overt metastatic disease at the time of initial surgery, and a further 30% have occult hepatic metastases.

Clonogenic cells derived in soft agar from colon adenocarcinomas have been established in culture and shown to bind 791T/36. Xenografts de-rived from these tumors also continue to bind 791T/36 (M. V. Pimm, unpublished findings). This has enabled the susceptibility of these tumor cells to MTX and MTX–antibody conjugates to be examined. Of particu-lar importance in these studies was the finding that the colon tumors were susceptible to the *in vitro* cytotoxic action of MTX–791T/36 conjugates, even though these target cells were insensitive to MTX. This implies that antibody–mediated pathways of drug internalization are important.

Therapeutic trials with MTX–HSA–791T/36 antibody conjugates have shown that the antibody conjugates are superior to free MTX in suppress-ing growth of sarcoma 791T xenografts in immunodeprived mice (Fig. 4). These trials validate the concept that anti-tumor monoclonal antibodies can be used to target therapeutic/cytotoxic agents to tumor deposits and to provide the basis for initiating clinical trials. It has to be recognized, however, that the therapeutic efficacy of monoclonal antibody conjugates is fundamentally dependent upon the majority of tumor cells expressing the relevant antigen(s). In some cases single antibody preparations may be sufficient, but "cocktails" of antibodies recognizing different tumor-associated antigens should improve drug targeting. This is illustrated by an analysis of the reactivity of five monoclonal antibodies with colon carcinoma cells from primary tumors (12). The antibodies used were 791T/36, which recognizes a 72-kDa integral membrane glycoprotein (11); C14/1/46/10, which recognizes difucosylated blood group chains (10); and anti-CEA antibodies (C24/1/39/11, 161/25, 11/285/14). Analyzing antigen expression on cells derived from 50 colorectal carcinomas showed that over 98% reacted with two or more of the monoclonal antibodies, with reactivity being enhanced with the aneuploid tumors (12).

Combinations of monoclonal antibodies also make possible the use of conjugates containing multiple cytotoxic agents. In this respect it has been shown that injection of monoclonal antibody 791T/36 and an anti-CEA monoclonal antibody (C24) leads to both localizing in colon carci-

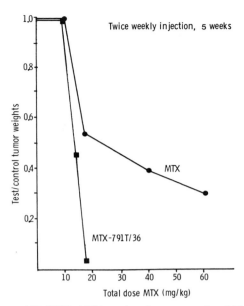

Fig. 4. Influence of 791T/36–MTX conjugate on growth of 791T osteogenic sarcoma xenografts. Groups of 8–10 athymic mice were injected subcutaneously with 791T cells, and twice weekly therapy with MTX or 791T/36–MTX conjugate was initiated 3 days later. Mice were killed after 7 weeks, and a test/control tumor weight was determined as

$$\frac{\dfrac{\text{Weight of all tumors in treated mice}}{\text{Total number of treated mice}}}{\dfrac{\text{Weight of all tumors in control mice}}{\text{Total number of control mice}}} \div$$

noma xenografts (22). Since conjugates have been synthesized with several cytotoxic agents including MTX, vindesine, and daunomycin as well as ricin A chain (6) monoclonal antibody–directed combination therapy is feasible.

Acknowledgments

These studies were supported by a grant from the Cancer Research Campaign, United Kingdom.

References

1. Armitage, N. C., Perkins, A. C., Pimm, M. V., Farrands, P. A., Baldwin, R. W. and Hardcastle, J. D. (1984). The localisation of an anti-tumour monoclonal antibody (791T/36) in gastrointestinal tumours. *Br. J. Surg.* **71,** 407–412.
2. Armitage, N. C., Perkins, A. C., Pimm, M. V., Baldwin, R. W., and Hardcastle, J. D. (1985). Imaging of primary and metastatic colorectal cancer using an ^{111}In-labelled anti-tumour monoclonal antibody (791T/36). *Nucl. Med. Commun.* **6,** 623–631.
3. Arnon, R. and Hurwitz, E. (1985). Monoclonal antibodies as carriers for immunotargeting of drugs. *In* "Monoclonal Antibodies for Tumour Detection and Drug Targeting" (R. W. Baldwin, and V. S. Byers, eds.), pp. 367–383. Academic Press, New York.
4. Baldwin, R. W. (1985). Design and development of drug-monoclonal antibody 791T/36 for cancer therapy. *In* "Monoclonal Antibody Therapy of Human Cancer" (K. Foon and A. C. Morgan, eds.), pp. 23–56. Martinus Nijoff Publishing, The Hague.
5. Baldwin, R. W., and Byers, V. S. eds. (1985). "Monoclonal Antibodies for Tumour Detection and Drug Targeting," pp. 1–395. Academic Press, New York.
6. Baldwin, R. W., and Byers, V. S. (1986). Monoclonal antibody targeting of anti-cancer agents. *Springer Semin. Immunopathol.* **9,** 39–50.
7. Baldwin, R. W., Durrant, L., Embleton, M. J., Garnett, M., Pimm, M. V., Robins, R. A., Hardcastle, J. D., Armitage, N. and Ballantyne, K. (1986). Design and therapeutic evaluation of monoclonal antibody 791T/36-methotrexate conjugates. *In* "Monoclonal Antibodies and Cancer Therapy" (R. A. Reisfeld and S. Sells, eds.), pp. 215–231. Alan R. Liss, New York.
8. Baldwin, R. W., Embleton, M. J., Gallego, J., Garnett, M., Pimm, M. V., and Price, M. R. (1986). Monoclonal antibody drug conjugates for cancer therapy. *In* "Monoclonal Antibodies for the Diagnosis and Therapy of Cancer" (J. Roth, ed.). Futura Publishing Co. (in press).
9. Ballantyne, K. C., Durrant, L. G., Armitage, N. C., Robins, R. A., Baldwin, R. W., and Hardcastle, J. D. (1986). Monoclonal antibody binding to primary and metastatic colorectal cancer. *Gut.* **26,** 1154.
10. Brown, A., Feizi, T., Gooi, H. C., Embleton, M. J., Picard, J. K., and Baldwin, R. W. (1983). A monoclonal antibody against human colonic adenoma recognises difucosylated type 2 blood group chains. *Biosci. Rep.* **3,** 163–170.
11. Campbell, D. G., Price, M. R., and Baldwin, R. W. (1984). Analysis of a human osteogenic sarcoma antigen and its expression on various human tumour cell lines. *Int. J. Cancer* **34,** 31–37.
12. Durrant, L. G., Robins, R. A., Armitage, N. C., Brown, A., Baldwin, R. W., and Hardcastle, J. D. (1986). Association of antigen expression and DNA ploidy in colorectal tumors. *Cancer Res.* **46,** 533.
13. Durrant, L. G., Robins, R. A., Pimm, M. V., Perkins, A. C., Armitage, N. C., Hardcastle, J. D., and Baldwin, R. W. (1986). Antigenicity of newly established colorectal cell lines. *Br. J. Cancer* **53,** 37–45.
14. Embleton, M. J., Gunn, B., Byers, V. S., and Baldwin, R. W. (1981). Antitumour reactions of monoclonal antibody against a human osteogenic sarcoma cell line. *Br. J. Cancer* **43,** 582–587.
15. Embleton, M. J., Rowland, G. F., Simmonds, R. G., Jacobs, E., Marsden, C. H., and Baldwin, R. W. (1983). Selective cytotoxicity against human tumour cells by a vindesine-monoclonal antibody conjugate. *Br. J. Cancer* **47,** 43–49.
16. Farrands, P. A., Perkins, A. C., Pimm, M. V., Hardy, J. G., Embleton, M. J., Baldwin,

R. W., and Hardcastle, J. D. (1982). Radioimmunodetection of human colorectal cancers using an anti-tumour monoclonal antibody. *Lancet* **2,** 397–400.

17. Garnett, M. C., and Baldwin, R. W. (1986). An improved synthesis of a methotrexate-albumin-791T/36 monoclonal antibody conjugate cytotoxic to osteogenic sarcoma cell lines. *Cancer Res.* **46,** 2407–2412.

18. Garnett, M. C., Embleton, M. J., Jacobs, E., and Baldwin, R. W. (1983). Preparation and properties of a drug-carrier-antibody conjugate showing selective antibody-directed cytotoxicity *in vitro*. *Int. J. Cancer* **31,** 661–670.

19. Perkins, A. C., Pimm, M. V., and Birch, M. K. (1985). The preparation and characterisation of ^{111}In-labelled 791T/36 monoclonal antibody for tumour immunoscintigraphy. *Eur. J. Nucl. Med.* **10,** 296–301.

20. Pimm, M. V., and Baldwin, R. W. (1984). Quantitative evaluation of the localization of a monoclonal antibody (791T/36) in human osteogenic sarcoma xenografts. *Eur. J. Cancer* **20,** 515–524.

21. Pimm, M. V., Embleton, M. J., Perkins, A. C., Price, M. R., Robins, R. A., Robinson, G. R., and Baldwin, R. W. (1982). *In vivo* localization of anti-osteogenic sarcoma 791T monoclonal antibody in osteogenic sarcoma xenografts. *Int. J. Cancer* **30,** 75–85.

22. Pimm, M. V., Perkins, A. C., and Baldwin, R. W. (1985). Simultaneous localization of two monoclonal antibodies in a human colon carcinoma xenograft. *IRCS Med. Sci.* **13,** 499–500.

23. Price, M. R., Pimm, M. V., Page, C. M., Armitage, N. C., Hardcastle, J. D., and Baldwin, R. W. (1984). Immunolocalization of the murine monoclonal antibody, 791T/36 within primary human colorectal carcinomas and identification of the target antigen. *Br. J. Cancer* **49,** 809–812.

24. Roe, R., Robins, R. A., Laxton, R. R., and Baldwin, R. W. (1985). Kinetics of divalent monoclonal antibody binding to tumour cell surface antigens using flow cytometry: Standardization and mathematical analysis. *Mol. Immunol.* **22,** 11–21.

25. Roth, J. A., Restropo, C., Scuderi, P., Baldwin, R. W., Reichert, C. M., and Hosoi, S. (1984). Analysis of antigenic expression by primary and autologous metastatic sarcomas using monoclonal antibodies. *Cancer Res.* **44,** 5320–5325.

26. Symonds, E. M., Perkins, A. C., Pimm, M. V., Baldwin, R. W., Hardy, J. G., and Williams, D. A. (1985). Clinical implications of immunoscintigraphy in patients with ovarian malignancy: A preliminary study using monoclonal antibody 791T/36. *Br. J. Obstet. Gynacol.* **92,** 270–276.

14

Antibody Ricin Immunotoxins in Allogeneic and Autologous Bone Marrow Transplantation

JOHN H. KERSEY, ALEXANDRA H. FILIPOVICH,
NORMA K. C. RAMSAY, PHILLIP McGLAVE, DAVID HURD,
TAE KIM, RICHARD YOULE, DAVID NEVILLE,
AND DANIEL VALLERA

Bone Marrow Transplantation Program
Departments of Pediatrics, Medicine, and Therapeutic Radiology
University of Minnesota
Minneapolis, Minnesota
and National Institutes of Health
Bethesda, Maryland

Bone marrow transplantation is now in widespread use for the treatment of a number of severe diseases including malignancies of the bone marrow. Marrow may be obtained from another individual in allogeneic transplantation or may be the patient's own marrow in autologous marrow transplantation (5,9). In allogeneic transplantation, immunocompetent cells capable of producing graft versus host disease (GVHD) contaminate the marrow; removal of these cells *ex vivo* prior to transplantation may be effective in reducing the incidence and severity of GVHD (13). In autologous transplantation for the treatment of the leukemias and lymphomas, the patient's marrow may contain not only the desired stem cells but also residual malignant cells. Unwanted leukemic cells may thus be reinfused to the patient. *Ex vivo* removal of these cells may result in reduced risk of relapse in these patients who receive their own marrow (4).

I. Antibody Ricin Immunotoxins

One approach to the removal of unwanted GVHD or leukemic cells in allogeneic and autologous transplantation, respectively, has been to utilize antibody ricin immunotoxins for *ex vivo* purging of marrow (15). We have utilized well-characterized antibodies which bind to specific cell surface molecules present on the unwanted cells but which are absent from normal marrow stem cells. Highly specific reagents can be used in this manner to treat marrow *ex vivo* without the need to administer potentially toxic substances *in vivo* after transplant.

II. Intact Ricin as a Potent Toxin

The toxic lectin ricin has been conjugated by ourselves and others to monoclonal antibodies to produce cell-type-specific toxins. The ricin molecule is a heterodimer made up of A and B chains, each about 30 kDa in size. Ricin kills cells via inhibition of protein synthesis at the level of the 60 S ribosome. Current data indicate that free A chain is responsible for cell killing via inhibition of protein synthesis; several groups have demonstrated that conjugates containing B chain kill more effectively than conjugates made with A chain alone (8,17). Ricin B chain binds to galactosyl residues on the cell surface; conjugates containing B chain are made specific for the target cell by blocking ricin binding to nontarget cells with lactose (8). In our clinical studies intact ricin is currently in use. Ricin for these clinical studies is conjugated to monoclonal antibody using a heterobifunctional cross-linker resulting in a thioether linkage (7,18).

III. Monoclonal T Cell Antibodies

In human studies we have utilized three T lymphocyte antibodies, each of which binds to a unique determinant on T cell surfaces. The TA-1 antibody binds to a 170- or 95-kDa cell surface glycoprotein (gp170/95) as previously described (3). The gp170/95 molecule is a member of the LFA-1 family. The antibody UCHT1 binds to a cell surface molecule which is a member of the CD3(T3) family of molecules physically associated with the T cell antigen receptor (1). The third antibody, T101, is a CD5 antibody which binds to a 65-kDa cell surface glycoprotein which has been previously described (11). All three antibodies are "pan T" in the sense that they bind to >95% of mature T lymphocytes. TA-1 is unique among the three in that it binds also to natural killer cells (3). The antibody ricin immunotoxin conjugates have been shown to effectively abolish T cell function in a mitogenic assay using PHA and in an assay for the generation of cytotoxic T lymphocytes (10,15). TA-1, UCHT1, and T101 antibody ricin immunotoxins singly and in combination are only minimally toxic to stem cells when studied *ex vivo* in mixed colony assays (15).

IV. Clinical Studies: Removal of Immunocompetent T Lymphocytes from Allogeneic Marrow for GVHD Prevention

In preclinical studies using a murine model of marrow transplantation we evaluated the efficacy of *ex vivo* treatment of donor marrow as a method of GVHD prophylaxis. These studies demonstrated that treatment of donor marrow with T cell antibody ricin is an effective method of GVHD prophylaxis even in mismatched donor–recipient combinations (6,14). Therefore, we proceeded to phase I–II studies in humans using a similar approach to that utilized in the murine model. Human studies to date have used a mixture of the three antibodies just described (TA-1, UCHT1, and T101) as whole ricin conjugates (2). Donor bone marrow mononuclear cells are prepared using a ficoll–hypaque density gradient. The resulting cell populations are treated with a total of 300–900 ng/ml of immunotoxin during a 2-hr incubation. Marrow is subsequently washed prior to administration to the recipient.

A. HLA-Matched Donors

Our largest experience with *ex vivo* immunotoxin treatment is with HLA-matched sibling donors (2a). A total of 17 patients with a minimum follow-up of 13 months was evaluable as of August 1985. All patients had leukemia; 7 had acute nonlymphocytic leukemia (ANL), 5 had acute lymphocytic leukemia (ALL), and 5 had chronic myelocytic leukemia (CML).

Patients in the acute leukemia group were very high risk for relapse since 3 patients were treated in relapse, 3 in third remission, 3 in second remission. The age range of patients was from 7 to 53 years, with 7 patients above the age of 30. The efficiency of removal of donor T lymphocytes was excellent, based on residual responses in the PHA and CTL assays (2). Thirteen patients had prompt and sustained engraftment of donor cells, whereas 4 patients had either primary graft failure or graft rejection. The typical course of graft rejection was one of initial engraftment followed by graft failure. These results suggest that *ex vivo* marrow treatment was not toxic to stem cells but instead eliminated cells from marrow which ordinarily prevent graft rejection. Acute GVHD developed in 5 of 17 patients; 1 patient had grade 1, 4 patients had grade 2, and no patients had grades 3 or 4 GVHD. Of the 12 patients with acute leukemia, 9 patients relapsed. None of the patients with CML relapsed; nonleukemic deaths were, however, more common in the CML group. Six patients in this group have survived from 13 to 29 months. In summary, we are encouraged by the lack of severe GVHD in this group of patients, many of whom were high risk for GVHD. We believe these results demonstrate effective removal of GVHD-producing lymphocytes from donor marrow. However, we are concerned by the cases of graft rejection/failure, since previous experience with conventional *in vivo* GVHD prophylaxis indicates that graft rejection/failure is unusual in leukemia patients who receive untreated HLA-matched marrow.

B. Non-HLA-Matched (Haploidentical) Donors

We have also used immunotoxin treatment of donor marrow in non–HLA identical, one haplotype–matched (haploidentical) donors. A total of 9 patients have been treated in this manner. Patients with several diseases including Wiskott-Aldrich syndrome (1 patient), Wolman disease (1 patient), severe combined immunodeficiency (1 patient), CML (3 patients), and ANL (3 patients) have been treated in this manner. Patients ranged in age from 1 to 29 years. All patients received conditioning regimens that included total body irradiation. Depletion of T lymphocytes from donor marrow was very effective as determined in PHA and CTL assays. While only 1 patient in this group experienced GVHD, 6 patients had graft rejection/failure. Two patients developed a posttransplant lymphoma. One of the patients is alive and in remission at >16 months. Thus, as in the case with HLA-matched donors, depletion of donor T lymphocytes reduced the incidence of GVHD while a high rate of graft failure/rejection was observed.

V. Immunotoxins in Autologous Marrow Transplantation for T Cell Leukemia/Lymphoma

In patients with leukemia and other malignancies, an alternative to allogeneic marrow transplantation is high-dose chemoradiotherapy followed by autologous marrow transplantation. Monoclonal antibody ricin immunotoxins can be used to purge marrow of leukemic cells. Preclinical studies suggested that such immunotoxins are very effective in destruction of tumor cells *ex vivo* and often result in a 5-log kill of tumor cells (12). We have utilized the same T cell immunotoxins described for allogeneic marrow transplantation in patients whose malignant cells are TA-1, UCHT1, or T101 positive. Six patients have been treated to date. Patients ranged in age from 5 to 23, and all had failed primary therapy and were high risk for relapse. Marrow was treated while patients were in remission and in a manner similar to that described for treatment of allogeneic donor marrow. All patients received total body irradiation and high-dose chemotherapy. All 6 had evidence of prompt engraftment of autologous marrow. Three patients have relapsed and died. Two patients are alive and disease free at >15 and >8 months. One patient died of infectious and other complications at 1 month. In summary, the prompt engraftment in all patients suggests that the T cell antibody ricin immunotoxin is not significantly toxic for stem cells. The lack of relapse in 2 patients suggests that the marrow treatment with immunotoxin is sufficient to remove residual tumor cells in the marrow.

VI. Summary and Future Prospects

Experience to date indicates that potent cell-type-specific immunotoxins may be produced with monoclonal T cell antibody covalently linked to intact ricin. Anti-human and anti-murine T cell immunotoxins have been produced and have been found to be potent for removal of immunocompetent T cells or leukemic T cells from bone marrow. Our experience with *ex vivo* treatment of bone marrow in patients undergoing allogeneic matched, allogeneic partially matched, or autologous transplantation suggests that this treatment is very effective in purging marrow of unwanted cells. These antibody ricin immunotoxins are therefore both highly potent and very specific.

Several problems remain to be solved before immunotoxins attain more widespread application to marrow transplantation and to cancer therapy in general. The effective removal of T lymphocytes from allogeneic marrow has suggested that certain T cells facilitate engraftment of allogeneic marrow in both matched and mismatched combinations. Studies in the murine model demonstrated the increased rate of graft rejection/failure in T-cell-depleted marrow transplantations (16). Further studies in basic transplantation biology are necessary to distinguish graft-facilitating cells from GVHD-producing T cells. Immunosuppressive conditioning of the recipient may be increased to reduce the risk of graft rejection.

At the level of immunotoxin production, development of safe, easily produced antibody toxin conjugates remains a high priority. The production of antibody ricin immunotoxins lacking the galactose binding site of the B chain would permit *in vivo* use of immunotoxins that utilize intact ricin. Ongoing and future attempts to chemically modify ricin or to produce antibody–toxin hybrids will require the use of the most sophisticated methods in cellular and molecular biology. Some of these approaches are discussed in other chapters in this volume. We are hopeful that ongoing developments in this important field will result in further success in the application of immunotoxins to the therapeutic challenges of marrow transplantation and cancer.

Acknowledgments

This research was supported in part by a grant from the National Institute of Health (CA-PO1-21737).

The authors gratefully acknowledge the assistance of Drs. Tucker LeBien, Peter Beverly, and Ivor Royston, as well as Hybritech, Inc., for providing monoclonal antibodies. We also thank the Minnesota Bone Marrow Transplant Database Group for assistance with the clinical data.

References

1. Beverley, P., and Callard, R. (1981). Distinctive functional characteristic of human T-lymphocytes by E-rosetting or a monoclonal anti-T-cell antibody. *Eur. J. Immunol.* **11,** 329.
2. Filipovich, A., Vallera, D., Youle, R., Quinones, R., Neville, D., Jr., and Kersey, J. (1984). *Ex vivo* treatment of donor bone marrow with anti-T-cell immunotoxins for the prevention of graft versus host disease. *Lancet* **1,** 469–471.
2a. Filipovich, A. *et al.* (1986). In preparation.
3. LeBien, T., and Kersey, J. (1980). A monoclonal antibody (TA-1) reactive with human T-lymphocytes and monocytes. *J. Immunol.* **125,** 2208–2214.
4. LeBien, T., Ash, R., Zanjani, E., and Kersey, J. (1983). *In vitro* destruction of leukemic cells using a cocktail of monoclonal antibodies. *In* "Modern Trends in Human Leukemia V" (R. Neth, ed.), pp. 112–116. Springer-Verlag, Berlin and New York.

5. McGlave, P., Ramsay, N., and Kersey, J. (1985). Allogeneic and autologous bone marrow transplantation. *In* "Recent Advances in Hematology" (V. Hoffbrand, ed.). Churchill-Livingstone, Edinburgh and London.

6. Neville, D., and Youle, R. Monoclonal antibody-ricin as a treatment of animal graft versus host disease. U.S. Patent 4,440,747.

7. Neville, D., and Youle, R. Anti-thy 1.2 monoclonal antibody-ricin hybrid utilized as a tumor suppressant. U.S. Patent 4,539,457.

8. Neville, D., Jr., and Youle, R. (1982). Monoclonal antibody-ricin or ricin A chain hybrids; kinetic analysis of cell killing for tumor therapy. *Immunol. Rev.* **62**, 135.

9. O'Reilly, R. (1983). Bone marrow transplantation; current status and future directions. *Blood* **62**, 941–964.

10. Quinones, R., Youle, R., Kersey, J., Zanjani, E., Azemove, S., Soderling, C., LeBien, T., Beverley, P., Neville, D., Jr., and Vallera, D. (1984). Anti-T-cell monoclonal antibodies conjugated to ricin as potential reagents for human GVHD prophylaxis: Effect on the generation of cytotoxic T-cells in both peripheral blood and bone marrow. *J. Immunol.* **132**, 678–673.

11. Royston, I., Majda, A., Baird, S., Meserve, B., and Griffiths, J. (1979). Monoclonal antibody specific for human T-lymphocyte identification of normal and malignant T-cells. *Blood* **54**, 1069.

12. Stong, R., Uckun, F., Youle, R., Kersey, J., and Vallera, D. (1985). Use of multiple T-cell directed intact ricin immunotoxins for autologous bone marrow transplantation. *Blood* (in press).

13. Vallera, D., Soderling, C., Carlson, G., and Kersey, J. (1981). Bone marrow transplantation across major histocompatibility barriers in mice: The effect of elimination of T-cells from donor grafts by treatment with monoclonal thy 1.2 plus complement or antibody alone. *Transplantation* **31**, 218–222.

14. Vallera, D., Youle, R., Neville, D., Jr., and Kersey, J. (1982). Bone marrow transplantation across major histocompatibility barriers. V. Protection of mice from lethal GVHD by pretreatment of donor cells with monoclonal anti-thy 1.2 coupled to the toxin lectin ricin. *J. Exp. Med.* **155**, 949–954.

15. Vallera, D., Ash, R., Zanjani, E., Kersey, J., LeBien, T., Beverley, P., Neville, D., Jr., and Youle, R. (1983). Anti-T-cell reagents for human bone marrow transplantation: Ricin linked to three monoclonal antibodies. *Science* **222**, 512–515.

16. Vallera, D., Soderling, C., Carlson, G., and Kersey, J. (1983). Bone marrow transplantation across major histocompatibility barriers in mice. II. T-cell requirement for engraftment in TLI-conditioned recipients. *Transplantation* **33**, 243–248.

17. Vitetta, E., and Uhr, J. (1985). Immunotoxins: Redirecting nature's poisons. *Cell (Cambridge, Mass.)* **41**, 653–654.

18. Youle, R., and Neville, D., Jr. (1980). Anti-thy 1.2 monoclonal antibody linked to ricin is a potent cell-type-specific toxin. *Proc. Natl. Acad. Sci. U.S.A.* **77**, 5483–5486.

15

Targeted Therapy *in Vitro* and *in Vivo*: Probing the Limits*

LEE D. LESERMAN, PATRICK MACHY, DENISE ARAGONAL,
AND SALVADOR ALINO

*Centre d'Immunologie INSERM-CNRS de Marseille-Luminy
Marseille, France*

BERNT ARNOLD

*Deutsches Krebsforschungszentrum
Heidelberg, Federal Republic of Germany*

1. Introduction

There are two basic problems common to all forms of targeted therapy. The first problem is that of access of the therapeutic agent to the cells which are the target of the therapy. It is necessary for the agent to contact

* This chapter is adapted from Reference 8 and Reference 45. Reprinted by permission of the author and the publisher.

NEW AVENUES IN DEVELOPMENTAL
CANCER CHEMOTHERAPY

its target in order for it to act. However, evolution has developed multiple systems of protection so that endothelia, basement membranes, and aggressive macrophages prevent interaction between the environment and the cells of the organism. In order to selectively bypass these defenses we must better understand them. The experiments in the first part of this chapter are directed towards that end. The study suggests that control of at least one of these mechanisms, that of uptake of targeted moieties by macrophages, may be possible. It summarizes work presented by Aragnol and Leserman (8).

The second fundamental problem with respect to targeted therapies is variability in expression of the target molecule by tumor cells. Specific delivery of drugs requires that cells express the targeted molecules. Even assuming that tumor-specific markers can be reliably exploited for many tumors despite the problems of access previously discussed, it is to be expected that variant cells exist that do not express the target molecule; these cells will be unaffected by the therapy. It is thus important to study the biological basis and control of tumor cell diversity with respect to the expression of target cell-surface determinants. A model system, using interferon to augment the level of expression of the target molecule for determinant-specific therapy, is the second topic to be presented. It summarizes work presented by Machy *et al.* (45).

II. Immune Clearance of Liposomes Inhibited by an Anti-Fc Receptor Antibody *in Vivo*

A. Introduction

The production of monoclonal antibodies (mAb) of defined specificity has stimulated clinical interest, notably in the identification of normal cellular subsets or tumor cells *in vitro,* in imaging *in vivo,* and in the elimination of tumor cells or T cells responsible for graft rejection, as discussed in detail in this volume. For these purposes, mAbs have been used alone or have been linked to radionuclides, toxins, or drugs. We have been oriented towards the use of liposomes bearing haptens or covalently coupled mAbs and containing conventional drugs, such as methotrexate (37,39,44).

Many of these treatment modalities have been shown to be effective *in vitro*. However, a major problem associated with these directed reagents *in vivo* is access to the target cells when the cells are not in the circulatory system. This access may be limited by physical barriers, such as vascular endothelia, and the extent to which any targeted reagents may efficiently leave the circulation remains to be determined (56). Important barriers exist even for interaction with those cellular targets which are accessible to the circulation. These barriers include cells of the reticuloendothelial system (RES) which are specialized in the removal of circulating complexes (56). This system is capable of recognizing elements to be cleared by virtue of receptors which, depending on the structure of the complex, are independent of (17), or dependent on (24), accessory molecules (opsonins) present in the blood. In addition to natural opsonins, preexisting antibodies may cross-react with the targeting ligand or with the product to be delivered. Moreover, the targeting ligands or substances coupled to them may induce immune responses in the recipient (68). These induced or preformed antibodies may compete with the cellular target molecules and may also augment uptake of the complex by receptors on cells of the RES, such as those for the Fc receptor (FcR) portion of immunoglobulin G (IgG) (51) or of complement (73), limiting subsequent usefulness of the complex.

Particulate carriers such as liposomes are especially affected by these factors. Depending to some extent on their composition and size, liposomes may be efficiently cleared from the circulation, notably by fixed macrophages of the liver, spleen, and lung (56). This property has been useful for the delivery of liposome-encapsulated drugs to the RES, as for the treatment of fungal (42) or parasitic infections (5) and for augmenting the tumoricidal activity of macrophages (21). This property, however, is an undesirable characteristic when the target cells are not macrophages. Natural antibodies to liposome components exist in some species (4), and liposomes may interact directly or via C-reactive protein with complement components (3) or with other uncharacterized serum proteins (30). Finally, liposomes are excellent adjuvants (2) and would be expected to stimulate immune responses directed against them or to ligands coupled to them. All of these circumstances may tend to reduce the capacity of liposomes to deliver molecules elsewhere than to phagocytes. However, the impact of such an immune response remains unknown, since no study has actually determined the effect of an anti-ligand immune response on the circulation of ligand-bearing liposomes.

Several *in vitro* studies have demonstrated that for efficient uptake of liposomes by FcR-bearing peritoneal macrophages (23) or macrophage-like tumor cells (37,40), it was necessary to opsonize liposomes with passively administered antibodies to liposome-bound ligands. As part of current experiments, mice passively received either anti-dinitrophenyl (anti-DNP) mAbs of different IgG subclasses or were immunized to respond to DNP. We evaluated the influence of passive or elicited anti-DNP antibodies on the circulation and tissue distribution of intravenous (i.v.) injected DNP-bearing liposomes (Figs. 1-6).

Recently, Kurlander *et al.* (33) showed that the anti-FcR mAb 2.4G2 (77) was able to augment the circulation of preformed complexes of human serum albumin/rabbit anti-human serum albumin (HSA/anti-HSA) in mice, principally by inhibiting the FcR-mediated uptake of injected complexes. This study suggested to us that it may be possible to prevent the alteration of the tissue distribution of liposomes, even in the presence of an ongoing immune response against them, by *in vivo* manipulation of the FcR. We thus evaluated the ability of the anti-FcR mAb 2.4G2 to influence the distribution of injected liposomes in the presence of accelerated immune elimination. The results demonstrate that it is possible *in vivo* to enhance FcR-mediated uptake of ligand-bearing liposomes by the use of liposome-specific mAbs or to reduce FcR-mediated uptake with an mAb to the FcR.

B. Materials and Methods

1. Preparation of Liposomes for in Vivo Studies

Liposomes for the *in vivo* studies were prepared as follows. Twenty micromoles of dipalmitoyl phosphatidylcholine (DPPC) (Sigma), 20 μmoles of cholesterol (Fluka), 0.4 μmoles of dinitrophenyl–caproyl–phosphatidylethanolamine (DNP–cap–PE) (Avanti Polar Lipids), and not more than 0.04 μmoles of [^{125}I]PE, prepared by the technique of Schroit (69) using dipalmitoyl phosphatidylethanolamine (DPPE) (Sigma) modified by the mono-iodo form of the Bolton-Hunter reagent (New England Nuclear), were mixed in benzene : methanol (9 : 1) and were evaporated from organic solvent. Small liposomes, prepared by probe sonication under nitrogen for 30 min at 50°C as described in detail (37), contained 80 mM purified (60) carboxyfluorescein (CF) (Kodak) in 100 mM NaHCO$_3$. Liposomes were ultracentrifuged at 100,000 g for 1 hr and were sterile-filtered (Millipore, 0.45 μm) before use.

2. Antibodies

Monoclonal antibodies used in this part of the study are described in Table I. Anti-DNP mAbs, resulting from fusion of spleen cells from BALB/c mice immune to DNP–keyhole limpet hemocyanin (DNP-KLH) and the NS-1 myeloma, were kindly provided by Z. Eshhar. Cells producing anti-FcR mAb 2.4G2, isolated by Unkeless (77), were a gift from D. Segal. The mAb B1.23.2 was from Malissen (61). Isotypes of the anti-DNP mAbs were confirmed by double diffusion in gel using subclass-specific goat anti-mouse Ig sera (Nordic Immunology). Monoclonal antibodies were ultracentrifuged before use to eliminate aggregates.

TABLE I

Monoclonal Antibodies Used in This Study[a]

Monoclonal antibody	Class	Specificity	Reference
U7.27	IgG$_{2a}$ (mouse)	DNP	Z. Eshhar (unpublished)
U12.5	IgG$_{2b}$ (mouse)	DNP	Z. Eshhar (unpublished)
2.4G2	IgG$_{2b}$ (rat)	FcR	77
B1.23.2	IgG$_{2a}$ (mouse)	HLA-B, -C	61

[a] All antibodies were purified from culture supernatants on Sepharose–protein A columns, except 2.4G2, which was from ascites of *nu/nu* Swiss mice, which was purified by $(NH_4)_2SO_4$ precipitation, DEAE-dextran ion exchange, and gel filtration chromatography.

3. Mice

BALB/c (Janvier, France) mice were age-matched (less than 16 weeks) and sex-matched in any given experiment; 4 or 5 mice were used for each test point. Values represent means ±S.D. for each group, except for cases in which the responses of individual mice are specified.

4. Antibody Injections

Variable amounts of anti-DNP and control mAbs or 120 μg of anti-FcR were injected intraperitoneally (i.p.) in a total volume of 0.2 ml 90 min before i.v. injection of liposomes. At this time the level of anti-DNP mAb in the blood was about 30% of the total quantity injected and remained at about this level for several hours (data not shown).

5. Immunization and Measurement of Antibodies

BALB/c mice were immunized by three i.p. injections of KLH substituted with 40–50 μmoles of trinitrophenyl (TNP) hapten per gram of KLH (100 μg per injection in saline at 10-day intervals). Liposome circulation and distribution were assayed 1 week after the third injection. The level of elicited antibodies cross-reactive with DNP was measured by an ELISA technique in which DNP-BSA was adsorbed to wells of 96-well microtiter plates, as described in detail by Reininger (62). Anti-DNP sera were measured by an alkaline phosphatase conjugated rabbit antiserum specific for mouse Ig (Sigma). The result presented in micrograms of antibodies per mililiter of serum was based upon a reference curve of known concentrations of the anti-DNP mAb U7.27.

6. Liposome Circulation

[^{125}I]DNP liposomes containing CF, diluted in Hepes (10 mM) buffered saline at pH 7.45, were i.v. injected with a total volume of 0.2 ml via the lateral tail vein so that each mouse received about 300 nmoles of lipid and 30 nmoles of CF. The analysis of liposome circulation was essentially as described by Kirby *et al.* (31). Fifty microliters of blood collected at intervals from the retroorbital plexus with a microcapillary tube was diluted into 0.5 ml of buffered saline containing 200 i.u. of heparin per mililiter and was centrifuged. Supernatant fluids were measured for ^{125}I and CF before and after lysis of liposomes with Triton X-100 detergent. The CF quenching ratio was calculated and compared to its value in the original liposome preparation, indicating that less than 10% of the fluorescence signal was due to free CF (78). The percentage of CF or ^{125}I remaining in the circulation is based on the dilution of liposomes into a blood volume assumed to be 8% of the weight determined for each mouse (31). The curves of liposome circulation were in a total agreement when measured for ^{125}I or CF; thus both of these levels are indicated on the figure ordinates (Figs. 1–3); the S.D. is based on the CF measurements.

7. [^{125}I]DNP-Liposome Tissue Distribution

Mice were killed by cervical dislocation 90 min after liposome injection. Tissue radioactivity is expressed as the percentage of the total injected.

8. ^{125}I-Labeled Anti-FcR mAb

To assess its tissue distribution in mice, the anti-FcR mAb was labeled with ^{125}I using iodogen (22). The specific activity of the ^{125}I-labeled and anti-FcR mAb was about 375 mCi/μmole. It was immediately mixed either with the control anti-human mAb (1 mg/ml in saline buffer) or with the nonradiolabeled homologous anti-FcR mAb (1 mg/ml) to a final concentration of 1 μCi/ml and was dialyzed against saline buffer. Mice received 0.2 ml of one or the other of these preparations. After 90 min, the radioactivity in the blood and in different organs was determined.

C. Results

1. Effect of Anti-FcR mAb on the Circulation of DNP Liposomes in Mice Injected with Anti-DNP mAbs of Different IgG Subclasses

Mice were divided into four groups and were injected i.p. with an IgG$_{2b}$ anti-DNP or a control anti-HLA mAb. Ninety minutes later DNP liposomes were injected i.v., and the mice were bled at intervals to assess

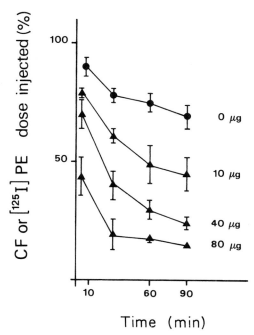

Fig. 1. Circulation of DNP liposomes in mice injected with different quantities of IgG$_{2b}$ anti-DNP. Mice marked as 0 μg received 80 μg of antibody B1.23.2 specific for HLA determinants. Data represent mean ±S.D. for five mice.

liposome circulation. Results of a representative experiment (Fig. 1) show that the injection of anti-DNP mAb reduced the circulation of DNP liposomes and that the reduction in the circulation of liposomes was proportional to the quantity of anti-DNP antibody injected. Injection of the control mAb had no effect on liposome circulation with respect to uninjected mice (not shown).

Other groups of mice were injected i.p. with 40 μg of IgG$_{2a}$ or IgG$_{2b}$ anti-DNP mAbs. As shown in Fig. 2 the reduction in circulation of DNP liposomes was practically identical for the two IgG subclasses. To evaluate the contribution of the FcR in the elimination of DNP liposomes opsonized with anti-DNP mAb, we also injected mice with the anti-FcR mAb. Figure 2 shows that liposome clearance curves were altered when mice received anti-FcR mAb together with anti-DNP mAb but not with the control anti-human mAb. In the presence of anti-DNP mAbs and independent of their subclass, injection of anti-FcR mAb reduced the blood clearance of DNP liposomes toward the value for mice not receiving anti-DNP mAbs.

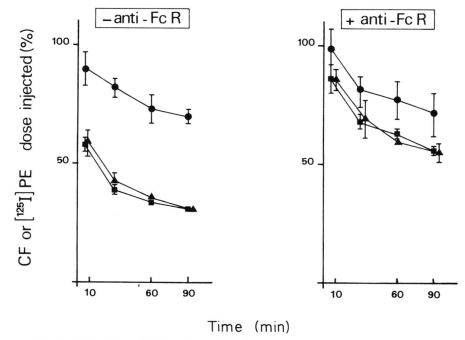

Fig. 2. Effect of anti-FcR mAb on DNP liposome circulation. Circulation of DNP liposomes in mice injected with IgG$_{2a}$ (■) or IgG$_{2b}$ (▲) anti-DNP, or control (●) mAbs, plus or minus 120 µg of anti-FcR mAb.

To assess the effect of anti-FcR mAb in a more physiological situation, we immunized mice with TNP-KLH, so that mice developed antibodies cross-reactive with DNP (Table II). Figure 3 shows that the circulation of DNP liposomes was reduced in immune mice, essentially in proportion to the magnitude of the immune response (see mice B1 and B2). We evaluated the effect of the anti-FcR mAb on the circulation of DNP liposomes in DNP-immune mice of group C. Despite the presence of anti-DNP antibodies in these mice (Table II), the circulation of DNP liposomes was nearly normal (Fig. 3), as previously observed when immunization was mimicked by passive injection of anti-DNP mAbs in the presence of the anti-FcR.

2. Effect of Anti-FcR mAb on the Tissue Distribution of DNP Liposomes in Passively Immune Mice

We determined the tissue distribution of DNP liposomes in the presence or absence of anti-DNP and anti-FcR mAbs. Figure 4 shows that in

TABLE II

Concentration of Anti-DNP Antibodies in Mice Immunized with TNP-KLH[a]

Group	Concentration (μg/ml serum)
A1[b]	0[c]
A2[b]	0[c]
A3[b]	0[c]
B1	6.7
B2	0.4
B3	3.3
B4	1.9
B5	ND[d]
C1	5.7
C2	2.9
C3	1.2
C4	1.2
C5	1.9

[a] The mice indicated in this table are those used to assess circulation and tissue distribution of [^{125}I]DNP liposomes in Figs. 3 and 5.
[b] Mice injected with saline.
[c] Less than the limit of detection of the technique (0.1 μg/ml serum).
[d] ND, not determined.

the presence of IgG_{2b} anti-DNP mAb, ^{125}I tissue levels were augmented in the liver and intestine. The percentage of ^{125}I in the spleen, kidney, lung, and also (not shown) heart and stomach were low, and the differences observed in the presence of the anti-DNP mAb are probably the consequence of reduced levels of ^{125}I-labeled liposomes in the blood in these organs at the time of sacrifice. In Fig. 4, the effect of anti-FcR mAb on the distribution of DNP liposomes is also presented. Infusion of anti-FcR mAb did not modify ^{125}I distribution in the absence of anti-DNP mAb. By contrast, in the presence of an anti-DNP mAb of the IgG_{2b} subclass, the anti-FcR mAb reduced ^{125}I sequestration in the liver and intestine to levels similar to those of mice not receiving anti-DNP mAb. Essentially the same tissue distribution and effect of the anti-FcR mAb was seen for mice receiving the IgG_{2a} anti-DNP (not shown). We obtained similar results for the distribution of [^{125}I]PE-labeled DNP liposome in immunized mice (Fig. 5). The quantity of ^{125}I sequestered in the liver and intestine correlated with the decrease in the circulation of DNP liposome and with the level of anti-DNP antibodies in each mouse.

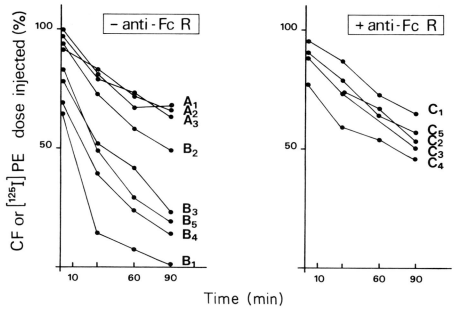

Fig. 3. Effect of anti-FcR mAb in immune mice. DNP liposome circulation in individual unimmunized (A) or TNP-KLH immune (B and C) mice. Group C mice received 120 μg of anti-FcR i.p. 90 min prior to liposome injection.

3. Tissue Distribution of ^{125}I-Labeled Anti-FcR mAb

We compared tissue distribution of i.v. injected ^{125}I-labeled anti-FcR mAb and opsonized ^{125}I-labeled DNP liposomes. Nonspecific binding was determined by mixing the ^{125}I-labeled mAb with an excess of nonradiolabeled homologous mAb. Figure 6 shows that the principal target for ^{125}I-labeled anti-FcR mAb is the liver and not, as in the case of opsonized DNP-liposomes, the intestine.

D. Discussion

Mice passively or actively immune to DNP had markedly accelerated blood clearance kinetics of DNP-bearing small liposomes with respect to nonimmune mice. This clearance was a function of the magnitude of the antibody level and resulted in increased tissue uptake by the liver, which also represents the principal site of deposition of injected liposomes in nonimmune mice (56). Passive immunization with antibodies specific for liposome-bound ligands may augment clearance kinetics of the liposomes,

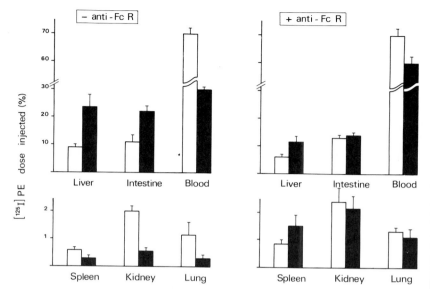

Fig. 4. Effect of anti-FcR mAb on [^{125}I]DNP liposome distribution in passively immune mice. The bars correspond to means ±S.D. (five mice) for ^{125}I in the indicated organs or via extrapolation from blood samples. Open bars, no anti-DNP; filled bars, 40 μg of IgG$_{2b}$ anti-DNP mAb i.p. 90 min. prior to i.v. liposome injection. Mice in the right panel also received 120 μg of anti-FcR mAb i.p. Mice were killed 90 min after liposome injection.

which may be of value in treatment of fungal (42) or parasitic infections (5) or for the activation of tumoricidal macrophages (21).

Prior administration of an antibody (2.4G2) directed against a murine IgG FcR almost totally inhibited this accelerated clearance. The nominal specificity of the 2.4G2 mAb is for the macrophage FcR for IgG$_1$ and IgG$_{2b}$, and not IgG$_{2a}$ (77). However, 2.4G2 inhibited clearance of liposomes opsonized with antibodies of the IgG$_{2b}$ or IgG$_{2a}$ subclasses. The cells responsible for the accelerated clearance of opsonized liposomes are probably the Kupffer cells of the liver (66). Inhibition by 2.4G2 suggests that these cells have FcRs which do not distinguish complexed IgG$_{2a}$ or IgG$_{2b}$, or, if these receptors are distinct, that they both have sites which will bind 2.4G2 and impair their function. It has previously been reported that immune complexes of IgG$_1$, IgG$_{2a}$, and IgG$_{2b}$, but not IgG$_3$, subclasses cross-inhibited each other's binding to murine lymphoid cells (71). Similarly, 2.4G2 inhibited binding to murine B cell tumors of erythrocytes opsonized with either IgG$_{2b}$ or IgG$_{2a}$ antibodies (75).

A comparison between the tissue distribution of ^{125}I-labeled liposomes

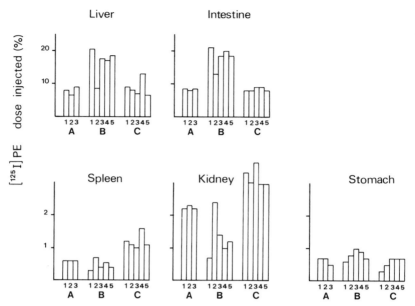

Fig. 5. Effect of anti-FcR mAb on [^{125}I]DNP liposome distribution in immune mice. Each bar represents indicated tissues of one mouse. (A) Nonimmunized. (B and C) Immunized with three injections TNP-KLH in saline. Group C mice received 120 μg of anti-FcR mAb 90 min prior to liposome injection; mice were killed 90 min after liposome injection. These are the mice for which circulation of liposomes was presented in Fig. 3.

in both passively (Fig. 4) and actively (Fig. 5) DNP-immune mice and the distribution of ^{125}I-labeled anti-FcR mAb 2.4G2 indicates concordance for the liver, but not the intestine, where the ^{125}I label from the mAb did not appear. There is no evidence for an IgG FcR in the intestine which is accessible to the circulation. The most probable cause for the apparently increased uptake of opsonized liposomes by the intestine is via FcR-mediated binding and digestion of liposomes by Kupffer cells, transfer of ^{125}I-labeled phospholipid to hepatocytes, as discussed by Scherphof (66), and excretion of label into the intestine via the bile. The anti-FcR mAb 2.4G2 almost completely inhibited this anti-DNP-mediated elimination of DNP-bearing liposomes, even in immune mice.

Liposomes are known to interact with complement in addition to, or in consequence of, fixation of antibody (3). Two studies indicate that Fc and complement C3b receptors of murine macrophage-like tumor cells (53) or of peritoneal macrophages (46) are functionally independent with respect to endocytosis, in that the internalization of the former did not affect the

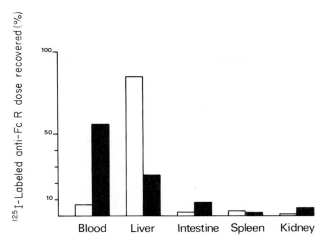

Fig. 6. Tissue distribution of ^{125}I-labeled anti-FcR. Mice were injected i.v. with 1 μCi of labeled anti-FcR mixed with a 2500–fold molar excess of unlabeled homologous mAb or a control mAb. Tissue radioactivity was measured 90 min after injection. Open bars, 2.4G2 mixed with control mAb; filled bars, 2.4G2 mixed with homologous mAb.

expression of the latter. However, a recent study showed that the Fc and the C3b receptors of human neutrophils co-capped following binding of ligands specific for one or the other molecules (29). In unpublished studies, we have observed that the antibody 2.4G2 completely inhibited binding and uptake of anti-DNP opsonized liposomes by P388D1 murine macrophage tumor cells *in vitro* but had no effect on binding or uptake of liposomes bearing mAbs specific for major histocompatibity complex–encoded determinants. Whether the Fc and C3b receptors are independent in the *in vivo* situation studied here or whether the C3b or other receptors are quantitatively unimportant in the absence of effective Fc receptor function remains to be determined.

Numerous reports of a blockage of "nonspecific" uptake of liposomes by cells of the RES exist. This blockade was mediated by an excess of empty liposomes, other particles, or dextrans (52). The effect of these reagents is transient. No information is available concerning nonspecific blockade in immune mice. The anti-FcR mAb 2.4G2 had no effect on circulation of liposomes in nonimmune mice (Fig. 1 and unpublished results). Given the efficiency of blockade of uptake by the anti-FcR in passively or actively immune mice, we conclude that natural antibodies with receptors corresponding to the specificity of the mAb 2.4G2 are not important in that "nonspecific" liposome clearance. However, it is not excluded that "nonspecific" uptake is mediated by receptors which will prove to be equally susceptible to immunological manipulation when those receptors are identified.

The inhibition by 2.4G2 of the *in vivo* uptake of preformed circulating immune complexes reported by Kurlander *et al.* (33) was confirmed, by us for antibody–ligand complexes which form *in vivo*. Preexisting antibodies which react with mouse immunoglobulins have been found in normal humans (72), and the level of these antibodies increased following administration of murine antibodies to immunocompetent individuals (14,68,72). Most of these antibodies would not be expected to interfere with the interaction of the targeting antibody and the target cell, as they do not have specificity for the combining site of the targeting antibodies, but they could augment the rate of clearance of the complex by an FcR-mediated mechanism. The DNP-bearing liposomes used in the present model study are not directed towards any target tissue, but maintenance of liposome circulation in the face of an immune response against a ligand present on the liposomes suggests that immunologic manipulation of the FcR may be of value in maintaining bioavailability of specifically targeted therapeutic reagents in similar circumstances.

Anti-idiotypic responses against injected murine antibodies have also been reported in humans (15,72). An anti-idiotypic response, if capable of blocking the antibody combining site, would prevent antibody-targeted particles from binding their target cells even if their circulation were prolonged. The same situation would apply to an antibody response directed against those determinants of carbohydrates or hormones used for targeting which were essential for target binding. In these circumstances, if the targeted particles carried drugs potentially toxic for the RES, then reduction of the rate of clearance of these particles may reduce their toxicity for phagocytic cells.

III. Interferon-Sensitive and -Insensitive MHC Variants of a Murine Thymoma Differentially Resistant to Methotrexate-Containing, Antibody-Directed Liposomes and Immunotoxin

A. Introduction

The role of the immune response in limiting tumor growth has long been postulated, and numerous studies indicate that cytotoxic T cells recognize tumor cells by virtue of antigens expressed in association with the class I molecules of the major histocompatibility complex (MHC) (18). These are the H-2 K, D, and L molecules in the mouse and the HLA-A, -B, and -C molecules of humans. Though other mechanisms exist for the elimination of tumor cells not expressing MHC determinants (81), the expression of class I molecules by tumor cells undoubtedly aids in generation of an optimal immune response against them. In consequence, nonexpression of class I molecules might confer a selective advantage on a tumor population (9,65).

This appears to be the situation for certain mouse and human tumors, such as embryonal cell carcinoma (11), neuroblastoma (35), and small-cell lung cancer (19), all of which fail to express class I molecules. Furthermore, infection of cells by the highly oncogenic adenovirus 2 or 12 resulted in diminished expression of class I molecules (7,67). The *in vivo* growth potential of these cells (74) and of other MHC deletion mutants (28) was reduced by the transfection of these cells with class I genes and their subsequent expression of class I molecules. Understanding of the control of expression of MHC molecules and the possibility of enhancement of MHC expression by pharmacologic manipulation may thus be of considerable interest in cancer therapy. Indeed, human small-cell lung cancer cells (19), and choriocarcinoma (6), which express low levels of MHC class I molecules, as well as adenovirus 12-transformed mouse cells (20) can be induced to augment their expression of these molecules in the presence of γ interferon (IFN-γ) (19).

Murine thymoma cells are known to be unstable with respect to MHC expression (25–27). In a model study evaluating the therapeutic potential of methotrexate- (MTX-)containing liposomes directed via surface-bound mAbs specific for murine MHC molecules, we found rare variant cells of the AKR thymoma RDM4 which expressed very low levels of the target H-2K^k molecule and escaped killing by the targeted drug (43). In the present study, we evaluated the ability of IFN-γ to render this population susceptible to killing by antibody-targeted liposomes or a chimeric toxin (immunotoxin) composed of antibody coupled to the α chain of ricin and began a study on the molecular basis for nonexpression of MHC molecules by these variant cells.

B. Materials and Methods

1. Preparation of Liposomes

Small, unilamellar liposomes containing 64 mol-% DPPC (Sigma), 35 mol-% cholesterol (Fluka), and 1 mol-% dipalmitoyl phosphatidylethanolamine (Calbiochem) modified with *N*-hydroxysuccinimidyl-3(2-pyridyldithio)propionate (SPDP) (Pharmacia) and containing 20 m*M* MTX

(Division of Cancer Treatment, U.S. National Cancer Institute) and 40 mM CF in 100 mM NaHCO$_3$ were prepared by probe sonication as previously described (12,38,43).

2. Antibodies

The anti-H-2K^k mAbs 100.5/28 and 100.30/33 (36) were obtained from cells provided by G. Hämmerling. The anti-H-2D^k mAb 15.5.5 (50) was supplied by K. Ozato. M. Pierres provided the rat anti-mouse kappa, anti-I-E^k mAb 39G (54), and rat anti-Thy-1 mAb 154.161.8 (55). Santo Landolfo kindly provided the rat anti-mouse IFN-γ mAb (59). Radiolabeled antibodies were iodinated using chloramine T to final specific activities of 100 mCi/μmole.

3. Immunotoxin

The ricin α chain immunotoxin was kindly provided by Jacques Barbet and was prepared using the anti-H-2K^k mAb 36.75 (64) modified with 10 moles of SPDP/mole of antibody, coupled to ricin α chain kindly supplied by F. Jansen. This immunotoxin inhibited [^{3}H]thymidine incorporation by RDM4 cells by 50% at a ricin concentration of 8 $\times$ 10^{-11} M.

4. Immunoselection of RDM4 Variants with Liposomes

For type 1 variants, RDM4 wild-type tumor cells were resuspended at 10^5 cells/ml. Cells (0.5 ml) were incubated in 24-well tissue-culture plates (Costar) with protein A–bearing, MTX-containing liposomes in the presence of anti-H-2K^k antibody 100.5/28 at a final antibody concentration of 4–8 μg/ml. Liposomes, which contained 20 mM MTX, were diluted so that the final concentration of MTX in culture was 60 nM. After 2 days of culture, cells were washed and incubated with liposomes containing MTX at a final concentration of 250 nM in the presence of 100.5/28 antibody for 2 days. The cells were washed and expanded (43). For type 2 variants, type 1 cells cloned by limiting dilution 1 month previously were incubated with 100 units of IFN-γ for 48 hr and then were exposed to liposomes as just described. Selection during the first 48 hr was also in the presence of IFN-γ.

5. Immunoselection with Immunotoxin

Type 3 cells were selected from wild-type RDM4 cells 3 months following cloning. Cells were incubated as described previously with ricin α chain coupled to the H-2K^k-specific mAb 36.75 at a ricin concentration of 10^{-9} M for 2 weeks, with changes of media and replacement of immunotoxin at 2- to 3-day intervals. After 2 weeks, the concentration of the immunotoxin was increased tenfold, and the selection continued 1 additional week. Cells were subsequently cultured in normal medium.

6. Interferon

γ-Interferon was kindly provided by Margaret Cooley from concanavalin A–stimulated supernatants of cloned CBA cytotoxic cells. These supernatants contained $10^{3.5}$ units/ml of IFN-γ (16).

7. Northern Blots

Northern blots were made using 5 μg of RNA isolated from RDM4 wild-type, type 1, or type 2 cells, uninduced or induced with IFN-γ for 48 hr, as previously described (80).

8. Dot–Blot Hybridization

Dot–blot hybridization was performed according to White and Bancroft (79), except that the RNA used was the purified RNA also used for the Northern blots.

9. Oligonucleotide Probe

A partial nucleotide sequence of the H-2K^k gene isolated from the AKR strain (10) and the corresponding H-2K^k-specific 23-base-pair oligonucleotide probe are as follows:

Amino acid:	61					65	
H-2K^k gene:	5′ GG GAG	CGG	AAC	ACG	CAG	ATC	GCC 3′
Oligonucleotide probe:	CC CTC	GCC	TTG	TGC	GTC	TAG	CGG

C. Results

1. γ-Interferon Augments Expression of H-2K^k

We have previously reported the selection of a variant cell type from RDM4 wild-type cells which expresses about tenfold fewer H-2K^k molecules than the parental type (about 1000–2000 H-2k^k molecules per cell, as compared to 25,000–30,000 molecules per cell) by using an anti-H-2K^k antibody and protein A–bearing, MTX-containing liposomes (43). RDM4 cells negatively selected for H-2K^k have stably maintained the nonexpressor phenotype.

Aliquots of these cells (called type 1 variants) were incubated with dilutions of IFN-γ-rich supernatants (from concanavalin A–stimulated CBA T cells) for 48 hr, and their expression of the H-2K^k molecule was compared to that of wild-type cells not stimulated by interferon. Results presented in Fig. 7A comparing the binding of the radiolabeled anti-H-2K^k antibody 100.5/28 show an interferon dose–dependent augmentation in H-

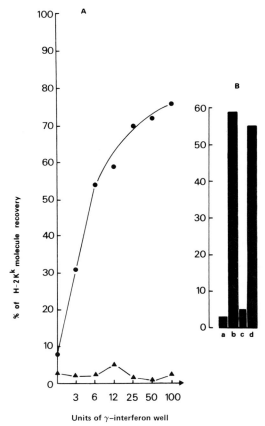

Fig. 7. Effect of γ interferon on the recovery of the H-2K^k molecule. Immunose-lected RDM4 low-expressor cells for the H-2k^k molecule (type 1) (10^5) were incubated in 0.5 ml of culture medium with different concentrations of γ interferon. After 48 hr of incubation at 37°C, cells were incubated with ^{125}I-radiolabeled 100.5/28 anti-H-2K^k monoclonal antibody (●) or with ^{125}I-radiolabeled B1.23.2 anti-HLA monoclonal anti-body (▲) in control experiments (3×10^5 cpm) (A). In a parallel experiment (B), cells were cultured either without IFN-γ (a), with 50 units of IFN-γ alone (b), with a rat anti-mouse IFN-γ monoclonal antibody (5 μg) and 50 units of IFN-γ (c), or with a rat anti-mouse immunoglobulin κ chain monoclonal antibody (5 μg) plus 50 units of IFN-γ as control (d) for 48 hrs at 37°C. The percentages were based on the counts per minute bound to cells after 1 hr of incubation with radiolabeled antibodies at 4°C and two washes in Hepes buffer (145 mM NaCl; 10 mM Hepes, pH 7.45). The control was RMD4 wild-type cells not incubated with IFN-γ. The percentage refers to a comparison with this control. RDM4 wild-type cells increased H-2K^k expression about tenfold when exposed to IFN-γ (not shown). ^{125}I-labeled 100.5/28 bound to RDM4 wild type: 10,000 cpm. ^{125}I-labeled B1.23.2 bound to RDM4 wild type: 400 cpm.

$2K^k$ expression. We tested the ability of a monoclonal rat anti-mouse IFN-γ antibody (59) to inhibit this augmentation. Figure 7B shows that this mAb, but not a control rat mAb at the same concentration, inhibited the effect of the supernatant. These results have been confirmed with recombinant IFN-γ (Genentech).

2. Immunoselection in the Presence of IFN-γ

Given an interferon-mediated augmentation in the expression of H-$2K^k$, we asked whether these cells might also have increased susceptibility to killing by liposomes directed at that molecule. We therefore exposed recently cloned H-$2K^k$ low-expressor cells to MTX-containing liposomes bearing protein A directed at the H-$2K^k$ molecule by 100.5/28 antibody for 48 hr in the presence of 100 units/ml of IFN-γ after 48 hr of incubation with IFN-γ at the same dose. As for our initial immunoselection (43), all cells appeared to have been killed, but after 2–3 weeks some cells grew. The selection was repeated; many cells died, but cells proliferated to the original density in 1 week. An additional cell selection in the presence of IFN-γ resulted in little or no cell death, even when the concentration of MTX-containing liposomes was increased.

We evaluated the expression of the H-$2K^k$ molecule by these cells (type 2) with reference to the population from which they were derived (type 1). Cells were incubated with two radiolabeled monoclonal anti-H-$2K^k$ antibodies recognizing different epitopes of that molecule (36) or with an anti-HLA antibody (B1.23.2) radiolabeled to the same specific activity as the control. Results are presented in Fig. 8. Maximal response by the initially selected population (type 1) was seen at 48 hr. By contrast, cells immunoselected in the presence of supernatants containing IFN-γ (type 2) failed to augment expression of the H-$2K^k$ molecule during that interval; neither an additional 12 hr of incubation nor incubation with higher concentrations of IFN-γ augmented expression (not shown). We also investigated the effect of affinity-purified IFN-α/β on these cells with analogous results; 2000 units/ml of IFN-α/β enhanced H-$2K^k$ expression by wild type and type 1 but not type 2 cells (not shown).

3. Expression of the IFN-γ Receptor by Selected Cells

The lack of sensitivity to interferon could be explained by a defect in the interferon receptor or in the biochemical consequences of interaction of that receptor with IFN-γ. First, the presence of IFN-γ receptors on the type 1 and 2 populations was evaluated. We incubated IFN-γ with me-

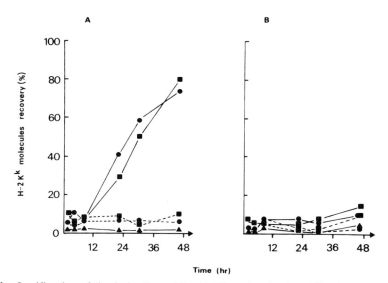

Fig. 8. Kinetics of the induction of the H-2K^k molecule. 4×10^5 cells in 0.5 ml of medium were incubated with (——) or without (————) 50 units of IFN-γ for different intervals. Cells were then incubated with ^{125}I-radiolabeled 100.5/28 (●) and 100.30/33 (■) anti-H-2K^k mAbs or with radiolabeled B1.23.2 (▲) anti-HLA mAb as control. After 1 hr of incubation at 4°C with 3×10^5 cpm of antibody, cells were washed two times in Hepes buffer and were counted in a γ-counter. The percentage refers to the counts per minute bound to RDM4 wild-type population. (A) RDM4H-2K^k low expressor, responder to IFN-γ (type 1). (B) RDM4 H-2K^k low expressor, nonresponder to IFN-γ (type 2).

dium alone, with human cells [expected to be able to bind mouse IFN-γ only nonspecifically, as the interferon effect is species specific (1)], or with the immunoselected cells. We then tested the ability of the absorbed interferon to stimulate the reappearance of H-2K^k on a fresh population of type 1 cells. As shown in Fig. 9, type 1 and type 2 cells absorbed interferon to the same extent, indicating equivalent expression of the IFN-γ receptor. The human cells did not absorb the activity.

4. Expression of Thy-1 and H-2D^k Molecules by Selected and Nonselected Cells in the Presence of IFN-γ

We verified that type 2 cells, nonresponsive to IFN-γ with respect to H-2K^k, responded normally to IFN-γ by augmentation of expression of the class I molecule H-2D^k (Fig. 10B). The level of H-2D^k expression by wild-type RDM4 cells is normally low (about 2000 molecules per cell), and the

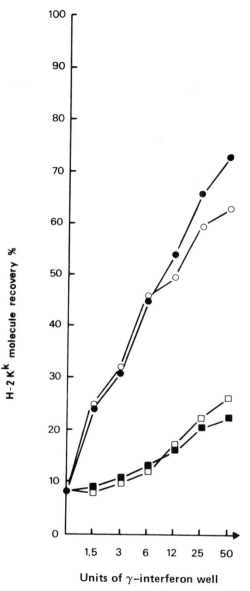

Fig. 9. Absorption of IFN-γ activity. 4×10^5 cells in 1 ml of medium were incubated with 100 units of IFN-γ for 48 hr. The supernatants were then incubated for 48 hr with RDM4 type 1 cells. These cells were then tested for their capacity to bind ^{125}I-radiolabeled 100-5/28 anti-H-2K^k mAb as described in Figs. 1 and 2. The percentage of the binding was based on the binding of the iodinated anti-H-2K^k antibody on RDM4 wild type. The absorption of IFN-γ activity was made on RDM4 H-2K^k low expressor, responder to IFN-γ (type 1) (■), on RDM4 H-2K^k low expressor, nonresponder to IFN-γ (type 2) (□), on the human cell line HeLa (○), or on nonabsorbed IFN-γ incubated in the same conditions without cells (●) as control.

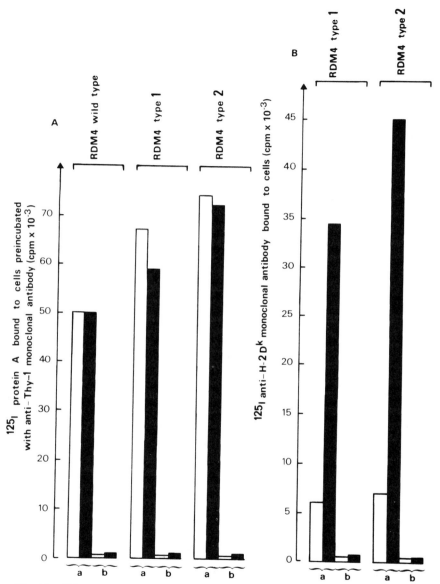

Fig. 10. Effect of IFN-γ on the modulation of other cell surface molecules. 4×10^5 cells in 0.5 ml of medium were cultured with (filled bars) or without (open bars) 50 units of IFN-γ for 48 hr. Cells were then tested for their capacity to bind anti-Thy-1 mAb (A) or anti-H-2D^k mAb (B). In Fig. 10A, cells were incubated with 154.161/8 anti-Thy-1 antibody for 1 hr at 4°C and washed two times in Hepes buffer. The cells were resuspended and

wild-type cells responded to IFN-γ by an augmentation of expression of H-2D^k to the same extent as the H-2K^k variants (not shown). The effect of IFN-γ was specific; Thy-1 expression was unchanged for any cell type as a consequence of interferon incubation (Fig. 10A). We also determined that a class II H-2 molecule (H-2 I-E^k), normally not expressed by RDM4, was not induced after IFN-γ exposure, as shown by the absence of binding with the H-2 I-E^k-specific antibody 39G (54) (not shown). These studies thus showed that the lack of expression of H-2K^k was not due to a lack of a normal response to IFN-γ nor to a loss of the chromosome(s) encoding H-2K^k, since the H-2D^k molecule, which is also present on the chromosome 17, was shown to augment its expression in response to IFN-γ.

5. Evaluation of Class I RNA Synthesis

Nonexpression of H-2K^k could be due to controls at both the transcriptional and translational levels. As an initial attempt to characterize the reason for the nonexpression of H-2K^k by type 2 cells we have isolated RNAs of the various cell types and used them in Northern blots with the class I–specific probe pH-2^d-4 (34) as well as in dot blots with a 23-base-pair oligonucleotide probe specific for a sequence of the H-2K^k molecule. Results of such a test are presented in Fig. 11. Wild-type RDM4 cells produced class I–specific RNA; type 1 and type 2 cells failed to express detectible class I RNA in the absence of interferon but did so in its presence (Northern blot, Fig. 11A). Analysis of the same RNAs with the H-2K^k-specific oligonucleotide probe showed H-2K^k RNA expression in wild-type and interferon-induced type 1 cells. By contrast, type 2 cells did not synthesize detectible H-2K^k RNA in the absence or presence of interferon, suggesting transcriptional control (Fig. 11B).

6. Selection with an H-2K^k-Specific Immunotoxin

The fact that RDM4 cells escaped killing by MTX-containing liposomes while still retaining normal MTX sensitivity (43) would not rule out the possibility that these cells might be susceptible to killing by other, perhaps

---

incubated with 3×10^5 cpm of ^{125}I-radiolabeled protein A. After an additional 1 hr of incubation at 4°C, cells were washed two times before being counted in a γ-counter. (a) Cells preincubated with anti-Thy-1 antibody before incubation with protein A. (b) Cells not preincubated with anti-Thy-1 antibody before incubation with protein A as control. In Fig. 10B, cells were incubated with 3×10^5 cpm of ^{125}I-radiolabeled 15.5.5 anti-H-2D^k mAb. After 1 hr of incubation at 4°C, cells were washed, and bound radioactivity was measured. (a) cpm of ^{125}I-labeled anti-H-2D^k antibody bound to cells. (b) cpm of ^{125}I-labeled anti-HLA antibody (B1.23.2) bound to cells as control. RDM4 type 1 = RDM4 H-2K^k low expressor, responder to INF-γ with respect to K^k. RDM4 type 2 = RDM4 H-2K^k low expressor, nonresponder to INF-γ with respect to K^k.

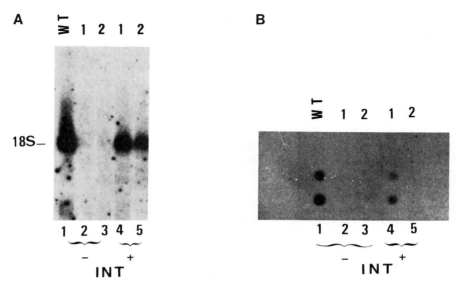

Fig. 11. Analysis of RNA from RDM4. Northern (A) and dot (B) blots of RNA from RDM4 wild type (lane 1) and immunoselected cells, type 1 (lanes 2 and 4) and type 2 (lanes 3 and 5). Cells were incubated in normal medium (lanes 1–3) or in medium supplemented with IFN-γ (100 units/ml) (lanes 4–5) for 48 hr prior to isolation of RNA. (A) 5 μg of RNA was applied to a 1% agarose gel. The position of the band corresponds to 17 S according to marker RNA (not shown). Hybridization was performed as described (80) using the nick-translated cDNA clone pH-2^d-4 which encodes sequences common to all murine class I molecules (34). (B) 1 μg (top) or 3 μg (bottom) of RNA isolated for the Northern blot for each cell type was applied to a nitrocellulose filter and was hybridized with the end-labeled H-2K^k oligonucleotide probe, according to White and Bancroft (79).

more potent techniques directed at the same target molecule. We therefore incubated both wild-type and immunoselected (type 2) RDM4 cells with an immunotoxin (76) of ricin α chain coupled to a specific anti-H-2K^k antibody. The immunotoxin was introduced into the cells, initially at a concentration of 10^{-9} M (with respect to the ricin α chain, as confirmed in a bioassay measuring ricin-mediated inhibition of [^{35}S]methionine incorporation in a cell-free translation system; not shown), for 2 weeks, then at 10^{-8} M for 1 week. Cells were subsequently cultured in normal medium. Extensive cell death was observed for the wild-type population; few cells died in the type 2 population. Surviving wild-type population cells (type 3) were then incubated with or without IFN-γ for 48 hr, and their expression of various cell surface molecules was studied in tests performed as described for Figs. 8 and 10. Type 3 cells augmented expression of H-2D^k and H-2K^k in response to IFN-γ and thus resemble type 1 cells.

D. Discussion

Phenotypic diversity with respect to cell surface molecules in tumor populations is undoubtedly of selective advantage for the tumors in the exploitation of local microenvironmental conditions or in their ability to escape from host defenses. In an immunocompetent host, changes in the primary sequence of class I MHC molecules are likely to lead to a strong, cell-mediated cytotoxic response against the cells which express the aberrant molecules (47), since the class I molecules represent privileged targets for immune surveillance. Consequently, changes in MHC expression are limited to quantitative differences.

Major histocompatibility complex molecules are sensitive to induction by the interferons (41). This has stimulated interest in the use of interferons or other potential agonists of MHC induction in order to augment host immune responses against tumors. In the present study we evaluated the ability of IFN-γ to augment the expression of H-2K^k in RDM4 wild-type or immunoselected cells. Exposure of immunoselected, low-expressor H-2K^k RDM4 cells to IFN-γ revealed that they remained sensitive to the interferon and that levels of the H-2K^k molecule, previously insufficient for kill, had increased, and that its expression was now sufficient so that most cells could be killed by H-2K^k-directed, MTX-containing liposomes. This is in contrast to the high-frequency, spontaneous H-2K^k-negative variants described by Holtkamp *et al.* (25,27), which were insensitive to the action of IFN-γ. However, in the present study, variant RDM4 cells could be isolated during negative selection which failed to express a sufficient amount of the H-2K^k molecule to be killed by liposomes, even in response to IFN-γ.

Though mutant cells nonresponsive to IFN (13) or expressing reduced levels of the IFN-α, β receptor have been reported (1), the failure to respond to IFN-γ was apparently not due to defects in expression of the IFN-γ receptor or in response to IFN interferons, since cells selected for nonexpression of H-2K^k were as efficient as H-2K^k expressors in absorbing IFN-γ. Similarly, these cells continued to respond to IFN-γ with increased expression of the H-2D^k molecule. The failure of MTX-containing liposomes to kill cells did not result from lack of sensitivity of the cells to MTX, nor could cells be killed by an H-2K^k-specific immunotoxin that is more potent than MTX-containing liposomes. Immunoselected type 2 but not wild-type RDM4 cells were also insensitive to the action of H-

2K^k-specific mAbs plus complement and to H-2K^k-specific cytotoxic T cells (not shown). There was a concordance of low expression observed by two independently obtained anti-H-2K^k monoclonal antibodies (Fig. 8) and by mRNA expression, as shown by dot blots with a synthetic H-2K^k-specific oligonucleotide probe (Fig. 11), ruling out the possibility that the antibody binding and hybridization techniques detect different species of MHC molecules (63).

Phenotypic variation with respect to MHC expression can occur even by different tumor metastases in the same individual (48). However, cells which normally fail to express MHC molecules constitute a minority of tumor or other cell types. We have used immunoselection techniques similar to those reported here and have been unable, in the absence of associated mutagenesis, to isolate MHC deletion variants from other cell types, including L cells and long-term cultured cytotoxic T cells (data not shown). There are some data to suggest that low levels of MHC expression are correlated with high levels of expression of the oncogene *C-myc* (19) and of the *C-myc*-related oncogene *N-myc* (32). Whether MHC expression has important physiologic functions independent of its role in immunological recognition is an interesting topic for further investigation.

Thymus-derived lymphocytes initially express low levels of MHC molecules, though high expression by mature T cells is stable (70). Instability of MHC molecules is frequently observed for T lymphomas. In the heterozygous (C3H × DBA/2) F$_1$ T cell lymphoma LDHB the frequency of spontaneous H-2K^k loss mutants was very high (about 10^{-1} to 10^{-2} per cell per generation) (27). A mutant of the homozygous *b* haplotype lymphoma EL4, which also fails to express the H2K molecule while maintaining expression of H-2D, has been reported (57). These cells have the K^b gene, as revealed by Southern blotting (58), but no detectible K^b-specific RNA is produced, as for K^k by RDM4. The EL4 H-2K^b-negative variant was found in a population of EL4 cells selected by BUdR for MTX resistance. The precise lesion accounting for the lack of H-2K^b production by the EL4 variant and the relation, if any, to BUdR selection has not been defined.

The homozygous AKR T lymphoma RDM4 normally expresses high levels of H-2K^k and low levels of H-2D^k. It gave rise to H-2K^k low or nonexpressor variants with a frequency of between 10^{-3} and 10^{-4} when cells were exposed to MTX-containing liposomes directed at the H-2K^k molecule (43). It is clear that for the lymphoid cell line used here, MHC expression shares with other characteristics, including drug or radiation sensitivity, the propensity for diversity which permits tumor cells to escape current treatment modalities (49). Thus, for this study, negative selection by liposomes or immunotoxin in the presence or absence of IFN-γ, despite eliminating the majority of tumor cells, did not prevent eventual outgrowth of tumor cells lacking the target molecule.

IV. Summary

The present studies are directed toward probing the limits of targeted therapy. To determine the potential for *in vivo* manipulation of the circulation and tissue distribution of injected liposomes, mice were passively injected with anti-dinitrophenyl monoclonal antibodies of the IgG$_{2a}$ or IgG$_{2b}$ subclasses or were immunized with the nitrophenyl hapten bound to a protein carrier. They were then injected intravenously with ^{125}I-labeled and carboxyfluorescein-labeled, dinitrophenyl-bearing liposomes. Circulation time of the dinitrophenyl-bearing liposomes was markedly reduced in both actively and passively immune mice, with increased deposition of liposomes in the liver. The increased clearance of liposomes could be abrogated by injection of a monoclonal antibody directed against the murine IgG Fc receptor (2.4G2). The results suggest that clearance of ligand-bearing reagent in the face of an immune response may be modified by specific immunologic manipulation *in vivo*.

In a second series of experiments we evaluated the ability of methotrexate-containing liposomes or a ricin α chain immunotoxin, both associated with monoclonal antibodies specific for the major histocompatibility complex–encoded class I molecule H-2K^k, to kill cells of the murine k haplotype thymoma RDM4. Cells were incubated with liposomes or immunotoxin in the presence or absence of interferon γ, which is known to augment the expression of the target class I molecules. The great majority of cells were killed by either of these reagents. Two types of mutant cells were obtained. Type 1 cells, selected by methotrexate-containing liposomes, failed to express sufficient target H-2^k molecules to be killed by liposomes in the absence of interferon γ. In the presence of interferon γ these cells increased expression of all H-2 class I molecules and could be killed by targeted liposomes. Type 2 cells were immunoselected by liposomes from cloned type 1 cells in the presence of interferon. These cells failed to respond to interferon with expression of the H-2K^k molecule but continued to augment H-2D^k expression in response to interferon. A third variant (type 3) selected from the wild-type population by an H-2K^k-specific immunotoxin in the absence of interferon phenotypically resembled type 1 cells. Type 1 but not type 2 cells respond to interferon by augmented synthesis of H-2K^k-specific mRNA. The results suggest that for interferon-sensitive cell surface molecules of tumor cells, use of interferon improves the efficacy of targeted chemotherapy but does not prevent development of mutants lacking the target molecule.

Acknowledgments

We thank B. Dalton for the purified IFN-α/β, G Victorero and G. Kübelbeck for technical assistance, M. J. Tucker and W. Falk for purification of the oligonucleotide probe, and C. Bellegarde for preparation of the manuscript. This work was supported by institutional grants from the Centre National de la Recherche Scientifique, the Institut National de la Santé et de la Recherche Médicale, and the Deutsches Forschungsgemeinschaft and by a grant from the Association pour le Développement de la Recherche contre le Cancer. P. Machy was supported by a fellowship from the Fondation pour la Recherche Médicale. D. Aragnol was a boursier of the Ligue Nationale Française contre le Cancer. S. Alino was supported by a short-term fellowship from the European Molecular Biology Organization.

References

1. Aguet, M. (1980). High affinity binding of ^{125}I-labeled mouse interferon to a specific cell surface receptor. *Nature (London)* **284,** 459–461.
2. Allison, A. C., and Gregoriadis, G. (1974). Liposomes as immunological adjuvants. *Nature (London)* **252,** 252–254.
3. Alving, C. R., and Richards, R. L. (1983). Immunologic aspects of liposomes. *In* "Liposomes" (M. Ostro, ed.), p. 209. Dekker, New York.
4. Alving, C. R. (1984). Natural antibodies against phospholipids and liposomes in human. *Biochem. Soc. Trans.* **12,** 342–344.
5. Alving, C. R., Weldon, J. S., Munnell, J. F., and Hanson, W. L. (1984). Liposomes in Leishmaniosis: The lysosome connection. *In* "Receptor Mediated Targeting of Drugs" (G. Gregoriadis, G. Poste, J. Senior, and A. Trouet, eds.), p. 317. Plenum, New York.
6. Anderson, D. J., and Berkowitz, R. S. (1985). Interferon-γ enhances expression of class I MHC antigens in weakly HLA$^+$ human choriocarcinoma cell line BeWo, but does not induce MHC expression in the HLA$^-$ chroiocarcinoma cell line Jar. *J. Immunol.* **135,** 2498–2501.
7. Anderson, M., Pääbo, S., Nilsson, T., and Peterson, P. A. (1985). Impaired intracellular transport of class I MHC antigens as a possible means for adenovirus to evade immune surveillance. *Cell* **43,** 215–222.
8. Aragnol, D., and Leserman, L. D. (1986). Immune clearance of liposomes inhibited by an anti-Fc receptor antibody *in vivo*. *Proc. Natl. Acad. Sci. U.S.A.* **83,** 2699–2703.
9. Arce-Gomez, B., Jones, E. A., Barnstable, C. J., Salomon, E., and Bodmer, W. F. (1978). The genetic control of HLA-A and B antigens in somatic cell hybrids: Requirement for β2-microglobulin. *Tissue Antigens* **11,** 96–112.
10. Arnold, B., Archibald, A., Burgert, H., and Kvist, S. (1984). Complete nucleotide sequence of the murine H-2K^k gene. Comparison of three H-2K locus alleles. *Nucleic Acids Res.* **12,** 9473–9487.

11. Artzt, K., Bennet, D., and Jacob, F. (1974). Primitive teratocarcinoma cells express a differentiation antigen specified by a gene at the T-locus in the mouse. *Proc. Natl. Acad. Sci. U.S.A.* **71**, 811–814.

12. Barbet, J., Machy, P., and Leserman, L. D. (1981). Monoclonal antibody covalently coupled to liposomes: Specific targeting to cells. *J. Supramol. Struct. Cell. Biochem.* **16**, 243–258.

13. Basham, T. Y., Bourgeade, M. F., Creasey, A. A., and Merigan, T. C. (1982). Interferon increases HLA synthesis in melanoma cells: Interferon resistant and sensitive lines. *Proc. Natl. Acad. Sci. U.S.A.* **79**, 3265–3269.

14. Chatenoud, L., Baudrihaye, M. F., Chkoff, N., Kreis, H., and Bach, J.-F. (1983). Immunologic follow up of renal allograft recipients treated prophylactically by OKT-3 alone. *Transplant. Proc.* **15**, 643–645.

15. Chatenoud, L., Baudrihaye, M. F., Kreis, H., Goldstein, G., and Bach, J.-F. (1985). The restricted human response to the murine monoclonal OKT 3 antibody. *Transplant. Proc.* **17**, 558–559.

16. Cooley, M. A., Blackman, M. J., and Morris, A. G. (1984). Production of type 1 (α/β) interferon after virus infection of cloned alloantigen-sensitized mouse T lymphocytes. *Eur. J. Immunol.* **14**, 376–379.

17. Czop, J., and Austen, K. F. (1985). Generation of leukotriene by human monocytes upon stimulation of their β-glucan receptor during phagocytosis. *Proc. Natl. Acad. Sci. U.S.A.* **82**, 2751–2755.

18. Doherty, P. C., Knowles, B. B., and Wettstein, P. J. (1984). Immunologic surveillance of tumors in the context of major histocompatibility complex restriction of T cell function. *Adv. Cancer Res.* **42**, 1–66.

19. Doyle, A., Martin, W. J., Funa, K., Gazdar, A., Carney, D., Martin, S. E., Linnoila, I., Cuttitta, F., Mulshine, J., Bunn, P., and Minna, J. (1985). Markedly decreased expression of class I histocompatibility antigens, protein and mRNA in human small-cell lung cancer. *J. Exp. Med.* **161**, 1135–1151.

20. Eager, K. B., Williams, J., Breiding, D., Knowles, P. B., Appella, E., and Ricciardi, R. (1985). Expression of histocompatibility antigen. H-2 K, -D and -L is reduced in adenovirus-12-transformed mouse cells and is restored by interferon γ. *Proc. Natl. Acad. Sci. U.S.A.* **82**, 5525–5529.

21. Fidler, I. J., Sone, S., Fogler, W. E., and Barnes, Z. L. (1981). Eradication of spontaneous metastases and activation of alveolar macrophages by intravenous injection of liposomes containing muramyl dipeptide. *Proc. Natl. Acad. U.S.A.* **78**, 1680–1684.

22. Fracker, P. J., and Speck, J. C., Jr. (1978). Protein and cell membrane iodinations with sparingly soluble chloroamide, 1, 3, 4, 6-tetrachloro-3a, 6a diphenylglycoluril. *Biochem. Biophys. Res. Commun.* **80**, 849–857.

23. Geiger, B., Gitler, C., Calef, E., and Arnon, R. (1981). Dynamics of antibody- and lectin-mediated endocytosis of hapten-containing liposomes by murine macrophages. *Eur. J. Immunol.* **11**, 710–716.

24. Griffin, F. M., Jr. (1977). Opsonins. *In* "Comprehensive Immunology" (N. K. Day and R. A. Good, Vol. 2, eds.), p. 85. Plenum, New York.

25. Holtkamp, B., Lindahl, K. F., Segall, M., and Rajewsky, K. (1979). Spontaneous loss and subsequent stimulation of H-2 expression in clones of a heterozygous lymphoma cell line. *Immunogenetics* **9**, 405–421.

26. Holtkamp, B., Cramer, M., Lemke, H., and Rajewsky, K. (1981). Isolation of a cloned cell line expressing variant H-2K^k using fluorescence activated cell sorting. *Nature (London)* **289**, 66–68.

27. Holtkamp, B., Cramer, M., and Rajewsky, K. (1983). Somatic variation of H-2K^k expression and structure in a T-cell lymphoma: Instability, stabilization, high production and structural mutation. *EMBO J.* **2**, 1943–1951.

28. Hui, K., Grosveld, F., and Festenstein, H. (1984). Rejection of transplantable AKR leukemic cells following MHC DNA-mediated cell transformation. *Nature (London)* **311**, 750–752.

29. Jack, R. M., and Fearon, D. T. (1984). Altered surface distribution of both C3b receptors and Fc receptors on neutrophils induced by anti-C3b receptor or aggregated IgG. *J. Immunol.* **132**, 3028–3033.

30. Juliano, R. L., and Lin, G. (1980). The interaction of plasma proteins with liposomes: Protein binding and effects on the clotting and complement systems. *In* "Liposomes in Immunobiology" (B. H. Tom and H. R. Six, eds.), p. 49. Am. Elsevier, New York.

31. Kirby, C., Clarke, J., and Gregoriadis, G. (1980). Effect of the cholesterol content of small unilamellar liposomes on their stability *in vivo* and *in vitro*. *Biochem. J.* **186**, 591–598.

32. Kohl, N. E., Kanda, N. N., Schrect, R. R., Bruns, G., Latt, S. A., Gilbert, F., and Alt, F. W. (1983). Transposition and amplification of oncogene related sequences in human neuroblastomas. *Cell (Cambridge, Mass.)* **35**, 359–367.

33. Kurlander, R. J., Ellison, D. M., and Hall, J. (1984). The blockade of Fc receptor-mediated clearance of immune complexes *in vivo* by a monoclonal antibody (24G2) directed against Fc receptors on murine leukocytes. *J. Immunol.* **133**, 855–862.

34. Lalanne, J. L., Brégérère, F., Delarbre, C., Abastado, J. P., Gachelin, G., and Kourilsky, P. (1982). Comparison of nucleotide sequences of mRNAs belonging to the mouse H-2 multigene family. *Nucleic Acids Res.* **10**, 1039–1049.

35. Lampson, L. A., Fisher, C. A., and Whelen, J. P. (1983). Striking paucity of HLA-A, β2-microglobulin on human neuroblastoma cell lines. *J. Immunol.* **130**, 2471–2478.

36. Lemke, H., and Hämmerling, G. J. (1981). Topographic arrangements of H-2 determinants defined by monoclonal hybridoma antibodies. *In* "Monoclonal Antibodies and T Cell Hybridomas" (G. J. Hämmerling, U. Hämmerling, and J. F. Kearney, eds.), pp. 102–109. Elsevier/North-Holland Biomedical Press, Amsterdam.

37. Leserman, L. D., Weinstein, J. N., Blumenthal, R., and Terry, W. D. (1980). Receptor-mediated endocytosis of antibody-opsonized liposomes by tumor cells. *Proc. Natl. Acad. Sci. U.S.A.* **77**, 4089–4093.

38. Leserman, L. D., Barbet, J., Kourilsky, F. M., and Weinstein, J. N. (1980). Targeting to cells of fluorescent liposomes covalently coupled with monoclonal antibody or protein A. *Nature (London)* **288**, 602–604.

39. Leserman, L. D., Machy, P., and Barbet, J. (1981). Cell-specific drug transfer from liposomes bearing monoclonal antibodies. *Nature (London)* **293**, 226–228.

40. Lewis, J. T., Hafeman, D. G., and McConnell, H. M. (1980). Kinetics of antibody-dependent binding of haptenated phospholipid vesicles to a macrophage-related cell line. *Biochemistry* **19**, 5376–5386.

41. Lindahl, P., Levy, P., and Gresser, I. (1973). Enhancement by interferon of the expression of surface antigens on murine leukemia L1210 cells. *Proc. Natl. Acad. Sci. U.S.A.* **70**, 2785–2788.

42. Lopez-Berestein, G., Mehta, R., Hopfer, R. L., Mills, K., Kasi, L., Mehta, K., Fainstein, V., Luna, M., Hersh, E. M., and Juliano, R. (1983). Treatment and prophylaxis of disseminated infection due to Candida albicans in mice with liposome-encapsulated Amphoteracin B. *J. Infect. Dis.* **5**, 939–945.

43. Machy, P., and Leserman, L. D. (1984). Elimination or rescue of cells in culture by

specifically targeted liposomes containing methotrexate or formyl-tetrahydrofolate. *EMBO J.* **3**, 1971–1977.

44. Machy, P., Barbet, J., and Leserman, L. D. (1982). Differential endocytosis of T and B lymphocyte surface molecules evaluated with antibody bearing fluorescent liposomes containing methotrexate. *Proc. Natl. Acad. Sci. U.S.A.* **79**, 4148–4152.

45. Machy, P., Arnold, B., Alino, S., and Leserman, L. D. (1986). Interferon sensitive and insensitive MHC variants of a murine thymoma differentially resistant to methotrexate-containing antibody-directed liposomes and immunotoxin. *J. Immunol.* **136**, 3110–3115.

46. Mellman, I. S., Plutner, H., Steinman, R. M., Unkeless, J. C., and Cohn, Z. A. (1983). Internalization and degradation of macrophage Fc receptors during receptor-mediated phagocytosis *J. Cell Biol.* **96**, 887–895.

47. Nairn, R., Yamaga, K., and Natheson, S. G. (1980). Biochemistry of the gene products from murine MHC mutants. *Annu. Rev. Genet.* **14**, 241–277.

48. Natali, P., Bigotti, M., Cavalière, R., Liao, S.-K., Taniguchi, M., Matsui, M., and Ferrone, S. (1985). Heterogeneous expression of melanoma-associated antigens and HLA antigens by primary and multiple metastatic lesions removed from patients with melanoma. *Cancer Res.* **45**, 2883–2889.

49. Olsson, L. (1983). Phenotypic diversity in leukemia cell populations. *Cancer Metastasis Rev.* **2**, 153–163.

50. Ozato, K., Mayer, N., and Sachs, D. H. (1980). Hybridoma cell lines secreting monoclonal antibodies to mouse H-2 and Ia antigens. *J. Immunol.* **124**, 533–540.

51. Paraskevas, F., Lee, S.-T., Orr, K. B., and Israels, L. G. (1972). A receptor for Fc on mouse B-lymphocytes. *J. Immunol.* **108**, 1319–1327.

52. Patel, K. R., Li, M. P., and Baldeschwieler, J. D. (1983). Suppression of liver uptake of lipsomes by dextran sulfate 500. *Proc. Natl. Acad. Sci. U.S.A.* **80**, 6518–6522.

53. Petty, H. R., Haefeman, D. G., and McConnell, H. M. (1980). Specific antibody-dependent phagocytosis of lipid vesicles by RAW 264 macrophages results in the loss of cell surface Fc but not C3b receptor activity. *J. Immunol.* **125**, 2391–2396.

54. Pierres, M., Devaux, C., Dosseto, M., and Marchetto, S. (1981). Clonal analysis of B- and T-cell responses to Ia antigens. *Immunogenetics* **14**, 481–495.

55. Pont, S., Regnier-Vigouroux, A., Naquet, P., Blanc, D., Pierres, A., Marchetto, S., and Pierres, M. (1985). Analysis of the Thy-1 pathway of T-cell hybridoma activation using 17 rat monoclonal antibodies reactive with distinctive Thy-1 epitopes. *Eur. J. Immunol.* **15**, 1222–1228.

56. Poste, G., and Kirsh, R. (1983). Site-specific (targeted) drug delivery in cancer therapy. *Bio/Technology* **1**, 869–878.

57. Potter, T. A., Boyer, C., Schmitt-Verhulst, A.-M., Golstein, P., and Rajan, T. V. (1984). Expression of H-2D^b on the cell surface in the absence of detectable β2-microglobulin. *J. Exp. Med.* **160**, 317–322.

58. Potter, T. A., Zeff, R. A., Schmitt-Verhulst, A.-M., and Rajan, T. V. (1985). Molecular analysis of an EL4 cell line that expresses H-2D^b but not H-2K^b or β2-microglobulin. *Proc. Natl. Acad. Sci. U.S.A.* **82**, 2950–2954.

59. Prat, M., Gribaudo, G., Comoglio, P. M., Cavallo, C., and Landolfo, S. (1984). Monoclonal antibodies against murine γ-interferon. *Proc. Natl. Acad. Sci. U.S.A.* **81**, 4515–4519.

60. Ralston, E., Hjemeland, L. M., Klausner, R. D., Weinstein, J. N., and Blumenthal, R. (1981). Carboxyfluorescein as a probe for liposome-cell interactions: Effect of impurities and purification of the dye. *Biochim. Biophys. Acta* **649**, 133–137.

61. Rebaï, N., and Malissen, B. (1983). Structural and genetic analyses of HLA class I molecules using monoclonal xenoantibodies. *Tissue Antigens* **22**, 107–117.
62. Reininger, L., Fueri, J., Boned, A., Prat, M., Landolfo, S., and Rubin, B. (1985). On the molecular basis of T-helper-cell function. IV. B-lymphocyte-promotor factors: On their mode of action, biochemical nature and possible relationship to molecules involved in specific T-helper-cell activity. *Cell. Immunol.* **92**, 85–104.
63. Rosa, F., and Fellous, M. (1984). The effect of γ-interferon on MHC antigens. *Immunol. Today* **5**, 261–262.
64. Sachs, D. H., Mayer, N., and Ozato, C. (1981). Hybridoma antibodies directed towards murine H-2 and Ia antigens. *In* "Monoclonal Antibodies and T Cell Hybridomas" (G. J. Hämmerling, V. Hämmerling, and J. F. Kearney, eds.), pp. 95–101. Elsevier/North-Holland Biomedical Press, Amsterdam.
65. Sanderson, A. R., and Beverley, P. C. L. (1983). Interferon, β2-microglobulin and immunoselection in the path to malignancy. *Immunol. Today* **4**, 211–213.
66. Scherphof, G., Roerdink, F., Dijkstra, J., Ellens, H., Zanger, R., and Wisse, E. (1983). Uptake of liposomes by rat and mouse hepatocytes and Kuppfer cells. *Biol. Cell.* **47**, 47–58.
67. Schrier, P. I., Bernards, R., Vaessen, R. T. M. J., Houweling, A., and Van der Eb, A. J. (1984). Expression of class I major histocompatibility antigens switched off by highly oncogenic adenovirus 12 in transformed rat cells. *Nature (London)* **305**, 771–775.
68. Shcroff, R. W., Foon, K. A., Beatty, S. M., Oldham, R. K., and Morgan, A. C., Jr. (1985). Human anti-murine immunoglobulin responses in patients receiving monoclonal antibody therapy. *Cancer Res.* **45**, 879–885.
69. Schroit, A. J. (1982). Synthesis and properties of an exchangeable radioiodinated phospholipid. *Biochemistry* **21**, 5323–5328.
70. Scollay, R., Jacobs, S., Jerabek, L., Butcher, E., and Weissman, I. (1980). T cell maturation: Thymocyte and thymus migrant subpopulations defined with monoclonal antibodies to MHC region antigens. *J. Immunol.* **124**, 2845–2853.
71. Segal, D. M., and Titus, J. A. (1978). The subclass specificity for the binding of murine myeloma proteins to macrophage and lymphocyte cell lines and to normal spleen cells. *J. Immunol.* **120**, 1395–1403.
72. Shawler, D. L., Bartholomew, R. M., Smith, L. M., and Dillman, R. O. (1985). Human immune response to multiple injections of murine monoclonal IgG. *J. Immunol.* **135**, 1530–1535.
73. Springer, T. A., and Unkeless, J. C. (1984). Analysis of macrophage differentiation and function with monoclonal antibodies. *Contemp. Top. Immunobiol.* **13**, 1–31.
74. Tanaka, K., Isselbacher, K. J., Khoury, G., and Jay, G. (1985). Reversal of oncogenesis by the expression of a major histocompatibility complex class I gene. *Science* **228**, 26–30.
75. Teillaud, J.-L., Diamond, B., Pollock, R. R., Fajtova, V., and Scharff, M. D. (1985). Fc receptor on cultured myeloma and hybridoma cells. *J. Immunol.* **134**, 1774–1779.
76. Uhr, J. W. (1984). Immunotoxins: Harnessing nature's poisons. *J. Immunol.* **133**, i–x.
77. Unkeless, J. C. (1979). Characterization of a monoclonal antibody directed against mouse macrophage and lymphocyte Fc receptors. *J. Exp. Med.* **150**, 580–595.
78. Weinstein, J. N., Ralston, E., Leserman, L. D., Klausner, R. D., Dragsten, P., Henkart, P., and Blumenthal, R. (1984). Self-quenching of carboxyfluorescein fluorescence: Uses in studying liposome stability and liposome cell interaction. *In* "Liposome Technology" (G. Gregoriadis, ed.), Vol. 3, p. 183. CRC Press, Boca Raton, Florida.
79. White, B. A., and Bancroft, F. C. (1982). Cytoplasmic dot hybridization. *J. Biol. Chem.* **257**, 8569–8572.

80. Xin, J.-H., Kvist, S., and Dobberstein, B. (1982). Identification of an H-2K^d gene using a specific cDNA probe. *EMBO J.* **1,** 467–471.
81. Zinkernagel, R. M., and Oldstone, M. B. A. (1976). Cells that express viral antigens but lack H-2 determinants are not lysed by immune thymus derived lymphocytes but are lysed by other anti-viral immune attack mechanisms. *Proc. Natl. Acad. Sci. U.S.A.* **73,** 3666–3670.

PART V

New Drugs in Development

16

Second-Generation Azolotetrazinones

MALCOLM F. G. STEVENS

Department of Pharmaceutical Sciences
Aston University
Birmingham, United Kingdom

I. Introduction

The first examples of the antitumor azolotetrazinones were originally synthesised in late 1980. The lead compound 8-carbamoyl-3-(2-chloroethyl)imidazo[5,1-*d*]-1,2,3,5-tetrazin-4(3H)-one (mitozolomide; **I**; Fig. 1), formerly known as azolastone, entered clinical trial in 1983 and at the time of writing of this chapter the first of the second-generation agents is at the preclinical toxicology stage prior to phase I evaluation.

The speed of development of this novel class of agent attests to the value of tackling drug discovery and development within an integrated research partnership involving the participation of chemists, biochemists, cell biologists, toxicologists, and pharmacists. Moreover, the program has been brought to fruition by the collaborative efforts of academia and

NEW AVENUES IN DEVELOPMENTAL
CANCER CHEMOTHERAPY

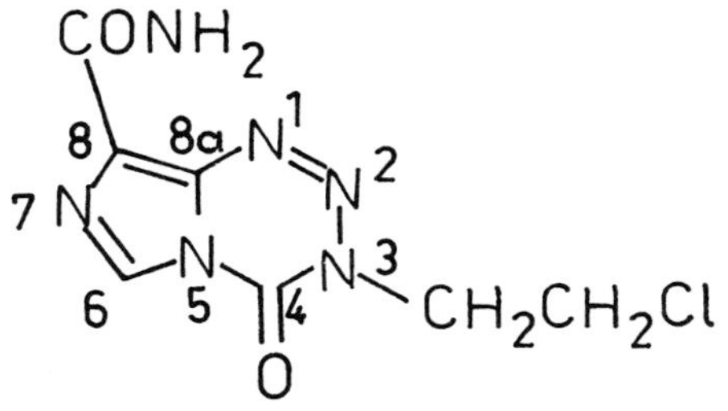

(I)

Fig. 1. Structure of 8-carbamoyl-3-(2-chloroethyl)imidazo[5,1-*d*]-1,2,3,5-tetrazin-4(3H)-one (mitozolomide; CCRG 81010; M&B 39565; NSC 353451) and numbering system.

industry with both parties—the Cancer Research Campaign Experimental Chemotherapy Group, Pharmaceutical Sciences Institute, Aston University, and May and Baker Ltd, Dagenham—combining their intellectual and managerial resources in a fruitful symbiosis. This account will focus on the chemical aspects of the development of second-generation azolotetrazinones.

II. Background to the Discovery of Mitozolomide

Nearly a hundred years ago, Finger (7) reported that 1,2,3-benzotriazin-4(3H)-one (**II**) underwent ring opening in the presence of aqueous alkali to afford anthranilic acid (**IV**). The mechanism of this reaction (Fig. 2) involving the unstable 1-aryltriazene (**III**) generated by nucleophilic attack at C-4 of the triazinone probably encompasses the essential chemical feature of the mode of action of mitozolomide (see Section V,B).

Compounds with NNN linkages in either a cyclic (1,2,3-triazine) or acyclic (triazene) arrangement have been the subject of detailed study by the author and colleagues since 1960. Some key structures which were

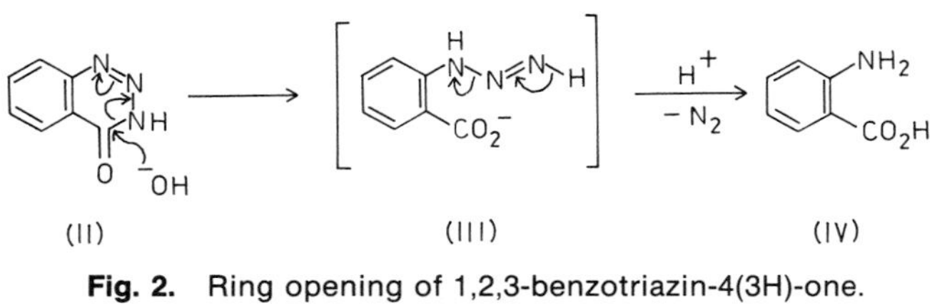

Fig. 2. Ring opening of 1,2,3-benzotriazin-4(3H)-one.

milestones in the evolution of the imidazotetrazinones are compiled in Fig. 3.

Although the 1,2,3-triazinones in general structure (**V**) possess versatile chemical reactivity dominated by cleavage of the 1,8a; 2,3; or 3,4 bonds, antitumor activity is not a feature of this series (37). In contrast, the acyclic triazenes possess a rich chemistry (43) and perplexing biological activity (18,39) and are represented in the clinic by the imidazotriazene DTIC (**VI**). DTIC is extremely photosensitive, and the red photoproduct formed in the formulated drug (DTIC-Dome) was identified as the imidazoazoimidazolium olate (**VII**) (22,23,38). The intermediate in this reaction is 5-diazoimidazole-4-carboxamide (**VIII**). The use of this valuable synthon in heterocyclic synthesis was exploited in 1977 to achieve a synthetic entry to the imidazo[5,1-c]-1,2,4-triazine system (**IX**). The imidazocarboxamide group was incorporated in these compounds in the hope that the bicyclic products might interfere in *de novo* purine biosynthesis (2). Imidazotriazines cleave with nucleophiles (e.g., hydrazine) at the 4,5 bond only (3) but are devoid of antitumor activity.

In 1979, Ege and Gilbert described a new general synthesis of azolote-

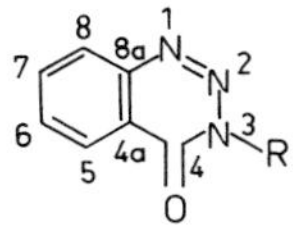

(V)

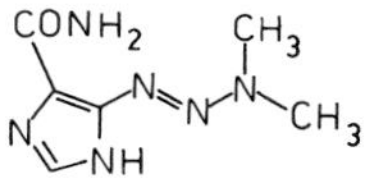

(VI)

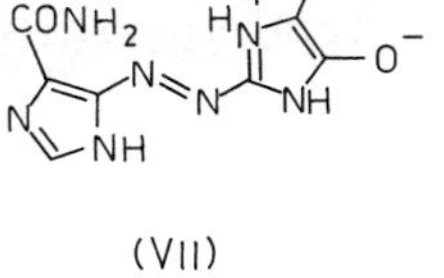

(VII)

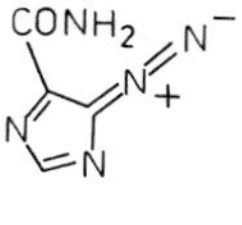

(VIII)

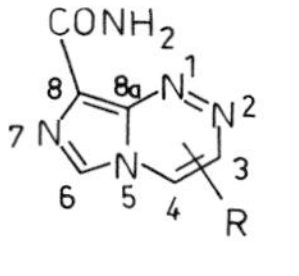

(IX)

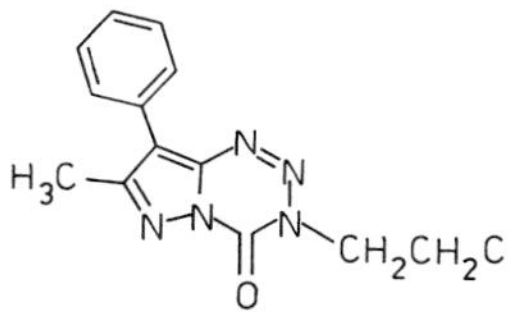

(X)

Fig. 3. Key structures in the development of antitumor azolotetrazinones.

trazinones by interaction of diazoazoles and isocyanates (6); one derivative prepared was the pyrazolo[5,1-*d*]-1,2,3,5-tetrazinone (**X**). This report provided the spur for the synthesis of imidazo[5,1-*d*]-1,2,3,5-tetrazinones at Aston University. Based on our knowledge of the chemistry of 1,2,3- and 1,2,4-triazines we predicted that incorporation of the extra heteroatom in a bicyclic 1,2,3,5-tetrazine such as mitozolomide would induce lability in four different bonds (1,8a; 2,3; 3,4; and 4,5). The prospect that these fragmentations might generate a cascade of reactive moieties, some of which are known to possess antitumor activity, was an enticing one. Reinforcing the eagerness to screen mitozolomide was the work of Gibson and Hickman (12), who showed that intracellular release of 2-chloroethyl isocyanate, a carbamoylating agent, may play a role in modulating the biological activity of the nitrosourea BCNU [1,3-*bis*-(2-chloroethyl)-1-nitrosourea] against the TLX5 lymphoma in mice. (Cleavage of the 2,3 and 4,5 bonds in mitozolomide would generate 2-chloroethyl isocyanate.) It transpires, however, that the antitumor activity of mitozolomide owes more to cleavage of the 3,4 or 4,5 bonds (Finger reaction) (see Section V,B) than isocyanate release.

Mitozolomide was the tenth compound screened by the Cancer Chemotherapy Research Group at Aston in 1981 (hence the code number CCRG 81010).

III. Synthesis of Mitozolomide and Its Analogs

Mitozolomide is prepared in good yield and in a high state of purity by stirring together 5-diazoimidazole-4-carboxamide (**VIII**) and 2-chloroethyl isocyanate in dichloromethane or ethyl acetate in the dark at room temperature (40). A single-crystal X-ray diffraction analysis of mitozolomide confirmed the structure and showed that the two independent molecules per asymmetric unit are rotamers about the C-8 to carboxamide bond. The orientation of the carbamoyl group in one rotamer facilitates an intramolecular H-bond of the type N—H. . .N. With the exception of the chloroethyl side chain both molecules are approximately planar (26).

The synthetic reaction is rewardingly adaptable to exploitation with a range of diazoimidazoles (**XI**) and isocyanates (**XII**) (4,31) (see Table I for a list of compounds). Suitable solvents include dichloromethane, ethyl acetate, or acetonitrile, and the mechanism probably involves an ionic process (Fig. 4) involving a dipolar intermediate (**XIII**), since the reaction can be accelerated by employing the polar solvent hexamethylphosphoramide as the reaction medium. Yields of imidazotetrazinones (**XIV**) were, in general, good except in the case of diazoimidazoles with a bulky

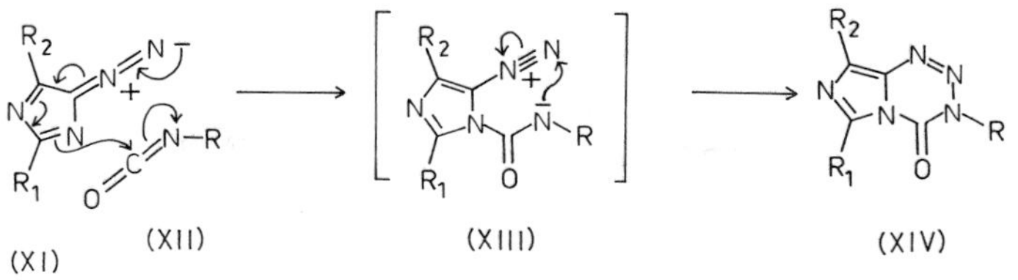

Fig. 4. Synthesis of imidazotetrazinones.

substituent in the 2 position (**XI**: R_1 = i-Pr, cyclohexyl, benzyl, phenethyl; R_2 = $CONH_2$) where the steric bulk of the substituent presumably hinders reaction with the isocyanate.

For the synthesis of the benzylamide (**XXXVII**) and anilide (**XXXVIII**) the amidic NH group was protected by a *p*-methoxybenzyl residue prior to synthesis of the diazoazole; the protecting group could be removed from the intact imidazotetrazinones with trifluoracetic acid–anisole (4). The nitroamide (**XL**) was prepared by nitration of mitozolomide in a concentrated sulfuric–nitric acid mixture. A series of 4-substituted-3-diazopyrazoles and 3-diazoindazole also participated in the reaction with 2-chloroethyl isocyanate to yield new pyrazolotetrazinones (**LIV–LVII**) and the indazolotetrazinone (**LVIII**), respectively.

IV. Antitumor Activity of Azolotetrazinones

Judicious choice of tumor used in screening studies can often provide preliminary information about the mode of action of novel agents. Compounds prepared in the imidazo- and pyrazolo-tetrazinone series were evaluated against the L1210 leukemia or TLX5 lymphoma in mice *in vivo*. These tumors were initially selected because of their inherent sensitivities to different biochemical classes of cytotoxic agents: the L1210 tumor responds to alkylating agents and antimetabolites, whereas the TLX5 lymphoma, although resistant to alkylating agents of the β-chloroethylamine type, is sensitive to electrophilic species generated from drugs of the triazene, nitrosourea, and hydrazine classes (1). In fact, in those cases in which sufficient compound was available for screening against both tumors, a remarkable consistency of response was observed (Table I).

The antitumor activity of mitozolomide against a broad spectrum of mouse tumors (19) and human tumor xenografts (8) has been reported; the drug exhibits curative activity against both L1210 and TLX5 tumors on a single-dose schedule. Of the 3-alkyl congeners of mitozolomide (**XV–XXV**; Table I) only the 3-methyl derivative (**XV**; CCRG 81045; M&B

TABLE I

Chemical Structures and Antitumor Activity of Imidazotetrazinones, Pyrazolotetrazinones, and an Indazolotetrazinone

Compounds (I) and (XV–LIII) [structure]

Compounds (LIV–LVIII) [structure]

Structure No.	R	R_1	R_2	Antitumor activity[a] L1210 leukemia[b]	TLX5 lymphoma[c]
(I)	$(CH_2)_2Cl$	H	$CONH_2$ (mitozolomide)	+++	+++
(XV)	Me	H	$CONH_2$ (CCRG 81045)	$+^d$	++
(XVI)	Et	H	$CONH_2$	—	—
(XVII)	$(CH_2)_2Br$	H	$CONH_2$	—	$+^e$
(XVIII)	$(CH_2)_2Me$	H	$CONH_2$	NT	—
(XIX)	$(CH_2)_2OMe$	H	$CONH_2$	NT	—
(XX)	$(CH_2)_3Cl$	H	$CONH_2$	—	—
(XXI)	$CH_2CH(Cl)CH_2Cl$	H	$CONH_2$	—	—
(XXII)	$CH_2CH=CH_2$	H	$CONH_2$	—	—
(XXIII)	$CH(Me)Et$	H	$CONH_2$	NT	—
(XXIV)	$(CH_2)_5Me$	H	$CONH_2$	NT	—
(XXV)	CH_2Ph	H	$CONH_2$	NT	—
(XXVI)	$(CH_2)_2Cl$	Me	$CONH_2$	++	+++
(XXVII)	$(CH_2)_2Cl$	Et	$CONH_2$	++	NT
(XXVIII)	$(CH_2)_2Cl$	n-Pr	$CONH_2$	+++	NT
(XXIX)	$(CH_2)_2Cl$	i-Pr	$CONH_2$	+	NT
(XXX)	$(CH_2)_2Cl$	n-But	$CONH_2$	+	NT
(XXXI)	$(CH_2)_2Cl$	CH_2Ph	$CONH_2$	+	NT
(XXXII)	$(CH_2)_2Cl$	C_6H_{11}	$CONH_2$	—	NT
(XXXIII)	$(CH_2)_2Cl$	$(CH_2)_2Ph$	$CONH_2$	—	NT
(XXXIV)	$(CH_2)_2Cl$	H	CONHMe	+++	+++
(XXXV)	$(CH_2)_2Cl$	H	$CONMe_2$	+++	+++
(XXXVI)	$(CH_2)_2Cl$	H	$CONC_5H_{10}$	++	+++
(XXXVII)	$(CH_2)_2Cl$	H	$CONHCH_2Ph$	++	NT
(XXXVIII)	$(CH_2)_2Cl$	H	CONHPh	NT	+
(XXXIX)	$(CH_2)_2Cl$	H	CON(Me)Ph	—	NT
(XL)	$(CH_2)_2Cl$	H	$CONHNO_2$	NT	+++
(XLI)	$(CH_2)_2Cl$	H	SO_2NH_2	+++	+++
(XLII)	$(CH_2)_2Cl$	Me	SO_2NH_2	+++	+++
(XLIII)	$(CH_2)_2Cl$	H	SO_2NHMe	+++	+++
(XLIV)	$(CH_2)_2Cl$	H	SO_2NMe_2	+++	+++
(XLV)	$(CH_2)_2Cl$	Me	SO_2NMe_2	+++	+++
(XLVI)	$(CH_2)_2Cl$	H	SO_2Me	+++	+++
(XLVII)	$(CH_2)_2Cl$	Me	SO_2Me	+++	+++

TABLE I (*Continued*)

Compounds (I) and (XV–LIII)				Compounds (LIV–LVIII)	

				Antitumor activity[a]	
Structure No.	R	R_1	R_2	L1210 leukemia[b]	TLX5 lymphoma[c]
(XLVIII)	(CH$_2$)$_2$Cl	Me	SO$_2$Et	+++	+++
(XLIX)	(CH$_2$)$_2$Cl	Me	SO$_2$n-Pr	+++	+++
(L)	(CH$_2$)$_2$Cl	Me	SOMe	+++	NT
(LI)	(CH$_2$)$_2$Cl	H	Ph	—	NT
(LII)	(CH$_2$)$_2$Cl	H	NO$_2$	—	NT
(LIII)	(CH$_2$)$_2$Cl	H	CN	NT	—
(LIV)	(CH$_2$)$_2$Cl	H	CONH$_2$	+++	++
(LV)	(CH$_2$)$_2$Cl	H	CONMe$_2$	+++	+++
(LVI)	(CH$_2$)$_2$Cl	H	SO$_2$Me	+++	NT
(LVII)	(CH$_2$)$_2$Cl	H	NO$_2$	—	NT
(LVIII)	(CH$_2$)$_2$Cl[f]	—CH=CH—CH=CH—		NT	—

[a] The antitumor assessment shown represents the optimal result on a single-dose schedule. Activity was rated according to the following scale: +++, T/C > 150% with cures at one or more dose levels; ++, T/C > 150% with no cures; +, T/C > 125%; —, T/C < 125%; and NT, not tested. Full details of the antitumor tests will be published elsewhere.

[b] The murine L1210 leukemia tests were conducted in accordance with the protocols described by the National Cancer Institute (10).

[c] The TLX5 lymphoma was passaged and used as described previously (11).

[d] On a repeat schedule CCRG 81045 rates ++ (see Table II).

[e] T/C 137% in one test at optimum dose in single-dose schedule.

[f] Sample prepared by Dr. R. Grayshan, Department of Pharmacy, Heriot-Watt University, Edinburgh.

39831; NSC 362856) exhibits pronounced activity, although the compound is not curative. All the other 3-alkyl derivatives, including the 3-ethylimidazotetrazinone (**XVI**) are less active or inactive against the TLX5 tumor on a single-dose schedule. These preliminary studies pointed to the 2-chloroethyl group being the substituent of choice at the 3 position.

Addition of a 6-alkyl group into the mitozolomide structure (**XXVI–XXXIII**) afforded a series of compounds with graded activity against the L1210 tumor. Small alkyl groups were tolerated without loss of activity, whereas a large hydrocarbon group, e.g., cyclohexyl (**XXXII**) and phenethyl (**XXXIII**) greatly reduced activity possibly because the bulky groups inhibit nucleophile-promoted ring opening at C-4 (see Section

V,B). Substitution of the hydrogens of the 8-carbamoyl group of mitozolomide by one alkyl or two small alkyl groups (**XXXIV–XXXVII**) gave compounds with high activity, whereas substitution with an aromatic residue (**XXXVIII–XXXIX**) reduced activity. The 8-nitroamide (**XL**) was equally active with mitozolomide against the TLX5 lymphoma.

Compounds with sulfur-containing 8-substituents—sulfonamides (**XLI–XLV**) and sulfones (**XLVI–XLIX**)—were all potently active against both tumors, and an 8-sulfoxide (**L**) displayed curative activity against the L1210 tumor. Although the 8-phenyl- (**LI**), 8-nitro- (**LII**), and 8-cyano- (**LIII**) derivatives were not tested in both tumor lines, these modifications in 3-(2-chloroethyl)-substituted imidazotetrazinones also have a dyschemotherapeutic effect.

A few examples of pyrazolo[5,1-*d*]-1,2,3,5-tetrazinones were also evaluated. 8-Carbamoylpyrazolotetrazinone (**LIV**), an isomer of mitozolomide, its *N, N*-dimethyl analog (**LV**), and the sulfone (**LVI**) all showed pronounced activity. Significantly, the inactivity of the 8-nitro-derivative (**LVII**) paralleled that in the imidazotetrazinone series; compound (**X**) originally prepared by Ege and Gilbert (6) and the indazolotetrazinone (**LVIII**) were also inactive.

In summary, the most active imidazotetrazines were those depicted in Figure 5.

The substitutent of choice at N-3 is the 2-chloroethyl group, at C-6 a hydrogen atom or small alkyl group is preferred, and at C-8 a rich vein of activity extends through a range of carboxamides, sulfonamides, and sulfones.

The dose-limiting toxicity encountered in the phase I clinical trial of mitozolomide was thrombocytopenia at doses >115 mg/m^2, and recovery from the thrombocytopenia was delayed for up to 8 weeks (32). No ideal model to mimic this condition is available which would be applicable for selecting a less myelosuppressive analog from the large portfolio of active azolotetrazinones. Although full data on the antitumor tests (i.e., opti-

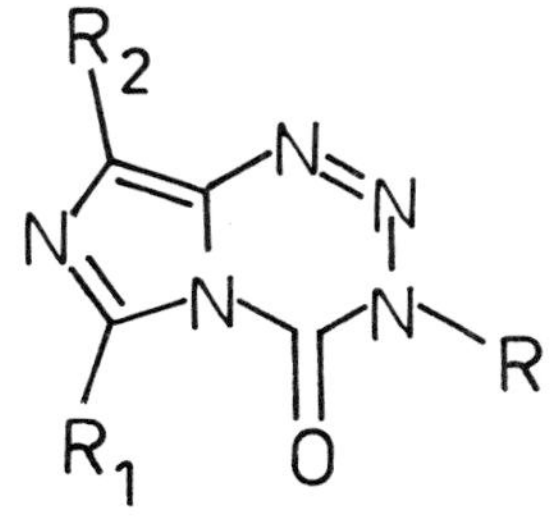

Fig. 5. Structural modifications in potent antitumor imidazotetrazinones.

TABLE II

Activity of 8-Carbamoyl-3-methylimidazo[5,1-d]-1,2,3,5-tetrazin-4(3H)-one (XV; CCRG 81045) against Murine Survival-Time Models[a] and Resistant Lines

Tumor	Schedule (day of injection)	Optimum dose (mg/kg/day)	Optimal T/C (%)	Assessment[b]
P388 leukemia	1	200	143	+[c]
	1–4	100	214	++[c]
	1–5	200	>214	+++[c]
P388/mitozolomide	1	200	110	—
	1–4	100	112	—
L1210 leukemia	1	200	149	+
	1–4	100	200	++
L1210/DTIC	1	200	116	—
	1–4	100	108	—
L1210/BCNU	1	200	148	+
	1–4	100	175	++
B16 melanoma	1–9	100	181	++
M5076 reticulum cell sarcoma	1,5,9,13	200	170	++
TLX5 lymphoma	3	160	151	++
	3,6,9	80	154	++
	3–7	40	181	++

[a] For reference to protocols, see footnote b, Table I.

[b] See footnote a, Table I.

[c] For the P388 tumor, +++, T/C > 175% with cures at one or more dose levels; ++, T/C > 175% with no cures; and +, T/C > 120%.

mum dose and schedule and toxic dose) are not reported in this account no obvious analog emerged with a dramatically improved therapeutic index. However one compound, 8-carbamoyl-3-methylimidazo[5,1-d]-1,2,3,5-tetrazin-4(3H)-one (**XV**; CCRG 81045) appeared to be qualitatively different in its activity and an attractive candidate for detailed study. Against a panel of survival time models (Table II) CCRG 81045 was potently active against the P388 and L1210 leukemias, the B16 melanoma, and M5076 reticulum-cell sarcoma. Whereas most of the 3-(2-chloroethyl)-azolotetrazinones display optimum activity on a single-dose schedule against the TLX5 lymphoma (Table I), CCRG 81045 was most active on a divided dose schedule (Table II). In addition, CCRG 81045 displays curative activity (data not shown) against three solid tumor models—the murine M5076 sarcoma and ADJ/PC6A plasmacytoma and the MX-1 human mammary xenograft. A P388 line resistant to mitozolomide and an L1210 variant resistant to DTIC are completely cross-resistant with CCRG

81045, but appreciable activity is still retained against a BCNU-resistant L1210 tumor.

V. Chemistry of Mitozolomide and Its Analogs

The chemistry of the imidazotetrazinones is exceedingly complex. Some reactions are predictable (see Section II); others are very unexpected.

A. Reactions in Nonaqueous Solvents

When mitozolomide is thermolyzed in hot acetonitrile the dominating fragmentation is cleavage of the 2,3 and 4,5 bonds to regenerate 5-diazoimidazole-4-carboxamide (**VIII**) and 2-chloroethyl isocyanate (40). The mechanism of this fragmentation, which is a reversal of the synthetic process, possibly involves an initial [1,5] sigmatropic shift to generate the unstable spirobicycle (**LIX**) which then undergoes an electrocyclic ring opening (Fig. 6). The products formed when mitozolomide is decomposed in the presence of a range of carbon, nitrogen, oxygen, and halogen nucleophiles can (formally) be considered to arise from ensuing interceptions of the diazoimidazole with the nucleophile. However, it is more likely, especially with the nitrogen and oxygen nucleophiles, that ring opening is initiated by attack of the nucleophile at C-4 of the tetrazine ring (see Section V,B) (40). When mitozolomide is heated with reactive methylenic esters in pyridine, imidazotriazinones (**LX**) are formed in high yields (5); when the reaction is accomplished in acetic acid the products are imidazotriazines (**LXI**). These reactions proceed via intermediate hydrazones (**LXII**), which have been prepared and characterized independently (2), and the overall reaction represents an interesting "one-pot" conversion of imidazo-1,2,3,5-tetrazines to imidazo-1,2,4-triazines. Decomposition of mitozolomide in cold ethanolic aniline leads to the formation of the triazene (**LXIII**). In the absence of other reactants, mitozolomide reacts with alcohols to form 2-azahypoxanthine (**LXIV**); under more forcing conditions the aminoimidazole esters (**LXV**) are formed as by-products (40). Mitozolomide reacts with cold hydrazine hydrate to yield 5-azidoimidazole-4-carboxamide (**LXVI**) and with sodium bromide or iodide in hot acetic acid to afford 5-halogenoimidazole-4-carboxamides (**LXVII**). In some cases 2-chloroethyl isocyanate was trapped by aniline to yield the urea (**LXVIII**) and by alcohols to produce carbamates (**LXIX**) (40).

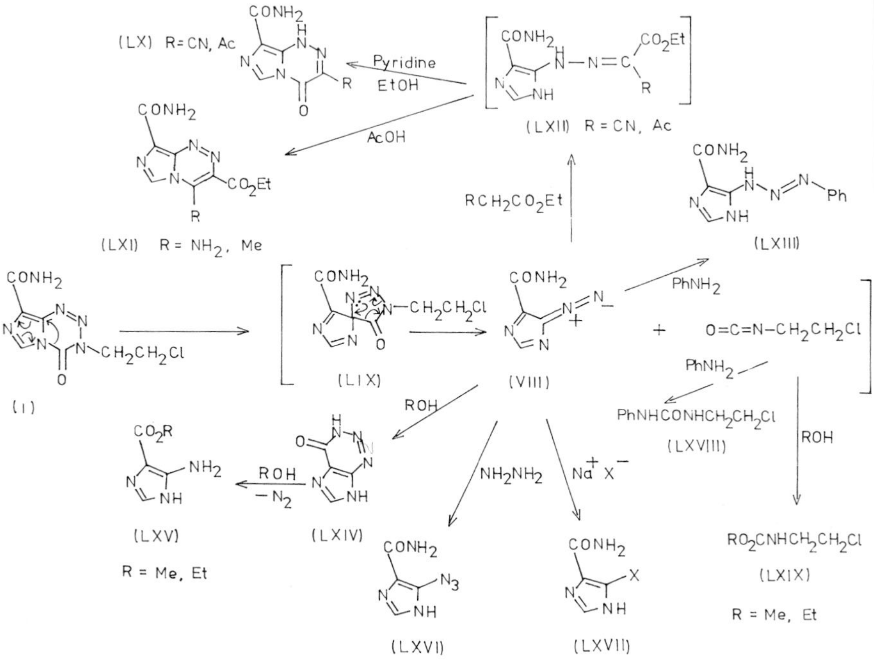

Fig. 6. Reactions of mitozolomide in nonaqueous conditions.

B. Reactions in Aqueous Conditions

The decomposition of mitozolomide and its analogs is strikingly pH dependent—the more basic the conditions the more unstable the compounds (Table III). In fact, mitozolomide can be crystallized quite satisfactorily from concentrated sulfuric acid, a most unexpected finding considering the acid sensitivity of 1,2,3-benzotriazines (37) and triazenes (43).

The major products from the decomposition of mitozolomide in phosphate buffer at pH 7.4 are 5-aminoimidazole-4-carboxamide (**LXXV**; AIC) and 2-chloroethanol. Significantly, the same products have been identified from the decomposition of 5-[3-(2-chloroethyl)triazen-1-yl]imidazole-4-carboxamide (**LXXII**; MCTIC) by Shealy et al. (35). Moreover, when mitozolomide is decomposed in 5% aqueous sodium carbonate on a preparative scale MCTIC can be isolated in 50% yield (40). Similarly, when CCRG 81045 (**XV**) and its 3-ethyl congener (**XVI**) were treated likewise the monoalkyltriazenes (**LXXIII**; MTIC) and (**LXXIV**; ETIC), respectively, were isolated (5).

TABLE III

Influence of pH on the Stability of Mitozolomide and Its Analogs in Buffers

Compound				$t_{1/2}$ at 37°C (hr)[a]						
No.	R	R_1	R_2	pH 4.0	pH 6.0	pH 7.0	pH 7.4	pH 7.5	pH 8.0	pH 9.0
(I)	$(CH_2)_2Cl$	H	$CONH_2$	240[b]	25.5	2.08	0.92[b]	0.9	0.37	0.15[b]
(XLI)	$(CH_2)_2Cl$	H	SO_2NH_2	—	8.95	1.27	—	0.6	0.27	—
(XLIII)	$(CH_2)_2Cl$	H	SO_2NHMe	—	7.53	0.90	—	0.32	0.15	—
(XLIV)	$(CH_2)_2Cl$	H	SO_2NMe_2	—	7.1	0.78	—	0.27	0.17	—
(LIII)	$(CH_2)_2Cl$	H	CN	—	3.48	0.38	—	0.13	0.042	—

[a] Determined by ultraviolet spectroscopy (21).
[b] Determined by high-performance liquid chromatography (36).

A mechanism to account for these observations is presented (Fig. 7): the mechanism has biological significance and its similarity to the Finger reaction (see Section II) should be noted. Attack by water at C-4 initiates the base catalyzed ring-opening process to give unstable carbamic acids (LXX) or (LXXI), depending on which bond (3,4 or 4,5) is cleaved. Decarboxylation then generates unstable monoalkyltriazenes which can be isolated in aqueous sodium carbonate. At pH 7.4 the triazenes alkylate water (in buffer) by an S_N2-type process leading to the formation of AIC, nitrogen, and an alcohol. It is possible that intramolecular H-bonding in the triazenes (LXXII–LXXIV) controls their reactivity by stabilizing the electrophilic alkylazotautomeric forms which alkylate (bio)nucleophiles.

Thus, chemically, mitozolomide and other imidazotetrazinones appear to be chemically activated pro-drug forms of monoalkyltriazenes, and their antitumor activity is fully explicable in terms of membership of the triazene lineage (39). Biological evaluation of mitozolomide against the DNA of L1210 cells (13), normal (IMR-90) and SV40-transformed (VA-13) human embryo cells (14), and a range of enzymes (20) points strongly to the agent acting as a pro-drug form of MCTIC which possibly crosslinks DNA (13,14). MCTIC itself has pronounced antitumor activity (35), but it is a very unstable moiety and not a realistic clinical candidate.

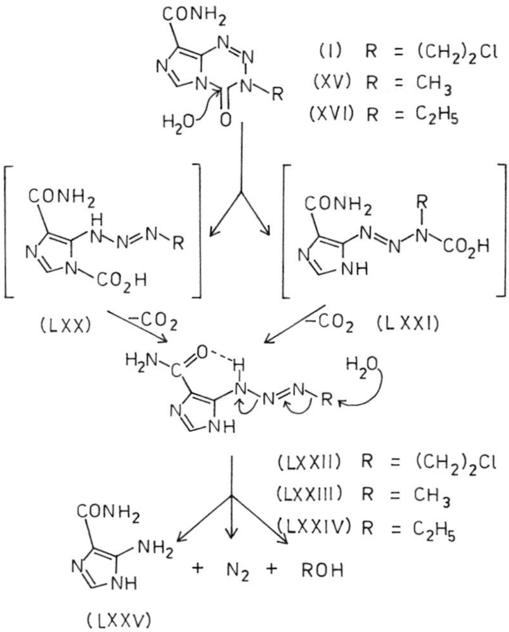

Fig. 7. Ring opening of imidazotetrazinones to imidazotriazenes in aqueous conditions.

VI. Structure–Activity Relationships

The hypothesis that mitozolomide operates by cross-linking DNA should be tempered somewhat by evaluation of the structure–activity relationships in the azolotetrazinone series (see Table I) and by closer scrutiny of the chemical, physical, and biological properties of key compounds. Mitozolomide (**I**), CCRG 81045 (**XV**), and the 3-ethylimidazotetrazinone (**XVI**) all ring-open to monoalkyltriazenes (**LXXII–LXXIV**) (see Fig. 7). Mitozolomide, which could ultimately cross-link DNA, is the most active; CCRG 81045, which cannot cross-link, is also very active but with a different antitumor profile; and the 3-ethyl analog is inactive against the tumors studied in a single-dose schedule. Other series of antitumor agents with N-alkyl groups display the same activity feature: chloroethyl > methyl ≫ ethyl. These agents include the 1-aryl-3,3-dialkyltriazenes, nitrosoureas, and hydrazines (1,18,39) but not N-alkylformamides (9). A full explanation for this phenomenon is awaited because, clearly, it has profound biological significance.

The propensity for ring opening appears to be general in imidazotetra-zinones. Experimentally determined bond lengths and interatomic angles for a series of active and inactive compounds (27,28) show the planar bicyclic ring to be quite unperturbed by structural modifications at N-3 and C-8. In mitozolomide C-4 is the most electron-deficient site in the ring skeleton and thus vulnerable to nucleophilic attack, and in a series of analogs the 4,5 bond is the longest and (presumably) the weakest.

The half-lives of five examples of imidazotetrazinones in the important pH range of 7–7.5 (straddling physiological pH) are broadly comparable (Table III). If $t_{\frac{1}{2}}$ values are considered a measure of the rate of ring open-ing, no obvious explanation is forthcoming as to why mitozolomide (**I**) and the sulfonamides (**XLI, XLIII,** and **XLIV**) but not the cyano deriva-tive (**LIII**) are antitumor compounds. Possibly, these 8-substituents vary in their abilities to participate in intramolecular H-bonding with the triazene side chain (see structures **LXXII–LXXIV** in Fig. 7) and so mod-ify the chemistry of the ring-opened forms and their reactivity towards nucleophiles. There may be a pharmacokinetic explanation for the inac-

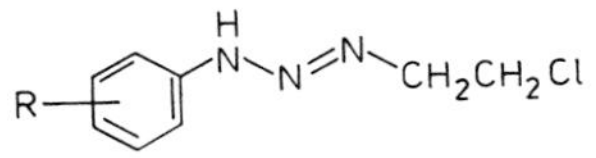

(LXXVI)

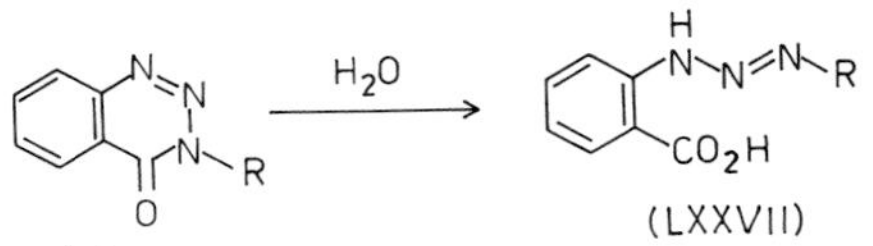

(V)   R = CH$_3$, C$_2$H$_5$, (CH$_2$)$_2$Cl

(LXXVII)

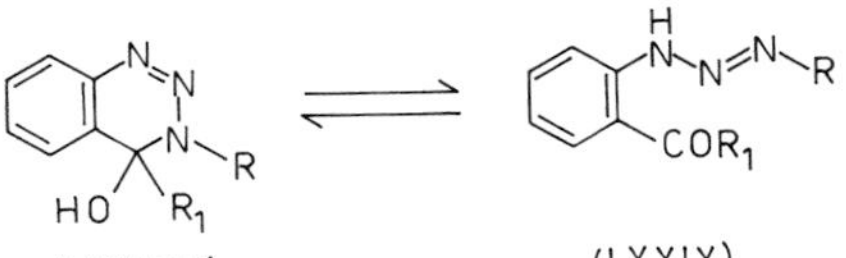

(LXXVIII)   (LXXIX)

R = CH$_3$, C$_2$H$_5$, (CH$_2$)$_2$Cl
R$_1$ = H, C$_6$H$_5$, o-FC$_6$H$_4$

Fig. 8. Ring opening of 3-alkyl-1,2,3-benzotriazines.

tivity of the 8-cyano derivative, although preliminary evidence indicates that this possibility is unlikely.

Alternatively, and most intriguingly, the 8-substituent may have a crucial role in targeting the imidazotetrazinone pro-drug (or its ring-opened active form) to specific nucleotide sequences in nucleic acids: this working hypothesis is presently attracting our attention at Aston.

In concluding this section, mention should be made of other molecules which are potential pro-drug forms of monochloroethyltriazenes (Fig. 8). Lown and Singh showed that 1-aryl-3-(2-chloroethyl)triazenes (**LXXVI**) have antitumor activity (29,30); however, like their imidazo counterparts they are unstable moieties likely to engender insurmountable formulation problems. The 1,2,3-benzotriazinones (**V**) are resistant to hydrolysis, do not ring-open to monoalkyltriazene carboxylic acids (**LXXVII**) under physiological conditions, and have no antitumor activity (41) against the TLX5 lymphoma.

A series of 3,4-dihydro-4-hydroxy-3-substituted-1,2,3-benzotriazines (**LXXVIII**) has been prepared by Vaughan and co-workers (44). These compounds are carbinolamines and exist in equilibrium with acyclic tautomers (**LXXIX**). Although it is possible to tune the equilibrium position to favor the ring-opened triazenes, no biological breakthroughs have rewarded this approach.

VII. CCRG 81045: A Clinical Alternative to DTIC

The recognition that the antitumor imidazotetrazinones are pro-drug forms of monoalkyltriazenes (see Sections V,B and VI) provides a basis for the rational selection of a second-generation clinical candidate— CCRG 81045.

It is generally recognized (24,39) that the antitumor activity of DTIC in rodents is dependent upon metabolic oxidation to the hydroxymethyl metabolite (**LXXX**) which then eliminates formaldehyde to afford the cytotoxic species MTIC (Fig. 9). Rutty *et al.* (34) have proposed that the disappointing clinical activity of DTIC may be explained by its being a poor substrate for oxidative demethylation in humans. Similarly, the metabolic activation of pentamethylmelamine to cytotoxic N-hydroxymethyl metabolites is species dependent (33). CCRG 81045 should be an ideal pro-drug of MTIC activated by a predictable chemical pathway rather than the vagaries of metabolism.

A range of biological and pharmaceutical properties commend CCRG 81045 as an agent worthy of clinical evaluation:

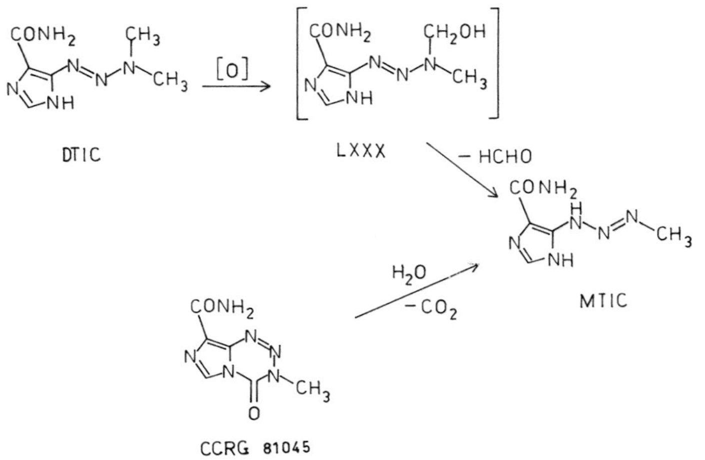

Fig. 9. Metabolic activation of DTIC and chemical activation of CCRG 81045 to MTIC.

1. The antitumor activity of CCRG 81045 is equal or superior to that of DTIC against a range of murine tumor models (25) (Table IV).

2. The compound promotes erythroid differentiation in K562 human erythroleukemia cells (42); this property is not shared by mitozolomide or the 3-ethylimidazotetrazinone (**XVI**). These results suggest that a methylating agent is more effective than a chloroethylating or ethylating agent in altering gene expression, a hypothesis supported by the observation that treatment of cells with CCRG 81045 causes a decrease in the concentration of 5-methylcytosine in the DNA of the treated cells.

3. CCRG 81045 is soluble in a range of pharmaceutically acceptable solvents and, unlike DTIC, is photostable.

4. The half-life of CCRG 81045 in 0.2 M phosphate buffer (pH 7.4) at 37°C is 1.24 hr (15). As expected, the main decomposition product is AIC (**LXXV**) (see Fig. 6).

5. CCRG 81045 has a plasma half-life in mice of 1.13 hr intraperitoneally (i.p.) and 1.29 hr orally (p.o.). These values are very close to the half-life in phosphate buffer at pH 7.4 and indicate that chemical degradation is the sole pathway for removal of intact drug (15).

6. CCRG 81045, like other imidazotetrazinones, is stable in acidic media and should be suitable for oral administration. Its oral bioavailability in mice (AUC p.o./AUC i.p.) is near unity (15).

TABLE IV

Comparison of 8-Carbamoyl-3-methylimidazo[5,1-d]-1,2,3,5-tetrazin-4(3H)-one (XV; CCRG 81045) and DTIC against Murine Tumor Systems

Model	Tumor	Optimal T/C (%) or therapeutic index	
		CCRG 81045	DTIC
Murine ascitic	TLX5 lymphoma[a]	181	180
survival time	L1210 leukemia[a]	200	160
	P388 leukemia[a]	>254	166
	B16 melanoma[a]	181	145[d]
	M5076 reticulum cell sarcoma[a]	200	NT[e]
Murine solid	M5076 reticulum cell sarcoma[b]	6.5	8.1
	ADJ/PC6A plasmacytoma[b]	>8	50
Murine human xenograft	MX-1 mammary[c]	15	37[d]

[a] Increase in survival time.
[b] Therapeutic index, LD_{50}/ID_{50}.
[c] Tumor volume change.
[d] Data from Goldin et al. (16).
[e] NT, not tested.

In 1978, Hansch and his colleagues (17) advised that "unless one had new biochemical or molecular biological information suggesting that a new triazene might be more effective in some specific way, we would not recommend the synthesis and testing of new congeners."

CCRG 81045 is a molecule which might exploit new information now available concerning the clinical (in)activity of DTIC and will test the hypothesis that DTIC could have been a successful drug if only humans had been able to metabolize it effectively.

Acknowledgments

The author thanks all his colleagues at Aston (J. A. Hickman, J. A. Slack, M. J. Tisdale, G. U. Baig, R. Stone, N. W. Gibson, S. P. Langdon, C. Goddard, C. M. T. Horgan, L. Vickers, and D. C. Chubb), at May & Baker Ltd (E. Lunt, C. G. Newton, R. J. A. Walsh, C. Smith, T. J. Warren, G. T. Stevens, and B. L. Pedgrift), and at Rhône-Poulenc Santé (F. Lavelle and C. Fizames) and has drawn freely from their work and ideas in the preparation of this chapter. The work has been partly supported financially by the Cancer Research Campaign and the Science and Engineering Research Council, United Kingdom.

References

1. Audette, R. C. S., Connors, T. A., Mandel, H. G., Merai, K., and Ross, W. C. J. (1973). Studies on the mechanism of action of tumor inhibitory triazenes. *Biochem. Pharmacol.* **22,** 1855–1864.

2. Baig, G. U., and Stevens, M. F. G. (1981). Triazines and related compounds. Part 22. Synthesis and reactions of imidazo[5,1-c][1,2,4]triazines. *J. Chem. Soc., Perkin Trans. 1,* pp. 1424–1432.

3. Baig, G. U., Stevens, M. F. G., Stone, R., and Lunt, E. (1982). Triazines and related compounds. Part 24. Synthesis of pyrazol-4-ylidenehydrazinoimidazoles by hydrazinolysis of imidazo[5,1-c][1,2,4]triazines and 2-arylazoimidazoles by diazonium coupling reactions. *J. Chem. Soc., Perkin Trans. 1,* pp. 1811–1819.

4. Baig, G. U., Stevens, M. F. G., Lunt, E., Newton, C. G., Pedgrift, B. L., Smith, C., Straw, C. G., Walsh, R. J. A., and Warren, P. J. (1984). New tetrazine derivatives. U. K. Patent Appl. 2,125,402A.

5. Baig, G. U., and Stevens, M. F. G. Antitumors imidazotetrazines. Part 12. Reactions of mitozolomide and its 3-alkyl congeners with oxygen, nitrogen, halogen and carbon nucleophiles. *J. Chem. Soc., Perkin Trans. 1,* (in press).

6. Ege, G., and Gilbert, K. (1979). [7+2]-and [11+2]-cycloaddition reactions of diazoazoles with isocyanates to azolo[5,1-d][1,2,3,5]tetrazine-4-ones. *Tetrahedron Lett.,* pp. 4253–4256.

7. Finger, H. (1888). Beiträge zur Kenntniss des o-Amidobenzamids. *J. Prakt. Chem.* **37,** 431.

8. Fodstad, Ø., Aamdal, S., Pihl, A., and Boyd, M. R. (1985). Activity of mitozolomide (NSC 353451), a new imidazotetrazine, against xenografts from human melanomas, sarcomas and lung and colon carcinomas. *Cancer Res.* **45,** 1778–1786.

9. Gate, E. N., Threadgill, M. D., Stevens, M. F. G., Chubb, D., Vickers, L. M., Langdon, S. P., Hickman, J. A., and Gescher, A. (1986). Structural studies on bioactive compounds. 4. A structure-antitumor activity study on analogs of N-methylformamide. *J. Med. Chem.* **29,** 1046–1052.

10. Geran, R. I., Greenberg, N. H., MacDonald, M. M., Schumacher, A. M., and Abbot, B. J. (1972). Protocols for screening chemical agents and natural products against animal tumors and other biological systems. *Cancer Chemother. Rep.* **3,** 1–104.

11. Gescher, A., Gibson, N. W., Hickman, J. A., Langdon, S. P., Ross, D., and Atassi, G. (1982). N-Methylformamide: Antitumor activity and metabolism in mice. *Br. J. Cancer* **45,** 843–850.

12. Gibson, N. W., and Hickman, J. A. (1982). The role of isocyanates in the toxicity of antitumour haloalkylnitrosoureas. *Biochem. Pharmacol.* **31,** 2795–2800.

13. Gibson, N. W., Erickson, L. C., and Hickman, J. A. (1984). Effects of the antitumor agent 8-carbamoyl-3-(2-chloroethyl)imidazo[5,1-d]-1,2,3,5-tetrazin-4(3H)-one on the DNA of mouse L1210 cells. *Cancer Res.* **44,** 1767–1771.

14. Gibson, N. W., Hickman, J. A., and Erickson, L. C. (1984). DNA cross-linking and cytotoxicity in normal and transformed human cells treated *in vitro* with 8-carbamoyl-3-(2-chloroethyl)imidazo[5,1-d]-1,2,3,5-tetrazin-4(3H)-one. *Cancer Res.* **44,** 1772–1775.

15. Goddard, C., Slack, J. A., Griffin, M. J., Baig, G. U., and Stevens, M. F. G. (1985). Preclinical studies on CCRG 81045. *Proc. Am. Assoc. Cancer Res.* **26,** 1396.

16. Goldin, A., Vendetti, J. M., MacDonald, J. S., Muggia, F. M., Henney, J. E., and DeVita, V. T. (1981). Current results of the screening program at the Division of Cancer Treatment, National Cancer Institute. *Eur. J. Cancer* **17,** 129–142.

17. Hansch, C., Hatheway, C. J., Quinn, F. R., and Greenberg, N. (1978). Antitumor 1-(X-

aryl)-3,3-dimethyltriazenes. 2. On the role of correlation analysis in decision making in drug modification. Toxicity quantitative structure-activity relationships of 1-(X-phenyl)-3,3-dialkyltriazenes in mice. *J. Med. Chem.* **21,** 574–577.

18. Hickman, J. A. (1978). Investigation of the mechanism of action of antitumor dimethy-ltriazenes. *Biochimie* **60,** 997–1002.

19. Hickman, J. A., Stevens, M. F. G., Gibson, N. W., Langdon, S. P., Fizames, C., Lavelle, F., Atassi, G., Lund, E., and Tilson, R. M. (1985). Experimental antitumor activity against murine tumor model systems of 8-carbamoyl-3-(2-chloroethyl)imi-dazo[5,1-d]-1,2,3,5-tetrazin-4(3H)-one (mitozolomide), a novel broad-spectrum agent. *Cancer Res.* **45,** 3008–3013.

20. Horgan, C. M. T., and Tisdale, M. J. (1984). Antitumor imidazotetrazines. IV. An investigation into the mechanism of antitumour activity of a novel and potent antitu-mour agent, mitozolomide (CCRG 81010; M&B 39565; NSC 353451). *Biochem. Phar-macol.* **33,** 2185–2192.

21. Horgan, C. M. T. (1985). Studies on mitozolomide (CCRG 81010), a new antineoplastic agent. Ph. D. Thesis, Aston University.

22. Horton, J. K., and Stevens, M. F. G. (1981). A new light on the photo-decomposition of the antitumour drug DTIC. *J. Pharm. Pharmacol.* **33,** 808–811.

23. Horton, J. K., and Stevens, M. F. G. (1981). Triazines and related compounds. Part 23. New photo-products from 5-diazoimidazole-4-carboxamide (Diazo-IC). *J. Chem. Soc., Perkin Trans. 1,* pp. 1433–1436.

24. Kolar, G. F., Maurer, M., and Wildschutte, M. (1980). 5-(3-Hydroxymethyl-3-methyl-1-triazeno)imidazole-4-carboxamide is a metabolite of 5-(3,3-dimethyl-1-triazeno)imida-zole-4-carboxamide (DIC, DTIC, NSC 45388). *Cancer Lett.* **10,** 235–241.

25. Langdon, S. P., Stone, R., Stevens, M. F. G., Gibson, N. W., Chubb, D., Hickman, J. A., Lavelle, F., and Fizames, C. (1985). CCRG 81045 - A novel imidazotetrazinone with broad-spectrum activity against murine tumors. *Proc. Am. Assoc. Cancer Res.* **26,** 1006.

26. Lowe, P. R., Schwalbe, C. H., and Stevens, M. F. G. (1985). Antitumour imidazotetra-zines. Part 5. Crystal and molecular structure of 8-carbamoyl-3-(2-chloroethyl)imi-dazo[5,1-d]-1,2,3,5-tetrazin-4-(3H)-one (Mitozolomide). *J. Chem. Soc., Perkin Trans. 2,* pp. 357–361.

27. Lowe, P. R., Schwalbe, C. H., Whiston, C. D., and Stevens, M. F. G. (1985). Antitu-mour imidazotetrazinones. The crystal and molecular structure of mitozolomide and five of its analogs. *J. Pharm. Pharmacol.* **37,** 1136P.

28. Lowe, P. R. (1985). A crystallographic study on some biologically important molecules. Ph.D. Thesis, Aston University.

29. Lown, J. W., and Singh, R. (1981). Synthesis of 3-(2-haloethyl)aryltriazenes and study of their reactions in aqueous solution. *Can. J. Chem.* **59,** 1347–1356.

30. Lown, J. W., and Singh, R. (1982). Mechanism of action of antitumour 3-(2-haloethy-l)aryltriazenes on deoxyribonucleic acid. *Biochem. Pharmacol.* **31,** 1257–1266.

31. Lunt, E., Stevens, M. F. G., Stone, R., and Wooldridge, K. R. H. (1983). Tetrazine derivatives. U. K. Patent Appl. 2,104,522B.

32. Newlands, E. S., Blackledge, G., Slack, J. A., Goddard, C., Brindley, C. J., Holden, L., and Stevens, M. F. G. (1985). Phase I clinical trial of mitozolomide (CCRG 81010; M&B 39565; NSC 353451). *Cancer Treat. Rep.* **69,** 801–805.

33. Rutty, C. J., Newell, D. R., Muindi, J. R. F., and Harrap, K. R. (1982). Comparative pharmacokinetics of pentamethylmelamine in man and mouse. *Cancer Chemother. Pharmacol.* **8,** 105–113.

34. Rutty, C. J., Newell, D. R., Vincent, R. B., Abel, G., Goddard, P. M., Harland, S. J., and Calvert, A. H. (1983). The species dependent pharmacokinetics of DTIC. *Br. J. Cancer* **48,** 140.

35. Shealy, Y. F., O'Dell, C. A., and Krauth, C. A. (1975). 5-[3-(2-Chloroethyl)-1-triazenyl]imidazole-4-carboxamide and a possible mechanism of action of 5-[3,3-bis(2-chloroethyl)-1-triazenyl]imidazole-4-carboxamide. *J. Pharm. Sci.* **64,** 177–180.
36. Slack, J. A., and Goddard, C. (1985). Antitumour imidazotetrazines. VII. Quantitative analysis of mitozolomide by high-performance liquid chromatography. *J. Chromatogr.* **337,** 178–181.
37. Stevens, M. F. G. (1976). The medicinal chemistry of 1,2,3-triazines. *Prog. Med. Chem.* **13,** 205–269.
38. Stevens, M. F. G., and Peatey, L. (1978). Photodegradation of solutions of the antitumour drug DTIC. *J. Pharm. Pharmacol.* **30S,** 47P.
39. Stevens, M. F. G. (1983). DTIC: A springboard to new antitumour agents. *In* "Structure-Activity Relationships of Anti-Tumour Agents" (D. N. Reinhoudt, T. A. Connors, H. M. Pinedo, and K. W. van de Poll, eds.), pp. 183–218. Martinus Nijhoff Publishers, The Hague.
40. Stevens, M. F. G., Hickman, J. A., Stone, R., Gibson, N. W., Baig, G. U., Lunt, E., and Newton, C. G. (1984). Antitumor imidazotetrazines. I. Synthesis and chemistry of 8-carbamoyl-3-(2-chloroethyl)imidazo[5,1-d]-1,2,3,5-tetrazin-4(3H)-one, a novel broad-spectrum antitumor agent. *J. Med. Chem.* **27,** 196–201.
41. Stevens, M. F. G. Unpublished results.
42. Tisdale, M. J. (1986). Antitumour imidazotetrazines. X. Effect of 8-carbamoyl-3-methylimidazo[5,1-d]-1,2,3,5-tetrazin-4(3H)-one (CCRG 81045; M&B 39831; NSC 362856) on DNA methylation during induction of haemoglobin synthesis in human leukaemic cell line K562. *Biochem. Pharmacol.* **35,** 311–316.
43. Vaughan, K., and Stevens, M. F. G. (1978). Monoalkyltriazenes. *Chem. Soc. Rev.* **7,** 377–397.
44. Vaughan, K., Lafrance, K. V., Tang, Y., and Hooper, D. L. Open-chain nitrogen compounds. Part VIII. 1-(2'-Acetylphenyl)-3-alkyltriazenes with reactive substituents in the alkyl group: Synthons for five- and six-membered nitrogen heterocycles. *Can. J. Chem.* **63,** 2455–2451.

17

5-Aminoanthrapyrazoles (CI-937, CI-941, CI-942): A Novel Class of DNA Binders with Broad-Spectrum Anticancer Activity

LESLIE M. WERBEL, EDWARD F. ELSLAGER, DAVID W. FRY,
ROBERT C. JACKSON, WILBUR R. LEOPOLD, AND
H. D. HOLLIS SHOWALTER

Departments of Chemistry and Chemotherapy
Warner-Lambert/Parke-Davis Pharmaceutical Research
Ann Arbor, Michigan

I. Introduction

Anticancer agents which exert their action primarily through binding to DNA are perhaps the most broadly active, available clinical agents for these diseases. Although the anthracyclines, particularly doxorubicin, are used widely to treat a variety of human neoplasms, their use is restricted by dose-limiting cumulative cardiotoxicity. Attempts to develop novel anthracyclines have been limited either by similar cardiotoxic liabilities or by more limited spectra of clinical efficacy (19).

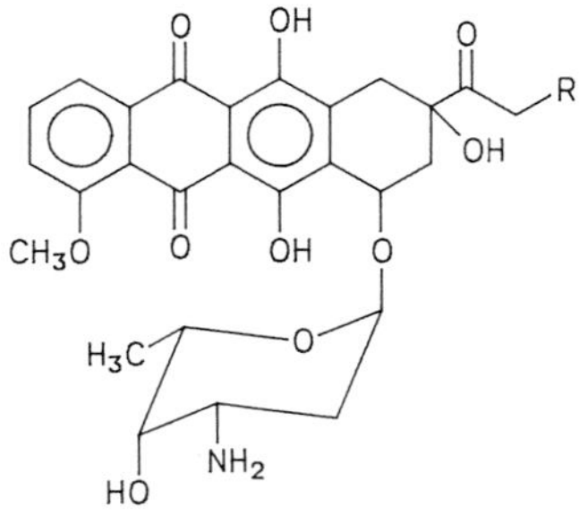

(I)

R = H; Daunorubicin
R = OH; Doxorubicin (Adriamycin)

Amsacrine **(II)** and mitoxantrone **(III)** are synthetic DNA binders developed in an effort to overcome the shortcomings of the anthracyclines. Both appear to be less cardiotoxic than doxorubicin; however, preliminary results suggest that neither agent retains the broad spectrum of activity of doxorubicin (8,17,20).

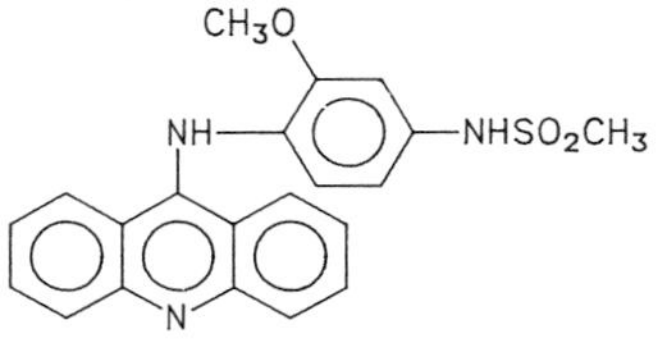

Amsacrine
(II)

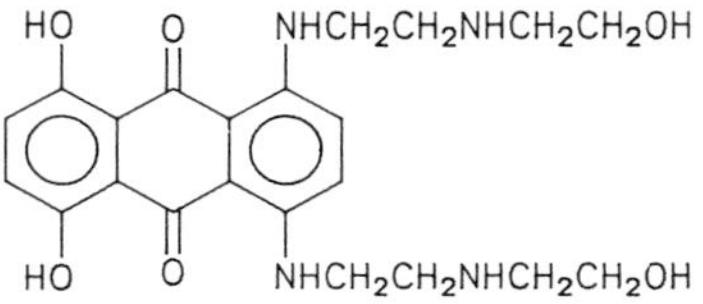

Mitoxantrone
(III)

II. Synthesis of Anthrapyrazoles

Our efforts to design a DNA binder structure which would retain high levels of broad-spectrum anticancer activity without the potential for cardiotoxicity by virtue of a reduced tendency to form semiquinone free radicals led to the anthrapyrazole system **(IV)** (15).

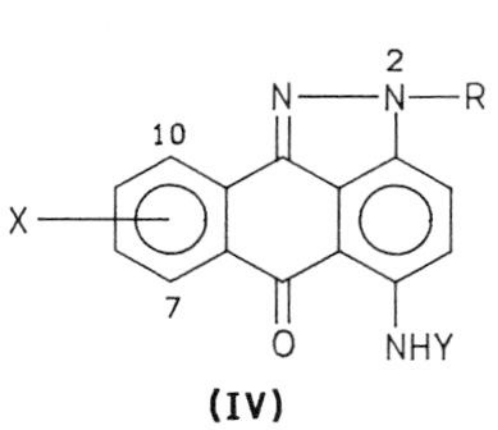

(IV)

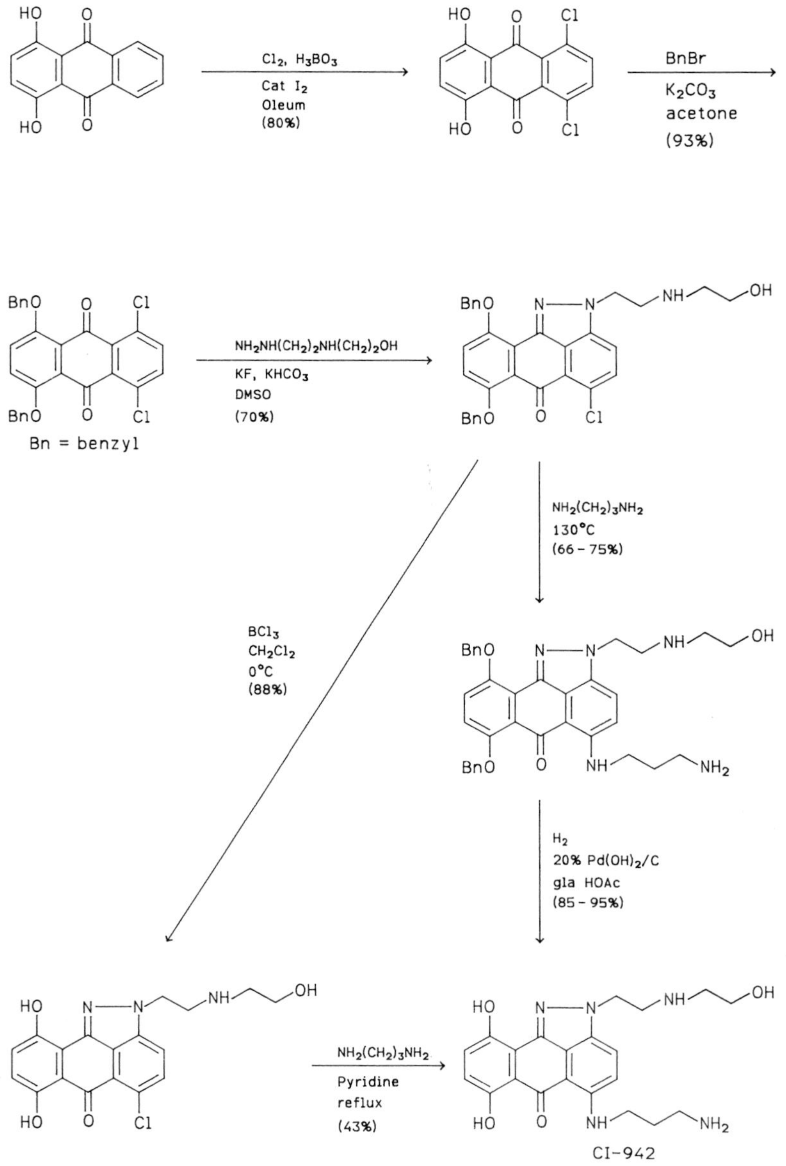

Fig. 1. Synthesis of CI-942.

Also inherent in the development rationale for this series were the possibilities of achieving a more favorable binding orientation to macromolecules, greater synthetic flexibility for the introduction of R and Y, reduced color liability, and ease of formulation.

A general synthetic sequence for the preparation of these compounds is shown in Fig. 1, which illustrates the preparation of CI-942.

III. Structure–Activity Relationships

Potent *in vitro* cytotoxicity (10^{-7} to 10^{-9} M) against the L1210 leukemia and a human colon adenocarcinoma line, as well as activity against the P388 leukemia in mice was demonstrated early on and led to a thorough exploration of structural variations within the series.

Among more than 100 analogs prepared and administered intraperitoneally (IP/IP) on days 1 and 5, at least 30 compounds exhibited lifespan increases in excess of 100%, with one or more cures at doses from 6.25–200 mg/kg against the murine P388. Structure–activity relationships derived from these data suggest that antitumor activity is maximized by the presence of basic side chains at both N-2 and C-5, by two to three carbon spacers between proximal and distal side-chain nitrogens, and by ring hydroxylation at positions 7, 8, and 10.

A variety of analogs were evaluated against the other tumors of the National Cancer Institute (NCI) panel, and high activity was not infrequently found against all of them, i.e., intraperitoneally implanted L1210 leukemia when administered intraperitoneally on days 1–9; B-16 melanoma, the M5076 sarcoma, and the MX-1 human mammary xenograft grown as a subrenal capsule implant in nude mice. To allow differentiation among these highly active compounds an expanded tumor panel was utilized that included mammary adenocarcinoma 16c, colon adenocarcinoma 11a, mammary adenocarcinoma 13c, and the Ridgway osteogenic sarcoma. All testing utilized intravenous treatment of subcutaneous tumor masses. These tumor models differ widely with respect to histology, growth rate, invasiveness, metastatic potential, and sensitivities to various classes of anticancer agents. Each has, however, been reported to be somewhat responsive to one or more of the clinically active intercalating drugs such as doxorubicin and mitoxantrone (2,3,10,14,18). Moreover, neither doxorubicin nor mitoxantrone were reported to be curative for either mammary 16c or colon 11a; hence superiority could theoretically be demonstrated. On the basis of these studies and others reported in a later section, three compounds (CI-937, CI-941, and CI-942) have been selected for development for clinical trial.

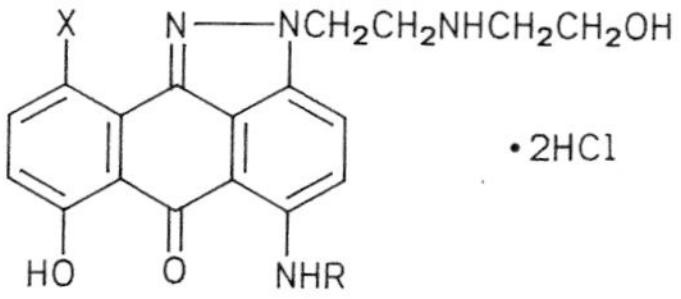

X N——NCH$_2$CH$_2$NHCH$_2$CH$_2$OH

• 2HCl

HO O NHR

CI	X	R
937	OH	CH$_2$CH$_2$NHCH$_3$
941	H	CH$_2$CH$_2$NHCH$_2$CH$_2$OH
942	OH	CH$_2$CH$_2$CH$_2$NH$_2$

A comparison of the three anthrapyrazole clinical candidates with doxorubicin and mitoxantrone in the tumors of the NCI panel is shown in Table I. A similar comparison in our expanded panel is shown in Table II.

Against mammary adenocarcinoma 16c relatively few compounds caused an actual net reduction in tumor burden at the end of the treatment regimen. CI-941 and CI-942 were among them, while treatment with CI-937 resulted in tumor stasis. Doxorubicin also produced a net reduction in tumor burden, while mitoxantrone produced only a slight inhibition of tumor growth relative to the controls but no net reduction in tumor burden.

Mammary adenocarcinoma 13c exhibits generally lower sensitivity to DNA binders. Neither doxorubicin nor mitoxantrone produced a net reduction in tumor burden, and only CI-942 had significant activity, producing tumor stasis when treated with the maximum tolerated dose of drug.

Colon adenocarcinoma 11a was considerably less sensitive to the anthrapyrazoles than was mammary 16c. For colon adenocarcinoma, only CI-937 produced as large a net reduction in tumor burden over the course of therapy as did doxorubicin. Mitoxantrone did not produce significant

TABLE I

Activity of Anthrapyrazoles in NCI Tumor Panel

	Increase in lifespan (%)				Tumor growth (%), MX-1 carcinoma
Compound	P388 Leukemia	L1210 Leukemia	B16 Melanoma	M5076 Sarcoma	
Doxorubicin	111 (0)[a]	47 (0)	138 (6/8)	76 (0)	−10 (0)
Mitoxantrone	191 (4/6)	95 (0)	226 (4/6)	160 (0)	+6 (1/6)
CI-937	176 (11/12)	200 (5/12)	163 (9/20)	124 (10/20)	−28 (3/12)
CI-941	254 (10/20)	261 (4/6)	178 (9/20)	153 (8/20)	Not tested
CI-942	163 (7/10)	235 (7/10)	177 (11/20)	86 (2/20)	−90 (12/18)

[a] Numbers in parentheses are proportions of cures.

TABLE II

Evaluation of Anthrapyrazoles in Expanded Tumor Panel

Compound	M16c[a]			C11a[a]			M13c[b]			ROS[b]	
	Dose	T-C (days)	Net change in tumor burden (logs)	Dose	T-C (days)	Net change in tumor burden (logs)	Dose	T-C (days)	Net change in tumor burden (logs)	Dose	T/C (day 35)
Doxorubicin	5	19	-2.5	5	19.8	-0.8	1.9	3.0	0.6	5	0
Mitoxantrone	2.5	4.4	1.2	1.25	4.1	0.4	1.2	1.0	0.8	1.2	50
CI-937	3	12	0.3	4.3	16.9	-0.9	1.5	3.5	0.5	4.0	0
CI-941	12.5	11.4	-0.9	6.25	9.2	-0.1	6.0	2.5	0.6	12.5	0
CI-942	15	12.3	-0.9	10	8.9	0	7.3	7.5	0.1	10.0	7
Controls		2.7			8.9	0.7			0.9		100

[a] Administered intravenously on days 1, 5, 9 (CI-937 d 1, 5, 9, 13).
[b] Administered intravenously on days 3, 7, 11. ROS, Ridgway osteogenic sarcoma.

tumor cell kill in this system, nor were any of the tested compounds curative against this tumor.

The Ridgway osteogenic sarcoma is sensitive to a wide variety of anti-cancer agents. All three clinical candidate anthrapyrazoles exhibited good activity in this system, as did doxorubicin. Mitoxantrone was active but not curative against the Ridgway tumor.

An early study of the cross-resistance of the anthrapyrazoles and dox-orubicin (ADR) indicated that a doxorubicin-resistant line of P388 leuke-mia (P388/ADR) which is pleiotropically cross-resistant to a number of structurally diverse anticancer agents was substantially cross-resistant to CI-942, producing net tumor cell kill at least four logs lower than that obtained against the parent P388 line. Tested intravenously on days 1, 5, and 9 against subcutaneous implants of mammary adenocarcinoma 16c or a doxorubicin-resistant line of mammary 16c (M16c/ADR), CI-937, CI-941, and CI-942 administered at 3.5, 9, and 12 mg/kg, respectively (the maximum tolerated doses of these drugs at this regimen), produced net change in tumor burden (logs) of -0.5, $+0.2$, and -0.5 against the sensi-tive line, and $+1.5$, $+1.6$, and $+0.8$ against the resistant line. The control tumors grew 2.4 logs under these conditions. Thus, although the anthra-pyrazoles exhibit partial cross-resistance to doxorubicin they clearly ex-hibit an effect against the cross-resistant tumor.

IV. Biochemical Properties

The biochemical effects of these compounds were studied in L1210 leukemia in relation to other clinically used DNA binders. Based on an ethidium displacement assay, CI-937, CI-941, and CI-942 bound strongly to DNA, reducing the fluorescence of an ethidium–DNA complex by 50% at concentrations of 23, 64, and 33 nM, respectively. This was comparable to mitoxantrone at 15 nM but much more potent than amsacrine, which required over 1.3 μM.

A common phenomenon in cells treated with intercalators is the ap-pearance of protein-linked single- and double-strand DNA breaks (13,21,22). This is quite likely related to the manner in which their antitu-mor effect is achieved. The anthrapyrazoles caused single- and, to a lesser extent, double-stranded DNA breaks in a concentration-dependent man-ner which appeared to be tightly associated with protein. Differences are observed, however, in the rate of formation of these breaks. For example, at a concentration of 1 μM, maximum DNA breakage was attained within 30 min with CI-937, while at least 3 hr were required in the presence of CI-942. Such differences in the rates of DNA strand scission could account for differences in cytotoxic potency *in vitro* and may reflect different transport rates into the intracellular compartment.

The cytotoxicity of a drug may also be related to the inability of a cell to recover from, or repair, the DNA breaks induced by intercalators, rather than the quantity of these lesions. If L1210 cells were treated with the anthrapyrazoles such that substantial strand breaks occurred and if the drug were removed, the breaks were repaired very slowly over the first 30 min, but then additional lesions occurred thereafter for at least 2 hr. Additional DNA damage after drug removal was also observed with doxorubicin and mitoxantrone.

Unlike other DNA binders such as doxorubicin and mitoxantrone which inhibit DNA and RNA synthesis equally at similar concentrations, the anthrapyrazoles exhibit a much more potent inhibitory effect on whole-cell DNA synthesis. Thus, after L1210 cells were exposed to drug for 2 hr, the drug concentration needed to inhibit DNA synthesis by 50% was 0.33, 0.30, and 0.59 μM for CI-937, CI-941, and CI-942, respectively, whereas 2.0, 4.5, and 11.3 μM were required to inhibit RNA synthesis to the same extent. Inhibition of these processes was not due to substrate depletion, since intracellular ribonucleoside and deoxyribonucleoside triphosphates either remained constant or were elevated after a 2-hr exposure to 1 or 10 μM of the drug. A similar discriminatory effect was observed on DNA and RNA polymerase in permeabilized cells and appeared to result entirely from the interaction with the DNA template, since this effect could be reversed by addition of exogenous primer DNA. Since little difference in the ability to displace ethidium from DNA existed between mitoxantrone and the anthrapyrazoles the discriminative effects of these classes of drugs on DNA and RNA synthesis are most likely to derive from properties distinct from differences in binding affinity.

The biochemical basis for the cardiotoxic liability observed with certain anthracyclines is still not completely understood. However, recent evidence has implicated the production of reactive oxygen species, including superoxide radical, hydroxyl radical, hydrogen peroxide, and lipid peroxides as a contributing factor (5). The capacity for many quinone anticancer agents to be reduced to semiquinone free radicals by intracellular reductive enzymes has been supported by electron spin resonance studies (9,11). Reports showing superoxide dismutase–sensitive oxygen consumption in the presence of liver microsomal or heart sarcosomal preparations (1,4) and the production of lipid peroxidation products (7,12) suggest that semiquinone free radicals are capable of donating electrons to molecular oxygen, thus forming superoxide radical, or to unsaturated lipids, thus producing lipid peroxides. The anthrapyrazoles induced five- to tenfold less superoxide dismutase–sensitive oxygen consumption than doxorubicin in the rat liver microsomal system, a property which may be indicative of a lower cardiotoxic potential. Recent studies of Fagan *et al.* (6), in which several anthrapyrazoles were compared to doxorubicin for toxicity to cultured fetal mouse hearts, also suggest that CI-937 and CI-942 have less cardiotoxic potential than doxorubicin.

Recent electrochemical studies by Lown *et al.* (16) on the anthrapyrazoles have confirmed that these compounds are very difficult to reduce. CI-941, for example, showed a reduction potential of -1.040 V, compared with -0.625 V for daunorubicin. CI-941 is also considerably more difficult to reduce than 5-iminodaunorubicin (-0.675 V) and mitoxantrone (-0.775 V). The reduction process, as observed by polarography, appears to involve two two-electron steps, the first of which may result from initial reduction at the quinone carbonyl and the imino nitrogen of the central ring, and the second may reflect subsequent reduction of the pyrazole ring.

V. Toxicology

The dose-limiting toxicity of the anthrapyrazoles appeared to be myelosuppressive in preliminary studies. Mice treated with lethal ($\geq LD_{10}$) levels died between 5 and 12 days after the last injection of an intermittent (every 4 days) treatment schedule. Intravenous administration produced little or no tail vein necrosis, no obvious sign of gastrointestinal toxicity such as diarrhea, and no sign of central nervous system toxicity. At dosage levels more than twice the LD_{10}, none of the anthrapyrazoles tested produced immediate lethality upon intravenous injection, and none caused delayed lethality (deaths occurring more than 20 days after the last treatment) in our studies. In other preliminary studies, the toxicity of selected anthrapyrazoles was not schedule dependent. Total maximum tolerated dosages were independent of the treatment schedule.

VI. Summary

Three members of this unique chemical class CI-937, CI-941, and CI-942 have thus been selected for toxicological evaluation and possible development for clinical trials. These agents exhibit exceptional *in vivo* anticancer activity, possible limited cross-resistance with the anthracyclines, and possible limited potential for cardiotoxicity in preclinical models. Their properties and performance in a wide variety of preclinical models confer exciting potential for these agents as useful clinical anticancer agents.

References

1. Bachur, N. R., Gordon, S. L., and Gee, M. V. (1977). Anthracycline antibiotic augmentation of microsomal electron transport and free radical formation. *Mol. Pharmacol.* **13,** 901–910.
2. Corbett, T. H., Griswold, D. P., Jr., and Roberts, B. J. (1978). Biology and therapeutic response of a mouse mammary adenocarcinoma (16/c) and its potential as a model for surgical adjuvant chemotherapy. *Cancer Treat. Rep.* **62,** 1471–1487.
3. Corbett, T. H., Roberts, B. J., Trader, M. W., Laster, W. R., Jr., Griswold, D. P., Jr., and Schabel, F. M., Jr. (1982). Response of transplantable tumors of mice to anthracenedione derivatives alone and in combination with clinically useful agents. *Cancer Treat. Rep.* **66,** 1187–1200.
4. Doroshow, J. H. (1983). Effect of anthracycline antibiotics on oxygen radical formation in rat heart. *Cancer Res.* **43,** 460–472.
5. Doroshow, J. H., and Hochstein, P. (1982). *In* Redox cycling and the mechanism of action of antibiotics in neoplastic diseases. "Pathology of Oxygen" (A. Autor, ed.), p. 245. Academic Press, New York.
6. Fagan, M. A., Hacker, M. P., and Newman, R. A. (1984). Cardiotoxic potential of substituted anthra (1,9-cd)pyrazole-6-(2H)ones (anthrapyrazoles) as assessed by the fetal mouse heart organ culture. *Proc. Am. Assoc. Cancer Res.* **25,** 302.
7. Goodman, J., and Hochstein, P. (1977). Generation of free radicals and lipid peroxidation by redox cycling of adriamycin and daunomycin. *Biochem. Biophys. Res. Commun.* **77,** 797–803.
8. Grove, W. R., Fortner, C. L., and Wiernik, P. H. (1982). Review of amsacrine, an investigational antineoplastic agent. *Clin. Pharmacol.* **1,** 320–326.
9. Kalyanaramon, B., Perez-Reyes, E., and Mason, R. P. (1980). Spin-trapping and direct electron spin resonance investigation of the redox metabolism of quinone anticancer drugs. *Biochim. Biophys. Acta* **630,** 119–130.
10. Laster, W. R., Jr. (1975). Ridgway osteogenic sarcoma—a promising laboratory model for special therapeutic trials against an advanced-stage drug-sensitive animal tumor system. *Cancer Chemother. Rep.* **5,** 151–168.
11. Lown, J. F., and Chen, H.-H. (1981). Electron paramagnetic characterization and conformation of daunorubicin semiquinone intermediate implicated in anthracycline metabolism, cardiotoxicity, and anticancer action. *Can. J. Chem.* **59,** 3212–3217.
12. Mimnaugh, E. G., Trush, M. A., Ginsburg, E., and Gram, T. E. (1982). Differential effects of anthracycline drugs on rat heart and liver microsomal reduced nicotinamide adenine dinucleotide phosphate-dependent lipid peroxidation. *Cancer Res.* **42,** 3574–3582.
13. Ross, W. E., Glaubiger, D. L., and Kohn, K. W. (1978). Protein-associated DNA breaks in cells with adriamycin or ellipticine. *Biochim. Biophys. Acta* **519,** 23–30.
14. Schabel, F. M., Jr., Corbett, T. H., Griswold, D. P., Jr., Laster, W. R., Jr., and Trader, M. W. (1983). Therapeutic activity of mitoxantrone and ametantrone against murine tumors. *Cancer Treat. Rev.* **10,** Suppl. B, 13–21.
15. Showalter, H. D. H., Johnson, J. L., Werbel, L. M., Leopold, W. R., Jackson, R. C., and Elslager, E. F. (1984). 5-[(Aminoalkyl)amino]-substituted anthra[1,9-*cd*]pyrazol-6(2*H*)ones as novel anticancer agents. Synthesis and biological evaluation. *J. Med. Chem.* **27,** 253–255.
16. Showalter, H. D. H., Fry, D. W., Leopold, W. R., Lown, J. W., Plambeck, J. A., and Reszka, K. (1986). Design, biochemical pharmacology, electrochemistry, and tumor biology of antitumor anthrapyrazoles. *Anticancer Drug Des.* **1,** 73–85.

17. Smith, I. E. (1983). Mitoxantrone (novantrone). A review of experimental and early clinical studies. *Cancer Treat. Rev.* **10,** 103–115.
18. Wallace, R. E., Murdock, K. C., Angier, R. B., and Durr, F. E. (1979). Activity of a novel anthracenedione, 1,4-dihydroxy-5,8-bis((2-[(2-hydroxyethyl)amino]ethyl]amino))-9,10-anthracenedione dihydrochloride, against experimental tumors in mice. *Cancer Res.* **39,** 1570–1574.
19. Young, R. C., Ozols, R. F., and Meyers, C. E. (1981). The anthracycline antineoplastic drugs. *N. Engl. J. Med.* **305,** 139–153.
20. Zee-Cheng, R. K. Y., and Cheng, C. C. (1983). Anthraquinone anticancer agents. *Drugs* **8,** 229–249.
21. Zwelling, L. A., Michaels, S., Erickson, L. C., Ungerleider, R. S., Nichols, M., and Kohn, K. W. (1981). Protein-associated deoxyribonucleic acid strand breaks in L1210 cells treated with the deoxyribonucleic acid intercalating agents 4'-(9-acridinyl-amino-)methan sulfon-*m*-anisidide and adriamycin. *Biochemistry* **20,** 6553–6563.
22. Zwelling, L. A., Michaels, S., Kerrigan, D., Pommier, Y., and Kohn, K. W. (1982). Protein-associated deoxyribonucleic acid strand breaks produced in mouse leukemia L1210 cells by ellipticine and 2-methyl-9-hydroxy ellipticinium. *Biochem. Pharmacol.* **31,** 3261–3281.

18

New Carbon–Carbon Linked Nucleosides with Potent Antitumor Activity

THOMAS L. AVERY

> St. Jude Children's Research Hospital
> Memphis, Tennessee

WILLIAM J. HENNEN

> Department of Chemistry
> Brigham Young University
> Provo, Utah

GANAPATHI R. REVANKAR AND ROLAND K. ROBINS

> Nucleic Acid Research Institute
> Costa Mesa, California

NEW AVENUES IN DEVELOPMENTAL
CANCER CHEMOTHERAPY

I. Introduction

Ribavirin (18,42,44) was first synthesized in our laboratory (53) as an analog of AICR (aminoimidazole carboxamide riboside). A broad-spectrum antiviral agent, ribavirin (**I**) inhibits the transformation of normal rat kidney cells by Rous sarcoma virus and more recently has been shown to inhibit T-lymphotropic virus type III, the human retrovirus responsible for acquired immunodeficiency syndrome (AIDS). As an anticancer agent ribavirin was slightly active against leukemia L1210 and adenocarcinoma 755 growing in mice (25) but was substantially more effective against leukemia-related splenomegaly (43) induced in mice by the Friend and Rauscher murine leukemia viruses. In 1977 we reported the chemical synthesis of 2-β-D-ribofuranosylthiazole-4-carboxamide (46) (**II**, tiazofurin), which is structurally similar to ribavirin (Fig. 1).

II. Animal Tumor Studies with Tiazofurin

For the treatment of intravenously inoculated Lewis lung carcinoma, tiazofurin was highly active over a broad range of dosages. Recent data (Table I) show as many as 10/10 mice cured by as little as 25 mg/kg/day when the drug was given for 9 consecutive days. On the same schedule of delivery, larger dosages (330, 500, and 750 mg/kg) produced a uniform T/C (treated/control) of 452, with 10/10 survivors at each dose level after 101 days. In similar experiments, another laboratory (Table II) obtained an increase in life-span (ILS) of 184%, with 12.5 mg/kg/day and 7/10 mice cured.

Recent testing of tiazofurin by the National Cancer Institute against L1210 leukemia in mice showed a T/C of 184 at 512 mg/kg/day for 9 days (Table III) and an ILS of 184%. Although L1210 responses to tiazofurin

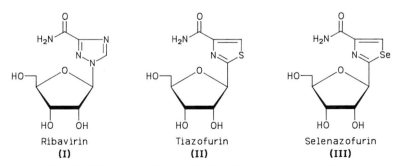

Fig. 1. Structures of ribavirin, tiazofurin, and selenazofurin.

TABLE I

Antitumor Activity of Tiazofurin against Lewis Lung Carcinoma in Mice[a]

Tox. surv.	Dos./inj.	BWD[b]	Median survival (days)	T/C	Cures
10/10	400.00	−0.7	60.0	326	10
10/10	200.0	−0.4	60.0	326	10
10/10	100.00	0.2	60.0	326	09
10/10	50.00	0.5	60.0	326	09
10/10	25.00	−0.1	60.0	326	10
40/40	Control		18.4		
10/10	400.00	−0.7	60.0	355	06
10/10	200.00	−0.5	60.0	355	06
10/10	100.00	−0.3	60.0	355	06
10/10	50.00	0.0	60.0	355	08
08/08	25.00	−0.1	60.0	355	05
40/40	Control		16.9		
10/10	750.00	−1.2	101.0	452	10
10/10	500.00	−1.4	101.0	452	10
10/10	330.00	−0.9	101.0	452	10
10/10	Control		22.3		

[a] Treatment schedule was every day for 9 days.
[b] Body weight difference.

TABLE II

Antitumor Activity of Tiazofurin for Lewis Lung Carcinoma in Mice

Dose[a] (mg/kg)	Median survival time/days	ILS (%)	60-Day survivors or cures
800.0	60/17	252	7/10
400.0	60/17	252	8/10
200.0	60/17	252	9/10
100.0	60/17	252	9/10
25.0	60/17	252	9/10
12.5	34/17	100	4/10
25.0	60/21	184	9/10
12.5	60/21	184	7/10
200	60/18.5	224	9/10
100	60/18.5	224	10/10
50	60/19.5	224	10/10
25	60/18.5	224	9/10

[a] Drug administered intraperitoneally, starting 24 hr post–tumor cell implantation. Dosage schedule was daily for 9 days.

TABLE III

Antitumor Activity of Tiazofurin against Leukemia L1210 and P388

Test system	Treatment schedule	Tox. surv.	Dos./inj. (mg/kg)	BWD	Cures	Days survival evaluation	T/C
L1210 leukemia	Every day for 9 days	10/10	512.00	−3.0	01	23.3	284
		10/10	256.00	−2.4	00	20.2	246
		10/10	128.00	−2.0	00	19.0	231
		10/10	64.00	−1.5	01	18.0	219
		10/10	32.00	−1.5	00	15.1	184
		10/10	16.00	−1.5	00	13.8	168
		10/10	8.00	−1.6	00	15.3	186
		10/10	4.00	−1.1	00	12.3	150
		30/30	Control			8.2	
P388 leukemia	Every day for 9 days	10/10	750.00	−3.8	00	28.3	277
		10/10	500.00	−2.5	00	24.8	243
		10/10	330.00	−1.9	00	21.8	213
		20/20	Control			10.2	

were dosage dependent, the drug was therapeutically effective at dosages as low as 4 mg/kg/day. Against P388 leukemia in mice, tiazofurin was similarly active with a T/C of 277 at 750 mg/kg/day for 9 days. On an extended schedule of intermittent bolus delivery, tiazofurin produced an ILS of 225% for L1210-inoculated mice (Table IV), and less frequent delivery of smaller dosages of the drug by intraperitoneal infusion was also highly effective (Table V).

Tiazofurin exhibited substantial activity *in vivo* against sublines of L1210 resistant to treatment with methotrexate or ara-C (Table VI) and also against those resistant to 6-mercaptopurine or 6-thioguanine (Table VII). Against ara-C-resistant P388 leukemia the drug was more active than against the parent line; this reflects collateral sensitivity (compare Tables III and VIII). Of 10 mice inoculated with P388/ara-C, 5 were cured when tiazofurin (700 mg/kg) was delivered once a day for 9 consecutive days. With similar treatment, the response of P388/cytoxan was comparable to that of the parent line (compare Tables III and IX).

Several additional models have been used to assess the therapeutic efficacy of tiazofurin *in vivo*. Against the ascites form of sarcoma 180, tiazofurin produced an ILS of 200% when given for 5 consecutive days at a daily dosage of 512 mg/kg. A single intraperitoneal injection of tiazofurin on day 1 reduced the mass of subcutaneous implanted $CD8F_1$ mammary tumors by 90% on the average, and 8 of 10 treated mice were long-term survivors. Additional striking results were obtained with the Glasgow

TABLE IV

Tiazofurin Bolus Treatment of L1210-Inoculated[a] BDF[1] Mice

Dosage (mg/kg/day)[b]	Schedule of administration	Postinoculation survival (days)	ILS (%)
156	Daily on days 1, 4, 7	7.83[c]	21
259	Daily on days 1, 4, 7	9.60[c]	48
432	Daily on days 1, 4, 7	10.90[c]	68
720	Daily on days 1, 4, 7	12.10[c]	86
1200	Daily on day 1	11.33[d]	65
	Daily on days 1, 4	13.33[d]	94
	Daily on days 1, 4, 7	15.00[c]	131
	Daily on days 1, 4, 7	15.71[d]	129
	Daily on days 1, 4, 7, 10, 13, 16	22.29[d]	225

[a] Mice were inoculated intraperitoncally with 1×10^6 cells on day zero.

[b] Tiazofurin was injected intraperitonically on each day indicated as a volume of 0.01 ml/g of mouse weight: Control mice were injected on days 1, 4, and 7 with equal volumes of 0.9% NaCl solution.

[c] Twelve control mice lived 6.50 days after leukemia cell inoculation.

[d] Fourteen control mice lived 6.86 days after leukemia cell inoculation.

osteogenic sarcoma. Delivered at a daily dosage of 600 mg/kg for 9 days, tiazofurin produced a T/C of 377, and 5 of 10 mice were cured (Table X). At 750 mg/kg/day a T/C (median survivor days) of 510 was obtained, with 7 of 10 animals cured. Such data strongly suggest the potential of tiazofurin for the treatment of human bone cancers. Weber and co-workers (30) have recently reported that tiazofurin treatment of rats bearing subcutaneously implanted hepatoma 3924A on a dosage schedule of 150 mg/kg every other day for 10 days, resulted in the reduction of this solid tumor to 6% (by volume) of that of the control animals. These data are particularly striking, since hepatomas are notoriously unresponsive to drug treatment. No *in vivo* antitumor activity was found with tiazofurin

TABLE V

**Tiazofurin Treatment of L1210-Inoculated[a]
BDF₁ Mice by Intraperitoneal Infusion[b]**

Dosage (mg/kg)	Postinoculation survival (days)	ILS (%)
156	15.70	142
259	15.90	145
432	16.10	148
720	17.00	162
1200	17.90	176
Control	6.5	

[a] Mice were inoculated intraperitoneally with 1×10^6 cells on day zero.

[b] Tiazofurin was infused intraperitoneally for 24-hr periods on days 1, 4, and 7. Control mice were infused with equal volumes of 0.9% NaCl solution.

TABLE VI

Tiazofurin Treatment of BDF₁ Mice[a] Inoculated with Drug-Resistant Sublines of L1210 Leukemia

Resistant subline of L1210	Treatment[b]		No. of mice	Postinoculation survival (days)	ILS (%)
	Drug	Dosage (mg/kg)			
L1210/MTX	None	—	12	7.75	—
	MTX	15	12	8.58	11
	Tiazofurin	720	7	13.71	77
	Tiazofurin	1200	7	16.71	116
L1210/ara-C	None	—	12	5.71	—
	Ara-C	720	12	6.00	5
	Tiazofurin	720	7	14.71	158
	Tiazofurin	1200	7	16.57	190

[a] Mice were inoculated intraperitoneally on day zero with 1×10^6 cells of L1210/MTX or 1×10^6 cells of L1210/ara-C.

[b] Drugs were administered intraperitoneally on days 1, 4, and 7 as a volume of 0.01 ml/g of mouse weight: Control mice were injected with equal volumes of 0.9% NaCl solution.

TABLE VII

In Vivo Activity of Tiazofurin against Leukemia L1210/MP and L1210/TG

Test system	Treatment schedule	Tox. surv.	Dos./inj.	Weight difference	Days survival evaluation	Control	T/C
L1210/MP	Daily for 5 days	06/06	600.00	−4.3	16.0	7.7	207
		05/06	300.00	−3.4	13.8	7.7	179
		06/06	150.00	−2.5	12.4	7.7	161
		05/06	75.00	−2.7	11.1	7.7	144
		06/06	37.50	−1.5	10.3	7.7	133
L1210/TG	Daily for 5 days	06/06	600.00	−3.5	17.8	9.0	197
		06/06	300.00	−2.9	16.0	9.0	177
		06/06	150.00	−1.7	14.8	9.0	164
		06/06	75.00	−2.5	13.0	9.0	144
		06/06	37.50	−1.6	12.8	9.0	142
		19/18					

TABLE VIII

In Vivo Tiazofurin Treatment of Leukemia P388/Ara C[a]

Tox. surv.	Dos./inj.	BWD	Median survival (days)	T/C	Cures
10/10	750.00	−3.7	45.0	387	5
10/10	500.00	−4.2	38.0	327	2
10/10	330.00	−3.0	33.0	284	1
20/20	Control		11.6		

[a] Treatment schedule was daily for 9 days.

TABLE IX

In Vivo Tiazofurin Treatment of Leukemia P388 Resistant to Cytoxan[a]

Tox. surv.	Dos./inj.	BWD	Median survival (days)	T/C	Cures
10/10	500.00	−2.0	26.0	265	0
10/10	330.00	−1.5	22.4	228	0
10/10	220.00	−1.1	21.0	214	0
20/20	Control		0.9		

[a] Treatment schedule was daily for 9 days.

TABLE X

Tiazofurin Treatment of Glasgow Osteogenic Sarcoma in Mice

Treatment schedule	Tox. surv.	Dos./inj.	Median survival (days)	T/C	Cures
Daily for	09/10	600.00	83.0	377	05
9 days	08/10	380.00	45.0	205	00
	09/09	240.00	42.0	191	00
	10/10	Control	22.0		
Daily for	10/10	750.00	109.0	510	07
12 days	07/10	500.00	62.5	298	04
	07/09	330.00	50.0	238	01
	10/10	Control	21.0		

against B16 melanoma, CX-1 human colon xenograft, or colon 38 tumors. Tiazofurin showed only weak activity against leukemia C1498 in mice.

III. Animal Tumor Studies with Selenazofurin

The synthesis of selenazofurin (2-β-D-ribofuranosylselenazole-4-carboxamide) (**III**) was reported by Srivastava and Robins (45) in 1983. Selenazofurin was similar to tiazofurin in its antitumor activity against Lewis lung carcinoma in mice but was active at lower doses (45). Against L1210 leukemia *in vivo* selenazofurin was as active as tiazofurin at about one-tenth the dose (7); a comparison of the two drugs is shown in Fig. 2. At doses of 500 mg/kg/day for each drug, selenazofurin produced an ILS approximately 100% greater than tiazofurin. Selenazofurin would appear to be the more potent of the two nucleosides for the treatment of L1210 leukemia *in vivo,* as judged by the lower dosage of the drug required to induce both optimal L1210 responses and lethality in mice (Fig. 2). Within the limits of dosage studied, selenazofurin also appeared to enjoy a degree of therapeutic advantage. Thus, an ILS of 184% was produced by the maximum nonlethal dosage (556 mg/kg) of this compound as compared with 131% that resulted from treatment with 1200 mg/kg (the maximum nonlethal dose) of tiazofurin. It may be noteworthy that the somnolent condition noted for tiazofurin was much less pronounced with selenazofurin and was not in evidence at dosages below 333 mg/kg.

A further study, involving two-drug combinations formed when either tiazofurin or selenazofurin was given in concert with each of 13 potent and clinically useful antitumor agents, showed that the selenazofurin

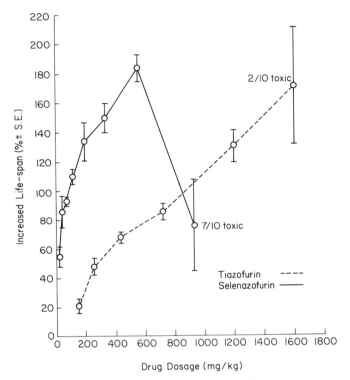

Fig. 2. Comparative responses of L1210-inoculated BDF₁ mice to treatment with tiazofurin or selenazofurin.

combinations were substantially less toxic, even though the delivered dosages of selenazofurin and tiazofurin produced equivalent increases in postinoculation life-span when given alone (Table XI). It is evident from the data in Table XI that selenazofurin combinations were less toxic (7 toxic deaths compared to 18 for tiazofurin) and in addition selenazofurin produced more cures (22 versus 11 for tiazofurin). In further combination studies, Schabel and co-workers (40) studying L1210 cells (1×10^7) inoculated intraperitoneally, obtained a 100% cure (60-day survivor) rate with the combination of tiazofurin and BCNU when the drugs were given on days 1–9. Given alone on the same schedule, these two drugs produced respective T/C values of 300 and 286 but were not curative at the dosages studied. Avery and Robins (3) have shown that combinations of tiazofurin and etoposide or tiazofurin and mitoxantrone are synergistic and curative against L1210 leukemia in animals over a wide range of dosage.

TABLE XI

Responses of L1210-Inoculated[a] BDF$_1$ Mice to Treatment with Tiazofurin or Selenazofurin Given Alone or in Two-Drug Combinations

Drug treatment[b]	No. of Mice treated	Tumor deaths occurence (days after inoculation)	Toxic deaths	Cures
Tiazofurin	7	13.66	0	0
Tiazofurin + drug panel[c]	91	18.51	18	11
Selenazofurin	7	13.80	0	0
Selenazofurin + drug panel	91	17.42	7	22
Control		6.83		

[a] Mice were inoculated intraperitoneally with 1×10^6 cells on day zero.

[b] Drugs were administered intraperitoneally. For combination chemotherapy, the drugs were given in rapid succession. Each of 26 2-drug combinations consisted of tiazofurin or selenazofurin plus one of 13 other drugs. Cyclophosphamide and carmustine were administered only on day 1. Each of the other drugs was given once daily on days 1, 4, and 7. The drugs were delivered as a volume of 0.01 ml/g of mouse weight. Controls received equal volumes of 0.9% NaCl solution.

[c] Panel consisted of 13 drugs: ara-C, MTX, 6MP, mitoxantrone, dactinomycin, cyclophosphamide, VCR, ADA, teniposide, etoposide, dacarbazine, carmustine, and *cis*-platinum.

IV. Mechanism of Action of Tiazofurin and Selenazofurin

Tiazofurin was shown by Robins and co-workers (46) to inhibit by 69% the synthesis of guanine nucleotides in Ehrlich ascites tumor cells. It was later revealed by Jayaram *et al.* (21) that tiazofurin caused a 15-fold increase in the concentration of inosine 5'-monophosphate (IMP) in P388 murine leukemia cells. Kuttan *et al.* (27) showed that tiazofurin is phosphorylated enzymatically in Chinese hamster ovary cells to tiazofurin 5'-phosphate, which in the presence of ATP and Mg^{2+} is further converted to the NAD analog (**IV**) which is a potent inhibitor of IMP dehydrogenase (Fig. 3). These studies were confirmed by Cooney *et al.* (10) in P388 leukemia cells in culture. The chemical synthesis of (**IV**) has been reported (13).

A comparative *in vitro* study of tiazofurin and selenazofurin in P388, L1210, B16 melanoma, and Lewis lung carcinoma cells in culture showed (49) that selenazofurin was consistently more cytotoxic by a factor of 5–17. The corresponding selenazofurin analog of NAD (**V**), which is formed

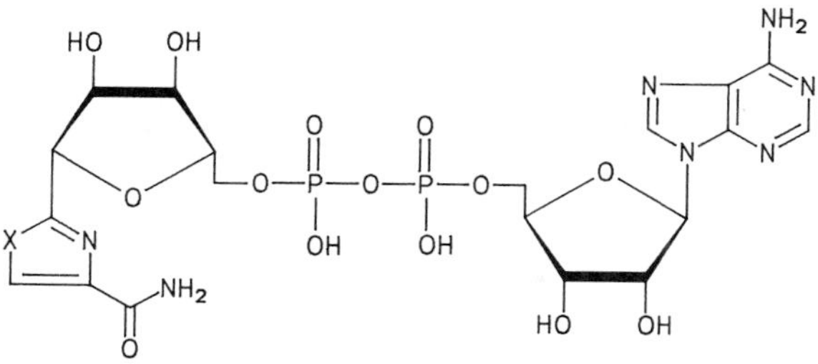

(IV)   X = S
(V)   X = Se

Fig. 3.   Metabolites of tiazofurin and selenazofurin.

in vitro from selenazofurin in P388 cells, is clearly a more potent inhibitor of IMP dehydrogenase (49) than the corresponding tiazofurin derivative (**IV**). This has recently been verified independently (14). The isolation of (**V**) from (**III**) in P388 cells was achieved, and the structure of (**V**) confirmed by mass spectra (22).

The NAD pyrophosphorylase in P388 lymphoblasts did not convert ribavirin or AICR to the corresponding NAD analog (14) which may explain why ribavirin has relatively weak antitumor activity compared to tiazofurin and selenazofurin.

Recently, D. G. Streeter (private communication) has studied (**IV**) and (**V**) as inhibitors of IMP dehydrogenase, glyceraldehyde-3-phosphate-dehydrogenase, glucose-6-phosphate dehydrogenase, malic dehydrogenase, and glutamate dehydrogenase. IMP dehydrogenase was the only dehydrogenase significantly inhibited by these NAD analogs.

Selenazofurin at a concentration of $1 \times 10^{-9} M$ decreases the proliferation of HL60 cells (human cell line of promyelocytic leukemia) and causes these cells to differentiate into mature myeloid cells (29). This cellular differentiation is believed to be due to inhibition of IMP dehydrogenase in this cell line (29). For a review of inhibitors of IMP dehydrogenase and their corresponding antitumor activity the reader is referred to a review by Robins (37). Weber (51) has also recently reviewed the importance of IMP dehydrogenase as a key enzyme in neoplasia. Sadee and co-workers (9) have shown that the inhibition of *de novo* synthesis of guanine nucleotides in S-49 cells results in the depletion of GTP, which inhibits DNA synthesis. Related studies (8) suggest that the biological consequences of purine starvation are primarily mediated by the depletion of guanine nucleotides rather than by adenine nucleotides. Earle and Glazer (11) studied tiazofurin inhibition of a number of human tumor cell lines and concluded that the antitumor effects of tiazofurin were related to guanine nucleotide depletion. In more recent studies, Johns and co-workers (1) have studied tiazofurin in a number of tumor cell lines sensitive and resistant to tiazofurin. In general, the levels of the NAD analog (**IV**), the percentage of inhibition of IMP dehydrogenase, the depression of guanine nucleotide pools, and the elevation of IMP correlated well with the sensitivity or resistance to tiazofurin in cell lines studied. Weber and co-workers (28) have recently shown that the tiazofurin-induced depletion of NAD pools in hepatoma 3924A–bearing rats was 20% of that of normal rat liver. The NAD analogs (**IV**) and (**V**) prepared chemically in our laboratory have been studied in a collaborative effort with Berger and co-workers (5), who have recently shown that (**IV**) and (**V**) in L1210 leukemia cells interfere with NAD synthesis apparently by blocking formation of nicotinamide mononucleotide. The NAD analogs are also inhibitors of poly(ADP-ribose) polymerase, which is an NAD-utilizing, chromatin-bound enzyme whose function is required for normal DNA repair processes. It would appear that tiazofurin and selenazofurin, as their NAD analogs, lower NAD levels and modulate poly(ADP-ribose) metabolism to synergistically potentiate the antitumor effects of DNA strand–disrupting agents (5), by inhibiting DNA repair. This would account for the considerable synergism of BCNU [*N,N*-Bis(2-chloroethyl)-*N*-nitrosourea] and tiazofurin reported by Schabel and co-workers (40) and strongly suggests the careful selection of antitumor agents which alkylate or cause breaks in DNA as potentially useful agents in combination with tiazofurin in future clinical trials.

There are a number of differences between the action of tiazofurin and selenazofurin. For example, selenazofurin possesses broad-spectrum, *in vitro* antiviral activity, 100-fold superior to tiazofurin (26). Interestingly enough, selenazofurin *in vitro* is highly synergistic in antiviral effects with ribavirin which, as the 5′-phosphate (54) also exerts significant inhibition of IMP dehydrogenase isolated from Ehrlich ascites cells.

A new synthesis of tiazofurin and selenazofurin has been achieved recently in our laboratory from ethyl-5-amino-2-β-D-ribofuranosyl-thiazole (or selenazole)-4-carboxylate via reductive removal of the 5-diazo group, followed by treatment of the product with methanolic ammonia to introduce the amide function (19). Tiazofurin 5′-phosphate is nearly as active against L1210 leukemia in mice as is tiazofurin. At 100 mg/kg/day Q01DX5 the T/C was 259 for L1210. Similarly, selenazofurin 5′-phosphate at 13 mg/kg/day against Lewis lung carcinoma showed a T/C of 315, with 4 out of 10 cures (45). This is slightly less active than selenazofurin, which at 12 mg/kg/day showed a T/C of 355, with 8 out of 10 cures against the same tumor (45). A single crystal x-ray study of tiazofurin (15) and selenazofurin (16) showed that the thiazole sulfur atom and the selenium atom in the selenazole ring each form a close intramolecular contact with the furanose ring oxygen, which is closer than the sum of their van der Waals radii. Such interaction may favor the *anti* form, which is similar to the more stable *anti* form of most purine nucleosides. This could be important in enzymatic phosphorylation of tiazofurin and selenazofurin to the 5'-phosphate form of the drugs. It is apparently not known which kinase is responsible for this phosphorylation. Unlike ribavirin, which is converted to the 5'-phosphate by adenosine kinase (52), Saunders and co-workers (39) have shown that tiazofurin is phosphorylated by crude extracts of Chinese hamster ovary (CHO) cells. Variant cell lines lacking adenosine kinase or deoxycytidine kinase, however, showed no resistance to tiazofurin, suggesting that adenosine kinase does not phosphorylate tiazofurin to any great extent. Recent data by Fridland and Connelly (12) suggest that tiazofurin may be phosphorylated by a cytoplasmic 5'-nucleotidase which catalyzes the phosphorylation of inosine (55).

Jackson and co-workers (6) have shown that in P388 leukemia cells the cytotoxicity of tiazofurin and selenazofurin is reversible by guanosine or guanine but not by other purine nucleosides or bases. Three human tumor cell lines selected for tiazofurin resistance showed cross-resistance between selenazofurin and tiazofurin (6).

V. Pharmacokinetics and Clinical Pharmacology of Tiazofurin

The pharmacokinetics of tiazofurin in the cerebral fluid of Rhesus monkeys shows significant penetration of the blood–brain barrier by the drug (17) and suggests a potential role of tiazofurin in the treatment of cancer of the central nervous system and brain tumors. The pharmacokinetics and metabolism of tiazofurin have been studied (2) in the mouse, rat, rabbit, and dog by use of tritiated drug as a marker. In all four species tiazofurin is removed from the circulation, with a generally prolonged terminal half-life of 3–16 hr. The major amount (90%) of the administered dose was excreted unchanged in the urine within 24 hr. Phosphorylation to tiazofurin 5'-phosphate was generally observed in most organs (2). Liver, kidney, and muscle catalyzed the synthesis of the NAD analogs (**IV**) and (**V**). Preclinical toxicology in mice and dogs revealed dose-related toxicity which was mild and reversible below the lethal doses (35) and absent at one-tenth the LD_{10} dose level. A procedure for assaying tiazofurin in plasma by reverse-phase, high-performance liquid chromatography has been reported (34). From toxicological studies with tiazofurin, the single-dose LD_{50} in mice is 3.5 g/kg, and with daily administration for 5 consecutive days becomes 2.2 g/kg/day (20).

Phase I clinical trials at 2200 mg/m^2/day over a 5-day treatment showed dose-limiting toxicity involving *headaches, fever, nausea,* and *diarrhea* (33). A phase I clinical trial of tiazofurin given by continuous infusion over a 5-day period showed neurotoxicity as the dose-limiting toxicity at 2350 mg/m^2/day (50). However, given as a bolus, tiazofurin has been administered at dosages as high as 4100 mg/m^2/day for 5 days (36).

The suggested dosage for phase II clinical trials is 1100–1200 mg/m^2/day intravenously for a 5-day treatment (33). Nineteen clinical centers in the United States and Canada are presently studying tiazofurin in phase II clinical trials against various types of human cancer.

VI. Structure–Activity Relationships

A number of specific modifications of the parent tiazofurin structure have been reported. The amide function has been replaced by thioamide (46) and amidine (48). The isomeric 2-β-D-ribofuranosylthiazole-5-car-

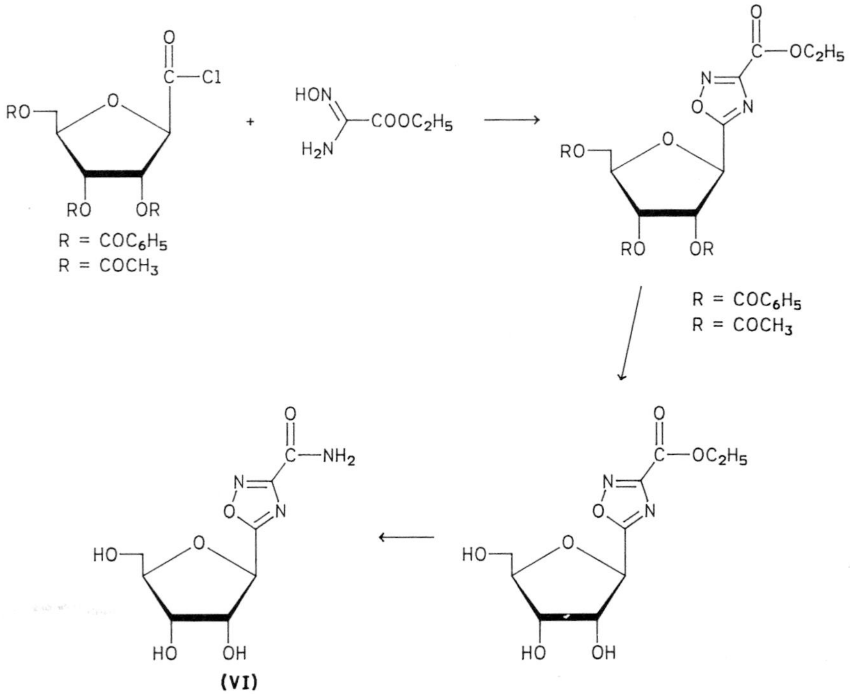

Fig. 4. Synthesis of 5-β-D-ribofuranosyl-1,2,4-oxadiazole-3-carboxamide (**VI**).

boxamide has also been synthesized (46). The sugar moiety has been altered to give the 5'-deoxy (46), 3'-deoxy (4), 2'-deoxy (47), arabino (24,31), and xylo (31) analogs of tiazofurin. None of these derivatives were significantly active against animal tumors. Recently, we introduced the amino group into the 5-position of the thiazole ring in tiazofurin and the selenazole ring of selenazofurin (19); these amino derivatives were totally inactive as antitumor agents. Most recently we have prepared the "C" nucleoside 5-β-D-ribofuranosyl-1,2,4-oxadiazole-3-carboxamide (**VI**) by a ring closure procedure of the β-D-ribofuranosyl acid chloride with the requisite amidoxime, followed by deblocking and amidation (19a) (Fig. 4). This novel "C" nucleoside is now being prepared in sufficient quantity for *in vivo* evaluation against a variety of animal tumors.

VII. Summary

Tiazofurin (**II**) and selenazofurin (**III**) have been synthesized as carbon-linked nucleoside analogs of the antiviral agent ribavirin (**I**). Both tiazofurin and selenazofurin are highly active against Lewis lung carcinoma and leukemias P388 and L1210 in mice. Tiazofurin is also active *in vivo* against ara-C and cytoxan resistant lines of P388 and against Glasgow osteogenic sarcoma. Selenazofurin has a spectrum of antitumor activity similar to that of tiazofurin at about one-tenth the dose. The "C" nucleosides (**II**) and (**III**) are converted *in vivo* to the corresponding NAD analogs (**IV**) and (**V**) which are excellent inhibitors of IMP dehydrogenase. These NAD analogs also reduce the formation of nicotinamide mononucleotide and are inhibitors of poly(ADP-ribose)polymerase which is a chromatin-bound, NAD-utilizing enzyme whose function is required for normal DNA repair processes. Thus, DNA damaging agents such as *N*-methylnitroso urea, BCNU, VP-16 (etoposide), and mitoxantrone show considerable synergism with tiazofurin or selenazofurin against L1210 cells in culture and against disseminated L1210 in mice due to the inhibition of DNA repair by metabolites (**IV**) and (**V**).

Phase I and phase II clinical studies of (**II**) and (**III**) are under way or are planned in a number of clinical centers throughout the United States and Europe. Studies with related "C" nucleosides suggest that the antitumor activities of tiazofurin and selenazofurin are quite specific.

Acknowledgment

The authors wish to thank the National Cancer Institute for supplying certain of the antitumor testing data included in this report.

References

1. Ahluwalia, G. S., Jayaram, H. N., Plowman, J. P., Cooney, D. A., and Johns, D. G. (1984). Studies on the mechanism of action of 2-β-D-ribofuranosylthiazole-4-caroxamide. *Biochem. Pharmacol.* **33,** 1195.

2. Arnold, S. T., Jayaram, H. N., Harper, G. R., Litterst, C. L., Malspeis, L., Desouza, J. J. V., Staubus, A. E., Ahluwalia, G. S., Wilson, Y. A., Cooney, D. A., and Johns, D. G. (1984). The distribution and metabolism of tiazofurin in rodents, rabbits, and dogs. *Drug Met. Dispos.* **2,** 165.

3. Avery, T. L., and Robins, R. K. (1984). Experimental antitumor activity of Tiazofurin. *Proc. Am. Assoc. Cancer Res.* **25,** 345.

4. Baur, R. H., and Baker, D. C. (1984). Synthesis of 2-(3-deoxy-β-D-*erythro*-pentofuranosyl-thiazole-4-carboxamide (3'-deoxytiazofurin). *Nucleosides Nucleotides* **3,** 77.

5. Berger, N. A., Berger, S. J., Catino, D. M., Petzold, S. J., and Robins, R. K. (1985). Modulation of nicotinamide adenine dinucleotide and poly-(adenosine diphosphoribose) metabolism by the synthetic "C" nucleoside analogs, tiazofurin and selenazofurin. *J. Clin. Invest.* **75,** 702.

6. Boritzki, T. J., Berry, D. A., Besserer, J. A., Cook, P. D., Fry, D. W., Leopold, W.R., and Jackson, R. C. (1985). Biochemical and antitumour activity of tiazofurin and its selenium analog (2-β-D-ribofuranosyl-4-selenazolecarboxamide). *Biochem. Pharmacol.* **34,** 1109.

7. Burchenal, J. H., Pancoast, T., Carroll, A., Elslager, E., and Robins, R. K. (1984). Antileukemic, antitumor and cross-resistance studies of 2-β-D-ribofuranosyl-selenazole-4-carboxamide (Selenazofurin). *Proc. Am. Assoc. Cancer Res.* **25,** 347.

8. Cohen, M. B., and Sadee, W. (1983). Contributions of the depletions of guanine and adenine nucleotides to the toxicity of purine starvation in the mouse T lymphoma cell line. *Cancer Res.* **43,** 1587.

9. Cohen, M. B., Maybaum, J., and Sadee, W. (1981). Guanine nucleotide depletion and toxicity in mouse T-lymphoma (S-4) cells. *J. Biol. Chem.* **256,** 8713.

10. Cooney, D. A., Jayaram, H. N., Gebeyehu, G., Betts, C. R., Kelley, J. A., Marques, V. E., and Johns, D. G. (1982). The conversion of 2-β-D-ribofuranosylthiazole-4-carboxamide to an analog of NAD with potent IMP dehydrogenase inhibitory properties. *Biochem. Pharmacol.* **31,** 2133.

11. Earle, M. F., and Glazer, R. I. (1983). Activity and metabolism of 2-β-D-ribofuranosylthiazole-4-carboxamide in human lymphoid tumor cells in culture. *Cancer Res.* **43,** 133.

12. Fridland, A., Connelly, M. C., and Robbins, T. J. (1985). Tiazofurin metabolism in human lymphoid cells: Evidence for phosphorylation by Adenosine and 5'-Nucleotidase. *Cancer Res.* **46,** 532.

13. Gebeyehu, G., Marques, V. E., Kelley, J. A., Cooney, D. A., Jayaram, H. N., and Johns, D. G. (1983). Synthesis of thiazole-4-carboxamide adenine dinucleotide. A powerful inhibitor of IMP dehydrogenase. *J. Med. Chem.* **26,** 922.

14. Gebeyehu, G., Marquez, V. E., Cott, A. V., Cooney, D. A., Kelley, J. A., Jayaram, H. N., Ahluwalia, S., Dion, R. L., Wilson, Y. A., and Johns, D. G. (1985). Ribavirin, tiazofurin, and selenazofurin: Mononucleotides and nicotinamide adenine dinucleotide analogues. Synthesis, structure and interactions with IMP dehydrogenase. *J. Med. Chem.* **28,** 99.

15. Goldstein, B. M., Takusagawa, F., Berman, H. M., Srivastava, P. C., and Robins, R. K. (1983). Structural studies of a new antitumour agent: Tiazofurin and its inactive analogues. *J. Am. Chem. Soc.* **105,** 7416.

16. Goldstein, B. M., Takusagawa, F., Berman, H. M., Srivastava, P. C., and Robins, R.

K. (1985). Structural studies of a new antitumour and antiviral agent: Selenazofurin and its α anomer. *J. Am. Chem. Soc.* **107,** 1394.

17. Grygiel, J. J., Balis, F. M., Collins, J. M., Lester, C. M., and Poplack, D. G. (1985). Pharmacokinetics of tiazofurin in the plasma and cerebrospinal fluid of Rhesus monkeys. *Cancer Res.* **45,** 2037.

18. Harris, S., and Robins, R. K. (1980). Ribavirin: Structure and antiviral activity relationships. *In* "Ribavirin: A Broad Spectrum Antiviral Agent" (R. A. Smith and W. Kirkpatrick, eds.), pp. 1–22. Academic Press, New York.

19. Hennen, W. J., Hinshaw, B. C., Riley, T. A., Wood, S. G., and Robins, R. K. (1985). Synthesis of 4-substituted 5-amino-2-(β-D-ribofuranosyl)thiazoles and their respective conversion into 2-(β-D-ribofuranosyl)thiazolo[5,4-d]pyrimidines and 2-(β-D-ribofuranosyl)selenazolo[5,4-d]pyrimidines. A new synthesis of tiazofurin and selenazofurin. *J. Org. Chem.* **50,** 1741.

19a. Hennen, W. J., and Robins, R. K. (1985). Synthesis of 5-β-D-ribofuranosyl-1,2,4-oxadiazole-3-carboxamide. *J. Heterocycl. Chem.* **22,** 1747.

20. Jayaram, H. N., and Johns, D. G. (1984). Metabolic and mechanistic studies with tiazofurin (2-β-D-ribofuranosylthiazole-4-carboxamide. *In* "Developments in Cancer Chemotherapy" (R. I. Glazer, ed.), p. 114. CRC Press, Boca Raton, Florida.

21. Jayaram, H. N., Dion, R. L., Glazer, R. I., Johns, D. G., Robins, R. K., Srivastava, P. C., and Cooney, D. A. (1982). Initial studies on the mechanism of action of a new oncolytic thiazole nucleoside, 2-β-D-ribofuranosylthiazole-4-carboxamide (NSC 286193). *Biochem. Pharmacol.* **31,** 2371.

22. Jayaram, H. N., Ahluwalia, G. S., Dion, R. L., Gebeyehu, G., Marquez, V. E., Kelley, J. A., Robins, R. K., Cooney, D. A., and Johns, D. G. (1983). Conversion of 2-β-D-ribofuranosylselenazole-4-carboxamide to an analogue of NAD with potent IMP dehydrogenase-inhibitory properties. *Biochem. Pharmacol.* **32,** 2633.

23. Jenkins, F. J., and Chen, Y. C. (1983). Effect of ribavirin on Rous sarcoma virus transformation. *Antimicrob. Agents Chemother.* **19,** 364.

24. Jiang, C., Baur, R. H., Dechter, J. J., and Baker, D. C. (1984). Synthesis and stereochemical assignments for 2-(α- and β-D-arabinofuranosyl)thiazole-4-carboxamides. *Nucleosides Nucleotides* **3,** 123.

25. Khwaja, T. A., Popovic, M. R., Witkowski, J. T., Robins, R. K., Halpern, R. M., and Smith, R. A. (1972). The antitumour activity of virazole, a new broad spectrum antiviral agent. *Proc. Am. Assoc. Cancer Res.* **13,** 91.

26. Kirsi, J. J., North, J. A., McKernan, P. A., Murray, B. K., Canonico, P. G., Huggins, J. W., Srivastava, P. C., and Robins, R. K. (1983). Broad-spectrum antiviral activity of 2-β-D-ribofuranosylselenazole-4-carboxamide, a new antiviral agent. *Antimicrob. Agents Chemother.* **24,** 353.

27. Kuttan, R., Robins, R. K., and Saunders, P. O. (1982). Inhibition of inosinate dehydrogenase by metabolites of 2-β-D-ribofuranosylthiazole-4-carboxamide. *Biochem. Biophys. Res. Commun.* **107,** 862.

28. Liepnieks, J. J., Faderan, M. A., Lui, M. S., and Weber, G. (1984). Tiazofurin-induced selective depression of NAD content in hepatoma 3924A. *Biochem. Biophys. Res. Commun.* **122,** 345.

29. Lucas, D. L., Robins, R. K., Knight, R. D., and Wright, D. G. (1983). Induced maturation of the human promyelocytic leukemia cell line, HL-60 by 2-β-D-ribofuranosylselenazole-4-carboxamide. *Biochem. Biophys. Res. Commun.* **115,** 971.

30. Lui, M. S., Faderan, M. A., Liepnieks, J. J., Natsumeda, Y., Olah, E., Jayaram, H. N., and Weber, G. (1984). Modulation of IMP dehydrogenase activity and guanylate metabolism by tiazofurin (2-β-D-ribofuranosylthiazole-4-carboxamide). *J. Biol. Chem.* **259,** 5078.

31. Mao, D. T., and Marquez, V. E. (1984). Synthesis of 2-β-D-ara and 2-β-D-xylofurano-sylthiazole-4-carboxamide. *Tetrahedron Lett.* **25**, 2111.
32. McCormick, J. B., Mitchell, S. W., Getchell, J. P., and Hicks, D. R. (1984). Ribavirin suppresses replication of lymphadenopathy-associated virus in cultures of human adult T lymphocytes. *Lancet* **2**, 1367.
33. Melink, T. J., Von Hoff, D. D., Kuhn, J. G., Hersh, M. R., Sternson, L. A., Patton, T. F., Siegler, R., Boldt, D. H., and Clark, G. M. (1985). Phase I evaluation and pharmaco-kinetics of tiazofurin (2-β-D-ribofuranosylthiazole-4-carboxamide, NSC 286193). *Cancer Res.* **45**, 2859.
34. Obeng, E. K., Vallner, J. J., and Gokhale, R. D. (1984). Determination of the antineo-plastic agent tiazofurin in plasma by high performance liquid chromatography. *Anal. Lett.* **17**, 607.
35. O'Dwyer, P. J., Shoemaker, D. D., Jayaram, H. N., Johns, D. G., Cooney, D. A., Marsoni, S., Malspeis, L., Plowman, J., Davingnon, J. P., and Davis, R. D. (1984). Tiazofurin: A new antitumour agent. *Invest. New Drugs* **2**, 79.
36. Roberts, J. D., Ackerly, C. A., Newman, R. A., Krakoff, I. H., and Stewart J. A. (1984). Phase I study of tiazofurin (2-β-D-ribofuranosylthiazole-4-carboxamide; NSC 286193). *Proc. Am. Assoc. Cancer Res.* **25**, 166 (Abstr. No. 655).
37. Robins, R. K. (1982). Nucleoside and nucleotide inhibitors of inosine monophosphate (IMP) dehydrogenase as potential antitumour inhibitors. *Nucleosides Nucleotides* **1**, 35.
38. Robins, R. K., Srivastava, P. C., Narayanan, V. L., Plowman, J., and Paull, K. D. (1982). 2-β-D-Ribofuranosylthiazole-4-carboxamide, a novel potential antitumor agent for lung tumors and metastases. *J. Med. Chem.* **25**, 107.
39. Saunders, P. O., Kuttan, R., Lai, M. M., and Robins, R. K. (1983). Action of 2-β-D-ribofuranosylthiazole-4-carboxamide (tiazofurin) in Chinese hamster ovary and variant cell lines. *Mol. Pharmacol.* **23**, 534.
40. Schabel, F. M., Jr., Griswold, D. P., Jr., Corbett, T. H., Laster, W. R., Jr., and Trader, M. W. (1983). Curative chemotherapy of advanced Pu-induced osteosarcoma in mice with 2-β-D-ribofuranosylthiazole-4-carboxamide (T-CAR) and of advanced leukemia L1210 with T-CAR plus BCNU. *Proc. Am. Assoc. Cancer Res.* **24**, 265.
41. Shannon, W. M. (1977). Selective inhibition of RNA tumor virus replication *in vitro* and evaluation of candidate antiviral agents *in vivo*. *Ann N. Y. Acad. Sci.* **284**, 472.
42. Sidwell, R. W., Huffman, J. H., Khare, G. P., Allen, L. B., Witkowski, J. T., and Robins, R. K. (1972). Broad-spectrum antiviral activity of virazole: β-D-ribofuranosyl-1,2,4-triazole-3-carboxamide. *Science* **117**, 705.
43. Sidwell, R. W., Allen, L. B., Huffman, J. H., Witkowski, J. T., and Simon, L. N. (1975). Effect of 1-β-D-ribofuranosyl-1,2,4-triazole-3-carboxamide (Ribavirin) on Friend leukaemia virus infections in mice (38647). *Proc. Soc. Exp. Biol. Med.* **148**, 854.
44. Sidwell, R. W., Robins, R. K., and Hillyard, I. W. (1979). Ribavirin: an antiviral agent. *Pharmacol. Ther.* **6**, 123.
45. Srivastava, P. C., and Robins, R. K. (1983). Synthesis and antitumor activity of 2-β-D-ribofuranosylselenazole-4-carboxamide and related derivatives. *J. Med. Chem.* **26**, 445.
46. Srivastava, P. C., Pickering, M. V., Allen, L. B., Streeter, D. G., Campbell, M. T., Witkowski, J. T., Sidwell, R. W., and Robins, R. K. (1977). Synthesis and antiviral activity of certain thiazole C-nucleosides. *J. Med. Chem.* **20**, 156.
47. Srivastava, P. C., Robins, R. K., Takusagawa, F., and Berman, H. M. (1981). Determi-nation of the anomeric configuration of 2'-deoxy-D-ribonucleosides by ^{1}H NMR and by crystallographic studies of a novel 2'-deoxy C-nucleoside. *J. Heterocycl. Chem.* **18**, 1659.
48. Srivastava, P. C., Revankar, G. R., and Robins, R. K. (1984). Synthesis and biological

activity of nucleosides and nucleotides related to the antitumor agent 2-β-D-ribofurano-sylthiazole-4-carboxamide. *J. Med. Chem.* **27,** 266.

49. Streeter, D. G., and Robins, R. K. (1983). Comparative *in vitro* studies of tiazofurin and a selenazole analog. *Biochem. Biophys. Res. Commun.* **115,** 544.

50. Trump, D. L., Tutsch, K. D., Koeller, J. M., and Tourmey, D. C. (1985). Phase I clinical study with pharmacokinetic analysis of 2-β-D-ribofuranosylthiazole-4-carbox-amide (NSC 286193) administered as a five-day infusion. *Cancer Res.* **45,** 2853.

51. Weber, G. (1983). Biochemical strategy of cancer cells and the design of chemotherapy. G. H. A. Clowes Memorial Lecture. *Cancer Res.* **43,** 3466.

52. Willis, R. C., Carson, D. A., and Seegmiller, J. E. (1978). Adenosine kinase initiates the major route of ribavirin activation in a cultured human cell line. *Proc. Natl. Acad. Sci. U.S.A.* **75,** 3042.

53. Witkowski, J. T., Robins, R. K., Sidwell, R. W., and Simon, L. N. (1972). Design, synthesis, and broad spectrum antiviral activity of 1-β-D-ribofuranosyl-1,2,4-triazole-3-carboxamide and related nucleosides. *J. Med. Chem.* **15,** 1150.

54. Witkowski, J. T., Khare, G. P., Sidwell, R. W., Bauer, R. J., Robins, R. K., and Simon, L. N. (1973). Mechanism of action of 1-β-D-ribofuranosyl-1,2,4-triazole-3-carboxamide (Virazole), a new broad-spectrum antiviral agent. *Proc. Natl. Acad. Sci. U.S.A.* **70,** 1174.

55. Worku, Y., and Newby, A. C. (1982). Nucleoside exchange catalysed by the cytoplas-mic 5'-nucleotidase. *Biochem. J.* **205,** 503.

19

Novel Phospholipid Analogs as Membrane-Active Antitumor Agents

EDWARD J. MODEST, LARRY W. DANIEL, ROBERT L. WYKLE,
MICHAEL E. BERENS

Department of Biochemistry, Department of Obstetrics and Gynecology,
and Oncology Research Center
Bowman Gray School of Medicine of Wake Forest University
Winston-Salem, North Carolina

CLAUDE PIANTADOSI, JEFFERSON R. SURLES,
AND SUSAN MORRIS-NATSCHKE

Department of Medicinal Chemistry and Natural Products
University of North Carolina
Chapel Hill, North Carolina

I. Introduction

Bioactive phospholipid analogs of platelet activating factor (PAF), which is 1-alkyl-2-acetyl-*sn*-glycero-3-phosphocholine (**I**) (13,34), represent a novel and little-studied class of potential cancer chemotherapeutic agents, worth further exploration. Reports in the literature and our own studies indicate that 1-alkyl-linked glycerophospholipids (ether lipids) possess an unusually broad range of biological properties, namely, neutrophil activation (25,26), macrophage activation (2,3), platelet aggregation (26,38), membrane interaction (37), antihypertensive action (8), protein kinase inhibition (14), malignant cell differentiation (16), cytotoxicity (3), and antitumor properties (3). It has been reported that two of these analogs are relatively nontoxic to normal cells and to the host (mouse, rabbit) and have no demonstrable mutagenic properties (3). More recently, Storme *et al.* related the antiinvasive effect of (**III**), 1-octadecyl-2-methyl-*rac*-glycero-3-phosphocholine (ET-18-OMe), to cellular membrane alteration in a mouse fibrosarcoma cell line (32), and Glasser *et al.* reported that this compound can successfully purge murine leukemic bone marrow, eliminating leukemic blasts and sparing sufficient normal stem cells to allow hematologic reconstitution (12). Thus ET-18-OMe has become the effective standard against which other analogs of this type are evaluated for antineoplastic activity.

Given this most interesting array of biological and inhibitory properties [reviewed recently by Berdel *et al.* (6)], together with the facts that (1) no concerted effort has been made in anticancer drug development of the highly limited number of available compounds and (2) there has not been time to exploit the very new and exciting biological properties of these phospholipid analogs, we have begun a comprehensive effort on the design and synthesis of new analogs, coupled with parallel biochemical, biological, and pharmacological studies on new and existing compounds.

II. Description of the Program

The focus of this program is on novel analogs of PAF. Earlier, these glycerophospholipids were examined primarily for platelet- and neutrophil-stimulating properties (26). These analogs are structurally related to alkyl lysophospholipids (ALP), a limited number of which have been examined for tumor inhibitory activity and other properties. Lysophospholipids contain an unsubstituted 2-hydroxyl group, whereas PAF contains a 2-acetyl group. Removal of the acetyl group of PAF results in formation of lyso PAF (**II,** Fig. 2), which is devoid of PAF activity. It should be noted that the general term ALP has been used in the earlier literature to denote ET-18-OMe and related compounds. We designate these novel inhibitors as ether lipids (EL).

In view of the unusually broad and most interesting spectrum of activity of the few ether lipids studied to date, we initiated a study of the relationship of various biochemical and biological parameters to antitumor ef-

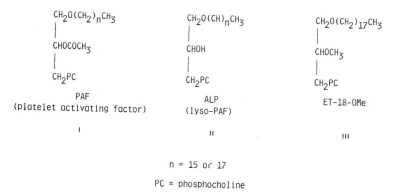

n = 15 or 17

PC = phosphocholine

Fig. 1. Structures of platelet-activating factor (PAF) and related ether lipids.

fects. Our major goals are to conduct a careful analysis of structure–activity relationships with our new analogs to relate specific chemical functionalities in these analogs to their diverse biological properties and to correlate antitumor properties of the active compounds with other biological effects—such that clinical antitumor predictability might be possible based on a set of laboratory data.

The analogs being synthesized and evaluated are thio and amino analogs, as well as oxy and deoxy compounds—all ether lipid analogs of

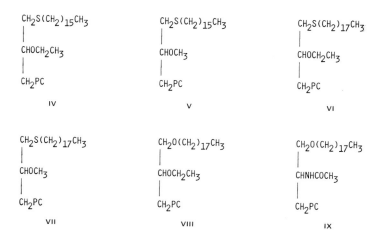

PC = phosphocholine

Fig. 2. Structures of thio and other analogs.

PAF. The phosphocholine residue is being varied, and selected analogs are under study as membrane probes. The biochemical and biological evaluation systems employed include inhibition of malignant cells *in vitro*, induction of differentiation in malignant cells *in vitro*, inhibition of protein kinase, activation of macrophages as mediators of antitumor properties, antitumor studies, membrane effects, and study of pharmacokinetics and toxicology of selected agents in mice.

Several analogs with thio substitution at position 1 (compounds **IV–VII,** Fig. 2) have been prepared in this program (23,24). Compound (**IV**) is the first representative of the 1-thio analogs that we have evaluated. During our studies, Berdel and co-workers described biologically active 1-thioether phospholipid analogs (4) that have reduced platelet aggregating activity, a highly desirable feature in a potential antitumor agent; the structure of the most active analog reported is shown as compound (**X**) (BM 41,440). Compound (**VIII**) has been studied for effects on platelets and neutrophils (26). We are also preparing and testing amino analogs. Hoffman *et al.* (15) reported that the amido compound (**IX**) was the most effective phospholipid analog to inhibit HL-60 human leukemic cells *in vitro*.

Berdel *et al.* (7) recently reported cytotoxic effects, cell membrane destruction, and loss of cell surface activity by compound **XI** (Fig. 3) (CP

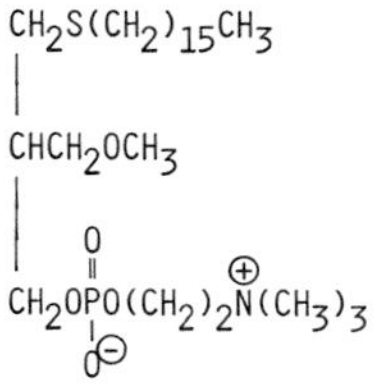

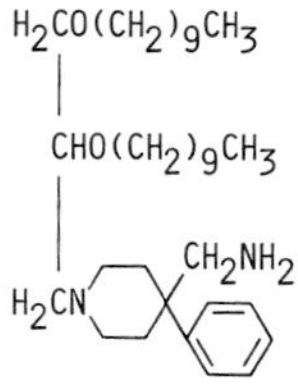

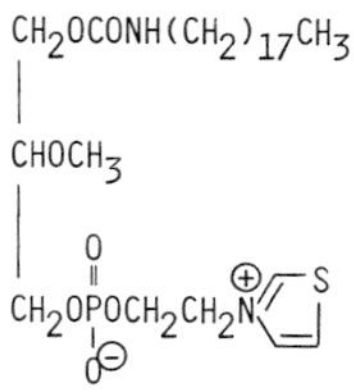

Fig. 3. Structures of other ether lipids.

46,665), an analog of glycerophosphocholine with a substituted amino group at position 3 in place of phosphocholine. Terashita *et al.* (35) have demonstrated that substitution of a thiazolio polar head group at the 3 position [(**XII**, CV 3988)] confers anti-PAF activity on the molecule. These latter two studies indicate that the biological activity can be modified by alterations in the phosphocholine group at position 3, an area we are investigating.

Compound (**III**) has been studied in a number of biological systems (3) and is being evaluated in all of our systems for comparative purposes as a positive control.

A. Mechanisms of Action

The selective activity of the ether lipid analogs against tumor cells has generally been attributed (1,5,15) to greater accumulation of these phospholipids in tumor cells compared with normal cells, because of the low activity of the alkyl cleavage enzyme in tumor cells (31). However, this explanation may be questionable, since one of the most active growth inhibitors (**III**) contains the *O*-methyl group in the 2 position, and other studies have shown that 1-alkyl phosphoglycerides containing substituents in the 2 position did not serve as substrates for the cleavage enzyme (21,30). For example, 1-alkyl-2-acetyl-*sn*-glycero-3-phosphocholine (PAF, **I**) is cleaved only after the acetyl group is removed to form 1-alkyl-2-lyso-*sn*-glycero-3-phosphocholine (**II**), which is readily cleaved (21).

Several recent studies indicate the importance of diacylglycerol as a regulatory molecule (18). These studies are summarized in Fig. 4. In this scheme, phospholipase C hydrolysis of phosphatidylinositol 4,5-bisphosphate (TPI) yields inositol 1,4,5-trisphosphate (IP$_3$) and diacylglycerol (DG) (10). Both IP$_3$ and DG have been suggested as intracellular second messengers in calcium-associated transmembrane signaling (17,19). At least some of the effects of the tumor promoter 12-*O*-tetradecanoyl-phorbol-13-acetate (TPA) appear to be due to the direct stimulation of a protein kinase (PKC) by TPA (9). Many of the biochemical effects of TPA are simulated by the addition of exogenous glycerides which activate PKC in intact cells. (11,20). One of the actions of TPA is the stimulation of HL-60 cells to differentiate into macrophage-like cells (27). We have recently shown that the glyceride analog 1-hexadecyl-2-acetyl-*sn*-glycerol (alkyl AG) also demonstrates this activity (22). Honma *et al.* found that ET-18-OMe induced HL-60 cells to develop some granulocyte characteristics (16). Therefore, it appears that exogenously added ether lipids can induce differentiation of HL-60 cells along different lineages. We have confirmed the report (14) that ether lipids inhibit PKC. This evidence further supports an involvement of PKC in the control of HL-60 cell differentiation, and HL-60 cells appear to be an appropriate model for evaluation of the bioactivity of ether lipids. Also, we anticipate the synthesis of phosphatidylinositol (PI) analogs which may interrupt the proliferation process at an early point and might block cellular proliferation through oncogene product inhibition at two points in the cycle (Fig. 4).

The ether lipids may act as anticancer agents in three ways: (1) by direct inhibition of mammalian cells through cytostatic or cytocidal action, (2) by immunomodulatory effects such as macrophage activation, and (3) by differentiation of malignant cells to the granulocyte type. It may be that all three of these observed effects are mediated through an initial interaction with the cell membrane. It is important to note that these agents do not interact with DNA.

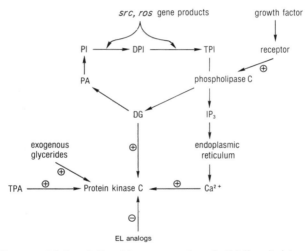

Fig. 4. Proposed interrelationship among phosphatidylinositol turnover, growth factor action, oncogene product activity, and protein kinase C activation. In this model, based on the results of others and our own studies, diacylglycerol (DG) is a central regulatory signal. DG is generated from the breakdown of phosphatidylinositol 4,5-bisphosphate (TPI) (10). The DG stimulates protein kinase C and is rapidly converted to phosphatidic acid (PA) and phosphatidylinositol (PI). TPI breakdown also results in the formation of inositol 1,4,5-trisphosphate, which appears to be an important regulator of intracellular Ca^{2+} concentration (17). The rise in intracellular free Ca^{2+} and the DG are synergistic stimuli for protein kinase C. Protein kinase C can also be stimulated by TPA (9) or exogenous glycerides (11,20) or inhibited by EL (14). Growth factors stimulate PI turnover (28) and the *src* and *ros* oncogene products have been reported to stimulate the turnover of inositol phospholipids (33). Thus, all these regulatory systems appear to be related; however, the relationships are at present unclear.

III. Growth Inhibition and Differentiation by Ether Lipids

The ether lipid analogs were evaluated for growth-inhibitory activity in the HL-60 cell system by hemocytometer counting of viable cells with trypan blue dye exclusion as the end point. Differentiation of HL-60 cells was determined by the morphological appearance of the cells in Wright-Giemsa-stained cytocentrifuge preparations and by nonspecific esterase staining as described previously (22). We found that PAF treatment of the cells resulted in a dose-dependent inhibition of HL-60 cell growth (Fig. 5). Treatment of the cells with 5 μM PAF resulted in no change in the number of viable cells during the 5 days of the experiment. However, 10 μM PAF caused significant cell killing. We also tested the ET-18-OMe analog (**III**) and ET-18S-OMe analog (**VII**) at a concentration of 5 μM and found both these compounds were more effective than PAF at the same molar concentration (Fig. 6). This may be due to the rapid conversion of PAF to 1-alkyl-2-radyl-*sn*-glycero-3-phosphocholine by the HL-60 cells (Fig. 7). Other lipid analogs were tested for growth-inhibitory properties; these are summarized in Table I. The cells were also assayed for the morphological differentiation by Wright-Giemsa staining of cytocentrifuge preparations and were tested for nonspecific esterase activity by staining as described previously (22). We found that the analogs with an *sn*-3 hydroxyl group caused the HL-60 cells to differentiate to cells which resemble macrophages (Fig. 8). These compounds also caused a marked increase in nonspecific esterase staining. For example, treatment with 1-hexadecyl-2-

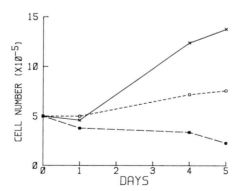

Fig. 5. Effect of PAF on HL-60 cell growth. HL-60 cells were incubated with PAF (racemic) or vehicle (ethanol) control for the times indicated, and viable cell numbers were determined by trypan blue dye exclusion. Control, X- - -X; 5 μM PAF, O- - -O; 10 μM PAF, ●- - -●.

TABLE I

Effect of Lipid Analogs on HL-60 Cell Growth[a]

Analog	Percentage of control (mean ±S.D.)[b]	n
ET-18-OMe	19.7 ± 3.6	13
ET-18-OEt	14.6 ± 3.0**	7
ET-16S-OMe	14.7 ± 5.4**	8
ET-16S-OEt	14.2 ± 3.2**	8
BM 41440	14.8 ± 4.5**	10
ET-18-H	32.2 ± 6.1**	6
CP 46665	43.7 ± 6.1**	12

[a] HL-60 cells (5×10^5 cells/ml) were treated with the compounds listed above. Each compound was tested at 5 μM, and the number of viable cells was determined by trypan blue dye exclusion at 48 hr after treatment. The data are expressed as percentage of vehicle control (ethanol 0.25%).

[b] Values followed by ** signify $p < 0.01$ versus ET-18-OMe.

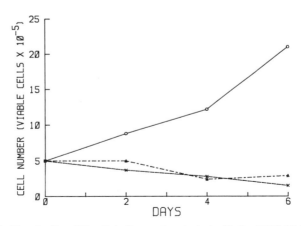

Fig. 6. HL-60 cells (5×10^5 cells/ml) were incubated with 5 μM ET-18-OMe, ▲- - -▲; with 5 μM ET-18S-OMe, X- - -X; or with ethanol (0.25%, vehicle control), ○- - -○. At the times indicated the number of viable cells was determined.

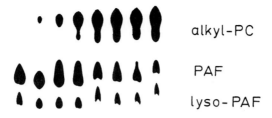

alkyl-PC

PAF

lyso-PAF

.5 1 2 5 10 20 30 60

minutes

Fig. 7. Catabolism of 1-O-[³H]alkyl-2-acetyl-*sn*-glycero-3-phosphocholine (PAF). HL-60 cells, 3 × 10⁷ cells/ml, were incubated with [³H]PAF, 10^{-8} *M* (45 Ci/mmole), in minimum essential medium containing 2.5% bovine serum albumin. At the indicated times the lipids were extracted with chloroform and methanol, and the extracted lipids were chromatographed on Silica Gel 60 plates (E. Merck, Darmstadt, Federal Republic of Germany) in a solvent system consisting of chloroform, methanol, acetic acid, and water (50 : 25 : 8 : 4). Products were identified by their comigration with authentic standards. The standards used were PAF, 1-alkyl-*sn*-glycero-3-phosphocholine (lyso-PAF), and 1-alkyl-2-acyl-*sn*-glycero-3-phosphocholine (alkyl-PC).

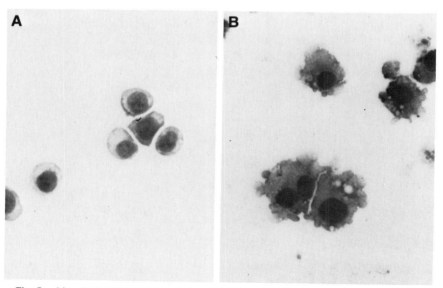

Fig. 8. Morphological changes induced by alkyl AG. HL-60 cells were prepared and stained as described (22). Undifferentiated HL-60 cells after 6-day incubation with vehicle control are shown at the left (A). HL-60 cells treated with 10 μg of alkyl AG/ml exhibited macrophage-like pseudopodia, eccentric nuclei, and condensed nucleoli, which appear at the right (B).

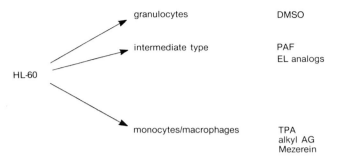

Fig. 9. Summary of the effects of tumor promoters and lipid mediators on HL-60 cell differentiation. See text for discussion.

acetyl-*sn*-glycerol resulted in an increase in nonspecific esterase (NSE) staining from 7 to 69% of the cells in 6 days. Cells treated with PAF or ET-18-OMe did not have an increased staining for nonspecific esterase and demonstrated some morphological changes which resemble granulocytes. A functional characteristic of HL-60 cells differentiated to granulocyte-like cells by dimethyl sulfoxide (DMSO) treatment is the ability to synthe-

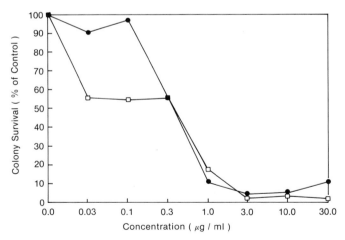

Fig. 10. Effect of ET-18-OMe (●) and ET-16S-OEt (□) on colony growth of human ovarian adenocarcinoma cell line, BG-1. Cells were initiated in soft agarose clonogenic culture, then treated by continuous exposure to the phospholipid analogs over a three-log range of concentrations (36). Untreated cultures served as controls. After 7-day incubation at 37°C at 7.5% CO_2, colony formation from the single cell suspension was evaluated by inverted microscopy and automated image analysis. All experiments were done in triplicate.

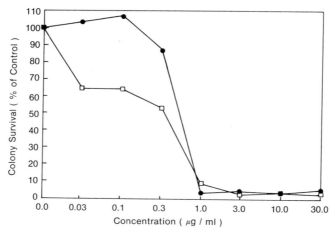

Fig. 11. Effect of ET-18-OMe (●) and ET-16S-OEt (□) on colony growth of human ovarian adenocarcinoma cell line, BG-3. Details of the experiment are as in Fig. 10.

size 5-hydroxyeicosatetraenoic (5-HETE) and leukotriene B_4 (LTB$_4$) in response to challenge with the Ca^{2+} ionophore A23187 (L. W. Daniel and S. C. Olson, unpublished data). ET-18-OMe-differentiated cells did not synthesize LTB$_4$ or 5-HETE (data not shown). Therefore these cells appear to be an intermediate type between those induced by DMSO and those induced by TPA (Fig. 9).

We have evaluated two analogs, compounds (**III**) and (**IV**), for inhibitory activity against two human ovarian carcinoma cell lines in soft agarose culture, in the BG-1 and BG-3 ovarian adenocarcinoma cell lines (36); the results are given in graphic form in Figs. 10 and 11. It is encouraging to note that the thio analog, compound (**IV**), is more active than the positive control, compound (**III**), in both cell lines. At concentrations of 0.03 and 0.1 μg/ml, the previously unreported thio analog compound (**IV**) is about twice as active as the widely studied compound (**III**), ET-18-OCH$_3$: Runge *et al.* (29) reported compound (**III**) to be the most active phospholipid analog tested against human ovarian carcinoma cells in culture.

IV. A Look to the Future

On the basis of carrying out and correlating multiple biological and preclinical studies as outlined previously, we hope to expand our mechanistic and pharmacologic studies and to identify a good candidate analog for clinical trial as a cancer chemotherapeutic agent—either alone or in combination with a DNA-interactive cytotoxic drug.

Acknowledgments

These studies are being supported by research grants CA 12197, CA 41314, and HL 28491 from the National Institutes of Health, U.S. Department of Health and Human Services, and by the Forsyth Cancer Service. Thanks are due to Dr. Alessandro Noseda, Department of Biochemistry, Bowman Gray School of Medicine, for his recent contributions to this program. Dr. Noseda is supported by a fellowship from Dr. Luciano Berti, Champion Industries, Winston-Salem, North Carolina.

References

1. Andreesen, R., Modolell, M., Weltzien, H. U., Eibl, H. H., Common, H. H., Lohr, G. W., and Munder, P. G. (1978). Selective destruction of human leukemic cells by alkyl-lysophospholipids. *Cancer Res.* **38**, 3894–3899.
2. Berdel, W. E., Fink, U., Egger, B., Reichert, A., Munder, P. G., and Rastetter, J. (1981). Growth inhibition of malignant hypernephroma cells by autologous lysophospholipid incubated macrophages obtained by a new method. *Anticancer Res.* **1**, 135–140.
3. Berdel, W. E., Bausert, W. R. E., Fink, U., Rastetter, J., and Munder, P. G. (1981). Anti-tumor action of alkyl-lysophospholipids. *Anticancer Res.* **1**, 345–352.
4. Berdel, W. E., Fromm, M., Fink, U., Pahlke, W., Bicker, U., Reichert, A., and Rastetter, J. (1983). Cytotoxicity of thioether-lysophospholipids in leukemias and tumors of human origin. *Cancer Res.* **43**, 5538–5543.
5. Berdel, W. E., Greiner, E., Fink, U., Stavrou, D., Reichert, A., Rastetter, J., Hoffman, D. R., and Snyder, F. (1983). Cytotoxicity of alkyl-lysophospholipid derivatives and low-alkyl-cleavage enzyme activities in rat brain tumor cells. *Cancer Res.* **43**, 541–545.
6. Berdel, W. E., Andreesen, R., and Munder, P. G. (1985). Synthetic alkyl-phospholipid analogs: A new class of antitumor agents. *In* "Phospholipids and Cellular Regulation" (J. F. Kuo, ed.), Vol. 2, pp. 41–73. CRC Press, Boca Raton, Florida.
7. Berdel, W. E., Schick, H. D., Fink, U., Reichert, A., Ulm, K., and Rastetter, J. (1985). Cytotoxicity of the alkyl-linked lipoidal amine 4-aminomethyl-1-[(2,3-di-*n*-decyloxy)*n*-propyl]-4-phenylpiperidine (CP-46,665) in cells from human tumors and leukemias. *Cancer Res.* **45**, 1206–1213.
8. Blank, M. L., Snyder, F., Byers, L. W., Brooks, B., and Muirhead, E. E. (1979). Antihypertensive activity of an alkyl ether analog of phosphatidylcholine. *Biochem. Biophys. Res. Commun.* **90**, 1194–1200.
9. Castagna, M., Takai, Y., Kaibuchi, K., Sano, K., Kikkawa, Y., and Nishizuka, Y. (1982). Direct activation of calcium-activated, phospholipid-dependent protein kinase by tumor-promoting phorbol esters. *J. Biol. Chem.* **257**, 7847–7851.
10. Daniel, L. W. (1985). Phospholipases. *In* "Prostaglandins, Leukotrienes and Cancer" (K. V. Honn and L. L. Marnett, eds.), Vol. 1, pp. 175–193. Martinus Nijhoff, Hingham, Massachusetts.

11. Ebeling, J. G., Vandenbark, G. R., Kuhn, L. J., Ganong, B. R., Bell, R. M., and Niedel, J. E. (1985). Diacylglycerols mimic phorbol diester induction of leukemic cell differentiation. *Proc. Natl. Acad. Sci. U.S.A.* **82**, 815–819.
12. Glasser, L., Somberg, L. B., and Vogler, W. R. (1984). Purging murine leukemic marrow with alkyl-lysophospholipids. *Blood* **64**, 1288–1291.
13. Hanahan, D. J., Demopoulos, C. A., Liehr, J., and Pinckard, R. N. (1980). Identification of platelet activating factor isolated from rabbit basophils as acetyl glyceryl ether phosphorylcholine. *J. Biol. Chem.* **255**, 5514–5516.
14. Helfman, D. M., Barnes, K. C., Kinkade, J. M., Jr., Vogler, W. R., Shoji, M., and Kuo, J. F. (1983). Phosopholipid-sensitive Ca^{2+}-dependent protein phosphorylation system in various types of leukemic cells from human patients and in human leukemic cell lines HL60 and K562, and its inhibition by alkyl-lysophospholipid. *Cancer Res.* **43**, 2955–2961.
15. Hoffman, D. R., Hajdu, J., and Snyder, F. (1984). Cytotoxicity of platelet activating factor and related alkyl-phospholipid analogs in human leukemia cells, polymorphonuclear neutrophils, and skin fibroblasts. *Blood* **63**, 545–552.
16. Honma, Y., Kasukabe, T., Hozumi, M., Tsushima, S., and Nomura, H. (1981). Induction of differentiation of cultured human and mouse myeloid leukemia cells by alkyl-lysophospholipids. *Cancer Res.* **41**, 3211–3216.
17. Joseph, S. K., Thomas, A. P., Williams, R. J., Irvine, R. F., and Williamson, J. R. (1984). *myo*-Inositol 1,4,5-trisphosphate: A second messenger for the hormonal mobilization of intracellular Ca^{2+} in liver. *J. Biol. Chem.* **259**, 3077–3081.
18. Kaibuchi, K., Sawamura, M., Katakami, Y., Kikkawa, V., Takai, Y., and Nishizuka, Y. (1985). Calcium and phospholipid degradation in signal transduction. *In* "Inositol and Phosphoinositides: Metabolism and Regulation" (J. E. Bleasdale, J. Eichberg, and G. Hauser, eds.), pp. 385–398. Humana Press, Clifton, New Jersey.
19. Lapetina, E. G., Watson, S. P., and Cuatrecasas, P. (1984). *myo*-Inositol 1,4,5-trisphosphate stimulates protein phosphorylation in saponin-permeabilized human platelets. *Proc. Natl. Acad. Sci. U.S.A.* **81**, 7431–7435.
20. Lapetina, E. G., Reep, B., Ganong, B. R., and Bell, R. M. (1985). Exogenous *sn*-1,2-diacylglycerols containing saturated fatty acids function as bioregulators of protein kinase C in human platelets. *J. Biol. Chem.* **260**, 1358–1361.
21. Lee, T-C., Blank, M. L., Fitzgerald, V., and Snyder, F. (1981). Substrate specificity in the biocleavage of the *O*-alkyl bond: 1-alkyl-2-acetyl-*sn*-glycero-3-phosphocholine (a hypotensive and platelet-activating lipid) and its metabolites. *Arch. Biochem. Biophys.* **208**, 353–357.
22. McNamara, M. J. C., Schmitt, J. D., Wykle, R. L., and Daniel, L. W. (1984). 1-*O*-Hexadecyl-2-acetyl-*sn*-glycerol stimulates differentiation of HL-60 human promyelocytic leukemia cells to macrophage-like cells. *Biochem. Biophys. Res. Commun.* **122**, 824–830.
23. Modest, E. J., Daniel, L. W., Berens, M. E., Morris-Natschke, S., Surles, J. R., and Piantadosi, C. (1986). Novel ether lipid analogs as membrane-active antitumor agents. *Proc. Am. Assoc. Cancer Res.* **27**, 275.
24. Morris-Natschke, S., Surles, J. R., Daniel, L. W., Berens, M. E., Modest, E. J., and Piantadosi, C. (1986). Synthesis of sulfur analogues of alkyl lysophospholipid and neoplastic cell growth inhibitory properties. *J. Med. Chem.* **29**, (in press).
25. O'Flaherty, J. T., Wykle, R. L., Miller, C. H., Lewis, J. C., Waite, M., Bass, D. A., McCall, C. E., and DeChatelet, L. R. (1981). 1-*O*-Alkyl-*sn*-3-phosphorylcholines: A novel class of neutrophil stimulants. *Am. J. Pathol.* **103**, 70–78.

26. O'Flaherty, J. T., Salzer, W. L., Cousart, S., McCall, C. E., Piantadosi, C., Surles, J. R., Hammett, M. J., and Wykle, R. L. (1983). Platelet activating factor and analogues: Comparative studies with human neutrophils and rabbit platelets. *Res. Commun. Chem. Pathol. Parmacol.* **39**, 291–309.

27. Rovera, G., Santoli, D., and Damsky, C. (1979). Human promyelocytic leukemia cells in culture differentiate into macrophage-like cells when treated with a phorbol diester. *Proc. Natl. Acad. Sci. U.S.A.* **76**, 2779–2783.

28. Rozengurt, E., Rodriguez-Pena, M., and Smith, K. A. (1983). Phorbol esters, phospholipase C and growth factors rapidly stimulate the phosphorylation of a Mr 80,000 protein in intact quiescent 3T3 cells. *Proc. Natl. Acad. Sci. U.S.A.* **80**, 7244–7248.

29. Runge, M. H., Andreesen, R., Pfleiderer, A., and Munder, P. G. (1980). Destruction of human solid tumors by alkyl lysophospholipids. *JNCI, J. Natl. Cancer Inst.* **64**, 1301–1306.

30. Snyder, F., Malone, B., and Piantadosi, C. (1973). Tetrahydropteridine-dependent cleavage enzyme for *O*-alkyl lipids: Substrate specificity. *Biochim. Biophys. Acta* **316**, 259–265.

31. Soodsma, J. F., Piantadosi, C., and Snyder, F. (1970). The biocleavage of alkyl glyceryl ethers in Morris hepatomas and other transplantable neoplasms. *Cancer Res.* **30**, 309–311.

32. Storme, G. A., Berdel, W. E., van Blitterswijk, W. J., Bruyneel, E. A., De Bruyne, G. K., and Mareel, M. M. (1985). Antiinvasive effect of racemic 1-*O*-octadecyl-2-*O*-methylglycero-3-phosphocholine on MO₄ mouse fibrosarcoma cells *in vitro*. *Cancer Res.* **45**, 351–357.

33. Sugimoto, Y., Whitman, M., Cantley, L. C., and Erickson, R. L. (1984). Evidence that the Rous sarcoma virus transforming gene product phosphorylates phosphatidylinositol and diacylglycerol. *Proc. Natl. Acad. Sci. U.S.A.* **81**, 2117–2121.

34. Tencé, M., Polonsky, J., Le Couedic, J. P., and Benveniste, J. (1980). Release, purification, and characterization of platelet-activating factor (PAF). *Biochimie* **62**, 251–259.

35. Terashita, Z.-i., Tsushima, S., Yoshioka, Y., Nomura, H., Inada, Y., and Nishikawa, K. (1983). CV-3988—a specific antagonist of platelet activating factor (PAF). *Life Sci.* **32**, 1975–1982.

36. Welander, C. E., Morgan, T. M., Homesley, H. D., Trotta, P. P., and Spiegel, R. J. (1985). Combined recombinant human interferon alpha₂ and cytotoxic agents studied in a clonogenic assay. *Int. J. Cancer* **35**, 721–729.

37. Weltzein, H. U. (1979). Cytolytic and membrane-perturbing properties of lysophosphatidylcholine. *Biochim. Biophys. Acta* **559**, 259–287.

38. Wykle, R. L., Surles, J. R., Piantadosi, C., Salzer, W. L., and O'Flaherty, J. T. (1982). Platelet activating factor (1-*O*-alkyl-2-*O*-acetyl-*sn*-glycero-3-phosphocholine): Activity of analogs lacking oxygen at the 2-position. *FEBS Lett.* **141**, 29–32.

New Preclinical Anticancer Leads in Development at the National Cancer Institute

V. L. NARAYANAN

Drug Synthesis and Chemistry Branch
Developmental Therapeutics Program
Division of Cancer Treatment
National Cancer Institute
Bethesda, Maryland

I. Introduction

The Division of Cancer Treatment of the National Cancer Institute (NCI) actively supports a continuing program to identify and develop novel anticancer leads with clinical potential. Comprehensive descriptions of the preclinical drug discovery and development program currently in place at NCI have recently become available (1,4). This chapter will describe the significant aspects of our new lead identification and development program from a preclinical perspective including (1) preselection, (2) the chemical structures and antitumor activity of the recent

NEW AVENUES IN DEVELOPMENTAL
CANCER CHEMOTHERAPY

leads, especially of synthetic origin that are under active development, and (3) screening new approaches.

II. Anticancer Screens

The majority of the new drug leads are discovered through the "semirational" approach of screening. Once a lead is identified, it can be optimized through congener synthesis and structure–activity fine tuning. However, the development of clinically predictable animal tumor models continues to be a major challenge. The biological systems that are used to evaluate compounds for anticancer activity are summarized in Table I. The mouse P388 leukemia model is used as a prescreen to select new compounds for secondary evaluation against a panel of tumors. Occasionally, the P388 prescreen is bypassed for compounds that have shown either (1) activity in antitumor screens not available at NCI or (2) other relevant biochemical or biological activities.

The tumor panel consisted of eight cancer models in mice—five transplanted mouse tumors (L1210 leukemia, B16 melanoma, colon, breast, and lung) and three human tumor xenografts (colon, breast, and lung) implanted under the kidney capsules of mice. As a result of retrospective analysis, the tumor panel has been modified recently; the current panel consisting of three transplanted mouse tumors, L1210 leukemia, B16 melanoma, and M5076 sarcoma, and the mammary human tumor xenograft implanted under the kidney capsule of mice. Two different parameters are used for evaluating the activity of a compound, namely, either the increase in life-span of the treated mice versus control or the reduction in tumor weight. An excellent discussion of *in vivo* anticancer screening experience at NCI has recently been published (9).

III. Preselection

We use a variety of criteria to select compounds for screening and extensively scan the literature to identify a rational basis for selecting compounds for screening, e.g., antitumor activity reported in other screening programs, compounds reported to exhibit relevant biochemical and other biological activities, and structural features suggestive of effects on enzymatic processes relevant to cancer chemotherapy. By and large, however, the majority of compounds come only with structural information. We have developed a computerized model that aids us in

TABLE I

Summary of *in Vivo* Anticancer Screens

Model	Code	Drug route/ schedule[a]	Parameter	Active T/C (%)	
				DN1 (+)	DN2 (++)
Prescreen					
IP P388 leukemia	3PS31	IP/Q1D × 5	Median survival time	≥120	≥175
Transplanted mouse tumors					
IP B16 melanoma	3B131	IP/Q1D × 9	Median survival time	≥125	≥150
SC B16 melanoma	3B132	IP/Q1D × 9	Median survival time	≥140	≥150
SC CD8F₁ mammary	3CDJ2	IP/Q1D × 1	Median tumor weight change	≤20	≤0
	3CD72	IP/Q7D × 5	Median tumor weight	≤42	≤10
IP colon 26	3C631	IP/Q4D × 2	Median survival time	≥130	≥150
SC colon 38	3C872	IP/Q7D × 2	Median tumor weight	≤42	≤10
IC ependymoblastoma	3EM37	IP/Q1D × 5	Median survival time	≥125	≥150
IV Lewis lung	3LL39	IP/Q1D × 9	Median survival time	≥140	≥150
IP L1210 leukemia	3LE31	IP/Q1D × 9	Median survival time	≥125	≥150
	3LE21	IP/Q1D × 9	Mean survival time	≥125	≥150
SC M5 ovarian	3M572	IP/Q2D × 11	Median survival time	≥125	≥150
Human tumor xenografts					
SRC CX-1 colon	3C2G5	SC/Q4D × 4	Mean tumor weight change	≤20	≤10
SC CX-1 colon	3C2H2	IP/Q4D × 3	Mean tumor weight change	≤20	≤10
SRC LX-1 lung	3LKG5	SC/Q4D × 3	Mean tumor weight change	≤20	≤10
SC LX-1 lung	3LKH2	IP/Q4D × 3	Mean tumor weight change	≤20	≤10
SRC MX-1 mammary	3MBG5	SC/Q4D × 3	Mean tumor weight change	≤20	≤10
SC MX-1 mammary	3MBH2	IP/Q4D × 3	Mean tumor weight change	≤20	≤10

[a] IP, intraperitoneally; SC, subcutaneously; Q1D, every day; Q2D every 2 days; etc.

selecting compounds for screening based on structural information alone (2,3). This model has been refined over the years.

A. Computer Model

The main features of the computer model are the following: (1) it evaluates a broad range of compounds; (2) it utilizes structural fragments (keys); (3) it utilizes the NCI screening experience with P388, L1210, and B16; and finally (4) the model integrates the massive volume of structural data and screening experience to predict novelty and activity for each compound under consideration.

The features used are those routinely generated as keys for the substructure inquiry system. The system incorporates an open-ended feature set as opposed to a dictionary (roughly 8000 structural features). The main types of keys are (1) augmented atom keys (AA), (2) ganglia augmented atom keys (GAA), (3) ring keys, (4) two kinds of nucleus keys, and (5) individual element keys (Fig. 1). The method assigns weight to each feature according to the statistical significance of its contribution to activity, using the P388, L1210, and B16 screening data. An unknown compound is scored by adding the weights of its dozen or so structure features. The score is not intended to estimate the strength of activity but only to provide some measure of the likelihood that the compound is active.

Another useful measure supplied by the computer is an indication of novelty based on the large number of compounds tested against P388, L1210, and B16, regardless of activity. Compounds are flagged as unique if they have a key which never occurred in all P388, L1210, and B16 testing. For each new compound, the feature that occurs least often is printed along with its frequency of occurrence. If the least occurring key in the compound occurred more than 100 times, the compound is considered adequately studied. Novelty scores are even more useful in selecting compounds for acquisition.

It must be emphasized that although this method is computerized, it is not designed to automatically pass or reject compounds. Rather, it is proposed as a tool to aid the medicinal chemist in selecting compounds. In practice, we find the method to be very useful in deselecting compounds from screening. The acquisition selection process is summarized in Fig. 2.

B. Structure–Activity Analysis

Detailed structure–activity analyses based on our large chemical–biological database are an integral part of our acquisition and synthesis activities. The large-scale analyses of NCI data files have become feasible

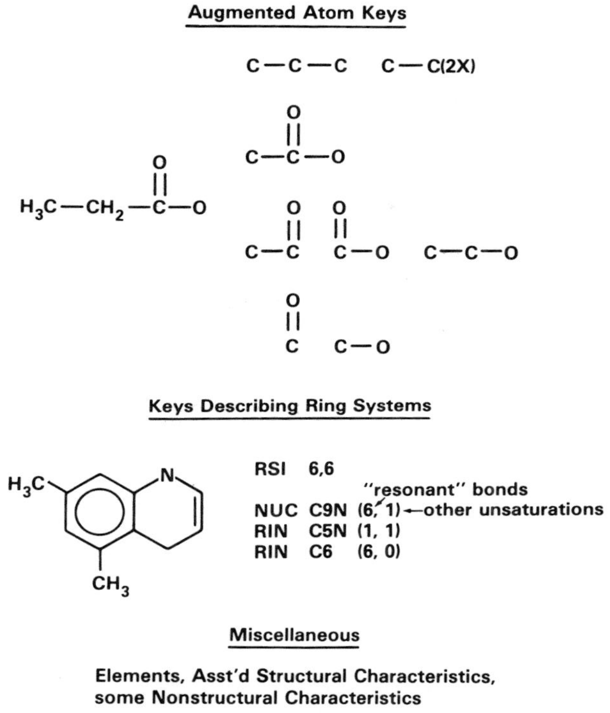

Augmented Atom Keys

$$C-C-C \quad C-C(2X)$$

$$C-\overset{\overset{\displaystyle O}{\|}}{C}-O$$

$$H_3C-CH_2-\overset{\overset{\displaystyle O}{\|}}{C}-O$$

$$C-\overset{\overset{\displaystyle O}{\|}}{C} \quad \overset{\overset{\displaystyle O}{\|}}{C}-O \quad C-C-O$$

$$\overset{\overset{\displaystyle O}{\|}}{C} \quad C-O$$

Keys Describing Ring Systems

RSI 6,6

"resonant" bonds

NUC C9N (6, 1) ←other unsaturations

RIN C5N (1, 1)

RIN C6 (6, 0)

Miscellaneous

Elements, Asst'd Structural Characteristics, some Nonstructural Characteristics

Fig. 1. Structural fragments (keys).

because of the development of the chemistry–biology interlink and its active implementation during the past couple of years. Such structure–activity analyses allow us to select compounds for screening by maximizing structural uniqueness and anticancer potential. It also allows us to identify gap areas for further research. We have recently published a few such structure–activity analyses on important classes of compounds (5–7).

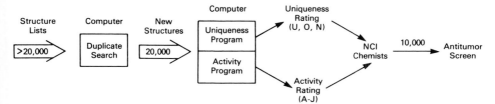

Fig. 2. Acquisition selection process.

IV. Current Preclinical Leads

Figure 3 illustrates several examples of novel synthetic compounds that are currently under active development. The chemical structure of each compound as well as its spectrum of anticancer activity is indicated. In

(A)

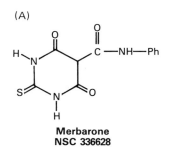

Merbarone
NSC 336628

Tumor Model	Activity
P_{388}	++
L_{1210} (i.p; s.c.)	++
B_{16}	++
M_{5076}	++

(B)

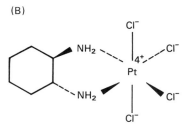

Tetraplatin
NSC 363812

Tumor Model	Activity
P_{388}	++
P_{388}/Cisplatin	++
L_{1210} (i.p.; s.c.)	++
L_{1210}/Cisplatin	++
B_{16}	++
M_{5076}	++
Mx1	++

(C)

Ara AC
NSC 281272

Tumor Model	Activity
P_{388}	++
L_{1210}	++
B_{16}	+
LL	++
Cx1	++
Lx1	++
Mx1	++

Fig. 3. Examples of novel synthetic compounds currently under active development.

(D)

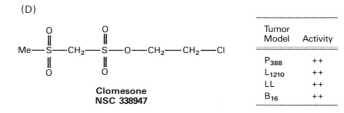

**Clomesone
NSC 338947**

Tumor Model	Activity
P$_{388}$	++
L$_{1210}$	++
LL	++
B$_{16}$	++

(E)

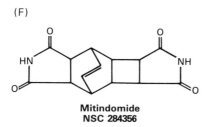

**Cyclodisone
NSC 348948**

Tumor Model	Activity
P$_{388}$	++
L$_{1210}$ (i.p.; s.c.; i.c.)	++
B$_{16}$	++
M$_{5076}$	++

(F)

**Mitindomide
NSC 284356**

Tumor Model	Activity
P$_{388}$	++
L$_{1210}$	++
B$_{16}$	+
CD8F$_1$	++
C38	+

(G)

**Diazohydroxide
NSC 361456**

Tumor Model	Activity
P$_{388}$	++
L$_{1210}$	++
B$_{16}$	++
Mx1	++
M$_{5076}$	++

Fig. 3. (*Continued*)

(H)

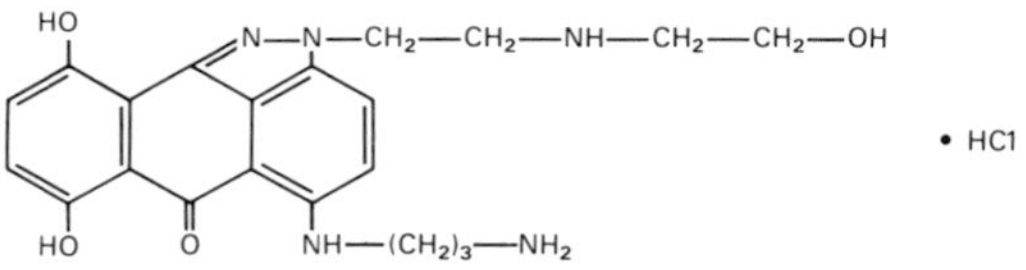

Anthrapyrazole Derivative
NSC 349174

• HCl

Tumor Model	Activity
P_{388}	++
L_{1210} (i.p.; s.c.)	++
B_{16}	++
M_{5076}	++
Mx1	++

(I)

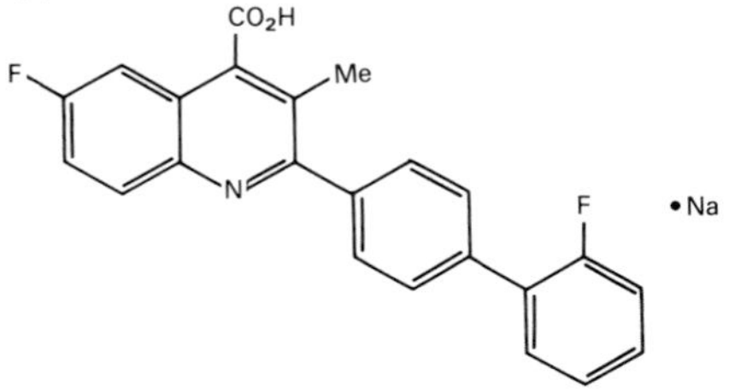

Bipenquinate
NSC 368390

• Na

Tumor Model	Activity
L_{1210} (i.p.; s.c.; p.o.)	++
B_{16}	+
C38	+
Lx1	++
Mx1	++

(J)

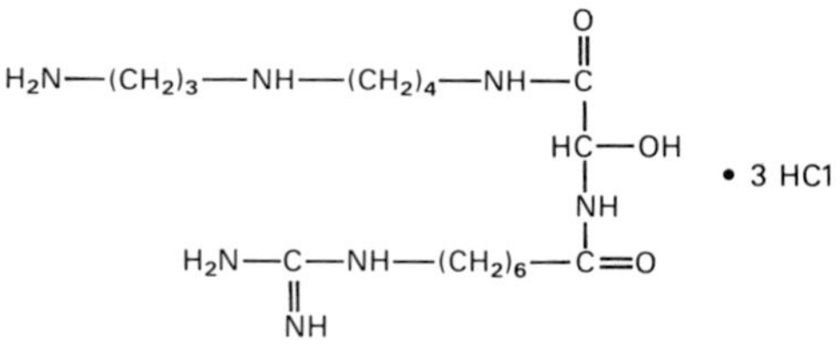

Deoxyspergualin
NSC 356894
Natural Product

• 3 HCl

Tumor Model	Activity
L_{1210} (i.p.; s.c.)	++

(K)

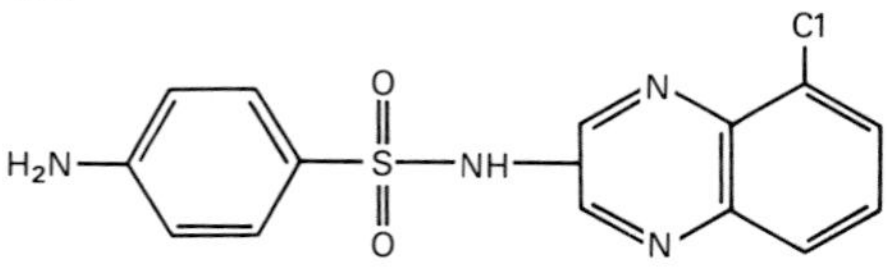

Quinoxaline Derivative
NSC 3390048

In vitro Model	Activity
HTCFA	++

Fig. 3.   (Continued)

(L)

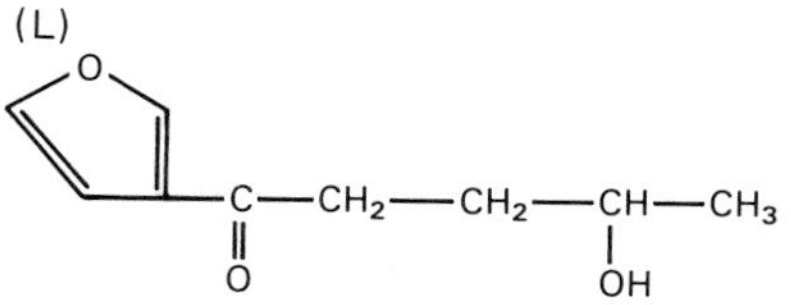

4-Ipomeanol
NSC 349438
Natural Product

Toxicity
Highly Specific Lung Toxin

(M)

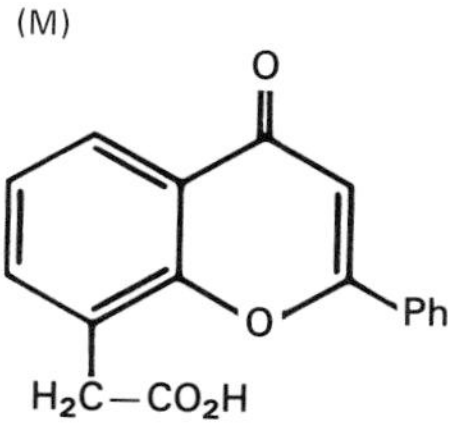

Flavone acetic acid
NSC 347512

Tumor Model	Activity
L_{1210}	+
B_{16}	++
C38	++

Fig. 3. (*Continued*)

particular, we would like to draw attention to flavone acetic acid (NSC 347512), whose antitumor activity is exceptional for both its specificity against subcutaneously implanted mouse colon 38, a tumor that has been refractory to most compounds tested, and its high degree of activity (8).

V. Future Directions

Recently NCI is undertaking a major restructuring of its anticancer drug screening program (10, 11). The restructuring represents a shift in emphasis from a "compound-oriented" strategy to a specific "disease-oriented" strategy focusing on major solid tumors for which there has been limited success in identifying active drugs. We will be replacing the mouse leukemia P388 prescreen with a new *in vitro* prescreen system consisting of panels of human tumor cell lines. The initial focus will be *in vitro* antitumor drug screening utilizing a panel of cell lines composed principally of human lung tumor cell lines. Compounds showing highly selective *in vitro* activity against a target tumor type would be earmarked for preclinical development and clinical trials in relevant target populations. Compounds showing a nonselective pattern of *in vitro* activity would be studied further in an "*in vivo*" tumor panel for antitumor activity. In order to provide a head-to-head comparison of the new "disease-oriented" strategy with the current strategy, compounds will be screened by both the systems for a period of 1 year. The emerging results will guide the future directions of the new anticancer drug screening program.

References

1. Driscoll, J. S. (1984). The preclinical new drug research program of the National Cancer Institute. *Cancer. Treat. Rep.* **68,** 63–76.
2. Hodes, L. (1981). Selection of molecular fragment features for structure-activity studies in antitumor screening. *J. Chem. Inf. Comput. Sci.* **21,** 132–136.
3. Hodes, L. (1981). Computer-aided selection of compounds for anti-tumor screening: Validation of a statistical - heuristic method. *J. Chem. Inf. Comput. Sci.* **21,** 128–132.
4. Narayanan, V. L. (1983). Strategy for the discovery and development of novel anticancer agents. *In* "Structure-Activity Relationships of Antitumor Agents" (D. H. Reinhoudt, T. A. Connors, H. M. Pinedo, and Van de Poll, eds.), pp 5–22. Martinus Nijhoff Publishers, The Hague.
5. Nasr, M., Paull, K. D., and Narayanan, V. L. (1984). Computer-assisted structure-activity correlations. *Adv. Pharmacol. Chemother.* **20,** 123–190.
6. Nasr, M., Paull, K. D., and Narayanan, V. L. (1984). Computer-assisted structure-anticancer activity correlations of carbamates and thiocarbamates. *J. Pharm. Sci.* **74,** 831–836.
7. Paull, K. D., Nasr, M., and Narayanan, V. L. (1984). Computer-assisted structure-activity correlations; evaluation of benzo (de) isoquinoline-1,3-diones and related compounds as antitumor agents. *Arzneim.-Forsch.* **34** (11), 1243–1246.
8. Plowman, J., Narayanan, V. L., Szarvasi, E., Briet, P., Yoder, O. C., and Paull, K. D. (1986). Flavone acetic acid (NSC 347512), a novel agent with preclinical antitumor activity against the colon adenocarcinoma 38 in mice. *Cancer Treat. Rep.* **70,** 631–635.
9. Venditti, J. M., Wesley, R. A., and Plowman, J. (1984). Current NCI preclinical antitumor screening *in-vivo:* Results of tumor panel screening, 1976–1982, and future directions. *Adv. Pharmacol. Chemother.* **20,** 1–20.
10. Boyd, M. R. (1986). NCI New drug development program. *In* "Cancer Therapy: Where Do We Go from Here?" (Frei and Freireich, eds.), Proceedings of the General Motors Cancer Research Foundation Conference, Jackson Hole, Wyoming, Sept. 14–15, 1984. Lippincott, Philadelphia, Pennsylvania. (In press.)
11. Boyd, M. R., McLemore, T., Johnston, M., Gazdav, A., Minna, J., and Shoemaker, R. (1986). Drug development. *In* "Thoracic Oncology" (Roth, Ruckdeschel, and Weisenburger, eds.), Chapter 51. Saunders, New York. (In press.)

PART VI

Oncogenes as a Target for Drug Design

21

Specific Genes Involved in Oncogenesis

ROBIN A. WEISS

The Institute of Cancer Research
Chester Beatty Laboratories
London, United Kingdom

I. Introduction

There is a sense of excitement in cancer research today about new findings and concepts that are arising from molecular biology. Most of the interest centers upon oncogenes, genes present in our normal genetic makeup that become altered in their structure or expression in cancer cells. A small number of identifiable genes, perhaps no more than 50 out of the 50,000 in the human genome, appear to be functionally involved in the neoplastic phenotype. Genes encode proteins, and by identifying the products of specific oncogenes and how they function as enzymes or structural components of the cell, we can begin to discern what makes tumor cells different from normal cells.

The oncogene concept of neoplasia has gained wide acceptance through studies made possible by laboratory manipulation of DNA and has brought together the hitherto disparate disciplines of cytogenetics, chemi-

NEW AVENUES IN DEVELOPMENTAL
CANCER CHEMOTHERAPY

cal carcinogenesis, and viral oncology. This new understanding opens the possibility of developing drugs and biological response modifiers that are directly targeted to those proteins in cells that become altered to produce the malignant state. Such drugs should be effective in specifically killing or blocking the growth of cancer cells while sparing normal tissues. However, these studies are only at their inception, and the differences between oncogenes and their counterparts in normal cells are so subtle that the development of selective drugs will require sustained effort based on a detailed understanding of the molecular genetics of cancer.

II. Somatic Mutation and Cancer

The notion that carcinogenesis involves somatic genetic change dates from the rediscovery of Mendelian genetics at the turn of the century. Theodor Boveri identified chromosomes as the repository of genetic material and speculated on chromosome imbalance causing cancer, though it was not until the discovery of the Philadelphia chromosome in 1960 that tumor-specific chromosomal deletions and translocations were recognized. The link between mutation and cancer was first drawn by H. J. Muller in 1927, who demonstrated the mutagenicity of ionizing radiation, and then by C. Auerbach in 1946, who showed that the chemical carcinogen mustard gas also induced mutations. Widescale screening by Ames and others more recently has shown that most carcinogens or their active metabolites are mutagens. Since the late 1970s recombinant DNA technology has provided the means to isolate individual genes, and attention began to focus on which genes are involved in oncogenesis.

The somatic mutation hypothesis of cancer presupposes the clonal origin of the tumor cell population. Where this has been amenable to investigation by isoenzyme analysis or recombinant DNA techniques, most tumors studied have indeed been found to be monoclonal, and studies on oncogenes have shown that one or more are altered in at least 20%, and probably the majority of human tumors are altered by somatic mutation or gene rearrangement. That cancer always involves irreversible genetic change has, however, been challenged by those who hold that cancer is epigenetic in character, being no more heritable than normal processes of cell differentiation, in which only lymphoid cells have been shown to undergo gene rearrangement (see Rabbitts *et al.,* Chapter 25). Cancer may be viewed as a clonal population of cells, which is partly arrested in maturation and in which the processes of proliferation and differentiation have become uncoupled (Sachs, Chapter 7). While such derangement is usually found to involve genetic change, mutation might not invariably be required for the development of neoplasia.

The epigenetic nature of cancer was strongly advocated by Smithers in the 1960s when he attacked what he called "cytologism," or the individual cellular basis of malignancy. "Cancer," he stated in 1962, "is no more a disease of cells than a traffic jam is a disease of cars. A lifetime of study of the internal-combustion engine would not help anyone to understand our traffic problems. A traffic jam is due to a failure of the normal relationship between driven cars and their environment and can occur whether they themselves are running normally or not." This holistic philosophy has recently been championed by Rubin and others. Moreover, studies on the incorporation of teratocarcinoma stem cells into normal tissues of the mouse after their inoculation into the embryo blastocyst give some credence to the view that cancer is reversible. Cancer cells are, of course, highly dependent on their environment within the body to express their malignant potential. Nevertheless, it is the reductionist analysis of the molecular genetics of tumor cells that has given us our recent insights into neoplasia and that promises a rational approach to new modes of treatment.

III. Identification of Oncogenes

Specific genes inducing neoplastic transformation were first identified in tumor viruses. Many of these viruses can transform cells in culture and are therefore amenable to genetic analysis by inducing mutations in the virus that affect cell transformation. For DNA tumor viruses, such as SV40 (discussed by Skene, Chapter 24), the transforming genes are essential genes for early steps in the replication of the virus, being required for the initiation of DNA synthesis and similar functions. But the products of these genes also interact with cellular DNA or with normal cellular proteins that in turn affect cellular DNA synthesis, and in this way the viral gene product promotes cell transformation. Analysis of the differential expression of cellular genes in cells transformed by tumor viruses has revealed a common set of genes, activated in cells transformed both by tumor viruses and by other carcinogens (see Skene, Chapter 24).

Some retroviruses also carry specific oncogenes, but these are not required for viral replication. Rather, they represent cellular genes that have been captured or transduced into the viral genome and then act as oncogenes when reintroduced into cells by infection, as they operate under the strong signals for gene expression from viral promoter and enhancer sequences. Transducing retroviruses are rare in nature but have proved to be invaluable as laboratory tools for exploring molecular carcinogenesis. Some 20 different retrovirus oncogenes have been described, each with its normal cellular homolog. These oncogenes have been captured by retroviruses after the insertion of the provirus into chromosomal DNA, resulting in the activation of adjacent cellular genes. If such a gene is a potential oncogene, its ectopic expression can lead to cell transformation.

Naturally occurring leukemogenic retroviruses, however, do not carry oncogenes themselves but exert their neoplastic effect when, by chance, they integrate next to a cellular protooncogene and enhance its expression.

IV. Oncogene Products

The products of retrovirus oncogenes and their cellular homologs act at different sites in the cell, connected in a complex network of control processes for cell proliferation (Fig. 1). Some oncogenes, such as *myc* and *fos,* encode proteins that become located in the nucleus and are thought to be involved in binding to DNA and to nuclear matrix proteins. This may result in the initiation of cellular DNA synthesis. Such oncoproteins will therefore drive the cell into a proliferative state without requiring any external stimuli for growth, whereas otherwise it would be in a quiescent

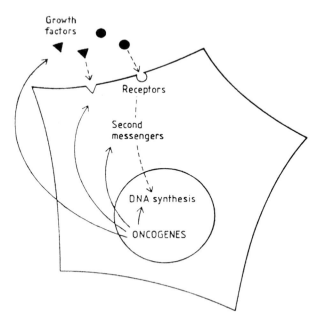

Fig. 1. Oncogene products disrupt normal regulation of cell growth at various levels of control.

state. Other oncogene products may mimic the external signals, such as growth factors, or the receptors on the cell surface for those factors. Thus the *sis* oncogene of simian sarcoma virus is derived from a cellular gene encoding one subunit of platelet-derived growth factor. This mitogenic factor is normally released by platelets aggregating in small lesions or blood clots, thereby stimulating mesenchymal cell proliferation locally to promote wound healing. Its production by a cell that also bears receptors for the factor would lead to "autocrine" or self-stimulated cell proliferation, as seen in fibroblasts transformed by the *sis* oncogene.

A large family of retrovirus oncogene products belong to a family of tyrosine kinase membrane proteins which are discussed in detail by Rayter *et al.* (Chapter 22). These proteins, of which the insulin receptor and the *src, abl,* and *erbB* oncogenes are best known, appear to act as receptors for growth factor and mitogenic hormones. For example, the *erbB* oncogene is a truncated form of the membrane receptor for epidermal growth factor (EGF). Although this oncogenic form of the receptor does not have the binding domain for EGF itself, it behaves as if it has been triggered by the mitogen, signaling internally into the cell to stimulate proliferation.

Intermediary cytoplasmic proteins act as secondary messages in the signaling pathways from membrane receptors to the nucleus. Among oncogene products, the *ras* proteins are believed to play this type of role. The 21,000-Da *ras* protein acts as a "G" protein, binding guanosine triphosphate (GTP) and exhibiting GTPase activity. The oncogenic form, frequently resulting from a mutation involving a single amino-acid residue, has reduced GTP-binding activity.

Oncogenes may act synergistically in promoting cell transformation. Retrovirus that carry two oncogenes, one encoding a nuclear protein and one a membrane protein, are particularly oncogenic. The introduction of molecularly cloned oncogenes of these two classes into normal primary cells in culture can lead to complete transformation, whereas one oncogene alone may act solely to "immortalize" the cell's proliferation potential or to transform a cell that is already immortalized in the sense of growing as an established cell line.

V. Human Oncogenes

The oncogenes first recognized in retroviruses, but sharing homology with cellular genes, have been highly conserved in evolution, indicating that their normal functions in cell physiology are important and universal. It was no surprise, therefore, to find that human cells have protooncogene homologs. An important question was whether these genes were altered or unusually active in human malignancy. In many cases, this has been demonstrated: virally induced animal tumors and naturally occurring human malignancies exhibit similar oncogene profiles.

Activated human oncogenes have been detected in several ways. First, it has become apparent that oncogenes are involved in specific chromosome translocations in certain human tumors. Thus the *abl* protooncogene, located on human chromosome 9, is brought into juxtaposition with a segment of chromosome 22 in chronic myeloid leukemia. In Burkitt's lymphoma, the *myc* gene on chromosome 8 is translocated to an active site of one of the immunoglobulin chain genes on chromosome 14, 2, or 22 (see Rabbitts *et al.,* Chapter 25). Just as the insertion of a retrovirus genome may activate an otherwise quiescent protooncogene, chromosome translocation can lead to proto-oncogene activation and mutation.

Second, oncogenes have been found in amplified numbers in several human malignancies. For example, the *myc* gene is amplified approximately 30-fold in HL60 promyelocytic leukemia cells, with associated double minute chromosomes or homogenous staining regions. Stark *et al.* (Chapter 26) and Housman *et al.* (Chapter 27) discuss mechanisms of gene amplification in respect to drug resistance, by which there is strong selection for increased amounts of the gene product to overcome the inhibitory effect of the cytotoxic drug. One may similarly infer that increased amounts of an oncogene product, in this case resulting from gene amplification rather than through unusual juxtaposition with expression enhancers, will allow the progression of a transformed cell to a more malignant phenotype.

Third, structural mutations in the coding regions of protooncogenes also result in increased oncogenic potential. This has been best exemplified in the *ras* genes already alluded to, in which single codon changes for amino acids in or around residues 12 and 61 change the properties of the protein. Mutant *ras* genes in human tumors were first detected through DNA "transfection" studies. DNA extracted from some human tumors, but not from normal human tissues, was shown to transform NIH-3T3 mouse cells in culture. By serial transfer of transforming DNA, a single human gene can be identified and molecularly cloned. In most cases of human tumor DNA transfer, the transforming genes identified belong to the *ras* family (Ha-*ras,* Ki-*ras,* and N-*ras* genes).

Some 20% of human tumors appear to have activated *ras* genes. It is the transforming forms of *ras* that have mutations in residues 12 or 61, resulting in conformational changes to the protein and reduced GTP binding or GTPase activity. Chemical mutagenization of normal cloned *ras* genes also results in the generation of transforming mutants with changes in one of these codons. Most human tumors with mutant *ras* genes express "normal" levels of the mutant product. In some tumors, however, amplification of the normal alleles can also result in cell transformation. Thus, either alteration in coding sequence or alteration in levels of expression of the normal protein may promote neoplastic transformation.

VI. Prospects for Intervention

How may the burgeoning knowledge of oncogenes and their products help in the treatment of cancer patients? To date, our new insight has not been translated into clinical application, but there is considerable optimism that this horizon is drawing closer.

First, a more detailed knowledge of the particular oncogenes active in individual human malignancies may offer more accurate prognostic indicators upon which treatment by existing regimes can be better suited to the patient. Some oncogenes may become mutated or activated in a wide variety of human neoplasms and at different stages in tumor progression, e.g., N-*ras* in carcinomas, sarcomas, melanomas and myeloid and lymphoid leukemias. Others, such as N-*myc,* are more specifically restricted, in this case to stage III and IV neuroblastomas. There has been little research so far to investigate whether activation of particular oncogenes is correlated with prognosis or with responsiveness to different treatment schedules.

Second, knowledge of the oncogenes expressed by the malignant cell may afford immunologically targeted attack directed to oncogene products themselves. The immunotherapy and immunotoxin regimes described in this volume are directed to markers of the tumor cells that can be modulated or reduced in expression without loss of malignancy. It is almost inevitable, therefore, that resistant tumors will arise. If, however, the target is an antigen essential for the cell to maintain its neoplastic phenotype, then modulation of expression by the cell would lead to reversion of malignancy, and hence a resistant population would be less likely to arise. Even in cases in which the oncogene product cannot be distinguished antigenically from its normal counterpart, its overexpression may allow preferential binding of an antibody or immunotoxin. This is currently being attempted with antibodies to the interleukin-2 receptor, which is overexpressed approximately 100-fold in adult T-cell leukemia cells transformed by human T-cell leukemia virus type I. Antibodies to the EGF receptor might similarly be useful for treating squamous carcinomas.

Third, the amplification of oncogenes seen in some tumors might possibly be turned to therapeutic advantage, in contrast to the resistance that gene amplification causes for conventional cytotoxic agents. Drugs that recognize the oncogene products might be selectively concentrated in the cancer cells overproducing the protein concerned. If the drug were linked to a suitable toxin or radionuclide, the cytotoxic effect might yield an enhanced therapeutic ratio based on the relative doses delivered to the cancer cells over the normal cells.

Fourth, where the oncogene product differs qualitatively from the normal product, as with *ras* genes, it may be possible to design drugs that bind preferentially and block the function of the oncoprotein while sparing the normal protein. Such drugs could be developed as cytotoxic agents or biological response modifiers.

Finally, it should be emphasized that the whole discussion of oncogenes deals with gene products whose activity promotes neoplasia. Very likely there are also proteins exerting a negative control on cell proliferation. Some of these may be the normal versions of oncogene products, but others may be encoded by "anti-oncogenes" that have not yet been identified. The recognition and isolation of such growth regulatory genes might allow us to intervene molecularly to promote the suppression of malignancy by noncytotoxic agents.

Suggested Readings

There is a vast literature on oncogenes from which the information for this overview chapter was drawn. In addition to the chapters by Rayter, Skene, Rabbitts, and Stark in this volume, the following sources of further reading are recommended:

1. Heldin, C.-H., and Westermark, B. (1984). Growth factors: Mechanism of action and relation to oncogenes. *Cell (Cambridge, Mass.)* **37,** 9–20.
2. Hunter, A. (1984). The proteins of oncogenes. *Sci. Am.* **251,** 60–69.
3. Tooze, J. (1983). "DNA Tumor Viruses," 2nd ed. Cold Spring Harbor Lab., Cold Spring Harbor, New York.
4. Weinberg, R. (1983). A molecular basis of cancer. *Sci. Am.* **249,** 126–142.
5. Weiss, R. A., and Marshall, C. J. (1984). Oncogenes. *Lancet* **2,** 1138–1142.
6. Weiss, R. A., Teich, N. M., Varmus, H. E., and Coffin, J. (1985). "RNA Tumor Viruses," 2nd ed. Cold Spring Harbor Lab., Cold Spring Harbor, New York.

22

Oncogene Function and Mechanism of Action

SYDONIA I. RAYTER, JOHN C. BELL, MICHAEL J. FRY,
AND J. GORDON FOULKES

Laboratory of Eukaryotic Molecular Genetics
National Institute for Medical Research
Mill Hill, London, United Kingdom

I. Oncogenes and Cell Transformation

Although originally defined by analysis of acutely transforming retroviruses, it is now apparent that the genomes of all eukaryotic species

NEW AVENUES IN DEVELOPMENTAL
CANCER CHEMOTHERAPY

421

contain a set of genes capable of transforming cells to the malignant state. Around 40 transforming genes, termed oncogenes, have been isolated so far, and current estimates suggest that as many as 200 may be found to exist (14,156).

Generation of oncogenes, from their nontransforming homologs, may be brought about in a variety of ways. For many animal species, except for humans, a major mechanism for protooncogene activation is transduction from the host cell genome by a retrovirus, such that the gene comes under transcriptional control of the strong retroviral promoter (84,107,115,144,151). This could result in a constitutive overproduction of the protein. For humans, spontaneous or evoked gene amplification could provide a similar mechanism to increase the concentration of a cellular oncogene product (15,90,138).

Mutations within the normal regulatory elements could also dissociate the gene from its usual transcriptional constraints. There are several examples whereby protooncogenes have become activated following the insertion of retroviral promoter/enhancer elements within the vicinity of the gene (38,64,123). Analogous mechanisms may again be applicable to human cancer in which many tumors show characteristic chromosomal translocations (90,109,166). In several cases protooncogenes have been mapped at, or close to, chromosomal break points, implicating those genes in tumorigenesis (2,7,94,129,135).

Mutations within coding regions are also known to be responsible for the generation of oncogenes. The most notable example is the human *ras* oncogene, in which a single point mutation in a 21,000-D protein is sufficient to activate the protooncogene and to induce cell transformation (19,52,131,149). Recent evidence with chemical carcinogens strongly implicates such mutations as being directly responsible for the generation of tumors, and not merely secondary consequences of the transformation event (146,167).

Regardless of the mechanism of protooncogene activation, the most important question for our laboratory is how a single gene, and hence a single protein, can actually transform cells. This clearly necessitates an understanding of the biochemistry of transforming proteins. In the following sections we will briefly review this area, in particular with regard to the *abl* oncogene, whose transforming protein encodes a tyrosine-specific protein kinase. In view of the fact that similar proteins may be encoded by one-third of all known oncogenes (Table I) (14) we have concluded this chapter by attempting to suggest ways in which an understanding of protein phosphorylation might lead to significant advances in cancer chemotherapy.

TABLE I

Oncogenes and Hormone Receptors

	Acronym	Molecular weight ($\times 10^{-3}$)
1. PROTEIN KINASES		
a. Protein-tyrosine kinases		
Viral		
1. Abelson murine leukemia virus (A-MuLV)	*abl*	120
2. Avian erythroblastosis virus (AEV)	*erb*-B	74
3. Gardner-Arnstein feline sarcoma virus (GA-FeSV)	*fes*	95
Snyder-Theilin feline sarcoma virus (ST-FeSV)	*fes*	85
Fujinami avian sarcoma virus (FSV)	*fps*	140
UR-1	*fps*	150
16L	*fps*	142
PRC11	*fps*	105
4. Gardner-Rasheed feline sarcoma virus (GR-FeSV)	*fgr*	72
5. Esh sarcoma virus (ESV)	*yes*	80
Y73	*yes*	90
6. McDonough feline sarcoma virus (SM-FeSV)	*fms*	140
7. Rous sarcoma virus (RSV)	*src*	60
8. UR-2 sarcoma virus	*ros*	68
9. HZ 4 feline sarcoma virus	*kit*	—
Nonviral		
1. —	*onc*D	—
2. —	*met*	—
3. —	*neu*	180
4. —	*lst*	56
Hormone receptors		
1. Epidermal growth factor (EGF)		170
2. Platelet-derived growth factor (PDGF)		175
3. Insulin-like growth factor-1 (IGF-1)		98
4. Insulin		95
5. Colony-stimulating factor-1 (CSF-1)		165
b. Protein-serine kinases		
1. Moloney murine urine sarcoma virus	*mos*	37
2. Reticuloendotheliosis virus	*rel*	60
3. Murine sarcoma virus 3611	*raf*	75
MH2 avian virus	*mil*	100
c. Protein kinase modulators		
1. Simian sarcoma virus	*sis*	28
2. Polyoma tumor virus	Polyoma middle T	55
2. Guaninenucleotide binding proteins		
1. Harvey murine sarcoma virus (rat)	Ha-*ras*	21
Kirsten murine sarcoma virus (rat)	Ki-*ras*	21
3. Nuclear proteins		
1. MC29 myelocytomatosis virus	*myc*	110
2. Avian myeloblastosis virus (AMV)	*myb(ets)*	50
3. FBJ osteosarcoma virus	*fos*	55
4. Avian SKV770 virus	*ski*	49

II. Biochemistry of Transforming Proteins

A single protein product capable of inducing the multitude of cellular alterations characteristic of the transformed phenotype must be capable of pleiotropic interactions. Although we understand little of the detailed biochemistry of such interactions, it appears that transforming proteins may be divided into at least three functional catagories (Table I): (1) nuclear proteins (2) guanine nucleotide binding proteins which may act within the plane of the plasma membrane, and (3) protein kinases, or their modulators, whose interactions at the plasma membrane may also prove essential for their transforming activity.

A. Nuclear Proteins

Oncogene products in this category are *fos, myc, myb, ski,* and p53, all of which are found in the nuclear matrix of the cell (14,91,157). Pulse–chase experiments have shown that the protein product (p110$^{gag-myc}$) of the MC29 myelocytomatosis virus migrates to the nucleus within 30–60 min following infection (22). The purified *gag-myc* polyproteins bind to DNA *in vitro* (40), although specific sequence binding has not yet been demonstrated (110). Nevertheless, this *in vitro* binding property correlates with transformation, since purified polyproteins from transformation-defective deletion mutants exhibit 10- to 20-fold reduced DNA binding ability (41). The action of the proteins encoded by cellular *myb* (c-*myb*) and viral *myb* (v-*myb*) appears to be directed toward hemopoietic tissues, since these are the principal tissues in which expression of the cellular gene has been found (140) and in which the viral gene induces tumors (46).

Expression of c-*myb* in early embryos of *Drosophila melanogaster* (89) and c-*fos* in mouse embryos (157) implicates a possible role for these protooncogenes in differentiation. Mouse embryos accumulate the highest concentration of c-*fos* transcripts in the day 18 amnion and also show c-*fos* protein located in the nucleus.

The mechanism by which these nuclear proteins induce transformation is unknown, although their subcellular localization suggest that they may act at the level of transcription or RNA processing.

B. Guanine Nucleotide Binding Proteins

A second class of oncogenes is the *ras* gene family, which express a 21,000-molecular-weight protein, p21^{ras}. The human cellular *ras* family consists of at least three functional protooncogenes, which are closely related at the nucleotide sequence level. Activation of *ras* oncogenes in human tumors is most commonly due to point mutations at one of several "hot spots" in the *ras* coding sequence (19,52,131,149). Activated *ras* oncogenes are found in 10–20% of human tumors and have been detected in carcinomas, sarcomas, and hematopoietic malignancies (37,50,128).

The first biochemical activity described for a p21^{ras} protein was the ability to phosphorylate itself on a threonine residue. This appears to be an intrinsic activity, but it is also a dispensable one, since certain actively transforming versions of p21^{ras} lack a threonine residue at the phosphorylation acceptor site (120). Although many protein kinases are capable of carrying out an autophosphorylation reaction, all attempts using the *ras* protein to phosphorylate exogenous substrates have, so far, proved unsuccessful.

A second biochemical activity described for proteins in the *ras* family is the ability to bind guanosine triphosphate (GTP) (142). Mammalian *ras* gene products are associated with the inner face of the plasma membrane, bind GTP, and exhibit a low GTPase activity (139,147). On the basis of sequence homology and biochemical properties it has been suggested that *ras* proteins may be members of the G protein family that serve to transduce information from cell surface receptors to internal effector molecules in a variety of systems (65,79), e.g., hormonal regulation of the adenylate cyclase system (66) and phosphoinositide turnover (10). Although there are few data concerning the normal function of p21^{ras} in mammalian cells, in yeast, one role of the *ras* proteins may be to integrate nutritional information with intracellular cAMP levels via the adenylate cyclase system (61,153). The GTPase activity of the oncogenic versions of p21^{ras} is considerably reduced compared to the normal product (65,147). Since the GTP–G protein complex is the active version of the G protein family, this could imply that the oncogenic version of p21 may transmit a continuous signal rather than a regulated, transient one. In the case of adenylate cyclase this would lead to alterations in the activity of the cAMP-dependent protein kinase and would thereby change the phosphorylation state of its protein substrates.

C. Protein Kinase Activities and Their Modulators

The idea that a transforming protein might act via protein phosphorylation is a particularly attractive one, as it provides a mechanism whereby a single protein could induce the multitude of altered cell parameters characteristic of the transformed phenotype. Since the discovery of the cAMP-dependent protein kinase in 1968 (158), reversible protein phosphorylation is now established as the major mechanism for the regulation of protein function in eukaryotic cells (25).

The previous section reviewed the possibility that the *ras* proteins might act as G proteins, thereby regulating protein phosphorylation via either cAMP levels (66) or phosphoinositide turnover (10; see also Section VI). The first evidence that oncogenes might directly encode protein kinases originated from work described in Erikson's laboratory, for the transforming protein of the Rous sarcoma virus, pp60[src] (26,48). Shortly after this discovery, Hunter and Sefton (77) identified phosphotyrosine as the novel phosphate acceptor.

In mammalian cells, the major amino acid phosphate acceptors are serine and threonine, with smaller amounts being linked to lysine, arginine, histidine, aspartic acid, glutamic acid, and cysteine (150,162). Phosphotyrosine is a rare modification in the normal cell (78) (0.02% of total phosphoamino acids), but is implicated by several recent findings as having an important role in the regulation of cell growth.

First, half of all known oncogenes have now been shown to encode protein–tyrosine kinase activities (Table I). Second, the plasma membrane receptors for several growth-stimulating hormones, namely, epidermal growth factor (EGF) (74,155), platelet-derived growth factor (PDGF) (116), insulin-like growth factor-1 (83), insulin (87,88), and colony stimulating factor-1 (CSF-1) (132), have been demonstrated to be associated with protein–tyrosine kinases (Table I). Third, the oncogene of the Simian sarcoma virus, *sis*, was shown to be derived from the cellular gene which encodes PDGF (161), and the oncogene of the avian erythroblastosis virus, *erb-B*, has been found to be homologous to the kinase domain of the EGF receptor (44). Finally, the glycoprotein encoded by the oncogene for McDonough feline sarcoma virus, *fms,* has recently been shown to be related to the CSF-1 receptor (141). Thus, protein–tyrosine kinases appear to be essential components in the regulation of both normal and abnormal cell growth.

III. The Role of Tyrosine Phosphorylation in Cell Transformation

A. Transformation as a Dynamic Equilibrium Process

Models of cell transformation based on tyrosine phosphorylation must take into account the fact that normal cells express homologous protein kinase activities without being transformed (58). This may be visualized in a number of ways. First, transformation may result from an overexpression of the kinase activity. This would increase the degree of phosphorylation of proteins which are substrates for the kinase encoded by the related protooncogene. Such a model is supported by the observation that cells transformed by viral oncogenes which encode protein–tyrosine kinases typically show a tenfold increase in total protein-bound phosphotyrosine when compared to normal cells (78). Several laboratories have reported that overexpression of the cellular c-*src* protein failed to transform cells (80,122). These cells, which expressed elevated levels of the c-*src* protein, however, did not show a corresponding increase in their total cell phosphotyrosine. These experiments, therefore, do not answer the question of whether a continuous increase in a protooncogene-encoded kinase activity would be sufficient to transform. An alternative model is to suggest that mutations alter the protein kinase specificity, thereby phosphorylating proteins or sites which are not phosphorylated by the normal enzyme. The fact that the $pp60^{v-src}$ kinase is more sensitive to inhibition by P^1,P^4-di(adenosine-5')tetraphosphate than $pp60^{c-src}$ (6,99) suggests these enzymes may possess at least some differences in substrate specificity. Mutations may also alter the ability of the kinase to be regulated, thus leading to an increase in functional kinase activity without elevating the actual concentration of the protein.

These models, however, ignore one important factor, namely, the role of the host cell phosphotyrosyl–protein phosphatases. An important role of these enzymes is suggested by observations involving tumor viruses with temperature-sensitive (ts) transforming proteins. Transformation of cells infected by either the Rous sarcoma virus (RSV) or by Fujinami sarcoma virus with ts transforming proteins undergo reversion to the normal phenotype in a temperature-dependent manner. In several cases, this has been correlated with a similar temperature-sensitive activity of the corresponding protein kinase *in vitro* (76,78,168). However, such cells do not revert to normal because the protein kinase becomes inactive per se, but because proteins are dephosphorylated by the phosphotyrosyl–protein phosphatases of the host cell. Clearly, the loss of kinase activity would have little effect if the already-phosphorylated proteins remained phosphorylated. Based on this analysis, transformation involving protein phosphorylation should be envisaged as a dynamic equilibrium process, the balance of the kinase–phosphatase activities. To date, little is known about phosphotyrosyl–protein phosphatases, but there appear to be multiple forms, all of which are distinct from the better-characterized phosphoseryl–phosphothreonyl phosphatases [reviewed by Foulkes (55)].

Recently, there has been considerable interest in the idea of anti-oncogenes, in which transformation would result from the functional loss of a gene product rather than the activation of a gene. Several human tumors, for example, Wilm's tumor (96) and hereditary retinoblastoma (24), are distinguished by characteristic chromosomal deletions. The DNA sequences encoding phosphotyrosyl–protein phosphatases may, therefore, represent a group of genes awaiting identification as anti-oncogenes.

Having established that cells contain oncogenes, that many oncogenes encode protein–tyrosine kinases, and that transformation by these proteins is a dynamic equilibrium process, the next question is to ask the identity of those proteins whose activity is modulated in response to tyrosine phosphorylation *in vivo.*

B. Physiological Targets versus Cellular Substrates

To understand how protein–tyrosine kinases regulate cell growth necessitates the identification of their substrates. To date, this quest has met with little success. The various approaches have included the use of one- and two-dimensional gel electrophoresis to analyze phosphoproteins found in normal versus transformed or growth factor–stimulated cells (28,29,31); the development of both poly- and monoclonal antibodies directed towards phosphotyrosine or its analogs (60); immunoprecipitation or isolation of specific proteins on an *a priori* prediction of their involvement (31); and the phosphorylation of candidate substrates *in vitro* (82).

There are several reasons for the slow progress in this area. Foremost is the complexity of the processes under investigation, namely, growth control and transformation. The best model for protein phosphorylation as a regulatory mechanism is that of glycogen metabolism. To date, at least six protein kinases, four protein phosphatases, and four heat-stable regulatory proteins have been isolated by analysis of this system. (25). If the cell employs such measures to control glycogen levels, it is daunting to imagine the networks which regulate cell proliferation. Second, phosphotyrosine is a rare modification, accounting for only 0.05–2.0% of the total phosphoamino acids, even in cells containing active protein–tyrosine kinases (28,30,32,33). The detection of such minor species is inherently difficult. Third, it is now clear that protein kinases, at least those found in association with retroviral oncogenes, are promiscuous, even *in vivo,* and phosphorylate proteins which are unrelated to the transformation event. It is necessary to distinguish between *in vivo* substrates, which include any protein phosphorylated by the appropriate kinase, and physiological targets, which refer only to those proteins that modify their biochemical activity in a physiologically relevant manner, both *in vivo* and *in vitro,* in response to phosphorylation of tyrosine. So far, no targets have been firmly established for any protein–tyrosine kinase. Recently, we have written an extended review of the published literature in this area (58), and reiterating the analysis which led to this conclusion seems unnecessary. Instead, we would like to present an outline of some of the various approaches our laboratory is currently employing to identify physiological targets. This work is focused on targets of the protein–tyrosine kinase encoded by the v-*abl* oncogene.

IV. Abelson Murine Leukemia Virus

The *abl* oncogene was first identified as the viral transforming gene (v-*abl*) of Abelson murine leukemia virus (A-MuLV) isolated from a chemically thymectomized mouse inoculated with Moloney murine leukemia virus (M-MuLV) (1). Instead of developing the typical, M-MuLV-induced T-cell leukemia, several mice developed acute B-cell leukemia. From one mouse, a virus was isolated which differed from M-MuLV in that although it was replication defective, it could transform both murine NIH3T3 fibroblasts and lymphoid cells *in vitro*. Subsequent analysis revealed that A-MuLV arose via a recombination event between M-MuLV and a cellular gene, c-*abl* (68,165). The v-*abl* genome codes for only one protein, which varies in size depending on the specific A-MuLV strain. Among the many A-MuLV variants, the one with the largest genome and the one assumed to be the product of the original recombination event, is termed A-MuLV p160, a virus that encodes a 160,000-molecular-weight protein (69). The v-*abl* sequences of this genome are colinear with exons of the normal c-*abl* cellular gene, although the normal gene has extra exon sequences on both the 5' and 3' ends. The c-*abl* gene encodes a 150,000 Da protein.

A. Characterization of the v-*abl* Oncogene

All naturally occurring A-MuLV variants thus far isolated encode *gag-abl* fusion proteins, in which the M-MuLV *gag* proteins, p15, p12, and part of p30, represent the N-terminus, and the rest of the protein is encoded by the v-*abl* sequences. Thus, the transforming protein p160 consists of 30 kDa of *gag* fused to 130 kDa of v-*abl*. Mutational analysis has established four functional regions of the p160 protein: (1) the p15 region of *gag*, (2) the 14 N-terminal amino acids of p15^{gag}, (3) the 5', 1.2-kilobase (1.2-kb) region of v-*abl*, and (4) the 3' half of v-*abl*.

1. The p15 Region of gag

Deletion of all of the *gag* sequences in A-MuLV, except for the first 34 amino acids in p15, results in a virus which still transforms NIH3T3 fibroblasts efficiently but totally abolishes the ability to transform lymphoid cells (125). Further analysis revealed that deletions in the p12 region of *gag* have no effect, whereas deletions in p15 abolish the lymphoid transforming activity (126,127). In transformed fibroblasts, the p15-deleted proteins and normal viral *gag-abl* proteins demonstrate a similar stability. When the p15-deleted genome was introduced into a chemically transformed lymphoid cell line, however, its protein product revealed a marked instability (126). Although the protein was synthesized efficiently, its steady-state level was less than 10% of the nondeleted protein. This specific instability of the p15-deleted protein in lymphoid cells may explain the requirement of these sequences for lymphoid but not fibroblast transformation.

2. The 14 N-Terminal Amino Acids of p15 ^{gag}

Further characterization of the *gag* region has established the requirement for fusion of sequences within the 14 amino acids of the N-terminal end of the p15 region to the beginning of the v-*abl* for A-MuLV transforming activity. A genome containing only two of the amino acids of *gag* is transformation defective even when NIH3T3 fibroblasts are used (R. Prywes and D. Baltimore, unpublished observations). One explanation may be a requirement for myristylation of the Abelson protein at the N-terminus.

Myristylation is an uncommon form of protein modification. In several instances it has been found that myristic acid is linked to the N-terminal glycine (3,23,73,119). In pp60^{src} it appears that myristylation of the protein is essential for its transforming activity (35,86).

3. The 5' 1.2-kb Region of v-abl

Only 1.2 kb at the 5' end of the 3.9-kb v-*abl* sequence is required for fibroblast transformation. This minimum transforming region has been delineated by using small 5' and 3' deletions (125,127). The mutant genes expressed in *Escherichia coli* were also assayed for protein–tyrosine kinase activity to confirm that the loss of transforming activity correlated with a loss of tyrosine-specific protein kinase activity. Insertion of four amino acids within this region abolishes both the kinase activity as well as the ability to transform, indicating that most of this domain plays a critical role in the transformation process.

4. The 3' Half of v-abl

The exact function of the 3' half of v-*abl* is unknown, but this region may regulate the protein–tyrosine kinase domain. Abelson proteins lacking the 3' half of v-*abl* transform fibroblasts efficiently but have a tenfold reduction in lymphoid transformation efficiency (125). In addition, this region appears to enhance the toxicity of the A-MuLV protein, although the 3' half of v-*abl* itself is not toxic (69,125,160).

B. Characterization of the v-*abl* Transforming Protein

To further characterize the minimal v-*abl* transforming gene, we decided to purify the corresponding protein using an expression vector system in *E. coli*. A variety of vectors have been used to express *abl* sequences in *E. coli* (Fig. 1) (53,56,93,159). Although each of these vectors had proved very effective in producing proteins in *E. coli*, *abl* sequences by themselves were very poorly expressed. By constructing fusion proteins (Fig. 1) large amounts of the v-*abl* polypeptide were produced. Under these conditions, the expressed proteins proved to be largley insoluble and possessed only very low levels of kinase activity. The problem of protein solubility is frequently encountered when proteins are expressed at high levels in *E. coli*. These constructs are still very useful, however, since large amounts of purified *abl* protein can be readily obtained (Fig. 2) and used to produce *abl*-specific antibodies. We hope to use these to facilitate our search for the role of the c-*abl* protein in the regulation of normal growth control and perhaps differentiation (see Section VII).

Fortunately, one construct, pt-*abl*50 (Fig. 1) produced a soluble, highly active form of the v-*abl* protein kinase. Although this protein is very poorly expressed, we have successfully purified this form of the kinase to homogeneity (56) using a combination of conventional chromatography, ion-exchange high-pressure liquid chromatography, and the use of an anti-phosphotyrosine monoclonal antibody. The Abelson kinase, like most protein kinases, is capable of carrying out an autophosphorylation reaction such that the protein phosphorylates itself on tyrosine residues. The Abelson kinase, therefore, binds to columns containing the anti-phosphotyrosine antibody and can be eluted gently by the addition of phenylphosphate, a phosphotyrosine analog (60).

The properties of the purified Abelson kinase have been reviewed (56). Two points are worth mentioning in the context of this chapter. First, the purified kinase has a turnover rate of 170 μmoles of phosphate. min$^-$$^1\mu$mole^{-1}. This is the highest specific activity so far recorded for any protein–tyrosine kinase; it is comparable to the specific activity of the cAMP-dependent protein kinase and demonstrates that the ability to phosphorylate tyrosine residues, at least for the Abelson kinase, is not a trace enzymatic activity. Having obtained a highly active, purified protein–tyrosine kinase, we can now test possible candidate target proteins

A-MuLV (3.9 Kb)

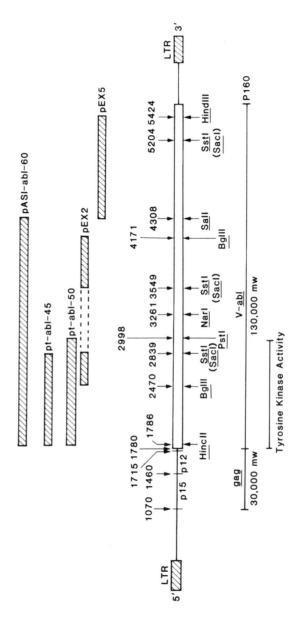

Construct	Promoter	Fusion	ABL–Sequences	Fusion Protein (mw)	Product	Kinase Activity
pASI–abl–60	λPL	7 Amino Acids Influenza Virus NSI	HincII–SalI	60,000	Insoluble Protein	±
pt–abl–45	λP$_R$	80 Amino Acids SV40 Small t	HincII–SacI	50,000 40,000	Insoluble Proteins	–
pt–abl–50	λP$_R$	80 Amino Acids SV40 Small t	HincII–PstI	50,000	Soluble Protein	+
pEX 2	trp L	558 Amino Acids E. coli trp E	BglII–BglII	48,000	Insoluble Protein	–
pEX 5	trp L	558 Amino Acids E. coli trp E	SalI–HindIII	54,000	Insoluble Protein	–

Fig. 1. Genome of A-MuLV showing fusion of *gag* to *v-abl* sequences. Regions of *v-abl* expressed as fusion proteins in *E. coli* are shown, as are the restriction sites used in construction of these plasmids.

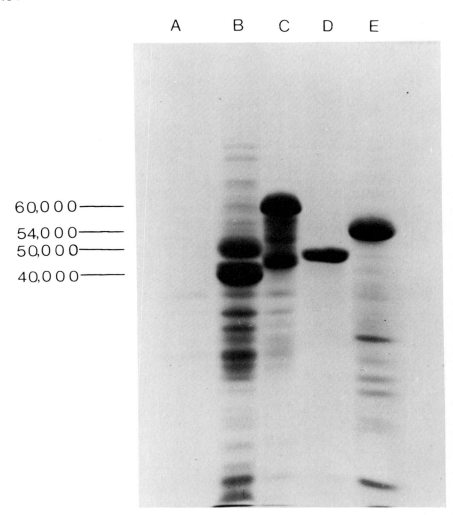

Fig. 2. Bacterial expression of *abl*-fusion proteins. Insoluble protein pellets were prepared from induced cultures harvested after 2.25 hr at 42°C for pAS1-*abl*-60 (lane C) and pt-*abl*-45 (lane B) and after an 8-hr induction for pEX2 (lane D) and pEX5 (lane E). Induction of pAS1-*abl*-60 and pt-*abl*-45 was carried out by a temperature shift to 42°C as described by Ferguson *et al.* (53). Induction of the *trp* operon by addition of 50 μg/ml of 3-β-indoleacrylic acid to cultures of pEX2 and pEX5 was carried out as described by Konopka *et al.* (93).

Insoluble protein pellets were prepared by resuspending the bacterial pellet in 50 m*M* Tris pH 8, 25% sucrose. Cells were lysed by addition of 2 mg/ml of lysozyme and were left on ice for 10 min. MgCl$_2$ was added to a final concentration of 5 m*M*, then DNAse (60 μg/ml) was added and left on ice for 15 min. Buffer 1 (10 m*M* Tris pH 7.2, 1

as substrates *in vitro*. If stoichiometric phosphorylation is obtained, one can then look for changes in the target protein's activity. If such changes are observed, however, one must look *in vivo* for the corresponding phosphorylation-induced activity change. *In vitro* data alone can be very misleading. A second interesting property of the Abelson kinase is its ability to phosphorylate peptides containing two or three amino acids. With respect to designing potential chemotherapeutic agents based on substrate analogs of protein kinases (see Section VIII) this observation may prove very useful.

V. Is the Tumor Phenotype Determined by the Protein Kinase Specificity?

Comparison of primary amino acid sequences of protein–tyrosine kinases reveals a high degree of homology within their kinase domains. This homology extends from the oncogene-encoded kinases of *abl, src, yes, fps, erb-B, fgr,* and *ros* to the hormone receptors for EGF and insulin (75,114). Despite this homology, oncogenic retroviruses induce distinct pathologies in their hosts. Rous sarcoma virus (RSV), for example, induces sarcomas in chickens, whereas A-MuLV causes lymphomas in mice. Under certain conditions, A-MuLV may also induce thymomas (27), but fibrosarcomas have never been observed, even though A-MuLV transforms NIH3T3 fibroblasts *in vitro* in addition to lymphoid cells (134, 137).

Such differences may reflect a host response, for example, perhaps sarcomas are not detected in Abelson-infected mice due to the rapidity with which animals die of lymphomas. Recently, several experiments have been carried out to address this problem. Anderson and Scolnick (5) reported the construction of a murine transforming retrovirus (MRSV) in which the *src* gene of RSV replaced the *env* gene of an amphotropic helper virus. When this virus was injected into the tail veins of 6-week-old mice, the animals developed erythroleukemia, characterized by splenic

---

mM EDTA, 100 mM NaCl, 1% NP40, 0.5% deoxycholate) was added, and insoluble protein was pelleted at 16,000 g for 30 min at 4°C. The pellet was washed again in buffer 1, once in buffer 2 (1 M NaCl, 0.1% NP40, 10 mM Tris pH 7.2), then three times in buffer 3 (1% Triton X-100, 1% deoxycholate, 150 mM NaCl, 10 mM Tris pH 7.2, 0.1% SDS, 1 M urea). The pellet was then boiled in 2X gel sample buffer for 10 min, debris was spun out, and the supernatant was electrophoresed on a 10% polyacryamide gel. Proteins were visualized by Coomassie brilliant blue staining. Lane A shows the pellet prepared from a control culture of pt-*abl*-45 grown at 32°C.

foci, splenomegaly, and anemia. A sarcoma was found in one case only. When newborn mice were injected intraperitoneally, fibrosarcomas and rhabdosarcomas were present in 8 out of 10 animals, in addition to erythroleukemia (124). In no instance, however, was transformation of pre–B cells, which is characteristic of the Abelson virus, observed. In the MRSV virus, the *src* gene is under the transcriptional control of an amphotropic long terminal repeat element (LTR). Enhancer sequences present in LTRs can result in tissue-specific expression of retroviral genes.

To avoid such problems, Mathey-Prevot and Baltimore (105) constructed a Moloney-based virus in which the *abl*-specific sequences were replaced by *src,* so that the resultant virus encoded a *gag-src* fusion protein, instead of *gag-abl.* This virus efficiently transformed fibroblasts *in vitro* but failed to transform lymphoid cells. Furthermore, the virus induced only fibrosarcomas *in vivo.* Similar results have been reported recently by Feuerman *et al.* (54).

We speculated, therefore, that structural differences between the protein–tyrosine kinases encoded by RSV and A-MuLV may explain the different pathology of these viruses *in vivo.* To test this hypothesis, we compared our purified Abelson kinase with pp60 ^{src}, using a variety of artificial substrates *in vitro* (57). Differences in their substrate specificities were clearly detected, with kinetic parameters varying between one and two orders of magnitude. These results, coupled with those of the distinct biological properties of the *gag-src* and *gag-abl* fusion proteins, suggest that small differences in amino acid sequences within the kinase domains of the *abl* and *src* proteins produce dramatic differences in their substrate specificity and are at least partly responsible for the different tumors produced by *src* and *abl* oncogenes *in vivo.* It will be interesting to analyze the differences between the v-*abl* oncogene in A-MuLV and the v-*abl* oncogene in the Hardy-Zuckerman feline virus, since this virus produces sarcomas in cats (12).

VI. Protein–Tyrosine Kinases: Interaction with Phosphoseryl Proteins and Phosphatidylinositol

Despite the fact that nearly half of the known oncogenes, as well as the membrane receptors for several growth factors, encode protein-tyrosine kinase activities. [reviewed by Foulkes and Rich Rosner (58)], physiologically important substrates for these enzymes have yet to be identified (see Section III,B).

Although all protein–tyrosine kinases appear to be specific for tyrosine residues *in vitro*, the addition of EGF (152), PDGF (117), or insulin (87,88,148,152) to responsive cells also results in the increased phosphorylation of certain proteins on serine residues. Similarly, in cells transformed by A-MuLV or RSV, both of which encode protein–tyrosine kinases, an increase in protein-bound phosphoserine has been observed (29,36,103). Among these phosphoseryl proteins, ribosomal protein S6 is of particular interest, because its phosphorylation is correlated with growth-promoting stimuli in a wide variety of systems (117,152). The exact role of S6 remains to be defined, but phosphorylated S6 may function to stimulate cell growth via the acquisition and preferential translation of growth-associated mRNAs (45,67,152).

Previously, we have shown that the phosphorylation of S6 in NIH3T3 fibroblasts is dependent on the presence of serum, but after transformation of these cells by A-MuLV S6 is highly phosphorylated on serine residues either in the absence or in the presence of serum. These results imply that the protein–tyrosine kinase encoded by A-MuLV can bypass the requirement for the growth factors in serum which normally regulate S6 phosphorylation (103). We decided, therefore, to use the phosphorylation of S6 on serine as a defined biochemical end point, and then to work backwards to determine how this process is regulated by a protein–tyrosine kinase.

In the course of these experiments, we had observed that the phorbol ester, TPA (phorbol 12-myristate 13-acetate), which is known to activate protein kinase C and to induce S6 phosphorylation (98,118,154), induces the phosphorylation of the same five S6 phosphopeptides as found in Abelson transformed cells (E. Erikson, J. Maller, and J. G. Foulkes, unpublished data). Furthermore, protein kinase C can phosphorylate S6 directly *in vitro* (98,121). This suggested that the Abelson kinase might regulate S6 phosphorylation by activation of protein kinase C. The most direct mechanism whereby the Abelson tyrosine kinase could regulate the phosphorylation of S6 on serine would be the activation of a serine-specific S6 kinase following phosphorylation of the S6 kinase on tyrosine. With this in mind, we immunoprecipitated protein kinase C from ^{32}P-labeled cells. In both NIH3T3 cells and Abelson transformed NIH3T3 cells protein kinase C was found to be phosphorylated. However, no difference was observed in the level of ^{32}P-labeled protein kinase C between these two cell types. Furthermore, phosphoamino acid analysis of protein kinase C isolated from Abelson transformed cells revealed only phosphoserine, with smaller amounts of phosphothreonine (62). Our lysis buffer appears to inactivate all protein phosphatase activities (55; J. G. Foulkes, unpublished observations), so it seems unlikely that phosphotyrosine would be lost during our isolation of protein kinase C. These data indicate that the Abelson transforming protein does not modulate the activity of protein kinase C by the direct phosphorylation of this enzyme on tyrosine residues. This suggested that we should search for alternative mechanisms by which the Abelson transforming protein might activate protein kinase C.

Recently, a large number of neurotransmitters, hormones, and growth factors have been shown to stimulate phosphoinositide turnover (20,34,43,71,130). It has been proposed that hydrolysis of phosphatidylinositol 4,5-bisphosphate by phospholipase C generates two potential second messengers (Fig. 3) (9), namely, diacylglycerol, which activates protein kinase C (118), and inositol 1,4,5-trisphosphate, which appears to release calcium from intracellular sites and to activate calmodulin-dependent pathways (10,81).

It has been suggested that the physiologically important targets for certain oncogenes may be components of phospholipid metabolism (10,11). In particular, data have been presented to suggest that protein–tyrosine kinases might phosphorylate phosphatidylinositol directly (101,102,145,163). It was possible that the Abelson transforming protein could stimulate protein kinase C indirectly via phosphatidylinositol phosphorylation. This perturbation might cause an increase in the level of

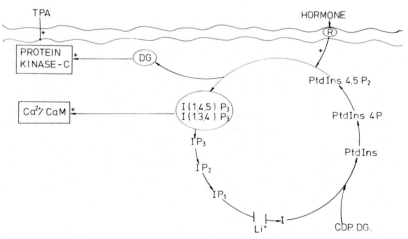

Fig. 3. Schematic representation of the phosphoinositide cycle. DG, Diacylglycerol; IP$_1$, inositol monophosphate; IP$_2$, inositol bisphosphate; IP$_3$ [I(1,4,5)P$_3$ or I(1,3,4)P$_3$], inositol trisphosphate; PtdIns, phosphatidylinositol; PtdIns4P, phosphatidylinositol 4-phosphate; PtdIns 4,5,P, phosphatidylinositol 4,5-bisphosphate; R, receptor for growth factor/hormone; TPA, phorbol ester.

diacylglycerol in Abelson transformed cells, which would activate protein kinase C and in turn regulate S6 phosphorylation.

A detailed analysis of the Abelson protein–tyrosine kinase, however, has demonstrated that the direct phosphorylation of phosphatidylinositol is highly unlikely to represent a physiologically significant enzymatic activity (62). At most, the Abelson kinase activity represents only 1/15,000 of the total potential phosphatidylinositol kinase activity present in transformed cell extracts.

A third mechanism by which the Abelson kinase might regulate protein kinase C could be the indirect activation of phosphoinositide turnover, for example, by the activation of one or more of the rate-limiting steps in phosphoinositide metabolism. We decided, therefore, to estimate the rate of phosphoinositide turnover *in vivo* by incubating cells for a short time in the presence of lithium chloride to block the conversion of inositol monophosphate to free inositol (8,42) (Fig. 3). Any stimulation of the phosphoinositide pathway is then reflected by an increase in the amount of inositol monophosphate. As shown previously, differences in S6 phosphorylation between normal and transformed cells are only apparent in the absence of serum (103). Under these conditions S6 is dephosphorylated in NIH3T3 cells but remains phosphorylated in Abelson transformed cells. If the Abelson kinase regulated S6 phosphorylation by the activation of phosphoinositide turnover and therby protein kinase C, differences in phosphoinositide turnover between normal and transformed cells might only be apparent in the absence of serum. Our approach, therefore, was to measure the rate of phosphoinositide turnover in the absence and presence of serum. In the absence of serum, inositol monophosphate levels were 2.5-fold higher in Abelson transformed cells than in NIH3T3 cells. Following the addition of serum for 10 min there was a rapid stimulation of inositol monophosphate levels in NIH3T3 cells, with no significant effect in Abelson transformed cells (62).

These data indicate that the phosphoinositide pathway is constitutively activated following transformation by A-MuLV. These results are supported by previous investigations of phosphatidylinositol metabolism in both UR2 virus and RSV transformed cell lines (39,101). This could lead to a sustained increase in the steady-state concentrations of both diacylglycerol, leading to the activation of protein kinase C, and inositol triphosphate, resulting in the release of intracellular calcium. Other phosphoinositide metabolites, e.g., arachidonic acid, might also act on systems potentially important in the transformation process. We are now determining the steady-state levels of each of the phosphoinositide metabolites in both NIH3T3 cells and Abelson transformed cells. This may indicate which step(s) is activated by the Abelson kinase. The phosphotyrosine content of the enzymes regulating phosphoinositide metabolism in Abelson transformed cells will then be examined. The relationship between protein kinase C activation and S6 phosphorylation also remains to be established, as it is unclear whether protein kinase C is directly responsible for the phosphorylation of S6 observed in Abelson transformed cells *in vivo*. This work suggests that a valuable approach in studying the mechanism of cell transformation by protein–tyrosine kinases will be to identify the physiological substrates of both protein kinase C and the Ca^{2+}-calmodulin-dependent kinases and phosphatases, since these may represent key targets in the transforming process. Finally, it is interesting to note that at least two oncogenes, namely *mos* (92) and *raf-mil* (111), may directly encode protein–serine kinases. How these oncogene products interact with protein–tyrosine kinases and phosphoinositide metabolism will be an important area for future investigation.

VII. Oncogenes and Differentiation

The proteins encoded by protooncogenes are thought to play essential roles in regulating the proliferation and differentiation of normal cells. The role of these proteins in differentiation is suggested by the observations that activated protooncogenes can arrest or interfere with cellular differentiation (13,51,104) and that high levels of expression of certain protooncogenes are found only in certain tissues (63,112,113) or at particular developmental stages (70,97,108).

Protein–tyrosine kinases constitute one group of oncogenes that appear to be able to disrupt the normal linkage between growth control and differentiation by posttranslational phosphorylation of tyrosine residues (29,47). Protein–tyrosine kinases may be envisaged to generate malignancies by "freezing" cells in the process of differentiation (47,133,136). The pp60[src] kinase can potentiate, inhibit, or reverse the differentiation program of infected cells, depending upon the developmental system under investigation (4,17,18). Furthermore, certain stem cells and differentiated cells appear to be totally refractory to the transforming effects of the v-*src* gene product (16,46). Taken together, these observations suggest that (1) particular protein–tyrosine kinases are integral components of the network regulating cell differentiation and growth and (2) protein–tyrosine kinases and their substrates are likely to be expressed (or activated) in a developmentally regulated fashion. We intend to test both of these predictions by investigating the role tyrosine phosphorylation plays in a normal, developmentally regulated system, focusing on the *abl* and *src* kinases. At present we are screening the tissues of the early mouse embryo by *in situ* hybridization with *abl*-specific probes to determine whether there is differential transcription of this gene at the cellular level. These studies are being complemented by double immunofluorescence staining of sectioned embryos with antibodies to the *abl* kinase and a monoclonal antibody to phosphotyrosine (59). We hope to be able to determine whether a relationship exists between the amount of *abl* kinase and the level of phosphotyrosine in individual embryonic cell types. Whole embryos at different stages in development are being analyzed by immunoblotting to determine if qualitative changes in the *abl* kinase and cellular phosphotyrosyl proteins can be correlated with embryonic cell differentiation.

Concomitant with these studies we have introduced the v-*abl* and v-*src* genes under the control of the glucocorticoid-responsive mouse mammary tumor virus (MMTV) promoter into the multi-potential mouse embryonal carcinoma cell line, P19 (106). Transgenic P19 cells harboring the MMTV-promoted tyrosine kinase genes will be induced to differentiate into a variety of different cell lineages *in vitro* (85). Glucocorticoids can then be added to the culture medium at discrete intervals during the differentiation process to induce expression of the mutant protein–tyrosine kinase. Using this regime we hope to identify windows of sensitivity during the developmental program when transitional cells are most susceptible to the transforming properties of the *abl* and the *src* gene products.

Bearing in mind that a large proportion of all human cancers develop in tissues involved in continuous self-renewal (21), the experiments just outlined will provide us with information pertinent to both the biological role protooncogenes play in normal differentiation and how oncogenes may perturb these processes to generate malignancies.

VIII. Approaches to Chemotherapy through Protein Phosphorylation

The establishment of a clear association between protein phosphorylation and cell transformation offers a number of novel approaches with regard to cancer chemotherapy. Until recently, a major approach adopted by many pharmaceutical companies in developing chemotherapeutic agents has involved screening compounds almost at random. This has been unavoidable, given the limited understanding of the transformation process. With the isolation of oncogenes, however, this situation has changed dramatically. For the first time we have a single protein with a defined biochemical activity capable of transforming cells. It should now be possible to develop specific inhibitors of protein–tyrosine kinases, for example, based on substrate analogs.

Since protein kinases show distinct substrate specificities [56,57; also reviewed by Foulkes and Rich-Rosner (58)], designing specific inhibitors should also be possible. The major difficulty will be to develop compounds which can distinguish between the mutated oncogenic version of a kinase and its normal cellular homolog. Further developments in this area will also require the identification of those human tumors which involve tyrosine phosphorylation. Although one-third of all known oncogenes encode protein–tyrosine kinases, to date there are very few data implicating these enzymes in human cancers (49,143). One notable exception is the *abl* oncogene which appears to be closely linked with chronic myelogenous leukemia (72,95). Our laboratory now intends to screen human tumors with an anti-phosphotyrosine antibody to detect those tumors which show an elevated level of phosphotyrosine-containing proteins. Another equally valid approach will be to study the host cell phosphotyrosyl protein phosphatases as potential anti-oncogenes. As discussed earlier, transformation by tyrosine-specific protein kinases is a dynamic equilibrium process. We need to purify tyrosine phosphatases and to find out how they are regulated. Instead of designing tyrosine kinase inhibitors, one could then think about chemotherapeutic agents based on protein phosphatase activators. Finally, once identified, relevant tyrosine kinase substrates could then become the target of chemotherapeutic drug design. Given the current cancer mortality figures of one in four people in the Western world (reviewed in "Cancer Research Campaign," 62nd Annual Report, 1984. Published by Sumfield and Day Ltd.), we must hope that such approaches will prove successful.

Acknowledgments

The plasmid pAS1-*abl*-60 was kindly provided by Dr. Lynn Pritchard and Dr. Martin Rosenberg from Smith, Kline and French Laboratories, Philadelphia, Pennsylvania. Plasmids pEX2 and pEX5 were obtained from Drs. Owen N. Witte and James Konopka (Department of Microbiology and Molecular Biology Institute, University of California, Los Angeles). This work was supported by the Medical Research Council (United Kingdom).

References

1. Abelson, H. T., and Rabstein, L. S. (1970). Lymphosarcoma: Virus-induced thymic-independent disease in mice. *Cancer Res.* **30,** 2213–2222.
2. Adams, J. M., Gerondakis, S., Webb, E., Corcoran, L. M., and Cary, S. (1983).

Cellular *myc* is altered by chromosome translocation to an immunoglobulin locus in murine plastocytomas and is rearranged similarily in human Burkitt lymphomas. *Proc. Natl. Acad. Sci. U.S.A.* **80**, 1982–1986.

3. Aitken, A., Cohen, P., Santikarn, S., Williams, D. H., Calder, A. G., Smith, A., and Klee, C. B. (1982). Identification of the NH$_2$-terminal blocking group of calcineurin B as Myristic acid. *FEBS Lett.* **150**, 314–318.

4. Alema, S., Casalbore, P., Agostini, E., and Tato, F. (1985). Differentiation of PC 12 phaeochromocytoma cells induced by v-*src* oncogene. *Nature (London)* **316**, 557–558.

5. Anderson, S. M., and Scolnick, E. M. (1983). Construction and isolation of a transforming murine retrovirus containing the *src* gene of RSV. *J. Virol.* **46**, 594–605.

6. Barnekow, A. (1983). Effect of several nucleotides on the phosphorylating activities of RSV transforming protein pp60$^{v\text{-}src}$ and its cellular homologue, pp60$^{c\text{-}src}$ *Biosci. Rep.* **3**, 153–162.

7. Bartram, C. R., Kleihauer, E., deKlein, A., Grosveld, G., Teyssier, J. R., Neisterkamp, N., and Groffen, J. (1985). c-*abl* and bcr are rearranged in a Ph' negative CML patient. *EMBO J.* **4**, 683–686.

8. Berridge, M. J. (1983). Rapid accumulation of inositol trisphosphate reveals that agonists hydrolyse polyphosphoinositides instead of phosphatidylinositol. *Biochem. J.* **212**, 849–858.

9. Berridge, M. J. (1984). Inositol trisphosphate and diacylglcerol as second messengers. *Biochem. J.* **220**, 345–360.

10. Berridge, M. J., and Irvine, R. F. (1984). Inositol trisphosphate, a novel second messenger in cellular signal transduction. *Nature (London)* **312**, 315–321.

11. Berridge, M. J., Brown, K. D., Irvine, R. F., and Heslop, J. P. (1985). Phosphoinositides and cell proliferation. *J. Cell Sci.* Suppl. **3**, 187–198.

12. Besmer, P., Hardy Jr., W. D., Zuckerman, E. E., Bergold, P., Lederman, L., and Snyder, H. W., Jr. (1983). The Hardy-Zuckerman 2-FeSV, a new feline retrovirus with oncogene homology to A-MuLV. *Nature (London)* **303**, 825–828.

13. Beug, H., Leutz, A., Kahn, P., and Graf, T. (1984). Ts mutants of E26 leukaemia virus allow transformed myeloblasts but not erythroblasts or fibroblasts, to differentiate at the non-permissive temperature. *Cell (Cambridge, Mass.)* **39**, 579–588.

14. Bishop, J. M. (1985). Viral oncogenes. *Cell* **42**, 23–38.

15. Blick, M., Westin, E., Gutterman, J., Wong-Staal, F., Gallo, R., McCredie, K., Keating, M., and Murphy, E. (1984). Oncogene expression in human leukaemia. *Blood* **64**, 1234–1239.

16. Boettiger D. (1985). Effect of oncogenes on stem cells. *BioEssays* **2**, 106–109.

17. Boettiger, D., and Durban, E. M. (1979). Progenitor-cell populations can be infected by RNA tumour viruses, but transformation is dependent on the expression of specific differentiated functions. *Cold Spring Harbor Symp. Quant. Biol.* **44**, 1249–1254.

18. Boettiger, D., Anderson, S. A., and Dexter, T. M. (1984). Effect of *src* infection on long term marrow cultures: Increased self renewal of hemopoietic progenitor cells without leukaemia. *(Cambridge, Mass.) Cell* **36**, 763–773.

19. Bos, J. L., Toksok, D., Marshall, C. J., Verlaan-de Vries, M., Veeneman, G. H., Van der Eb, A., van Boom, J. H., Janssen, J. W. G., and Steenvoorden, A. C. M. (1985). Amino-acid substitutions at codon 13 of the N-*ras* oncogene in human acute myeloid leukaemia. *Nature (London)* **315**, 726–730.

20. Brown, K. D., Blay, J., Irvine, R. F., Heslop, J. P., and Berridge, M. J. (1984). Reduction of EGF receptor affinity by heterologous ligands: Evidence for a mechanism involving the breakdown of phosphoinositides and activation of protein kinase C. *Biochem. Biophys. Res. Commun.* **123**, 377–384.

21. Buick, R. N., and Pollack, M. A. (1984). Perspectives on clonogenic tumour cells, stem cells and oncogenes. *Cancer Res.* **44,** 4909–4918.
22. Bunte, T., Greiser-Wilke, I., Donner, P., and Moelling, K. (1982). Association of *gag-myc* proteins from avian myelocytomatosis virus wild-type and mutants with chromatin. *EMBO J.* **1,** 919–927.
23. Carr, S. A., Biemann, K., Shoji, S., Parmelee, D. C., and Titani, K. (1982). *n*-Tetradecanoyl is the NH_2-terminal blocking group of the catalytic subunit of cyclic AMP-dependant protein kinase from bovine cardiac muscle. *Proc. Natl. Acad. Sci. U.S.A.* **79,** 6128–6131.
24. Cavenee, W. K., Dryja, T. P., Phillips, R. A., Benedict, W. F., Godbout, R., Gallie, B. L., Murphree, A. L., Strong, L. C., and White, R. L. (1983). Expression of recessive alleles by chromosomal mechanisms in retinoblastoma. *Nature (London)* **305,** 779–784.
25. Cohen, P. (1982). The role of protein phosphorylation in neural and hormonal control of cellular activity. *Nature (London)* **296,** 613–619.
25a. Colledge, W. H., Edge, M., and Foulkes, J. C. (1986). A comparison of topoisomerase activity in normal and transformed cells. *Biosci. Rep.* **6,** 301–307.
26. Collett, M. S., and Erikson, R. L. (1978). Protein kinase activity associated with the avian sarcoma virus *src* gene product. *Proc. Natl. Acad. Sci. U.S.A.* **75,** 2021–2024.
27. Cook, W. (1982). Rapid thymomas induced by A-MuLV. *Proc. Natl. Acad. Sci. U.S.A.* **79,** 2917–2921.
28. Cooper, J. A., and Hunter, T. (1981). Changes in protein phosphorylation in RSV-transformed chicken embryo cells. *Mol. Cell. Biol.* **1,** 165–178.
29. Cooper, J. A., and Hunter, T. (1983). Identification and characterisation of cellular targets for tyrosine protein kinases. *J. Biol. Chem.* **258,** 1108–1115.
30. Cooper, J. A., Bowen-Pope, D. F., Raines, E., Ross, R., and Hunter, T. (1982). Similar effects of PDGF and EGF on the phosphorylation of tyrosine in cellular proteins. *Cell (Cambridge, Mass.)* **31,** 263–273.
31. Cooper, J. A., Reiss, N. A., Schwartz, R. J., and Hunter, T. (1983). Three glycolytic enzymes are phosphorylated at tyrosine in cells transformed by RSV. *Nature (London)* **302,** 218–223.
32. Cooper, J. A., Esch, F. S., Taylor, S. S., and Hunter, T. (1984). Phosphorylation sites in enolase and lactate dehydrogenase utilised by tyrosine protein kinases *in vivo* and *in vitro*. *J. Biol. Chem.* **259,** 7835–7841.
33. Cooper, J. A., Sefton, B. M., and Hunter, T. (1984). Diverse mitogenic agents induce the phosphorylation of two related 42,000 dalton proteins on tyrosine in quiescent chick cells. *Mol. Cell. Biol.* **4,** 30–37.
34. Creba, J. A., Downes, C. P., Hawkins, P. T., Brewster, G., Michell, R. H., and Kirk, C. J. (1983). Rapid breakdown of phosphatidylinositol 4-phosphate and phosphatidylinositol 4,5-bisphosphate in rat hepatocytes stimulated by vasopressin and other Ca^{2+}-mobilising hormones. *Biochem. J.* **212,** 733–747.
35. Cross, F. R., Garber, E. A., Pellman, D., and Hanafusa, H. (1984). A short sequence in p60^{src} N terminus is required for p60^{src} myristylation and membrane association and for cell transformation. *Mol. Cell. Biol.* **4,** 1834–1842.
36. Decker, S. (1981). Phosphorylation of ribosomal protein S6 in avian sarcoma virus-transformed chicken embryo fibroblasts. *Proc. Natl. Acad. Sci. U.S.A.* **78,** 4112–4115.
37. Der, C. J., Krontiris, T. G., and Cooper, G. M. (1982). Transforming genes of human bladder and lung carcinoma cell lines are homologous to the *ras* genes of harvey and Kirsten sarcoma viruses. *Proc. Natl. Acad. Sci. U.S.A.* **79,** 3637–3640.
38. Dickson, C., Smith, R., Brookes, S., and Peters, G. (1984). Tumorigenesis by mouse mammary tumor virus. *Cell (Cambridge, Mass.)* **37,** 529–536.

39. Diringer, H., and Friis, R. R. (1977). Changes in phosphatidylinositol metabolism correlated to growth state of normal and RSV-transformed Japanese quail cells. *Cancer Res.* **37,** 2979–2984.
40. Donner, P., Greiser-Wilke, I., and Moelling, K. (1982). Nuclear localisation and DNA-binding of the transforming gene product of avian myelocytomatosis virus. *Nature (London)* **296,** 262–266.
41. Donner, P., Bunte, T., Greiser-Wilke, I., and Moelling, K. (1983). Reduced DNA-binding ability of purified transformation-specific proteins from deletion mutants of the acute avian leukaemia virus MC29. *Proc. Natl. Acad. Sci. U.S.A.* **80,** 2861–2865.
42. Downes, C. P., and Michell, R. H. (1981). The polyphosphoinositide phosphodiesterase of erythrocyte membranes. *Biochem. J.* **198,** 133–140.
43. Downes, C. P., and Wusteman, M. M. (1983). Breakdown of polyphosphoinositides and not phosphatidylinositol accounts for muscarinic agonist-stimulated inositol phospholipid metabolism in rat parotid glands. *Biochem. J.* **216,** 633–640.
44. Downward, J., Yarden, Y., Mayes, E., Scrace, G., Totty, N., Stockwell, P., Ullrich, A., Schlessinger, J., and Waterfield, M. D. (1984). Close similarity of EGF receptor and v-*erb-B* oncogene protein sequences. *Nature (London)* **307,** 521–527.
45. Duncan, R., and McConkey, E. H. (1982). Preferential utilisation of phosphorylated 40S ribosomal subunits during initiation complex formation. *Eur. J. Biochem.* **123,** 535–538.
46. Durban, E. M., and Boettiger, D. (1981). Differential effects of transforming avian RNA tumour virus on avian macrophages. *Proc. Natl. Acad. Sci. U.S.A.* **78,** 3600–3604.
47. Eniretto, P. J., and Wyke, J. A. (1983). The pathogenesis of oncogenic avian retroviruses. *Adv. Cancer Res.* **39,** 269–309.
48. Erikson, R. L., Purchio, A. F., Erikson, E., Collett, M. S., and Brugge, J. S. (1980). Molecular events in cells transformed by RSV. *J. Cell Biol.* **87,** 319–325.
49. Eva, A., Robbins, K. C., Anderson, P. R., Srinivasan, A., Tronick, S. R., Reddy, E. P., Ellimore, N. W., Galen, A. T., Lautenberger, J. A., Papas, T. S., Westin, E. H., Wong-Staal, F., Gallo, R. C., and Aaronson, S. A. (1982). Cellular genes analogous to retroviral *onc* genes are transcribed in human tumour cells. *Nature (London)* **295,** 116–119.
50. Eva, A., Tronick, S. R., Gol, R. A., Pierce, J. M., and Aaronson, A. S. (1983). Transforming genes of human hematopoietic tumours: Frequent detection of *ras*-related oncogenes whose activation appears to be independent of tumour phenotype. *Proc. Natl. Acad. Sci. U.S.A.* **80,** 4926–4930.
51. Falcone, G., Tato, F., and Alemo, S. (1985). Distinctive effects of the viral oncogenes *myc, erb, fps,* and *src* on the differentiation program of quail myogenic cells. *Proc. Natl. Acad. Sci. U.S.A.* **82,** 426–430.
52. Fasano, O., Aldrich, T., Tamanoi, F., Taparowsky, E., Furth, M., and Wigler, M. (1984). Analysis of the transforming potential of the human H-ras gene. *Proc. Natl. Acad. Sci. U.S.A.* **81,** 4008–4012.
53. Ferguson, B., Pritchards, M. L., Feild, J., Rieman, D., Greig, G., Poste, G., and Rosenberg, M. (1985). Isolation and analysis of an A-MuLV encoded tyrosine-specific kinase produced in *E. coli. J. Biol. Chem.* **260,** 3652–3657.
54. Feuerman, M. H., Davis, B. R., Pattengate, P. K., and Fang, H. (1985). Generation of a recombinant moloney murine leukaemia virus. *J. Virol.* **54,** 804–816.
55. Foulkes, J. G. (1983). Phosphotyrosyl-protein phosphatases. *Curr. Top. Microbiol. Immunol.* **107,** 163–180.
56. Foulkes, J. G., Chow, M., Gorka, C., Frackelton, R., and Baltimore, D. (1985).

Purification and characterisation of a protein-tyrosine kinase encoded by the Abelson murine leukaemia virus. *J. Biol. Chem.* **260**, 8070–8077.

57. Foulkes, J. G., Mathey-Prevot, B., Guild, B. C., Prywes, R., and Baltimore, D. (1985). A comparison of the protein-tyrosine kinases encoded by A-MuLV and RSV. *Cancer Cells* **3**, 329–337.

58. Foulkes, J. G., and Rich-Rosner, M. (1985). Tyrosine-specific protein kinases as mediators of growth control. *In* "Molecular Aspects of Cellular Regulation" Vol. 4 (P. Cohen and M. D. Housley, eds.), pp. 217–252. Elsevier North-Holland, New York.

59. Frackelton, A. R., Ross, A. H., and Eisen, H. N. (1983). Characterisation and use of monoclonal antibodies for isolation of phosphotyrosyl proteins from retrovirus transformed cells and growth factor stimulated cells. *Mol. Cell. Biol.* **3**, 1343–1352.

60. Frackelton, A. R., Tremble, P. M., and Williams, L. T. (1984). Evidence for the PDGF-stimulated tyrosine phosphorylation of the PDGF receptor *in vivo:* Immunopurification using a monoclonal antibody to phosphotyrosine. *J. Biol. Chem.* **259**, 7909–7915.

61. Fraenkel, D. G. (1985). On *ras* gene function in yeast. *Proc. Natl. Acad. Sci. U.S.A.* **82**, 4740-4744.

62. Fry, M. J., Gebhardt, A., Parker, P. J., and Foulkes, J. G. (1985). Phosphatidylinositol turnover and transformation of cells by A-MuLV. *EMBO J.* **4**, 3173–3178.

63. Fults, D. W., Towle, A. C., Kauder, J. M., and Maness, P. F. (1985). pp60^{c-src} in the developing cerebellum. *Mol. Cell. Biol.* **5**, 27–32.

64. Fung, Y. K. T., Lewis, W. G., denCritten, L. B., and Kung, H. J. (1983). Activation of the cellular oncogene c-erbB by LTR insertion. *Cell (Cambridge, Mass.)* **33**, 357–368.

65. Gibbs, J. B., Sigal, I. S., Poe, M., and Scolnick, E. M. (1984). Intrinsic GTPase activity distinguishes normal and oncogenic *ras* p21 molecules. *Proc. Natl. Acad. Sci. U.S.A.,* **81**, 5704–5708.

66. Gilman, A. G. (1984). G proteins and dual control of adenylate cyclase. *Cell (Cambridge, Mass.)* **36**, 577–579.

67. Glover, C. V. C. (1982). Heat shock induces rapid dephosphorylation of a ribosomal protein in *Drosophila*. *Proc. Natl. Acad. Sci. U.S.A.* **79**, 1781–1785.

68. Goff, S. P., Giboa, E., Witte, O. N., and Baltimore, D. (1980). Structure of the A-MuLV genome and the homologous cellular gene: Studies with cloned viral DNA. *Cell (Cambridge, Mass.)* **22**, 777–785.

69. Goff, S. P., Tabin, C. J., Wang, J. Y. J., Weinberg, R., and Baltimore, D. (1982). Transfection of fibroblasts by cloned A-MuLV DNA and recovery of transmissible virus by recombination with helper virus. *J. Virol.* **41**, 271–285.

70. Gonda, T. J., and Metcalf, D. (1984). Expression of *myb, myc,* and *fos* proto-oncogenes during the differentiation of a murine myeloid leukemia. *Nature (London)* **310**, 249–251.

71. Habernicht, A. J. R., Glomset, J. A., King, W. C., Nist, C., Mitchell, C. D., and Ross, R. (1981). Early changes in phosphatidylinositol and arachidonic acid metabolism in quiescent Swiss 3T3 cells stimulated to divide by PDGF. *J. Biol. Chem.* **256**, 12329–12335.

72. Heisterkamp, N., Groffen, J., Stephenson, J. R., Spurr, N. K., Goodfellow, P. N., Solomon, B., Garritt, B., and Bodmer, W. F. (1982). Chromosomal localisation of human cellular homologues of two viral oncogenes. *Nature (London)* **299**, 747–749.

73. Henderson, L. E., Krutzsch, H. C., and Oroszlan, S. (1983). Myristyl amino-terminal acylation of murine retrovirus proteins: An unusual post-translational protein modification. *Proc. Natl. Acad. Sci. U.S.A.* **80**, 339–343.

74. Hunter, T. (1984). The EGF receptor gene and its product. *Nature (London)* **311**, 414–416.
75. Hunter, T., and Cooper, J. A. (1985). Protein-tyrosine kinases. *Annu. Rev. Biochem.* **54**, 897–930.
76. Hunter, T., Sefton, B. M., and Beemon, K. (1979). Studies on the structure and function of the avian sarcoma virus transforming gene product. *Cold Spring Harbor Symp. Quant. Biol.* **44**, 931–941.
77. Hunter, T., and Sefton, B. M. (1980). Transforming gene product of Rous sarcoma virus phosphorylates tryosine. *Proc. Natl. Acad. Sci. U.S.A.* **77**, 1311–1315.
78. Hunter, T., and Sefton, B. M. (1981). Protein kinases and viral transformation. *In* "Molecular Aspects of Cellular Regulation" (P. Cohen and S. Van Heyningen, eds.), Vol. 2, pp. 337–370. Elsevier North-Holland, New York.
79. Hurley, J. B., Simon, M. I., Teplow, D. B., Robinson, J. D., and Gilman, A. G. (1984). Homologies between signal transducing proteins and *ras* gene products. *Science,* **226**, 860–862.
80. Iba, H., Takeya, T., Cross, F. R., Hanafusa, T., and Hanafusa, H. (1984). Rous sarcoma variants that carry c-*src* instead of v-*src* cannot transform chicken embryo fibroblasts. *Proc. Natl. Acad. Sci. U.S.A.* **81**, 4424–4428.
81. Irvine, R. F., Brown, K. D., and Berridge, M. J. (1984). Specificity of inositol trisphosphate-induced calcium release from permeabilized Swiss-mouse 3T3 cells. *Biochem. J.* **221**, 269–272.
82. Ito, S., Richert, N., and Pastan, I. (1982). Phospholipids stimulate phosphorylation of vinculin by the tyrosine specific protein kinase of RSV. *Proc. Natl. Acad. Sci. U.S.A.* **79**, 4628–4631.
83. Jacobs, S., Kull, F. C., Earp, H. S., Svoboda, M. E., Van Wyk, J. J., and Cuatrecasas, P. (1983). Somatomedin C stimulates the phosphorylation of the subunit of its own receptor. *J. Biol. Chem.* **258**, 9581–9584.
84. Jakobovits, E. B., Majors, J. E., and Varmus, H. E. (1984). Hormonal regulation of the Rous sarcoma virus *src* gene defines a threshold dose for cellular transformation. *Cell (Cambridge, Mass.)* **38**, 757–765.
85. Jones-Villeneuve, E. M. V., McBurney, M. W., Rogers, K. A., and Kalnins, V. I. (1982). Retinoic acid induces embryonal carcinoma cells to differentiate into neurons and glial cells. *J. Cell. Biol.* **94**, 253–262.
86. Kamps, M. P., Buss, J. E., and Sefton, B. M. (1985). Mutation of NH_2-terminal glycine of p60^{src} prevents myristilation and morphological transformation. *Proc. Natl. Acad. Sci. U.S.A.* **82**, 4625–4628.
87. Kasuga, M., Zick, Y., Blith, D. L., Karlsson, F. A., Haring, H. U., and Kahn, C. R. (1982). Insulin stimulation of phosphorylation of the subunit of the insulin receptor. *J. Biol. Chem.* **257**, 9891-9894.
88. Kasuga, M., Zick, Y., Blithe, D. L., Crettaz, M., and Kahn, C. R. (1982). Insulin stimulates tyrosine phosphorylation of the insulin receptor in a cell-free system. *Nature (London)* **298**, 667–669.
89. Katzen, A. L., Kornberg, T. B., and Bishop, J. M. (1985). Isolation of the protooncogene c-*myb* from *D. melanogaster*. *Cell (Cambridge, Mass.)* **41**, 449–456.
90. Klein, G., and Klein, E. (1985). Evolution of tumors and the impact of molecular oncology. *Nature (London)* **315**, 190–195.
91. Klempnauer, K. H., Symonds, G., Evans, G. I., and Bishop, J. M. (1984). Subcellular localisation of proteins encoded by oncogenes of avian myeloblastosis virus and avian leukaemia virus E26 and by the chicken c-*myb* gene. *Cell (Cambridge, Mass.)* **37**, 537–547.

92. Kloetzer, W. S., Maxwell, S. A., and Arlinghaus, R. B. (1983). p85$^{gag-mos}$ has an associated protein kinase activity. *Proc. Natl. Acad. Sci. U.S.A.* **80,** 412–416.
93. Konopka, J. B., Davis, R. L., Watanabe, S. M., Ponticelli, A. S., Schiff-Maker, L., Rosenberg, N., and Witte, O. N. (1984). Only site-directed antibodies reactive with the highly conserved *src*-homologous region of the v-*abl* protein neutralize kinase activity. *J. Virol.* **51,** 223–232.
94. Konopka, J. B., Watanabe, S. M., Singer, J. W., Collins, S. J., and Witte, O. N. (1985). Cell lines and clinical isolates derived from Ph'-positive chronic myelogenous leukemia patients. *Proc. Natl. Acad. Sci. U.S.A.* **82,** 1810–1814.
95. Konopka, J. B., and Witte, O. N. (1985). Activation of the *abl* oncogene in murine and human leukaemias. *Biochim. Biophys. Acta* **823,** 1–17.
96. Koufos, A., Hansen, M. F., Lampkin, B. C., Workman, M. L., Copeland, N. G., Jenkins, N. A., and Cavenee, W. K. (1984). Loss of alleles at loci on human chromosome 11 during genesis of Wilm's tumour. *Nature (London)* **309,** 170–172.
97. Lachman, H. M., and Skoultchi, A. I. (1984). Expression of c-*myc* changes during differentiation of mouse erythroleukemia cells. *Nature (London)* **310,** 592–594.
98. LePeuch, C. J., Ballester, R., and Rosen, I. (1983). Purified rat brain calcium- and phospholipid-dependent protein kinase phosphorylates ribosomal protein S6. *Proc. Natl. Acad. Sci. U.S.A.* **80,** 6858–6862.
99. Levy, B. T., Sorge, L. K., Dram, C. C., and Manes, P. F. (1983). Differential inhibition of cellular and viral pp60^{v-src} kinase by P^1,P^{4}di(adenosine-5^1) tetraphosphate. *Mol. Cell. Biol.* **3,** 1718–1723.
100. Little, C. D., Nau, M. M., Carney, D. N., Gazdar, A. F., and Minn, J. D. (1983). Amplification and expression of the c-*myc* oncogene. *Nature (London)* **306,** 194–196.
101. Macara, I. G., Marinetti, G. V., and Balduzzi, P. C. (1984). Transforming protein of avian sarcoma virus UR2 is associated with phosphatidylinositol kinase activity: Possible role in tumorigenesis. *Proc. Natl. Acad. Sci. U.S.A.* **81,** 2728–2732.
102. Macara, I. G. (1985). Oncogenes, ions, and phospholipids. *Am. J. Physiol.* **248,** c3–c11.
103. Maller, J. L., Foulkes, J. G., Erikson, E., and Baltimore, D. (1985). Phosphorylation of ribosomal protein S6 on serine after microinjection of the Abelson murine leukaemia virus tyrosine-specific protein kinase into *Xenopus* oocytes. *Proc. Natl. Acad. Sci. U.S.A.* **82,** 272–276.
104. Maltzman, W., and Levine, A. J. (1981). Viruses as probes for development and differentiation. *Adv. Virus Res.* **26,** 65–116.
105. Mathey-Prevot, B., and Baltimore, D. (1985). Specific transforming potential of oncogenes encoding protein-tyrosine kinases. *EMBO J.* **4,** 1769–1774.
106. McBurney, M. W., and Rogers, B. J. (1982). Isolation of male embryonal carcinoma cells and their chromosome replication patterns. *Dev. Biol.* **89,** 503–508.
107. Miller, A. D., Curran, T., and Verma, I. M. (1984). c-*fos* protein can induce cellular transformation. *Cell (Cambridge, Mass.)* **36,** 51–60.
108. Mitchell, R. L., Zokas, L., Schreiber, R. D., and Verma, I. M. (1985). Rapid induction of the expression of proto-oncogene *fos* during human monocytic differentiation. *Cell (Cambridge, Mass.)* **40,** 209–217.
109. Mitelman, F. (1984). Restricted number of chromosomal regions implicated in the aetiology of human cancer. *Nature (London)* **310,** 325–327.
110. Moelling, K., Bunte, T., Greiser-Wilke, I., Donner, P., and Pfaff, E. (1984). Properties of the avian viral transforming proteins *gag-myc, myc,* and *gag-mil. Cancer Cells* **2,** 173–180.
111. Moelling, K., Heimann, B., Beimling, P., Rapp, H. R., and Sander, T. (1984). Serine-

and threonine-specific protein kinase activities of purified *gag-mil* and *gag-raf* proteins. *Nature (London)* **312,** 558–561.

112. Muller, R., and Wagner, E. F. (1984). Differentiation of F9 teratocarcinoma stem cells after transfer of c-*fos* proto-oncogenes. *Nature (London)* **311,** 438–442.

113. Muller, R., Slamon, D. J., Tremblay, J. M., Cline, M. J., and Verma, I. M. (1982). Differential expression of cellular oncogenes during pre- and post-natal development of the mouse. *Nature (London)* **299,** 640–644.

114. Neckameyer, W. S., and Wang, L. H. (1985). Nucleotide sequence of avian sarcoma virus UR2. *J. Virol.* **53,** 879–885.

115. Neil, J. C., Hughes, D., McFarlane, R., Wilkie, N. M., Onions, D. E., Lees, G., and Jarrett, O. (1984). Transduction and rearrangement of the *myc* gene by feline leukaemia virus. *Nature (London)* **308,** 814–820.

116. Nishimura, J., Huang, J. S., and Deuel, T. F. (1982). PDGF stimulates tyrosine - specific protein kinase activity in Swiss mouse 3T3 cell membranes. *Proc. Natl. Acad. Sci. U.S.A.* **79,** 4303–4307.

117. Nishimura, J., and Deuel, T. F. (1983). PDGF stimulates the phosphorylation of ribosomal protein S6. *FEBS Lett.* **156,** 130–134.

118. Nishizuka, Y. (1984). The role of protein kinase C in cell surface signal transduction and tumour production. *Nature (London)* **308,** 693–698.

119. Ozols, J., Carr, S. A., and Strittmatter, P. (1984). Identification of the NH$_2$-terminal blocking group of NADH-cytochrome b$_5$ reductase as myristic acid and the complete amino acid sequence of the membrane-binding domain. *J. Biol. Chem.* **259,** 13349–13354.

120. Papageorge, A., Lowy, D., and Scolnick, E. M. (1982). Comparative biochemical properties of p21^{ras} molecules. *J. Virol.* **44,** 509–519.

121. Parker, P. J., Katan, M., Waterfield, M. D., and Leader, D. P. (1985). The phosphorylation of eukaryotic ribosomal protein S6 by protein kinase C. *Eur. J. Biochem.* **148,** 579–586.

122. Parker, R. C., Varmus, H. E., and Bishop, J. M. (1984). Expression of v-*src* and chicken c-*src* in rat cells demonstrates qualitative differences between pp60^{v-src} and pp60^{c-src}. *Cell (Cambridge, Mass.)* **37,** 131–139.

123. Payne, G. S., Bishop, J. M., and Varmus H. E. (1982). Multiple arrangements of viral DNA and an activated host oncogene in bursal lymphomas. *Nature (London)* **295,** 209–217.

124. Pierce, J. H., Aaronson, S. A., and Anderson, S. M. (1984). Hematopoietic cells transformation by a murine recombinant retrovirus containing the *src* gene of RSV. *Proc. Natl. Acad. Sci. U.S.A.* **81,** 2374–2378.

125. Prywes, R., Foulkes, J. G., Rosenberg, N., and Baltimore, D. (1983). Sequences of the A-MuLV protein needed for fibroblast and lymphoid cell transformation. *Cell (Cambridge, Mass.)* **34,** 569–579.

126. Prywes, R., Hoag, J., Rosenberg, N., and Baltimore, D. (1985). Protein stabilisation explains the *gag* requirement for transformation of lymphoid cell by Abelson murine leukaemia virus. *J. Virol.* **54,** 123–132.

127. Prywes, R., Foulkes, J. G., and Baltimore, D. (1985). The minimum transforming region of v-*abl* is the segment encoding protein-tyrosine kinase. *J. Virol.* **54,** 114–122.

128. Pulciani, S., Santos, E., Lauver, A. V., Long, L. K., Robbins, K. C., and Barbacid, M. (1982). Oncogenes in human tumour cell lines: Molecular cloning of a transforming gene from human bladder carcinoma cells. *Proc. Natl. Acad. Sci. U.S.A.* **79,** 2845–2850.

129. Rabbitts, T. H., Forster, A., Hamlyn, P., and Baer, R. (1984). Effect of somatic

mutation within translocated c-*myc* genes in Burkitt's lymphoma. *Nature (London)* **309**, 592–597.

130. Rebecchi, M. J., and Gershengorn, M. C. (1983). Thyroliberin stimulates rapid hydrolysis of phosphatidylinositol 4,5-bisphosphate by a phosphodiesterase in rat mammotropic pituitary cells. *Biochem. J.* **216**, 287–294.

131. Reddy, E. P., Reynolds, R. K., Santos, E., and Barbacid, M. (1982). A single point mutation is responsible for the acquisition of transforming properties of the T24 bladder carcinoma oncogene. *Nature (London)* **300**, 149–152.

132. Rettenmier, C. W., Chen, J. H., Roussel, M. F., and Sherr, C. J. (1985). The product of the c-*fms* proto-oncogene: A glycoprotein with associated tyrosine kinase activity. *Science,* **228** 320–322.

133. Risser, R. (1982). The patheogenesis of Abelson virus lymphomas of the mouse. *Biochim. Biophys. Acta* **651**, 213–244.

134. Rosenberg, N., Baltimore, D., and Scher, C. D. (1975). *In vitro* transformation of lymphoid cells by A-MuLV. *Proc. Natl. Acad. Sci. U.S.A.* **72**, 1932–1936.

135. Saito, H., Hayday, A. C., Wiman, K., Hayward, W. S., and Tonegawa, S. (1983). Activation of the c-*myc* gene by transduction. *Proc. Natl. Acad. Sci. U.S.A.* **80**, 7476–7480.

136. Samurat, J., and Gazylo, L. (1982). Target cells infected by AEV differentiate and become transformed. *Cell (Cambridge, Mass.)* **28**, 921–929.

137. Scher, C. D., and Siegler, R. (1975). Direct transformation of 3T3 cells by A-MuLV. *Nature (London)* **253**, 729–731.

138. Schwab, M., Varmus, H. E., and Bishop, J. M. (1984). Amplification of cellular oncogenes in tumor cells. *Cancer Cells* **2**, 215–220.

139. Sefton, B. M., Trowbridge, I. S., Cooper, J. A., and Scolnick, E. M. (1982). The transforming proteins of RSV, Harvey sarcoma virus, and A-MuLV contain tightly bound lipid. *Cell (Cambridge, Mass.)* **31**, 465–474.

140. Sheiness, D., and Gardinier, M. (1984). Expression of a proto-oncogene (proto-*myb*) in hemopoietic tissues of mice. *Mol. Cell. Biol.* **4**, 1206–1212.

141. Sherr, C. J., Rettenmier, C. W., Sacca, R., Roussel, M. F., Look, A. T., and Stanley, E. R. (1985). The c-*fms* proto-oncogene product is related to the receptor for the mononuclear phagocyte growth factor, CSF-1. *Cell (Cambridge, Mass.)* **4**, 665–676.

142. Shih, T. Y., Papageorge, A. G., Stokes, P. E., Weeks, M. O., and Scolnick, E. M. (1980). Guanine nucleotide-binding and autophosphorylation activities associated with p21^{src} protein of Harvey murine sarcoma virus. *Nature (London)* **287**, 686–691.

143. Slamon, D. J., deKernion, J. B., Verma, I. M., and Cline, M. J. (1984). Expression of cellular oncogenes in human malignancies. *Science,* **224**, 256–262.

144. Srinivasan, A., Reddy, E. P., Dunn, C. Y., and Aaronson, S. (1984). Molecular dissection of transcriptional control elements. *Science* **223**, 286–289.

145. Sugimoto, Y., Whitman, M., Cantley, L. C., and Erikson, R. L. (1984). Evidence that the RSV transforming gene product phosphorylates phosphatidylinositol and diacylglycerol. *Proc. Natl. Acad. Sci. U.S.A.* **81**, 2117–2121.

146. Sukumar, S., Notario, V., Martin-Zanca, D., and Barbacid, M. (1983). Induction of mammary carcinomas in rats by nitroso-methyl urea involves malignant activation of H-*ras*-1 by single point mutations. *Nature (London)* **306**, 658–661.

147. Sweet, R. W., Yokoyama, S., Kamata, T., Fermisco, J. R., Rosenberg, M., and Gross, M. (1984). The product of *ras* is a GTPase and the T24 oncogenic mutant is deficient in this activity. *Nature (London)* **311**, 273–275.

148. Swergold, G. D., Rosen, O. M., and Rubin, C. S. (1982). Hormonal regulation of the phosphorylation of ATP citrate lyase in 3T3-L1 adipocytes. Effects of insulin and isoproterenol. *J. Biol. Chem.* **257**, 4207–4215.

149. Tabin, C., Bradley, S., Bargmann, C., Weinberg, R., Papageorge, A., Scolnick, E., Dhar, R., Lowy, D., and Chang, E. (1982). Mechanism of activation of a human oncogene. *Nature (London)* **300**, 143–149.

150. Taborsky, G. (1974). Phosphoproteins. *Adv. Protein Chem.* **28**, 1–210.

151. Temin, H. M. (1982). Function of the retrovirus long terminal repeat. *Cell (Cambridge, Mass.)* **28**, 3–5.

152. Thomas, G., Martin-Perez, J., Siegmann, M., and Otto, A. M. (1982). The effect of serum, EGF, PGF$_2$ and insulin on S6 phosphorylation and initiation of protein and DNA synthesis. *Cell (Cambridge, Mass.)* **30**, 235–242.

153. Toda, T., Uno, I., Ishikawa, T., Powers, S., Kataoka, T., Broek, D., Cameron, S., Broach, J., Matsumoto, K., and Wigler, M. (1985). In yeast, RAS proteins are controlling elements of adenylate cyclase. *Cell (Cambridge, Mass.)* **40**, 27–36.

154. Trevillyan, J. M., Kulkarni, R. K., and Byus, C. V. (1984). Tumor-promoting phorbol esters stimulate the phosphorylation of ribosomal protein S6 in quiescent Reuber H35 Hepatoma cells. *J. Biol. Chem.* **259**, 897–902.

155. Ushiro, H., and Cohen, S. (1980). Identification of phosphotyrosine as a product of the EGF-activated protein kinase in A431 cell membranes. *J. Biol. Chem.* **255**, 8363–8365.

156. Varmus, H. E. (1982). Form and function of retroviral proviruses. *Science*, **216**, 812–820.

157. Verma, I. M., Curran, T., Muller, R., Van Straaten, F., MacConnell, W. P., Miller, A. D., and Van Beveren, C. (1984). The *fos* gene: Organization and expression. *Cancer Cells* **2**, 309–321.

158. Walsh, D. A., Perkins, J. P., and Krebs, E. G. (1968). An adenosine 3′,5′-monophosphate-dependant protein kinase from rabbit skeletal muscle. *J. Biol. Chem.* **243**, 3763–3774.

159. Wang, J., Queen, C., and Baltimore, D. (1982). Expression of an A-MuLV-encoded protein in *E. coli* causes extensive phosphorylation of tyrosine residues. *J. Biol. Chem.* **257**, 13181–13184.

160. Watanabe, S. M., and Witte, O. N. (1983). Site-directed deletions of A-MuLV define 3′ sequences essential for transformation and lethality. *J. Virol.* **45**, 1028–1036.

161. Waterfield, M. D., Scrace, G. T., Whittle, N., Stroobant, P., Johnsson, A., Wasteson, A., Westermark, B., Heldin, C-H., Huang, J. S., and Deuel, T. F. (1983). PDGF is structurally related to the putative transforming protein p28^{sis} of Simian sarcoma virus. *Nature (London)* **304**, 35–39.

162. Weller, M. (1979), "Protein Phosphorylation." Pion Ltd., London.

163. Whitman, M., Kaplan, D. R., Schaffhausen, B., Cantley, L., and Roberts, T. M. (1985). Association of phosphatidylinositol kinase activity with polyoma middle-T competent for transformation. *Nature (London)* **315**, 239–242.

164. Wigler, M., Fasano, O., Taparowsky, E., Powers, S., Kataoka, T., Birnbaum, D., Shimizu, K., and Goldfarb, M. (1984). Structure and activation of *ras* genes. *Cancer Cells* **2**, 419–423.

165. Witte, O. N., Rosenberg, N., and Baltimore, D. (1979). A normal cell protein cross-reactive to the major A-MuLV gene product. *Nature (London)* **281**, 396–398.

166. Yunis, J. J. (1983). Chromosomal basis of human neoplasia. *Science* **221**, 227–235.

167. Zarbl, H., Sukumar, S., Arthur, A. V., Martin-Zanca, D., and Barbacid, M. (1985). Direct mutagenesis of Ha-*ras*-1 oncogenes by N nitroso-N methyl urea. *Nature (London)* **315**, 382–385.

168. Ziemiecki, A., and Friis, R. R. (1980). Phosphorylation of pp60^{src} and the cycloheximide insensitive activation of the pp60^{src} associated kinase activity of transformation-defective temperature-sensitive mutants of RSV. *Virology* **106**, 391–394.

23

Major Histocompatibility Complex Class I Expression and Malignancy

MICHAEL J. CHORNEY, RAKESH SRIVASTAVA, JULIAN PAN, AND SHERMAN M. WEISSMAN

Department of Human Genetics
Yale University School of Medicine
New Haven, Connecticut

YURI BUSHKIN* AND YVON CAYRE†

* Laboratory of Molecular Immunology
† Laboratory of Molecular Immunogenetics
Memorial Sloan-Kettering Cancer Center
New York, New York

I. Introduction

The major histocompatibility complex (MHC) of the mouse is composed of an assemblage of diverse genes whose products participate directly in the regulation of both humoral and cellular immune responses (23). The murine MHC has recently been divided into two main regions by

NEW AVENUES IN DEVELOPMENTAL
CANCER CHEMOTHERAPY

molecular immunogeneticists, one termed *H-2* and the other known as *Qa/Tla*. The genes of the *H-2* complex region have been divided into three classes designated I, II, and III (64). Class I genes include those whose structurally similar protein products [45-kDa, β2-microglobulin- (β2M-) associated] were first observed to trigger tissue graft rejection (35,42). Expressed on all somatic cells, these glycoproteins, termed K, D, and L, are now known to direct the killing of cells bearing foreign antigens by syngeneic immune T cells, a process known as restriction (75). Class II genes, encoded in the *I* region, were originally termed *Ir* (for immune response) and were directly linked to an individual mouse strain's ability to mount an antibody response to a variety of antigens (1). *I* region genes encode α and β glycoprotein chains which are expressed on B cells, activated T cells, and macrophages; together they function as signals ensuring effective cooperation among the cells of the lymphoid system. Unlike class I and II molecules which exist at the cell surface, class III products function in the blood where they partially comprise the complement system. In summation, the *H-2* gene products are intimately involved in the coordination and implementation of the antibody and cellular responses to foreign antigens.

Molecules encoded in the *Qa/Tla* region (telomeric distal to *H-2*) are, by virtue of their protein structure, placed within the class I category. However, unlike *H-2* class I products, these cell surface glycoproteins are not expressed by all somatic cells (most are limited to a very narrow range of tissue expression) and do not serve as restriction elements in T-cell-mediated immune recognition. Their most interesting attribute is their anomalous expression on malignant cells and hence their possible association with the process of leukemogenesis in the mouse (5).

Although *H-2*-encoded class I gene products are involved in self recognition, the question of an association between class I expression in general and cancer is becoming increasingly intriguing. Although little information exists on the direct interaction between class I genes and the genes involved in malignant transformation, changes in the expression of the classical transplantation antigens in tumor cells may alter their tumorigenicity. Further investigations into the nature of class I gene regulation, especially with respect to the genes of the *Qa/Tla* region, may well lead to a clearer understanding of the changes occurring during malignant transformation.

II. Thymus-Leukemia Antigen

Thymus-leukemia antigen (TL) was discovered by Old and co-workers at Memorial Sloan-Kettering Cancer Center in 1963 while they were looking for leukemia-specific cell surface molecules (37). Using C57BL/6 mice and immunizing with spontaneous and X-ray-induced A strain leukemias they were able to show, after *H-2* antibodies were absorbed, reactivities against some leukemias and against thymocytes of some mouse strains. The most surprising findings were that TL may be expressed in leukemias from strains of mice phenotypically TL negative (C57BL/6), and that leukemias expressing TL and arising from certain strains (i.e. BALB/c and DBA/2) could express TL serological specificities not normally found on their thymocytes (38). These findings suggested that the TL structural gene is present in all strains although repressed in the thymuses of some mice (only to be derepressed during some stage of leukemogenesis) and that TL may be encoded by more than one structural gene allowing for the phenotypic representation of leukemia-specific serologic determinants.

Biochemically, TL differs from *H-2* by occurring not as a single heavy chain but as a doublet of two closely migrating heavy chains (both β2M-associated) derived from a common precursor of approximately 40,000 Da (48). This doublet situation is invariant among all thymocyte TL molecules thus far examined. In addition to the TL doublet proteins (which arise from differences in posttranslational glycosylation or possibly fatty-acylation), certain strains of mice express additional TL-like molecules of higher molecular weight precipitable by anti-TL monoclonal antibodies (10) (Fig. 1). B10.M and A.CA mice possess a single, 53-kDa TL-like molecule more negatively charged than their TL doublet proteins. Strains representative of the *Tla^e* genotype possess two additional TL-like molecules of 52,000 and 53,000 Da, similar but different in primary structure from the doublet TL molecules (11). These findings support the original hypothesis of multiple functional TL genes.

Molecular studies have recently shown the *Tla* region to be much more genetically complex than originally anticipated. Winoto *et al.* (72) have shown that in the BALB/c mouse the majority of class I genes map to *Qa/Tla*. In their report they state that a total of 31 of 36 class I genes are linked in this extensive region, while 5 genes map to *H-2*. The exact number of BALB/c class I genes has now been amended to include 7 *H-2* region genes, 8 *Qa* region genes, 18 *Tla* region genes, and pseudogenes (44,64a). It remains to be seen as to how many of these genes are expressed as distinct proteins.

Fisher *et al.* (15) have sequenced one BALB/c TL gene (*T13^c*) contained in the λ clone 17.3; this gene is believed to be responsible for thymocyte TL expression. In addition, they have identified three other *Tla* genes which show strong homology to 5' and 3' probes obtained from *T13^c*. It is not known, however, whether these genes are expressed. At the nucleotide level, *T13^c* and *H-2K^d* genes share approximately 73% homology in the regions spanning both exons 2 and 3 (encoding the two external

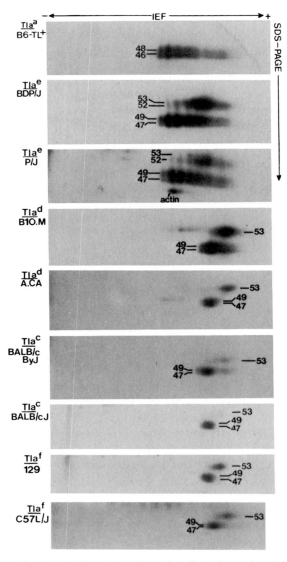

Fig. 1. Two-dimensional isoelectric focusing (first dimension pH 5–8; second dimension 12% acrylamide) of TL immunoprecipitated from ^{125}I-labeled thymocyte lysates. The inbred mouse strains and their *Tla* genotypes are according to Shen *et al.* (54). All genotypes presented, with the exception of *Tla^a^*, encode TL molecules of higher molecular weight than their TL doublet proteins (10,11).

protein domains), while their fourth exons (which encode the β2M-binding domains) show 91% homology. The exon 5 sequences, encoding the transmembrane domains, diverge significantly (64% homology), while exons encoding the cytoplasmic domains are even more divergent.

Obata *et al.* (36) have recently published the sequence of a TL gene (*T3^b*) derived from a C57BL/6 leukemia (ERLD). This gene was isolated from a cosmid library using a probe derived from the 3' coding region of the *T13^c* gene. In general, this gene is as divergent from *H-2K^b* as BALB/c *T13^c* is from *H-2K^d*; both TL genes show a high percentage of overall homology in their coding sequences (approximately 90–96%), which is consistent with the relatively limited polymorphism observed at the tryptic peptide level between TL products in general (10,73,74). The *T3^b* gene previously isolated by Weiss *et al.* (70) from a C57BL/6 genomic library has also been recently sequenced by Pontarotti *et al.* (42a).

Serum from C57BL/6 mice immunized with the B6 leukemia ERLD originally identified the leukemia-specific TL.4 determinant (4). The region of the ERLD TL molecule encoding the TL.4 determinant is as yet uncertain; however, the expression of TL in the ERLD line represents the most striking example of class I gene derepression. Using probes from the *T13^c* and *T3^b* genes, no TL RNA has been observed in B6 thymocytes whose serological phenotype is TL$^-$ (9a,36,42a). In contrast, Michaelson *et al.* (34) have recently claimed that very low amounts of TL are immunoprecipitable from labeled C57BL/6 thymocyte lysates, a protein perhaps encoded by one of the remaining 12 C57BL/6 *Tla* region genes (and not *T3^b*). Unfortunately, because of the exceedingly low amounts of TL present in the lysates, no biochemical data can be obtained to evaluate the possibility that two different *Tla* genes are functioning, one expressed in normal cells and one expressed solely in leukemias, both of which diverge from each other at the nucleotide level. The situation is further complicated by the finding of Chorney *et al.* (10) which suggests that there are in fact two ERLD surface TL molecules, one (50 kDa) expressed at high levels and the other (53 kDa) expressed at lower levels. In any event, the induction of large quantities of surface TL in some leukemias derived from serologically TL-negative strains warrants further investigation at the molecular level.

The question as to whether there are indeed leukemia-specific TL gene products has been investigated by Chorney *et al.*, who looked at TL immunoprecipitated from ^{125}I-labeled lysates of X-ray-induced BALB/c leukemias (11). SDS-PAGE gels revealed two TL molecules equally precipitable by both TL and leukemia-specific TL.4 alloantisera, one of which was 47,000 Da and clearly represented the TL molecule normally expressed on BALB/c thymocytes. The other molecule of approximately

50,000 Da revealed a two-dimensional isoelectric focusing (IEF) profile and a two-dimensional chymotryptic peptide map, both of which were different from those of 47-kDa TL (Fig. 2). Although both molecules were precipitable by anti-TL and anti-TL.4 antisera, the 47 kDa molecule was well recognized by monoclonal anti-TL.2 antibodies which recognize thymocyte TL, whereas the 50 kDa molecule was weakly recognized by the monoclonal antibodies, suggesting serological as well as biochemical differences. Although the authors are cautious to claim that the 50 kDa molecule indeed represents a leukemia-specific TL molecule induced during leukemogenesis, the phenotypic differences observed between thymocyte and leukemia TL make it quite possible that 50 kDa TL may well be limited to expression only on leukemia cells. It may be noted that normal BALB/c thymocytes express a 53 kDa molecule which is precipitable by

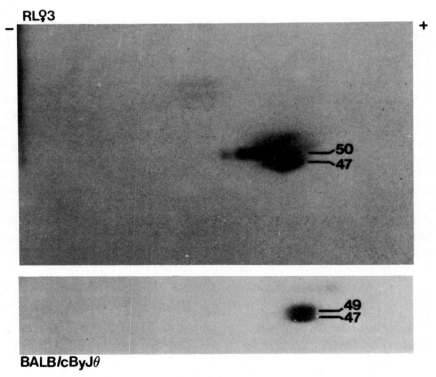

Fig. 2. Two-dimensional IEF comparison of TL immunoprecipitated from BALB/c thymocytes and an X-ray-induced leukemia, RL♀3. The biochemical and serological differences between thymocyte and leukemia TL molecules support the hypothesis that the 50-kDa TL product may be limited to expression on leukemia cells.

anti-TL serum. However, because of the very low amounts of this molecule present on the thymocyte surface no biochemical data have been obtained which could either confirm or refute the possibility that the 50 kDa leukemia molecule represents a modified form of the thymocyte 53 kDa TL-like protein.

There is little doubt that the *Tla* region of the mouse is complex, both at the structural and functional levels. The changes occurring during leukemogenesis raise a multitude of questions as to the involvement of TL expression in malignant transformation. (1) Is TL derepression involved directly in the process of transformation, or is it just one of many ancillary epigenetic events? (2) Does the expression of TL lead to any selective advantages for the survival of the leukemia cells *in vivo?* We hope that these questions, along with the identification of a possible function of TL molecules during normal T-cell differentiation, may be answered in the ensuing years.

III. *Qa*

Like the *Tla* region, the *Qa* region encodes an array of glycoproteins and is genetically complex (17). However, unlike the *Tla* region whose products are limited to cortical lymphoblasts of the thymus (50), certain leukemias, and ConA-stimulated lymphoblasts (12), *Qa* products are expressed both at the cell surface of a variety of lymphoid cell types and as secretory proteins in the blood.

The first *Qa* antigen described was termed *Qa-2* and was found to be expressed in a wide range of lymphoid tissues and cell types as well as in leukemias (16,17). The molecule is approximately 40,000 Da and is associated with β2M (32); interestingly, although the molecules isolated from the spleens from a variety of mouse strains lack discernable polymorphism as judged by isoelectric focusing (33), a diversity in pI and M_r was recently observed for *Qa-2* isolated from cloned CTL (55). The extent of homology between *Qa-2* and *H-2* as observed by tryptic peptide mapping and by amino acid sequencing has suggested that *Qa-2* and *H-2K^b/D^b* have arisen relatively recently from a common ancestral gene (58,59). Indeed, using probes derived from the flanking regions of *Qa* genes, Flavell and his co-workers have concluded that the *Qa* region genes arose by a pair duplication process, and that the *K* region and certain *Qa* region class I genes are related evolutionarily (18). This hypothesis is further supported by the observation that some monoclonal antibodies cross-react with both *K* and *Qa* region class I products (53).

Although the range of *Qa* tissue distribution surpasses TL, *Qa-2* shares with TL the property of undergoing a derepression; that is, certain strains of mice which are *Qa2*⁻ (notably the BALB substrain BALB/cBy) express the antigen on some of their leukemias (47). Evidence presented by Flaherty *et al.* (17a) and Mellor *et al.* (31) suggests that the *Qa-2*⁻ phenotype in BALB/cBy mice has arisen through a deletion in the *Qa* region generated by unequal crossing-over and resulting in the formation of a hybrid class I *Qa* gene (31). However, the induction of the *Qa-2*⁺ BALB/cBy leukemia phenotype just described remains a mystery.

In addition to *Qa-2*, the *Qa* region contains genes encoding *Qa-1*, a molecule found on thymocytes and on mature lymphoid cell types (49,62). Qat4 and Qat5 molecules are other recently identified *Qa* region products found on natural killer cells (19). As yet, the occurrence of anomalous expression of the genes encoding these proteins comparable to those described for TL and *Qa-2* is unknown.

Molecularly, the *Qa* region has been studied extensively in both BALB/c and C57BL/6 mice (18). Weiss *et al.* (70), using C57BL/6 mice, have identified 10 genes mapping to this region, spanning approximately 320 kilobases (kb). One of these genes, termed *Q10,* has been sequenced and expresses a nonpolymorphic liver-specific secretory protein (25). The allele of the *Q7* gene identified in the C57BL/6 linkage map has been isolated from BALB/c mice and sequenced by Steinmetz *et al.* (63). This gene, termed 27.1, was originally thought to be a pseudogene due to the presence of a stop codon in exon 5, a hydrophilic amino acid in the transmembrane domain, and an abnormal 3′ acceptor splice site next to exon 7. Recently, Stroynowski *et al.* (65) have shown that an experimental hybrid gene composed of 5′ sequence of 27.1 (exons 1, 2, and 3) joined to 3′ sequence of an *H-2* class I gene was expressed and that the 5′ end encoded a protein sequence recognizable by a monoclonal antibody which defines an antigen known as CR (53). These results led the authors to conclude that the 27.1 gene is actually expressed in the mouse and that it may encode the CR protein which resides at the cell surface.

We have isolated and studied a gene believed to be allelic to 27.1 from 129 mice and have determined the nucleotide sequence of most of its coding regions. In support of allelism, we have found that the entire coding sequence diverges only 1–2% from that of the BALB/c 27.1 gene just discussed; in fact, exon 5, which has only a single base substitution, has retained the stop codon found in exon 5 of 27.1 at an identical position (Fig. 3). Lalanne *et al.* (27) have identified the transcript of yet another allele of 27.1, in this case derived from the DBA/2 strain of mouse. Like the *Q10* gene, the "27.1" transcript was found only in the liver; the authors suggest that the protein product of this transcript may be secre-

BALB/c 27.1   AGCCTCCTCCATACACTGTCTCCAACATGGCGACCATTGCTGTTGTGGTTGACCTTGGAGC

    129   AGCCTCCTCCATACACTGTCTCCAACATGGCGACCAGTGCTGTTGTGGTTGACCTTGGAGC

  BALB/c   TGTGGCCATCATTGGAGCTGTGGTGGCTTTTGTGATGAATAGGAGGTGAAACACAG

    129   TGTGGCCATCATTGGAGCTGTGGTGGCTTTTGTGATGAATAGGAGGTGAAACACAG

Fig. 3. Comparison of the nucleotide sequences of exon 5 from the *Qa* region gene 27.1 from the BALB/c mouse (63) and an allele of 27.1 isolated from the 129 strain. Only one nucleotide difference is observed between the two sequences. Identical TGA termination codons are located seven nucleotides from the 3′ exon-intron splice junction.

tory. They also showed that the liver produces eight different class I transcripts, more than originally expected.

We have transfected Ltk⁻ cells with a cloned, 13-kb *Eco*RI DNA fragment containing the allelic "27.1" gene from the 129 strain. This fragment apparently contains the 3′ portion of yet another closely linked *Qa* gene. The 13-kb *Eco*RI fragment was subcloned in the plasmid vector pBR322 containing the gene for neomycin resistance. Upon transfection and selection with G418, we have observed a significant decrease in the quantity of class I products at the transfected L-cell surface, judged by immunoprecipitation with anti-H-2K^K and anti-β2M antisera (Fig. 4). The molecular events leading to such an inhibition of class I expression are unknown, although it is possible that the controlling elements reside within this 13-kb fragment. Using anti-CR monoclonal antibody, we could not detect any specific binding to the transfected cells.

Reports have appeared suggesting that a *Qa/Tla* gene may play a more active role in transformation than merely directing the appearance of a protein at the cell surface ancillary to the transformation event. Lane *et al.* (28) have recently isolated a 4.7-kb *Hind*III- *Bam*Hi fragment from a BALB/c library cloned in λ Charon 30 which possesses transforming activity (termed *Tlym-1*). The gene was found to hybridize to transcripts of 0.6, 0.7, and 1.6 kb in both T and B cells and to a 1.8-kb transcript in a suppressor T-cell line. The fragments share homology with MHC genes, and the authors present suggestive evidence that the gene may be localized to the *Qa/Tla* region. In this regard, it may be noted that Brickell *et al.* (6) reported the presence of what appeared to be a *Qa/Tla* transcript in all murine tumor cells examined; however, the sequence of the cDNA upon further examination was recently found to be an *H-2* class I gene.

All of the products encoded by the genes of the *Qa/Tla* region are far from identification. Even our limited knowledge, however, has already uncovered a varied and intriguing pattern of tissue expression. The most interesting facet may be the anomalous expression of class I genes on the surface of malignant cells. An important question is this: Does this phe-

UNTRANSFECTED

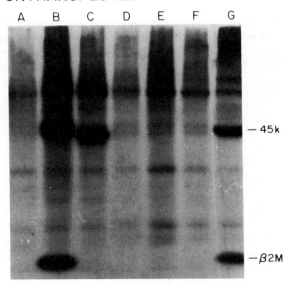

A   B   C   D   E   F   G

— 45k

—β2M

TRANSFECTED

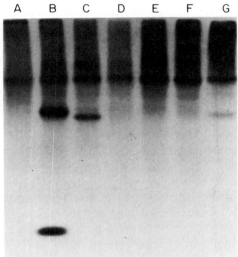

A   B   C   D   E   F   G

Fig. 4. Analysis of ^{125}I-labeled class I molecules immunoprecipitated from transfected Ltk$^-$ cells (upper) and Ltk$^-$ cells transfected with the 129 strain 27.1 *Qa* region gene (lower). The TCA-precipitable counts per minute in all lysates prior to the start of each immunoprecipitation were identical (3.0×10^6). The amount of H-2K^k and β2M-associated class I heavy chains precipitated from lysates of labeled transfected cells versus untransfected cells (lanes B and G, respectively) was significantly lowered. An

nomenon occur in human beings? If so, these proteins could serve as targets for immunotherapeutic monoclonal antibodies in the future.

IV. Novel Class I Products on Tumor Cells

Our group is currently studying a novel 43-kDa class I–like molecule from a spontaneous variant of mouse Ltk⁻ cells, which does not appear to be in association with β2M (Fig. 4). This characteristic is reminiscent of a class I protein previously identified in the rabbit (71). Unexpectedly, the protein was precipitated by an antiserum made in BALB/c mice against human T- and B-cell leukemias; as yet, we have not been able to identify a comparable molecule from C3H thymocyte and spleen lysates which suggests that this molecule may undergo an unmasking in tumor cells comparable to that discussed previously for TL. Two-dimensional chymotryptic peptide mapping has shown that the molecule possesses peptides common to H-2K^k but contains additional peptides unique to this protein. Like H-2, the level of expression of this protein in L-cells upon transfection with the 13-kb RI fragment containing the "27.1" gene was significantly lowered.

Recently, Phillips et al. (41) have described a novel tumor-specific class I molecule isolated from a ultraviolet-induced fibrosarcoma (designated 1591) from the C3H/HeN strain of mouse. This molecule, unlike the one previously described is β2M-associated. An extremely interesting finding by this group of investigators was that the loss of this tumor-specific class I molecule resulted in rapid tumor growth of the cell line in syngeneic hosts; this suggests that the molecule acts as a tumor-specific transplantation antigen in the strictest sense. McMillan et al. (30) observed the appearance of two novel class I molecules in the same tumor line; one was a mosaic of H-2K^k and H-2D^k while one was related to H-2L^d. The mechanism(s) underlying their expression are still uncertain.

Other reports have repeatedly appeared in the literature regarding the occurrence of altered H-2 molecules on the surface of tumor cells (46,57). These and other reports demand greater attention in view of the observation concerning the occurrence of hybrid class I products on the cell

anti-human leukemia antiserum also precipitated a novel class I from both cell lysates which is not associated with β2M (lane C). Qa-2 monoclonal antibody and Qa-2 polyclonal antiserum served as negative controls (lanes E and F, respectively); monoclonal antibody recognizing the CR antigen (lane D) did not specifically precipitate any protein from the transfected cell lysates. Lane A: goat anti-mouse agarose beads (background control).

surface of the 1591 line and the generation of a hybrid *Qa* gene in Qa-2⁻ BALB/cBy mice (31). The results *in toto* suggest that the genes of the MHC may readily undergo recombination or a genetic reshuffling during both ontogeny and phylogeny. The generation of novel class I proteins on tumor cells which are incapable of serving as restriction elements by CTL may provide a way in which cancer cells evade host recognition (29). Alternatively, novel and putative foreign class I molecules displayed at the tumor cell surface may be advantageous to the host considering the strength of the murine alloreactive response (18a).

V. Changes in *H-2* Expression and Malignancy

Similar to the association between repression of the novel class I gene in the 1591 tumor line and its heightened tumorigenicity just described, a diminution in or elimination of the expression of transplantation antigens on tumor cells in certain instances increases the cells' malignant properties. This has been observed for carcinomas (51), teratocarcinomas (21), and metastatic melanomas (S. Sarkar, personal communication). The reduced level of MHC antigens capable of serving as restriction elements in the aforementioned tumors may aid in their escape from immunosurveillance. However, the underlying causes of MHC switch-off in these cases remain enigmatic.

Schrier *et al.* (52) observed that infection of baby rat kidney cells with the highly oncogenic adenovirus 12 (Ad12) caused the disappearance of rat MHC products and a 32-kDa protein from [³⁵S]methionine-labeled cell lysates. Ad5 virus, a nononcogenic adenovirus, did not elicit the same phenomenon. Transfection of cells with a plasmid containing the Ad12 early region, termed *E1a,* also caused the disappearance of precipitable MHC molecules and of the 32-kDa moiety from cell lysates (the transfection of the *E1a* region from Ad5 had no similar effect). An accompanying paper demonstrated the lack of a cytotoxic T-cell response to the Ad12 *E1a*-transfected cells (2); therefore, the authors concluded that the lack of detectable MHC determinants which serve as restriction elements negated the cellular immune response.

Recently, Vaessen *et al.* (67b) demonstrated that Ad12 infection was clearly responsible for the shutoff of class I transcription and that the adenovirus did not selectively infect cells expressing reduced levels of class I products. The authors also showed that the level of class I transcripts in Ad12-infected cells could return to normal upon infection with Ad5. The dominant effect of the Ad5 *E1a* region is quite interesting and suggests the occurrence of a specific recognition sequence(s) for the *E1a-*

encoded proteins in the promoter regions of the affected class I genes. Whether these site(s) overlap enhancer sequences comparable to those described by Kimura *et al.* (22a) in the *H-2K^b* promoter region will be of interest.

Conclusive evidence that MHC expression lost during Ad12 infection is responsible for enhanced tumorgenicity was supplied by Tanaka *et al.* (66). These authors infected embryonic cells from C57BL/6 (C57AT1) and C3H (C3AT1) mice with Ad12 virus and found a suppression of class I transcripts in one line (C57AT1) and a 20-fold decrease of class I transcripts in another line (C3AT1). Both cell lines were highly tumorigenic when injected into both syngeneic and H-2-incompatible hosts. DNA-mediated transfer of an *H-2L^d* gene into C57AT1 cells generated cell surface H-2L^d as assayed with monoclonal anti-H-2L^d antibody. Introduction of the transfected cells into BALB/c mice syngeneic with the *H-2L^d*-encoded restriction element caused a significant lowering of tumorigenicity.

It has been shown that in the case of adenovirus 2 (Ad2) infection there is a physical association between MHC antigens and the adenovirus-encoded glycoprotein E3/19K. This association was first shown by Kvist *et al.* (26) in rat cells and by Signäs *et al.* (56) in human (HeLa) and mouse cells (YAC1); similar findings were presented by Kämpe *et al.* (22). Pääbo *et al.* (40) constructed a recombinant plasmid containing the *E19* gene placed under the control of the SV40 early promoter. In addition, the virus gene contained at its 3' end the second β-globin intron and its polyadenylation site. Upon transfection of the recombinant plasmid into HeLa cells, synthesis of the *E19*-encoded protein and its subsequent association with the human class I antigens were observed. The results clearly indicate that the *E19* gene alone is responsible for the class I–viral protein association.

Burgert and Kvist (7) extended these studies and showed that the physical association between HLA and E3/19K results in an inhibition in the processing of the HLA protein to the cell surface by specifically impeding terminal glycosylation. The reason for the difference between Ad12 and Ad2 infections, that is, the shutting off of MHC transcripts versus inhibition of HLA terminal glycosylation, is not clear.

Hui *et al.* (20), using a subline of the AKR leukemia cell K36 which lacks detectable H-2K^K, observed that transfection of the line with an *H-2K^K* gene reversed the inability of the cell to be recognized by cytotoxic T cells. In addition, the tumor line's ability to grow *in vivo* was decreased upon transfection. As with the adenovirus-infected cells, the loss of MHC antigens seems to serve as a very successful tumor-escape mechanism. The generality of this phenomenon, however, it still uncertain.

It has been known for some time that class I genes may by alternatively spliced [reviewed in (28a)]. Kourilsky and his colleagues (67a) have shown that 5' alternate splicing may occur within the *H-2K^d* gene although these transcripts are produced at $\frac{1}{10}$ the level of normal transcripts. The biological role of alternately spliced transcripts and their protein products, which have remained uncharacterized, is unknown. However, Krangel (24a) has now shown that many human cell lines (notably HPB-ALL) and normal peripheral blood leukocytes produce HLA class I proteins which are secreted, water-soluble, and β2M-associated. Isolated cDNA clones have shown that these products, produced by alternate splicing, lack exon 5 sequence encoding the transmembrane domain. Although not every line examined produced secretory class I products, it now appears that the secretion of class I proteins may be a quite general phenomenon. Similarly, the secretion of molecules carrying Qa-2 determinants from activated murine T cells has very recently been observed by Soloski *et al.* (59a). The role of secreted MHC proteins in immunoregulation is uncertain, although it is tempting to suggest that secretion of class I glycoproteins may be a component of the mechanism(s) whereby tumor cells escape immunological detection and destruction by CTL.

VI. Human MHC Genes

Our laboratory has focused on the study of the structure and expression of the human MHC. In efforts to enumerate and to localize the genes of the MHC, we have carried out extensive cloning of this region from JY (homozygous for HLA-A2 and B7) and 3.1.0. (hemizygous for the entire HLA locus) cell lines and from the placental DNA of an untyped individual. As a result, several human class I genes have been identified and fully sequenced; these include the genes encoding HLA-A2, HLA-B7, an HLA-C-like gene termed 328, and a pseudogene termed LN11A (3,60,61).

Unlike the mouse MHC, which over the past 20 years has been well characterized at the product level, we have faced a difficult situation in identifying functional class I gene products, due to a dearth of available monoclonal antibodies. In addition, the number of Qa/TL-like human class I products that have been identified is very limited; monoclonal antibodies recognizing such proteins include OKT6 (43), m241 (24), 4A7.6 (39), OKT10 (13), and C21 (9). The T6 glycoprotein has been the most well characterized biochemically (67,68), and it superficially resembles murine TL due to its expression on thymocytes and leukemias. However, T6 is also expressed on dendritic cells of the skin (69). Biochemically, the T6 protein shows no similarity to murine TL isolated from all of the various genotypes (8). The gene encoding T6 has not been identified to date.

Our own approach toward the identification of functional class I genes has centered around the DNA-mediated transfer of isolated class I genes into mouse Ltk⁻ cells followed by Northern blotting of transcripts and serological analysis of the transfected cells. Even in view of the difficulties cited previously, this approach has allowed us to identify an HLA-C-like gene from a JY genomic library (14), which interestingly directs the synthesis of a considerable amount of transcript in L cells (greater than that observed for the HLA-B7 gene; R. Srivastava, personal observation). We have also observed the transcription of another JY class I clone termed RS20. At the product level, no serological reagent has reacted specifically with L cells transfected with this clone. Another class I gene, contained in the cosmid clone cos-RS5 derived from the 3.1.0. cell line, yielded a positive ELISA result (upon transfection into mouse cells) using the monoclonal anti-HLA antibody W6/32; however, the molecule became undetectable at the cell surface after several passages. This gene, which is also currently undergoing sequence analysis, possesses considerable homology to HLA but resembles a mouse gene in the 5' promoter region (60).

As yet, the composition of the human *Qa/Tla* region is uncertain. In fact, the existence of human genes homologous to those encoded in *Tla* has been questioned (45). The large number of class I genes isolated from human genomic libraries does support the possibility of the existence of a region comparable (but perhaps vestigial) to the extensive *Qa/Tla* region of the mouse. We have been developing several methods, such as "chromosome hopping," pulse field gradient electrophoresis combined with Southern blotting, and use of recA complexes to isolate large DNA fragments, to more rapidly characterize and clone extended gene families such as the MHC. Unraveling of the genetic structure of the human MHC in its entirety will, it is hoped, allow for investigations into the expression and regulation of this multigene family during normal development and malignancy.

Acknowledgments

The authors wish to thank Ann M. Mulvey for preparation of this manuscript. We would also like to thank Drs. H. Vasavada, E. A. Boyse, F. W. Shen, and J. S. Tung for many helpful discussions. M. J. C. is a recipient of NIH Postdoctoral Fellowship GM09964. S. M. W. acknowledges support from NIH grant CA30938.

References

1. Benacerraf, B. (1981). Role of MHC gene products in immune regulations. *Science* **212,** 1229–1238.
2. Bernards, R., Shrier, P. I., Houweling, A., Bos, J. L., Van der Eb, A. J., Zijlstra, M., and Melief, C. J. M. (1983). Tumorgenicity of cells transformed by adenovirus type 12 by evasion of T-cell immunity. *Nature (London)* **305,** 776–779.
3. Biro, P. A., Reddy, V. B., Sood, A., Pererira, D., and Weissman, S. M. (1981). Isolation and analysis of human major histocompatibility complex genes. *In* "Recombinant DNA, Proceedings of the Third Cleveland Symposium on Macromolecules" (A. Walton, ed.), pp. 41–49. Elsevier, Amsterdam.
4. Boyse, E. A., Stockert, E., and Old, L. J. (1969). Properties of four antigens specified by the *Tla* locus: Similarities and differences. *In* "International Convocation on Immunology" (N. R. Rose and F. Milgram, eds.), pp. 353–357. Karger, Basel.
5. Boyse E. A. (1984). The biology of *Tla. Cell (Cambridge, Mass.)* **38,** 1–2.
6. Brickell, P. M., Latchman, D. S., Murphy, D., Willison, K., and Rigby, P. W. J. (1983). Activation of a *Qa/Tla* class I major histocompatibility antigen gene is a general feature of oncogenesis in the mouse. *Nature (London)* **306,** 756–760.
7. Burgert, H.-G., and Kvist, S. (1985). An adenovirus type 2 glycoprotein blocks cell surface expression of human histocompatibility class I antigens. *Cell (Cambridge, Mass)* **41,** 987–997.
8. Bushkin, Y., Chorney, M. J., Diamante, E., Fu, S. M., and Wang, C. Y. (1984). Biochemical characterization of the human T6 antigen: A comparison between T6 and murine TL. *Mol. Immunol.* **21,** 821–829.
9. Bushkin, Y., Chorney, M. J., Diamante, E., Lane, C., Fu, S. M., and Wang, C. Y. (1985). Biochemical characterization of a p43,12 complex: Comparison with human and murine class I molecules. *Mol. Immunol.* **22,** 695–703.
9a. Chen, Y.-T., Obata, Y., Stockert, E., and Old, L. J. (1985). Thymus-leukemia (TL) antigens of the mouse. Analysis of TL mRNA and TL cDNA from TL⁺ and TL⁻ strains. *J. Exp. Med.* **162,** 1134–1148.
10. Chorney, M. J., Tung, J.-S., Bushkin, Y., and Shen, F.-W. (1985). Structural characteristics of *Tla* products. *J. Exp. Med.* **162,** 781–789.
11. Chorney, M. J., Shen, F.-W., Tung., J.-S., and Boyse, E. A. (1985). Additional products of the *Tla* locus of the mouse. *Proc. Natl. Acad. Sci. U.S.A.* **82,** 7044–7047.
12. Cook, R. G., and Landolfi, N. F. (1983). Expression of the thymus leukemia antigen by activated peripheral T lymphocytes. *J. Exp. Med.* **158,** 1012–1017.
13. Cotner, T., Mashino, H., Kung, P. C., Goldstein, G., and Strominger, J. L. (1981). Human T cell surface antigens bearing a structural relationship to HLA antigens. *Proc. Natl. Acad. Sci. U.S.A.* **78,** 3858–3862.
14. Duceman, B. W., Ness, D., Rende, R., Chorney, M. J., Srivastava, R., Greenspan, D. S., Pan, J., Weissman, S. M., and Grumet, F. C. (1985). HLA-JY328: Mapping studies and expressions of a polymorphic HLA class I gene. *Immunogenetics* **23,** 90–99.
15. Fisher, D. A., Hunt, S. W., and Hood, (1986). The structure of a gene encoding a murine thymus leukemia antigen and the organization of *Tla* genes in the BALB/c mouse *J. Exp. Med.* **162,** 528–545.
16. Flaherty, L. (1976). The Tla region of the mouse: Identification of a new serologically defined locus, Qa-2. *Immunogenetics* **3,** 533–539.
17. Flaherty, L. (1981). *Tla*-region antigens. *In* "The Role of the Major Histocompatibility Complex in Immunobiology" (M. Dorf, ed.), pp. 33–57. Garland Press, New York.
17a. Flaherty, L., Dibiase, K., Lynes, M. A., Seidman, J. G., Weinberger, O., and Rinchik,

E. M. (1985). Characterization of a Q subregion gene in the major histocompatibility complex. *Proc. Natl. Acad. Sci. (USA)* **82**, 1503–1507.

18. Flavell, R. A., Allen, H., Huber, B., Wake, C., and Widera, G. (1985). Organization and expression of the MHC of the C57BL/10 mouse. *Immunol. Rev.* **84**, 29–50.

18a. Goodenow, R., Vogel, R. M., and Linsk, R. L. (1985). Histocompatibility antigens on murine tumors. *Science* **230**, 777–783.

19. Hämmerling, G. J., Hämmerling, U., and Flaherty, L. (1979). Qat-4 and Qat-5, new murine T-cell antigens governed by the *Tla* region and identified by monolonal antibodies. *J. Exp. Med.* **150**, 108–116.

20. Hui, K., Grosveld, F., and Festenstein, H. (1984). Rejection of transplantable AKR leukemia cells following MHC DNA mediated cell transformation. *Nature (London)* **311**, 750–752.

21. Jacob, F. (1977). Mouse teratocarcinomas and embryonic antigens. *Immunol. Rev.* **33**, 3–32.

22. Kämpe, O., Bellgrau, D., Hämmerling, V., Lind, P., Pääbo, S., Severinsson, L., and Peterson, P. A. (1983). Complex-formation of class I transplantation antigens and viral glycoprotein. *J. Biol. Chem.* **258**, 10594–10598.

22a. Kimura, A., Israel, A., LeBail, O., and Kourilsky, P. (1986). Detailed analysis of the mouse H-2K^b promoter: Enhancer-like sequences and their role in the regulation of class I gene expression. *Cell* **44**, 261–272.

23. Klein, J., and Figueroa, F. (1981). Polymorphism of the mouse H-2 loci. *Immunol. Rev.* **60**, 23–57.

24. Knowles, R. W., and Bodmer, W. F. (1982). A monoclonal antibody recognizing a human thymus leukemia-like antigen associated with β_2-microglobulin. *Eur. J. Immunol.* **12**, 676–681.

24a. Krangel, M. S. (1986). Secretion of HLA-A and -B antigens via an alternate RNA splicing pathway. *J. Exp. Med.* **163**, 1173–1190.

25. Kress, M., Cosman, D., Khoury, G., and Jay, G. (1983). Secretion of a transplantation-related antigen. *Cell (Cambridge, Mass.* **43**, 189–196.

26. Kvist, S., Östberg, L., Persson, H., and Philipson, L. (1978). Molecular association between transplantation antigens and cell surface antigen in adenovirus-transformed cell line. *Proc. Natl. Acad. Sci. U.S.A.* **75**, 5674–5678.

27. Lalanne, J.-L., Transy, C., Guerin, S., Darche, S., Meulien, P., and Kourilsky, P. (1985). Expression of class I genes in the major histocompatibility complex: Identification of eight distinct mRNAs in DBA/2 mouse liver. *Cell (Cambridge, Mass.)* **41**, 469–478.

28. Lane, M.-A., Stephens, H. A. F., Doherty, K. M., and Tobin, M. B. (1984). Tlym-I, a stage specific transforming gene shares homology with MHC I region genes. *Curr. Top. Microbiol. Immunol.* **113**, 31–33.

28a. Lew, A. M., Lillehoh, E. P., Cowan, E. P., Maloy, W. L., van Schravendijk, M. R., and Coligan, J. E. (1986). Class I genes and molecules: an update. *Immunology* **57**, 3–18.

29. Martin, W. J. (1983). Structural and functional alterations in H-2 antigen expression on tumor cells. *Transplant. Proc.* **15**, 2097–2100.

30. McMillan, M., Lewis, K. D., and Rovner, D. M. (1985). Molecular characterization of novel H-2 class I molecules expressed by a UV-induced fibrosarcoma. *Proc. Natl. Acad. Sci. U.S.A.* **82**, 5485–5489.

31. Mellor, A. L., Antoniou, J., and Robinson, P. J. (1985). Structure and expression of genes encoding murine Qa-2 class I antigens. *Proc. Natl. Acad. Sci. U.S.A.* **82**, 5920–5924.

32. Michaelson, J., Bushkin, Y., Flaherty, L., and Boyse, E. A. (1981). Further biochemical data on Qa-2. *Immunogenetics* **14,** 129–140.
33. Michaelson, J., Flaherty, L., Hutchinson, B., and Yudkowitz, H. (1982). Qa-2 does not display structural genetic polymorphism detectable on isoelectric-focusing gels. *Immunogenetics* **16,** 363–366.
34. Michaelson, J., Boyse, E. A., Chorney, M., Flaherty, L., Fleissmen, E., Hammerling, U., Reinisch, C., Rosenson, R., and Shen, F.-W. (1983). The biochemical genetics of the *Qa-Tla* region. *Transplant. Proc.* **15,** 2033–2038.
35. Nathenson, S. G., Uehara, H., and Ewenstein, B. M. (1981). Primary structural analysis of the transplantation antigens of the murine H-2 major histocompatibility complex. *Annu. Rev. Biochem.* **50,** 1025–1052.
36. Obata, Y., Chen, Y.-T., Stockert, E., and Old, L. J. (1985). Structural analysis of TL genes in the mouse. *Proc. Natl. Acad. Sci. U.S.A.* **82,** 5475–5479.
37. Old. L. J., Boyse, E. A., and Stockert, E. (1963). Antigenic properties of experimental leukemias. I. Serological studies *in vitro* with spontaneous and radiation-induced leukemias. *J. Natl. Cancer Inst. (U.S.)* **31,** 977–986.
38. Old, L. J., and Stockert, E. (1977). Immunogenetics of cell surface antigens of mouse leukemia. *Annu. Rev. Genet.* **17,** 127–160.
39. Olive, D., Dubreuil, P., and Mawas, C. (1984). Two distinct TL-like molecular subsets defined by monoclonal antibodies on the surface of human thymocytes with different expression on leukemia lines. *Immunogenetics* **20,** 253–264.
40. Pääbo, S., Weber, F., Kämpe, O., Schaffner, W., and Peterson, P. A. (1983). Association between transplantation antigens and a viral membrane protein synthesized from a mamalian expression vector. *Cell (Cambridge, Mass.)* **33,** 445–453.
41. Phillips, C., McMillan, M., Flood, P. M., Murphy, D. B., Forman, J., Lancki, D., Womack, J. E., Goodenow, R. S., and Schreiber, H. (1985). Identification of a unique tumor specific antigen as a novel class I major histocompatibility molecule. *Proc. Natl. Acad. Sci. U.S.A.* **82,** 5140–5144.
42. Ploegh, H. L., Orr, H. T., and Strominger, J. L. (1981). Major histocompatibility antigens: The human (HLA-A-B-C) and murine (H-2K, H-2D) class I molecules. *Cell (Cambridge, Mass.)* **24,** 287–299.
42a. Pontarotti, P. A., Mashimo, J., Zeff, R. A., Fisher, D. A., Hood, L., Mellor, A., Flavell, R. A., and Nathenson, S. G. (1986). Conservation and diversity of class I genes of the major histocompatibility complex: sequence analysis of a *Tla*ᵇ gene and comparison with a *Tla*ᶜ gene. *Proc. Natl. Acad. Sci. U.S.A.* **82,** 1782–1786.
43. Reinherz, E. L., Kung, P. C., Goldstein, G., Levey, R. H., and Schlossman, S. F. (1980). Discrete stages of human intrathymic differentiation: Analysis of normal thymocytes and leukemic lymphoblasts of T-cell lineage. *Proc. Natl. Acad. Sci. U.S.A.* **77,** 1588–1592.
44. Rogers, J. H. (1985). Family organization of mouse H-2 class I genes. *Immunogenetics* **21,** 343–353.
45. Rogers, J. H. (1985). Mouse histocompatibility-related genes are not conserved in other mammals. *EMBO J.* **4,** 749–753.
46. Rogers, M. J. Appella, E., Pierotti, M. A., Invernizzi, G., and Parmiani, G. (1979). Biochemical characterization of alien H-2 antigens expressed on a methylcholanthrene induced tumor. *Proc. Natl. Acad. Sci. U.S.A.* **76,** 1415–1419.
47. Rosenson, R. S., Flaherty, L., and Reinisch, C. L. (1981). Induction of surface Qa2 on lymphoid cells. *J. Immunol.* **126,** 2253–2257.
48. Rothenberg, E., and Boyse, E. A. (1979). Synthesis and processing of molecules bearing thymus leukemia antigen. *J. Exp. Med.* **150,** 777–791.

49. Rothenberg, E., and Triglia, D. (1981). Structure and expression of glycoproteins controlled by the Qa-1ᵃ allele. *Immunogenetics* **14**, 455–468.
50. Rothenberg, E. (1982). A specific biosynthetic marker for immature thymic lymphoblasts. *J. Exp. Med.* **155**, 140–154.
51. Sanderson, A. R., and Beverley, P. C. L. (1983). Interferon, β-2-microglobulin and immunoselection in the pathway to malignancy. *Immunol. Today* **4**, 211–213.
52. Schrier, P. I., Bernards, R., Vaessen, R. T. M. J., Houweling, A., and Van der Eb, A. J. (1983). Expression of class I major histocompatibility antigens switched off by highly oncogenic adenovirus 12 in transformed rat cells. *Nature (London)* **305**, 771–775.
53. Sharrow, S. O., Flaherty, L., and Sachs, D. H. (1984). Serologic cross-reactivity between class I MHC molecules and an H-2-linked differentiation antigen as detected by monoclonal antibodies. *J. Exp. Med.* **159**, 21–40.
54. Shen, F. W., Chorney, M. J., and Boyse, E. A., (1982). Further polymorphism of the *Tla* locus defined by monoclonal TL antibodies. *Immunogenetics* **15**, 573–578.
55. Sherman, D. H., Kranz, D. M., and Eisen, H. N. (1984). Expression of structurally diverse Qa-2-encoded molecules on the surface of cloned cytotoxic T lymphocytes. *J. Exp. Med.* **160**, 1421–1430.
56. Signäs, C., Katz, M. G., Persson, H., and Philipson, L. (1982). An adenovirus glycoprotein binds heavy chains of class I transplantation antigens from man and mouse. *Nature (London)* **299**, 175–178.
57. Siwarski, D. F., Prat, M., and Rogers, M. J. (1985). A novel H-2ˢ class I molecule expressed on a B-cell leukemia from SJL/J mice. *Mol. Immunol.* **22**, 961–966.
58. Soloski, M. J., Urh, J. W., Flaherty, L., and Vitetta, E. S. (1981). Qa-2, H-2K and H-2D alloantigens evolved from a common ancestral gene. *J. Exp. Med.* **153**, 1080–1093.
59. Soloski, M. J., Uhr, J. W., and Vitetta E. S. (1982). Primary structural studies of the Qa-2 alloantigen: Implications for the evolution of the MHC. *Nature (London)* **296**, 759–761.
59a. Soloski, M., Vernachio, J., Einhorn, G., and Lattimore, A. (1986). Qa gene expression: biosynthesis and secretion of Qa-2 molecules in activated T cells. *Proc. Natl. Acad. Sci. (USA)* **83**, 2949–2953.
60. Srivastava, R., Duceman, B. W., Biro, P. A., Sood, A. K., and Weissman, S. M. (1985). Molecular organization of the class I genes of human major histocompatibility complex. *Immunol. Rev.* **84**, 93–120.
61. Srivastava, R., Duceman, B. W., Biro, P. A., Chorney, M. J., Sood, A. K., Greenspan, D. S., Pan, J., and Weissman, S. M. (1985). New approaches and results in cloning of the human major histocompatibility complex. *In* "Cell Biology of the Major Histocompatibility Complex" (B. Pernis and H. J. Vogel, eds.). Academic Press, New York.
62. Stanton, T., and Boyse, E. A. (1976). A new serologically defined locus, *Qa-1*, in the *Tla* region of the mouse. *Immunogenetics* **3**, 525–531.
63. Steinmetz, M., Moore, K. W., Frelinger, J. G., Sher, B. T., Shen, F.-W., Boyse, E. A., and Hood, L. (1981). A pseudogene homologous to mouse transplantation antigens: transplantation antigens are encoded by eight exons that correlate with protein domains. *Cell (Cambridge, Mass.)* **25**, 683–692.
64. Steinmetz, M., and Hood, L., (1983). Genes of the major histocompatibility complex in mouse and man. *Science* **222**, 727–733.
64a. Stephan, D., Sun, H., Fischer Lindahl, K., Meyer, E., Hammerling, G., Hood, L., and Steinmetz, M. (1986). Organization and evolution of D region class I genes in the mouse major histocompatibility complex. *J. Exp. Med.* **163**, 1227–1244.
65. Stroynowski, I., Forman, J., Goodenow, R. S., Schiffer, S. G., McMillan, M., Scharrow, S. O., Sachs, D. H., and Hood, L. (1985). Expression and T cell recognition of

hybrid antigens with amino-terminal domains encoded by Qa-2 region of major histocompatibility complex and carboxyl termini of transplantation antigens. *J. Exp. Med.* **161,** 935–952.

66. Tanaka, K., Isselbacher, K. J., Khoury, G., and Jay G. (1985). Reversal of oncogenesis by the expression of a major histocompatibility complex class I gene. *Science* **228,** 26–30.

67. Terhorst, C., Van Agthoven, A., Leclair, K., Snow, P., Reinherz, E., and Schlossman, S. (1981). Biochemical studies of the human thymocyte cell-surface antigens T6, T9 and T10. *Cell (Cambridge, Mass.)* **23,** 771–780.

67a. Transy, C., Lalanne, J.-L., and Kourilsky, P. (1984). Alternative splicing in the 5′ moiety of the H-2K^d gene transcript. *EMBO J.* **3,** 2383–2386.

67b. Vaessen, R. T. M. J., Houweling A., Israel, A., Kourilsky, P., and van der Eb, A. J. (1986). Adenovirus E1A-mediated regulation of class I MHC expression. *EMBO J.* **5,** 335–341.

68. Van Agthoven, A., and Terhorst, C. (1982). Further biochemical characterization of the human thymocyte differentiation antigen T6. *J. Immunol.* **128,** 426–432.

69. Van de Rijn, M., Lerch, P. G., Bronstein, B. R., Knowles, R. W., Bhan, A. K., and Terhorst, C. (1985). Human cutaneous dendritic cells express two glycoproteins T6 and m241, which are biochemically identical to those found on cortical thymocytes. *Hum. Immunol.* **9,** 201–210.

70. Weiss, H., Golden, T., Fahrner, K., Mellor, A. T., Devlin, J. J., Bullman, H., Tiddens, H., Bud, H., and Flavell, R. A. (1984). Organization and evolution of the class I gene family in the major histocompatibility complex of the C57BL/10 mouse. *Nature (London)* **310,** 650–655.

71. Wilkinson, J. M., Tykocinski, M. J., Coligan, J. E., Kimball, E. S., and Kindt, T. J. (1982). Rabbit MHC antigens: Occurrence of non-β-2-microglobulin-associated class I molecules. *Mol. Immunol.* **19,** 1441–1451.

72. Winoto, A., Steinmetz, M., and Hood, L. (1983). Genetic mapping in the major histocompatibility complex by restriction enzyme site polymorphisms: Most mouse class I genes map to the *Tla* complex. *Proc. Natl. Acad. Sci. U.S.A.* **80,** 3425–3429.

73. Yokoyama, K., Stockert, E., Old, L. J., and Nathenson, S. G. (1982). Structural comparisons of TL antigens derived from normal and leukemia cells of TL$^+$ and TL$^-$ strains and relationship to genetically linked *H-2* major histocompatibility complex products. *Proc. Natl. Acad. Sci. U.S.A.* **78,** 7078–7082.

74. Yokoyama, K., Stockert, E., Pease, L., R., Obata, Y., Old, L. J., and Nathenson, S. G. (1983). Polymorphism and diversity in the *Tla* gene system. *Immunogenetics* **81,** 445–451.

75. Zinkernagel, R. M., and Doherty, P. C. (1974). Restriction of *in vitro* T cell-mediated cytotoxicity in lymphocytic choriomeningitis within a syngeneic or semiallogeneic system. *Nature (London)* **248,** 701–702.

24

The Regulation of Cellular Transcription by Viral Transforming Proteins

BARBARA I. SKENE, NICHOLAS B. LA THANGUE, DAVID MURPHY, AND PETER W. J. RIGBY

Cancer Research Campaign
Eukaryotic Molecular Genetics Research Group
Department of Biochemistry
Imperial College of Science and Technology
London, United Kingdom

I. Introduction

A single viral or cellular oncogene, and thus a single transforming protein, is sufficient to transform established lines of cultured cells [reviewed by Marshall and Rigby (15)]. However, transformed cells differ from their normal parents in a large number of biochemical and biological properties, and it is difficult to imagine how these changes can be achieved without significant reprograming of the pattern of cellular gene expression. We have been interested in identifying and characterizing cellular genes which are regulated as a result of transformation. We hoped that by obtaining molecular clones of such genes we would be able to approach two types of questions. First, by making hybrid genes in which the transformation-regulated gene is transcribed from a strong promoter and by reintroducing such genes into normal cells we would be able to determine

NEW AVENUES IN DEVELOPMENTAL
CANCER CHEMOTHERAPY

whether overexpression of the gene induced any of the properties characteristic of transformed cells. Second, we could study the transcriptional
control region of the regulated gene in both gene transfer and *in vitro*
transcription systems in order to elucidate the biochemical mechanisms
involved in the regulation. This latter type of experiment requires that the
biochemical activities of the transforming protein are understood.

Viral transformation systems are ideal for this type of work, because a
number of oncogenic viruses encode proteins which are known to be both
required for transformation and capable of regulating transcription (12,
27, 30). Most of our work has been concerned with the DNA tumor virus
Simian virus 40 (SV40). The transforming protein of SV40, large T-antigen, is a nuclear, sequence-specific, DNA-binding protein [reviewed by
Rigby and Lane (18)]. Large T-antigen is known to be able to regulate the
transcription of rDNA by RNA polymerase I, both *in vivo* and *in vitro* (13,
25), and when we began our work there was indirect evidence that it could
regulate the transcription of protein-coding genes by RNA polymerase II
(17, 31). Many other DNA tumor viruses are now known to encode such
transcriptional trans-activators. The *E1a* region of human adenoviruses
encodes proteins which can both activate and repress polymerase II transcription of viral and cellular genes (3, 8, 9, 11, 21, 28, 29), whereas the E2
of Bovine papillomavirus (BPV) type 1 protein can trans-activate the
enhancer of BPV itself as well as heterologous enhancers (26). Such proteins are not confined to DNA viruses. The retrovirus HTLVI encodes
within the *tat*I gene a protein which stimulates viral transcription, and
activation of cellular genes by this protein probably will play a role in
HTLVI-induced leukemogenesis (24).

We have used differential cDNA cloning techniques to isolate a number
of genes which are expressed at elevated levels in SV40-transformed
mouse fibroblasts relative to the normal parental line (22). In this chapter,
we will review our knowledge of these genes and of the mechanisms by
which they are activated.

II. Results

The scheme used to isolate the transformation-regulated genes is shown
in Fig. 1. Large, plasmid-based cDNA libraries were constructed from
normal BALB/c 3T3 A31 fibroblasts and from an SV40-transformed derivative, SV3T3 C138. From the normal cell library 50,000 clones were
pooled and grown in bulk culture; plasmid DNA was isolated and covalently coupled to cellulose to generate a solid-phase, reusable hybridiza-

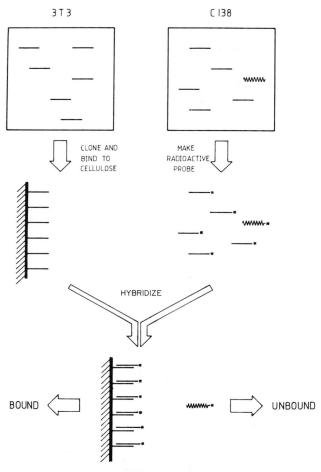

Fig. 1. Protocol for subtractive cDNA cloning to isolate genes activated in SV40-transformed mouse fibroblasts. For further details see text and Scott *et al.* (22).

tion probe. Radioactive cDNA was synthesized on SV3T3 Cl38 mRNA and then hybridized reiteratively against the immobilized normal cell cDNA library. After five cycles of hybridization and a further solution hybridization step, we obtained a probe that was significantly enriched in sequences activated by transformation and used this to screen the SV3T3 Cl38 cDNA library. In this way we obtained 42 clones (22), which are summarized in Table I.

TABLE I

cDNA Clones Corresponding to Genes Activated in SV40-Transformed Cells

				Designation			
	Set 1	Set 2	Set 3	Set 4	Set 5	Set 6	Set 7
Prototype	pAG64	pAG59	pAG82	pAG88	pAG10	pAG23	pAG38
Insert length (kb)	1.55	1.8	1.58	0.70	1.2	0.7	0.5
pAG Clones related to prototype	15,71,85, 86,104	37,57,58, 69	1,31,75,	13,47,48, 74,77,97, 98,105,109	—	—	pAG22
Identity	Class I MHC antigen	Endogenous retrovirus	Cytochrome oxidase subunit I (COI)	Cytochrome oxidase subunit II (COII)	Related to COII	Unknown	B2 repeat non-Class-I

Most of these clones have now been identified by determining their nucleotide sequences and comparing these with the data bases (4,5; P. M. Brickell, D. S. Latchman, M. R. D. Scott, and P. W. J. Rigby, unpublished data; see Table I). The prototype cDNA clone of Set 1, pAG64, encodes the H-2D^d class I antigen of the major histocompatibility complex (MHC). Figure 2 shows that this gene is expressed at high levels in mouse cells transformed by a variety of agents, including DNA and RNA tumor viruses and chemical carcinogens. Within its 3′ untranslated region the *H-2D^d* gene contains a member of the B2 family of mouse repetitive sequences. It is because of this repetitive element that pAG64 also hybridizes to small, polydisperse RNAs which are present at elevated levels in many transformed cell lines (4,22,23). These RNAs are transcribed by the cellular RNA polymerase III (19,23).

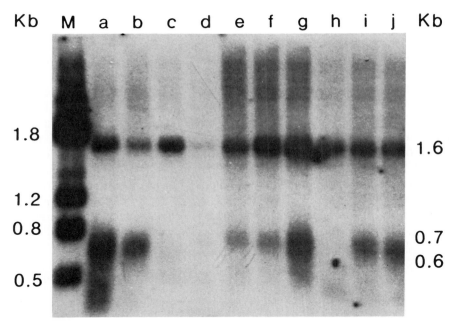

Fig. 2. Expression of class I MHC antigen mRNAs in transformed mouse cell lines. This Northern blot analysis was probed with pAG64, the prototype clone of Set 1. The samples were M, DNA size markers; a, SV3T3 Cl38; b, Py3T3; c, Py*tsa*3T3; d, BALB/c N; e, RSV TK3 BXB4; f, RSV3T3 BC6; g, ANN-1; h, BALB/c AMuLV AIRl; i, BALB/c lOME HD A5Rl; j, BALB/c Cr MC A2R1. The 1.6-kb transcript corresponds to the class I MHC mRNA. The small RNAs, which migrate as if they are between 0.6 and 0.7 kb, are detected by virtue of their homology to the B2 element in pAG64. [Reproduced, with permission, from Scott *et al.* (22), which gives further details. Copyright MIT Press, 1983.]

We have begun to study the mechanisms by which large T-antigen regulates the expression of the *H-2D^d* gene and the B2 repetitive elements using both DNA-mediated gene transfer and *in vitro* transcription systems. We have constructed a chimeric gene in which transcription of the bacterial gene encoding chloramphenicol acetyl transferase is driven by the upstream sequences of the *H-2D^d* gene. When this construct, called 64-*cat,* is transfected into BALB/c 3T3 cells we observe a low level of expression, consistent with the low level at which the endogenous gene is expressed in these cells (Fig. 3). However, when 64-*cat* is cotransfected with pTSV3, a plasmid which encodes large T-antigen, there is a marked stimulation of expression (Fig. 3). This induction is also observed in stable transfectants, and we have used primer extension to show that the mRNAs in stable transfectants initiate at the RNA polymerase II cap site of the *H-2D^d* gene. By deletion analysis we have located at least some of the sequences involved in this induction to a region 4 kilobases (kb) upstream of the transcription start site (19; B. I. Skene and P. W. J. Rigby, unpublished data). In similar cotransfection experiments we have also demonstrated activation of the *H-2D^d/cat* chimeric gene by the *E1a/E1b* regions of human adenovirus types 5 and 12.

Figure 4 shows the results of an *in vitro* transcription experiment in which the template is a B2 repetitive element from the upstream region of the *H-2D^d* gene. Comparison of lanes 1 and 2 shows that large T-antigen stimulates this transcription, while lanes 3 and 4 show that this stimulation is not seen with a control RNA polymerase III promoter, that of the VA$_1$ RNA gene of adenovirus type 2. Singh *et al.* (23) have shown that the levels of 5S rRNA, another polymerase III transcript, are not altered in transformed cell lines which contain elevated levels of the B2-homologous RNAs, further suggesting that there is some specificity to the ability of large T-antigen to regulate polymerase III transcription.

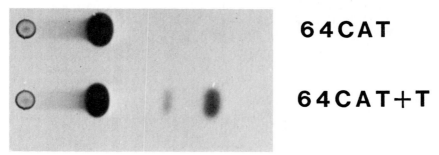

Fig. 3. Activation by SV40 large T-antigen of expression directed by the upstream region of *H-2D^d*. The construct 64*cat* contains the bacterial *cat* gene driven by the upstream region of the *H-2D^d* gene. It was transfected into BALB/c 3T3 cells either alone or with a plasmid, pTSV3, which encodes large T-antigen. For further details see Rigby *et al.* (19).

Fig. 4. Activation by SV40 large T-antigen of RNA polymerase III transcription of a B2 repetitive element. A cloned B2 element was used to program a HeLa cell *in vitro* transcription system. Lane B shows the RNA synthesized in an unsupplemented system. Lane A shows the RNA synthesized in a system supplemented with pure large T-antigen. For further details see Rigby *et al.* (19).

III. Discussion

The use of subtractive cDNA cloning techniques has allowed us to isolate and identify a number of cellular genes which are expressed at elevated levels in SV40-transformed cells (22). Some of these genes are also activated in cells transformed by other agents (4,22). We have so far been unable to link the overexpression of any of these genes to any feature of the transformed phenotype, but we have made some progress in elucidating the mechanisms by which the transforming protein of SV40, large T-antigen, regulates the transcription of these genes.

Our finding that one of the activated genes is that encoding the H-2D^d class I MHC antigen is of considerable interest. Class I antigens are involved in the recognition of tumor cells by cytotoxic T cells, and thus alterations in the expression of these genes may have implications for the ability of the host organism to reject transformed cells. High levels of class I MHC antigen mRNA are found in a wide variety of transformed cells (4,14,22), but in cells transformed by adenovirus type 12, class I expression is repressed by an activity of the *E1a* region (21). It has been argued that this repression accounts for the fact that adenovirus type 12 is oncogenic whereas the very similar type 5 adenovirus, which does not repress class I expression, is not (2). However, acute infection of mouse cells by adenovirus type 12 results in activation of class I mRNA transcription (20), and our experiments using cotransfection of the *H-2D^d-cat* gene and adenovirus *E1a* genes also indicate that these viral proteins can activate the expression of class I genes. It is thus clear that the interactions of viral transforming proteins with these genes are complex.

It is, moreover, noteworthy that even nononcogenic adenoviruses have another mechanism for affecting the expression of class I antigens in which the 19 kD glycoprotein encoded in the E3 region of the viral genome complexes with class I molecules and interferes with their processing (1,6). It seems unlikely that different classes of virus would have evolved both transcriptional and posttranscriptional mechanisms for regulating class I antigen expression if this ability were not of selective advantage, but at present the nature of this advantage is not known. It should be noted, however, that many of the viruses studied by molecular biologists, including SV40 and the adenoviruses, are not known to be oncogenic in their natural hosts (27), and thus it is likely that the interactions with class I antigen expression are relevant, for example, to latency rather than to tumorigenesis.

Nonetheless the experiments described here pave the way for a detailed study of the mechanisms by which SV40 large T-antigen and the adenovirus *E1a* proteins regulate the expression of class I antigen genes. Further deletional analysis should precisely define the cis-acting DNA sequences involved, and we are presently attempting to mimic this regulation of polymerase II transcription by large T-antigen in *in vitro* systems so as to be able to characterize the trans-acting protein factors involved.

We do not know the function, if any, of the small RNAs transcribed by polymerase III from the B2 repetitive elements. However, we have shown that pure large T-antigen is capable of activating this transcription in *in vitro* systems. Moreover, we and others have shown that the expression of these small RNAs is also regulated by the proliferation state of fibroblasts (7,23; K.-H. Westphal and P. W. J. Rigby, unpublished data) and during the differentiation of embryonal carcinoma cells (16). It will thus be of considerable interest to define the biochemical mechanisms involved in controlling the transcription of these repetitive elements. Large T-antigen is not the only viral transforming protein capable of regulating polymerase III transcription. Adenovirus E1a products can also do this, and Hoeffler and Roeder (10) have shown that this is mediated by an increase in the activity of the polymerase III transcription factor TFIIIC in infected cells. Our results, which show that pure large T-antigen can directly activate polymerase III transcription, suggest strongly that in this case another mechanism is involved.

It is thus clear that viral transforming proteins have the ability to regulate transcription by all three cellular RNA polymerases. It remains highly likely although unproven that such transcriptional regulation is involved in the mechanism of transformation, and further studies of the type described here should resolve this issue. It must, however, be said that transcriptional regulation is unlikely to be an easy target for therapeutic intervention against virus-induced tumors, since any drug which inhibited the transcriptional regulatory activities of the viral transforming protein would probably also interfere with essential processes in normal cells.

Acknowledgments

We are very grateful to Julian Gannon and David Lane for providing us with pure SV40 T antigen. B. I. Skene and N. B. La Thangue were supported by a Research Studentship and a Training Fellowship, respectively, from the Medical Research Council. P. W. J. Rigby held a Career Development Award from the Cancer Research Campaign, which also paid for this work.

References

1. Andersson, M., Paabo, S., Nilsson, T., and Peterson, P. A. (1985). Impaired intracellular transport of class I MHC antigens as a possible means for adenoviruses to evade immune surveillance. *Cell (Cambridge, Mass.)* **43,** 215–222.
2. Bernards, R., Schrier, P. I., Houweling, A., Bos, J. L., van der Eb, A. J., Zjilstra, M., and Melief, C. J. M. (1983). Tumorigenicity of cells transformed by adenovirus type 12 by evasion of T-cell immunity. *Nature (London)* **305,** 776–779.
3. Borrelli, E., Hen, R., and Chambon, P. (1984). Adenovirus-2 Ela products repress enhancer stimulation of transcription. *Nature (London)* **312,** 608–612.
4. Brickell, P. M., Latchman, D. S., Murphy, D., Willison, K., and Rigby, P. W. J. (1983). Activation of a *Qa/Tla* class I major histocompatibility antigen gene is a general feature of oncogenesis in the mouse. *Nature (London)* **306,** 756–760.
5. Brickell, P. M., Latchman, D. S., Murphy, D., Willison, K., and Rigby, P. W. J. (1985). The class I major histocompatibility antigen gene activated in a line of SV40-transformed mouse cells is *H2D^d*, not *Qa/Tla*. *Nature (London)* **316,** 162–163.
6. Burgert, H.-G., and Kvist, S. (1985). An adenovirus type 2 glycoprotein blocks cell surface expression of human histocompatibility class I antigens. *Cell (Cambridge, Mass.)* **41,** 987–997.
7. Edwards, D. R., Parfett, C. L. J., and Denhardt, D. T. (1985). Transcriptional regulation of two serum-induced RNAs in mouse fibroblasts; equivalence of one species to B2 repetitive elements. *Mol. Cell. Biol.* **5,** 3280–3288.
8. Gaynor, R., Hillman, D., and Berk, A. (1984). Adenovirus early region 1A protein activates transcription of a nonviral gene introduced into mammalian cells by infection or transfection. *Proc. Natl. Acad. Sci. U.S.A.* **81,** 1193–1197.
9. Green, M. R., Treisman, R., and Maniatis, T. (1983). Transcriptional activation of cloned human β-globin genes by viral immediate-early gene products. *Cell (Cambridge, Mass.)* **35,** 137–148.
10. Hoeffler, W. K., and Roeder, R. G. (1985). Enhancement of RNA polymerase III transcription by the ElA gene product of adenovirus. *Cell (Cambridge, Mass.)* **41,** 955–963.
11. Kao, H.-T., and Nevins, J. R. (1983). Transcriptional activation and subsequent control of the human heat shock gene during adenovirous infection. *Mol. Cell. Biol.* **3,** 2058–2065.
12. Kingston, R. E., Baldwin, A. S., and Sharp, P. A. (1985). Transcription control by oncogenes. *Cell (Cambridge, Mass.)* **41,** 3–5.
13. Learned, R. M., Smale, S. T., Haltiner, M. M., and Tjian, R. (1983). Regulation of human ribosomal RNA transcription. *Proc. Natl. Acad. Sci. U.S.A.* **80,** 3558–3562.
14. Majello, B., La Mantia, G., Simeone, A., Boncinelli, E., and Lania, L. (1985). Activation of major histocompatibility complex class I mRNA containing an *Alu*-like repeat in polyoma virus-transformed rat cells. *Nature (London)* **314,** 457–459.
15. Marshall, C. J., and Rigby, P. W. J. (1984). Viral and cellular genes involved in oncogenesis. *Cancer Surv.* **3,** 183–214.
16. Murphy, D., Brickell, P. M., Latchman, D. S., Willison, K., and Rigby, P. W. J. (1983). Transcripts regulated during normal embryonic development and oncogenic transformation share a repetitive element. *Cell (Cambridge, Mass.)* **35,** 865–871.
17. Postel, E. H., and Levine, A. J. (1976). The requirement of Simian virus 40 gene A product for the stimulation of cellular thymidine kinase activity after viral infection. *Virology* **73,** 206–215.

18. Rigby, P. W. J., and Lane, D. P. (1983). Structure and function of the Simian virus 40 large T-antigen. *Adv. Viral Oncol.* **3**, 31–57.
19. Rigby, P. W. J., La Thangue, N. B., Murphy, D., and Skene B. I. (1985). The regulation of cellular transcription by Simian virus 40 large T-antigen. *Proc. R. Soc. London, Ser. B* **226**, 15–23.
20. Rosenthal, A., Wright, S., Quade, K., Gallimore, P., Cedar, H., and Grosveld, F. (1985). Increased MHC *H2K* gene transcription in cultured mouse embryo cells after adenovirus infection. *Nature (London)* **315**, 579–581.
21. Schrier, P. I., Bernards, R., Vaessen, R. T. M. J., Houweling, A., and van der Eb, A. J. (1983). Expression of class I major histocompatibility antigens switched off by highly oncogenic adenovirus 12 in transformed rat cells. *Nature (London)* **305**, 771–775.
22. Scott, M. R. D., Westphal, K.-H., and Rigby, P. W. J. (1983). Activation of mouse genes in transformed cells. *Cell (Cambridge, Mass.)* **34**, 557–567.
23. Singh, K., Carey, M., Saragosti, S., and Botchan, M. (1985). Expression of enhanced levels of small RNA polymerase III transcripts encoded by the *B2* repeats in Simian virus 40-transformed mouse cells. *Nature (London)* **314**, 553–556.
24. Sodroski, J. G., Rosen, C. A., and Haseltine, W. A. (1984). *Trans*-acting transcriptional activation of the long terminal repeat of human T lymphotropic viruses in infected cells. *Science* **225**, 381–385.
25. Soprano, K. J., Galanti, N., Jonak, G. J., McKercher, S., Pipas, J. M., Peden, K. W. C., and Baserga, R. (1983). Mutational analysis of Simian virus 40 T-antigen:stimulation of cellular DNA synthesis and activation of rRNA genes by mutants with deletions in the T-antigen gene. *Mol. Cell. Biol.* **3**, 214–219.
26. Spalholz, B. A., Yang, Y.-C., and Howley, P. M. (1985). Transactivation of a bovine papilloma virus transcriptional regulatory element by the E2 gene product. *Cell (Cambridge, Mass.)* **42**, 183–191.
27. Tooze, J. (1981). "Molecular Biology of Tumor Viruses. DNA Tumor Viruses," 2nd rev. ed. Cold Spring Harbor Lab., Cold Spring Harbor, New York.
28. Treisman, R., Green, M. R., and Maniatis, T. (1983). *Cis*- and *trans*-activation of globin gene transcription in transient assays. *Proc. Natl. Acad. Sci. U.S.A.* **80**, 7428–7432.
29. Velcich, A., and Ziff, E. (1985). Adenovirus Ela proteins repress transcription from the SV40 early promotor. *Cell (Cambridge, Mass.)* **40**, 705–716.
30. Weiss, R., Teich, N., Varmus, H., and Coffin, J. (1985). "Molecular Biology of Tumor Viruses. RNA Tumor Viruses," 2nd rev. ed. Cold Spring Harbor Lab., Cold Spring Harbor, New York.
31. Williams, J. G., Hoffman, R., and Penman, S. (1977). The extensive homology between mRNA sequences of normal and SV40 transformed human fibroblasts. *Cell (Cambridge, Mass.)* **11**, 901–907.

25

Joining of the Human T-Cell Receptor α Chain Gene with an Immunoglobulin Gene in a Chromosome 14 Inversion (q11;q32) of T-Cell Leukemia

T. H. RABBITTS, R. BAER, A. FORSTER, M.-P. LEFRANC,
AND M. A. STINSON

Medical Research Council
Laboratory of Molecular Biology
Cambridge, United Kingdom

K.-C. CHEN

Department of Haematological Medicine
University of Cambridge
Clinical School
Cambridge, United Kingdom

S. SMITH

Department of Pediatrics
Stanford University
Stanford, California

NEW AVENUES IN DEVELOPMENTAL
CANCER CHEMOTHERAPY

I. Introduction

T-cells have at least three loci with gene segments which rearrange during T-cell differentiation, these are α and β genes [which make up the T-cell antigen receptor (TCR) (5,8,10,13,15,16,18)] and a third gene, called γ (11,13), whose function is unknown. Studies on the β-chain locus have shown that like the immunoglobulin genes, the β-chain locus carries separate variable (V), diversity (D), joining (J), and constant (C) region gene segments which undergo chromosomal rearrangement to create the active β-chain gene. The γ-rearranging locus in humans has been assigned to chromosome 7 (12), and the α locus to chromosome 14q11 (3,6,7,12). Since these genes rearrange, it was possible that specific cytogenetic abnormalities would be associated with those loci analogous to those observed in Burkitt's lymphoma which involve the immunoglobulin (Ig) genes and the c-myc oncogene. One consistent marker chromosome which does appear in T-cell leukemia is an inversion (inv) of a segment of the long arm of chromosome 14 in which the break points are at 14q11 and 14q32 (9,19). This was interesting, because the TCR α gene maps to 14q11, and the Ig heavy (H) chain genes to 14q32, raising the possibility of association of α-chain genes with another gene after inversion.

In this chapter we describe experiments on the structure and rearrangement of the human T-cell receptor α-chain locus and the molecular cloning of the break point in one case of inv14, which fuses an Ig H-chain V-gene to a TCR Jα segment.

II. Material and Methods

DNA filter hybridizations (17) were performed as previously described (12). Nucleotide sequencing was carried out in M13 vectors using the dideoxy chain termination method (14).

III. Results

A. The Human TCR Cα Gene Segment and Adjoining Jα Segments

Using a mouse α cDNA clone (4) (kindly provided by Dr. M. Davis), we isolated human genomic clones containing the Cα gene. Comparing restriction fragment sizes in the clones (Fig. 1) and in the genomic hybridizations confirms that only one Cα gene exists per haploid genome. Nucleotide sequences of the Cα gene showed that there are four exons, as shown in Fig. 1. The first, large exon contains most of the coding region, with the rest split into two small exons. The putative transmembrane/cytoplasmic tail portion is present as a separate exon. Interestingly, the 3' noncoding region of this gene is also contained in a separate exon, there being an RNA splice site immediately after the protein termination codon.

An α chain J segment was localized 4 kilobases (kb) upstream from the Cα gene (Fig. 1) by hybridization with a J probe from the α cDNA, pJM3E11 (12). The nucleotide sequence of a 2-kb region around this J segment revealed only one active Jα segment (1), which is the one (here designated J$_\alpha^{SP}$) used in the productive rearrangement of the cell line JM (12). The J$_\alpha^{SP}$ in the unrearranged state possesses the characteristic conserved nanomer and heptamer sequences (separated by 12 base pairs) which are thought to be involved in the V–J or V–D–J joining process.

When probes from this region [pUCJαBS or pUCJαSP (Fig. 2)] were used in genomic hybridization experiments with a panel of 53 T-cell lines and primary T-cell tumors, we found only a small proportion had detectable rearrangements at J$_\alpha^{SP}$ (Fig. 2). However, other rearrangements could be detected using various restriction enzymes; for example, PstI digestion of patient 4 (P4) DNA hybridized with pUCJαSP indicated the presence of further Jα segments upstream of J$_\alpha^{SP}$ and within the indicated PstI fragment.

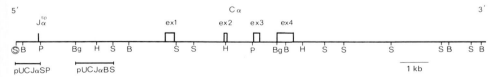

Fig. 1. Structure of human TCR Cα gene. The partial restriction map and exon structure of the human T-cell receptor α chain constant region is shown with the location of the J$_\alpha^{SP}$ segment. The restriction enzymes are S, SacI; B, BamHI; P, PstI; H, HindIII; Bg, BglII. (The SacI site circled at the end of the clone is from the λ2001 vector).

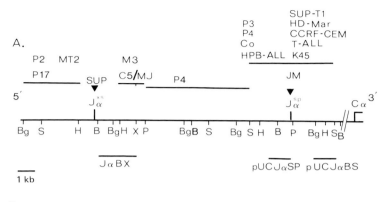

B.

CELL LINE or TUMOR	T3	pUCJ$_\alpha$BS/SacI	pUCJ$_\alpha$SP/PstI	J$_\alpha$BX/HindIII	J$_\alpha$BX/BglII	OVERALL STATUS
P2	−	G/G	G/G	G/G	R/G	R/G
P3	+	R/G	R/G	D/G	D/G	R/G
P4	n.d.	R/G	R/R	D/D	n.d.	R/R
P17	n.d.	G/G	G/G	G/G	R/G	R/G
JM	+	R/G	R/G	D/G	D/G	R/G
MT2	−	G/G	G/G	G/G	R/G	R/G
Co	+	R/G	R/G	D/G	D/G	R/G
C5/MJ	−	G/G	G/G	D/D	n.d.	R/R
HPB-ALL	+	R/R	R/D?	D/D	n.d.	R/R
HD-Mar	+	R/G	R/G	D/G	D/G	R/G
CCRF-CEM	+	R/G	R/G	D/G	D/G	R/G
T-ALL	+	R/G	R/G	D/G	D/G	R/G
MOLT3	−	G/G	G/G	R/G	D/G	R/G
K45	+	R/G	R/G	D/G	D/G	R/G
SUP-T1	+	R/G	R/G	R/D	n.d.	R/R

Fig. 2. Restriction map of part of Jα locus and DNA rearrangement data on T-cell lines. (A) Partial restriction map of a region of the human Jα locus. Enzyme sites are Bg, *Bgl*II; S, *Sac*I; H, *Hind*III; B, *Bam*HI; X, *Xho*I; P, *Pst*I. (B) State of rearrangement in T-cell DNAs using the indicated probes (see Fig. 2A) and restriction enzymes. R, Rearrangement; G, germ line; D, deleted; n.d., not determined. The bars indicate location of putative Jα segments as deduced by hybridization experiments.

Further analysis of the complexity of the Jα region was carried out by isolating genomic clones using pUCJαSP from a phage library prepared from DNA of the SUPT1 cell line (9). Two sets of clones were isolated. One set extended upstream of the J_α^{SP} and was found to include a rearranged region at its very end. The restriction map of this clone (λSα9) appears in Fig. 3. Sequence analysis of the rearrangement in λSα9 shows that a Vα gene (here designated V_α^{XS}) has joined to another Jα segment (J_α^{XS}), and the sequence at the junction of the V and J regions shows that this rearrangement has occurred nonproductively because it produced an in-frame protein termination codon (Fig. 4).

The two Jα segments thus identified by sequence analysis (J_α^{SP}) are about 10 kb apart. This is unusual, since other known rearranging genes with multiple J segments occur in clusters. Evidence for more Jα segments both upstream of J_α^{XS} and between J_α^{XS} and J_α^{SP} comes from patterns of rearrangement seen in the panel of T cells used in Fig. 2. With the various probes and combinations of restriction enzyme digestion of genomic DNA, we were able to detect a set of different rearrangements. This strongly indicates that additional Jα segments occur in these regions (Fig. 2). Many other T cells failed to show any α gene rearrangements at all, implying the existence of, as yet, undetected Jα segments upstream of J_α^{XS}.

The human Jα segments occur, therefore, over more than 15 kb of DNA. This is unusual among the known genes which undergo rearrangement and may imply special requirements of the α chain system. Expression patterns of the various Jα segments are needed before a full picture will emerge on this point, but it may be significant that all the T cells in

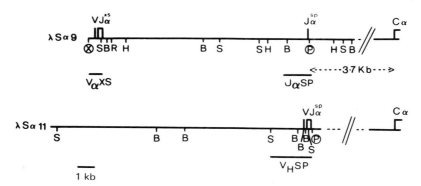

Fig. 3. Partial restriction maps of SUPT1 rearranged α chain genes. The sites of rearranged V genes with J_α^{XS} and J_α^{SP} are indicated (designated V_α^{XS} and V_H^{SP}, respectively) (see text). Restriction enzymes are X, *Xho*I (the circles Xho site in λSα9 comes from λ2001 polylinker); S, *Sac*I; B, *Bam*HI; R, *Eco*RI; H, *Hind*III; P, *Pst*I.

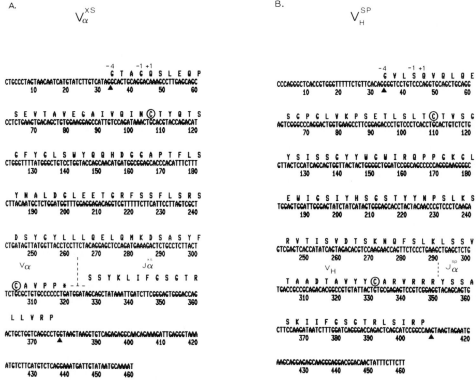

Fig. 4. Nucleotide sequences of the rearranged V gene in SUPT1. (A) Sequence of V-J segments of λSα9 (V_α^{XS}). (B) Sequence of V-J segments of λSα11 (V_H^{SP}).

this study which rearranged to J_α^{SP} are positive for surface expression of the T3 antigen (1).

B. Molecular Cloning of an inv14 Break Point

The λ phage clones made from the cell line SUPT1 (which is derived from a patient with T-cell lymphoma (9)) included a group which was found to have a rearrangement at J_α^{SP} (e.g., λSα11). This cell line, therefore, has both α chain alleles rearranged, one to J_α^{XS} and one to J_α^{SP}, of which the V_α^{XS} is joined nonproductively (see above). The restriction map of λSα11 is shown in Fig. 3, together with λSα9. Nucleotide sequence analysis of the rearrangement at J_α^{SP} showed that a variable region sequence was joined productively with the Jα segment (Fig. 4). When the sequence of the Vα joined to J_α^{XS} was compared with the V joined to J_α^{SP} in SUPT1, it was found that the V joined to J_α^{SP} was, in fact, an immunoglobulin VH segment and not a Vα segment. Detailed sequence analysis showed that the joined VH segment (called V_H^{SP}) comes from the Ig VH subgroup II having about 85% homology with this group (2). An understanding of the events occurring at the chromosomal level was obtained by *in situ* hybridization (2). The results of these experiments (summarized in Fig. 5) showed that V_H^{SP} localized to 14q32 in both the normal and inverted chromosome 14 (i.e., the position of the Igh locus). Further, the TCR Cα gene is at 14q12 in the normal chromosome but moves to q32 in the inverted chromosome 14 (Fig. 6). The Igh Cμ segment, on the other hand, moves from its normal position at q32 to q12 in the inverted chromosome. Therefore, the TCR Cα segment moves from its normal centromere position to join with the Ig VH segment at the 14q32.

Therefore, λSα11 is a clone which contains the junction of the inversion chromosome 14 from SUPT1 and shows that at least in this cell line, the inversion results in fusion of an Ig VH segment and a TCR Jα segment. This fusion results in the productive rearrangement of VH and may involve a diversity or Dα segment (2). The mechanism of the inversion is interesting but cannot be deduced from the present data. This will need to await further studies such as the cloning of the reciprocal event, if this is possible.

C. Does the Ig-TCR Fusion Gene (IgT) Have a Bearing on T-CLL Etiology?

Unlike Burkitt's lymphoma, the case of inv14 described here does not involve an oncogene aberrantly rearranged to a new genetic locus. Instead, we find an Ig VH joined to a Jα segment. A diagrammatic represen-

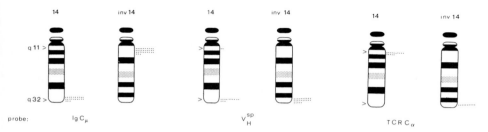

Fig. 5. Summary of *in situ* hybridization data. The figure illustrates banded metaphase chromosomes of normal 14 (14) or inverted 14 (inv14) plus distribution of silver grains associated with each position. Immunoglobulin Cμ, TCR Cα and V_H^{SP} probes were used as indicated. The break points of inv14 are arrowed at q11 and q32.

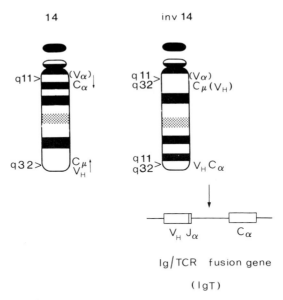

Fig. 6. Diagram of arrangement of immunoglobulin heavy chain and T-cell receptor genes in normal and inverted chromosome 14.

tation of the various gene segments on the two types of chromosomes appears in Fig. 6. Since this fusion (which we call the IgT gene) occurs productively, the gene can potentially generate a functional protein (which would be VH-Cα) which might form into heterodimers with the β chain and be produced at the cell surface. At this point we can only speculate about the relationship of this putative chimeric receptor protein and tumor etiology. It is possible that the putative chimeric receptor (perhaps because of abnormal folding or because of specific unusual antigen recognition) causes the T cell to be continuously triggered or activated. Such a constitutively dividing T cell might ultimately become malignant as a result of secondary oncogenic changes. Clearly we need to know more of the generality of the phenomenon in inv14 to see whether these chimeric genes are a common feature of this abnormality.

Acknowledgments

M.P.L. was a recipient of an EMBO fellowship, and R.B. of a Lady Tata fellowship.

References

1. Baer, R., Lefranc, M.-P., Minowada, J., Forster, A., Stinson, M. A., and Rabbitts, T. H. (1986). Organization of the T-cell receptor α chain gene and rearrangement in human T cell leukaemias. *Mol. Biol. Med.* **3**, 265–277.
2. Baer, R., Chen, K.-C., Smith, S. D., and Rabbitts, T. H. (1985). Fusion of an immunoglobulin variable gene and a T cell receptor constant gene in the chromosome 16 inversion associated with T cell tumours. *Cell* **63**, 705–713.
3. Caccia, N., Bruns, G. A. P., Kirsch, I. R., Hollis, G. F., Bertness, V., and Mak, T. W. (1985). T cell receptor α-chain genes are located on chromosome 14 at 14q11-14q12 in humans. *J. Exp. Med.* **161**, 1255–1260.
4. Chien, Y.-H., Becker, D. M., Lindsten, T., Okamura, M., Cohen, D. I., and Davis, M. M. (1984). A third type of murine T-cell receptor gene. *Nature* (London) **312**, *31–35*.
5. Clark, S. P., Yoshikai, Y., Siu, G., Taylor, S., Hood, L., and Mak, T. W. (1984). Identification of a diversity segment of human T-cell receptor β-chain, and comparison with the analogous murine element. *Nature* (*London*) **311**, 387–389.
6. Collins, M. K. L., Goodfellow, P. N., Spurr, N. K., Solomon, E., Tanigawa, G., Tonegawa, S., and Owen, M. J. (1985). The human T-cell receptor α-chain gene maps to chromosome 14. *Nature* (London) **314**, *273–274.*
7. Croce, C. M., Isobe, M., Palumbo, A., Puck, J., Ming, J., Tweardy, D., Erikson, J., Davis, M., and Rovera, G. (1985). Gene for a chain of human T cell receptor: Location of chromosome 14 region involved in t cell neoplasms. *Science* **227**, *1044–1047.*
8. Gascoigne, N. R. J., Chien, Y.-H., Becker, D. M., Kavaler, J., and Davis, M. M. (1984). Genomic organisation and sequence of T-cell receptor β-chain constant- and joining-region genes. *Nature* (*London*) **310**, 387–391.
9. Hecht, F., Morgan, R., Kaiser-McCaw Hecht, B., and Smith, S. D. (1984). Common region on chromosome 14 in T-cell leukaemia and lymphoma. *Science* **226**, 1445–1447.
10. Hedrick, S. M., Nielsen, E. A., Kavaler, J., Cohen, D. I., and Davis, M. M. (1984). Sequence relationships between putative T-cell receptor polypeptides and immunoglobulins. *Nature* (*London*) **308**, 153–158.
11. Lefranc, M.-P., and Rabbitts, T. H. (1985). Two tandemly organised human genes encoding the T-cell γ constant-region sequences show multiple rearrangement in different T-cell types. *Nature* (*London*) **316**, 464–466.
12. Rabbitts, T. H., Lefranc, M. P., Stinson, M. A., Sims, J. E., Schroder, J., Steinmetz, M., Spurr, N. L., Solomon, E., and Goodfellow, P. N. (1985). The chromosomal location of T-cell receptor genes and a T cell rearranging gene: possible correlation with specific translocations in human T cell leukaemia. *EMBO J.* **4**, 1461–1465.
13. Saito, H., Kranz, D. M., Takagaki, Y., Hayday, A. C., Eisen, H., and Tonegawa, S. (1984). Complete primary structure of a heterodimeric T-cell receptor deduced from cDNA sequences. *Nature* (*London*) **309**, 757–762.
14. Sanger, F., Coulson, A. R., Barrell, B. G., Smith, A. J. H., and Roe, B. A. (1980). Cloning in a single-stranded bacteriophage as an aid to rapid DNA sequencing. *J. Mol. Biol.* **143**, 161–178.
15. Sims, J. E., Tunnacliffe, A., Smith, W. S., and Rabbitts, T. H. (1984). Complexity of human T-cell antigen receptor β-chain constant- and variable-region genes. *Nature* (*London*) **312**, 541–545.
16. Siu, G., Clark, S. P., Yoshikai, Y., Malissen, M., Yanagi, Y., Strauss, E., Mak, T. W., and Hood, L. (1984). The human T-cell antigen receptor is encoded by variable, diversity, and joining gene segments that rearrange to generate a complete V gene. *Cell* (*Cambridge, Mass.*) **37**, 393–401.

17. Southern, E. M. (1975). Detection of specific sequences among DNA fragments separated by gel electrophoresis. *J. Mol. Biol.* **98,** 503–517.

18. Yanagi, Y., Yoshikai, Y., Leggett, K., Clark, S. P., Aleksander, I., and Mak, T. W. (1984). A human T cell-specific cDNA clone encodes a protein having extensive homology to immunoglobulin chains. *Nature (London)* **308,** 145–149.

19. Zech, L., Gahrton, G., Hammarström, L., Juliusson, G., Mellstedt, H., Robert, K. H., and Smith, C. I. E. (1984). Inversion of chromosome 14 marks human T-cell chronic lymphocytic leukaemia. *Nature (London)* **308,** 858–860.

26

DNA Amplification in Tumors and Drug-Resistant Cells

GEORGE R. STARK, ELENA GIULOTTO, AND IZUMU SAITO

Imperial Cancer Research Fund
Lincoln's Inn Fields
London, United Kingdom

I. Amplification in Tumors

Populations of tumor cells and populations of individual organisms evolve in ways that are somewhat analogous. As postulated by Darwin, two essential elements in evolution are natural selection and a means of generating variation within a population. For a tumor growing in an animal, host defense mechanisms provide the means of selection, and DNA amplification provides a major means of generating individual variation. The karyotypic hallmarks of amplification are small extrachromosomal elements, termed double minute chromosomes, and homogeneously staining regions within otherwise normal chromosomes. These abnormal structures have been noted in tumor cells for many years. Now, using DNA probes, it is revealed that they contain amplified DNA. Using probes derived from retroviruses, it has been found that the cellular counterparts of viral oncogenes ("cellular oncogenes") are often amplified in primary tumors and in cell lines derived from tumors. Some examples are presented in Table I.

NEW AVENUES IN DEVELOPMENTAL
CANCER CHEMOTHERAPY

TABLE I

Amplified Cellular Oncogenes

Oncogene	Tumor	Reference
c-myc	Lung, breast, colon, Burkitt's lymphoma	Alitalo *et al.* (1), Saksela *et al.* (14), Shibuya *et al.* (17)
c-Ki-ras	Adrenocortical tumor (mouse)	George *et al.* (7)
c-abl	Chronic myelogenous leukemia	Collins and Groudine (5)
N-myc	Neuroblastoma, retinoblastoma	Brodeur *et al.* (4), Lee *et al.* (10), Shiloh *et al.* (18)
EGF receptor	Glioma, squamous carcinoma	Libermann *et al.* (11)

If overexpression of a particular gene confers a selective advantage upon a variant cell, the proportion of that variant within a growing population will increase. Oncogenes are amplified in tumors because their overexpression contributes to survival in the selective environment of the host. Expression of an amplified gene is usually proportional to the number of copies of that gene; therefore, proteins and mRNAs corresponding to amplified cellular oncogenes are overproduced in tumors. It is reasonable to conclude that overproduction of the protein products of cellular oncogenes must contribute to tumor generation, tumor progression, or both. In one study (4), the *N-myc* oncogene was found to be amplified in 24 out of 63 untreated neuroblastomas, and the degree of amplification was as great as 300-fold. Poor prognosis was correlated with a high degree of amplification.

II. Amplification and Drug Resistance

DNA amplification in mammals was discovered in studies of drug-resistant cells in which overproduction of a specific protein, often but not always the direct target of the selective drug, allows the resistant cell to survive. We now know of about 20 different situations in which amplification is responsible for drug resistance, and it seems certain that additional examples will be uncovered in the future: see Stark and Wahl (20) for details and references. In recent work, the gene for dihydrofolate reductase, the target enzyme for the drug methotrexate, has been found to be amplified in tumor cells derived from methotrexate-treated patients (15). Furthermore, mammals are not the only species capable of amplifying their DNA—the phenomenon is widespread throughout nature, and there are many examples from bacteria, yeast, plants, and other organisms. Of clinical relevance, the parasite *Leishmania tropica* can acquire resistance to methotrexate by amplifying its gene for a bifunctional enzyme, dihydrofolate reductase–thymidylate synthetase (2).

Multiple-drug cross-resistance is a particularly interesting and clinically important situation in which DNA amplification leads to overproduction of a membrane protein of molecular weight about 170,000. The presence of large amounts of this protein, often more than 100-fold above normal, leads by an unknown mechanism to a substantial decrease in the intracellular accumulation of many different drugs, often unrelated in structure and mechanism of action. Examples are vincristine, maytansine, adriamycin, colchicine, actinomycin D, emetine, melphalan, puromycin, dactinomycin, cytochalasin B, daunorubicin, epipodophyllotoxin, and taxol. Selection with one of these drugs leads to resistance to many. Since double minute chromosomes are often present in cross-resistant cells, it was strongly suspected that amplification was involved. Recently, a probe for the 170K protein has been cloned by Riordan *et al.* (12) and used to show that the degree of amplification correlates with the degree of cross-resistance.

III. Parameters of Amplification

We know something about the details of DNA amplification from studies of cells in culture. It is clear that many different regions of the genome can be amplified, perhaps most of it. At a single locus, the frequencies are often as high as 10^{-4}. Although DNA amplification occurs spontaneously at high frequency, the frequency may be increased after application of certain drugs which interfere with DNA synthesis, such as hydroxyurea, or by a treatment, such as exposure to ultraviolet radiation, which damages DNA and leads to induction of repair mechanisms. The average amount of DNA coamplified along with the selected gene is often very large, typically about 10^6 bases of flanking DNA per selected gene (about 10^{-4} of the entire genome). Often genes which happen to lie near the selected gene are coamplified and correspondingly overexpressed. If such coordinate overexpression is deleterious to the cell, amplification of such a region may be selected against. If a frequency typical of amplification of genes for drug resistance, say 10^{-5}, is also typical of the amplification of most regions of the DNA of tumor cells, a tumor of, say, 10^9 cells may well contain 10^4 cells already resistant to a given drug before that drug is administered. The frequent observation that tumors often respond to cytotoxic drugs but then grow back in a drug-resistant form is consistent with this model. In a straightforward case such as resistance to metho-

trexate due to amplification of the dihydrofolate reductase gene, exposure
to a maximally tolerated dose of drug, rather than prolonged treatment
with a low dose, and use of several drugs simultaneously are reasonable
strategies aimed to destroy the small cohort of preexisting resistant cells.
Multiple-drug cross-resistance presents a more difficult problem, because
accumulation of many different drugs is inhibited within the resistant
cells. Since the 170K protein is exposed on the cell surface, it may be
possible to destroy the resistant cells selectively, using antibodies linked
to toxins or radionuclides. Since DNA amplification is such a pervasive
phenomenon, it may well be responsible for drug resistance in cases in
which the mechanisms remain unknown at present. For example, resistance to alkylating agents can easily be imagined to arise through amplification of genes for DNA repair enzymes. A general method to screen
drug-resistant cells for amplified genes would be of help in studying such a
situation, and such methods are being developed [see Brison *et al.* (3) and
Roninson *et al.* (13)].

IV. Amplification in Normal Cells

If amplification at a single locus usually involves 0.01% of the genome
and if the frequences of 10^{-4} that have been determined for some cases
were to be typical of most regions of genome, then it follows that most
cells would carry an amplification somewhere in their genome. It is hard
to imagine that this situation can be true for normal somatic cells and
impossible that it could be true for germ-line cells. Analyses of amplification in normal cells are exceedingly difficult to perform for several reasons, such as the limited life-span of normal cells in culture and their
propensity to survive exposure to some cytotoxic drugs by entering G_o
arrest. Thus at the moment, we have no information about amplification
in normal cells within any mammalian organism, and there have been only
a few analyses of amplification in normal cells in culture. Srivastava *et al.*
(19) have found that the cellular oncogene *c-Ha-ras-1* undergoes up to
fourfold amplification during the limited replicative life-span of normal
human diploid fibroblasts in culture, and Turner *et al.* (21) have found that
the X-linked HPRT gene undergoes amplification and other rearrangements during proliferation of normal human lymphocytes in culture, under thioguanine selection.

If amplification is rare in most normal cells and common in most tumors
and cell lines, the following question arises: What step in the origin or
progression of tumors allows widespread amplification to occur at high
frequency? From a limited analysis of cell lines, it seems that the fre-

quency of amplification at several loci is not substantially different in nontumorigenic lines such as BHK or 3T3 than it is in highly malignant lines transformed by viruses or carcinogens. This correlation suggests that the propensity to amplify may be linked to immortalization of cells rather than to their transformation, and it is tempting to speculate about possible mechanistic connections between loss of control of the number of times replication can be repeated in a cell lineage (immortalization) and loss of control of the number times replication can be repeated within a single cell cycle (amplification).

V. Some Ideas about Mechanism

Studies on mechanism have been frustrated by the fact that amplification at any particular locus is a rare event and, up to now, no way has been found to cause it to occur synchronously in a majority of cells in a culture, so that biochemical aspects might be studied. Virtually all the work that has been done, as summarized in several recent reviews, has of necessity been limited to analyses of the structure of amplified DNA in drug-resistant cells, studied many generations after the primary event, and analyses of the rate or frequency of spontaneous amplification at a particular locus or of amplification after treatment with cytotoxic drugs, tumor promoters, ultraviolet radiation, and the like. The most likely model to emerge from such studies is one in which multiple rounds of replication during a single cell cycle can lead to an onionskin structure (Fig. 1), which can then resolve by recombination into intrachromosomal or extrachromosomal amplified elements. Although this model has many attractive features, it still must be regarded as a working hypothesis for which there is little direct evidence. The work of Kavathas and Herzenberg (9) and Wahl et al. (22) has suggested the possible existence in DNA of cis-acting elements which favor amplification. For example, such elements could be origins of replication which are particularly prone to multiple initiation events during a single cell cycle. Movement of amplified DNA has been observed often, and chromosomal translocations are often found at or near amplified regions of chromosomes [see Flintoff et al. (6) for an example]. Neither of these observations are predicted by the basic "onionskin" model as illustrated in Fig. 1, and their explanation will require additions to the model or new hypotheses.

For very good practical reasons, initial studies of the structure of amplified DNA were focused on cases in which the degree of amplification was large, resulting from multiple, independent events selected in several discrete steps. Because of improved methods, it has recently become possi-

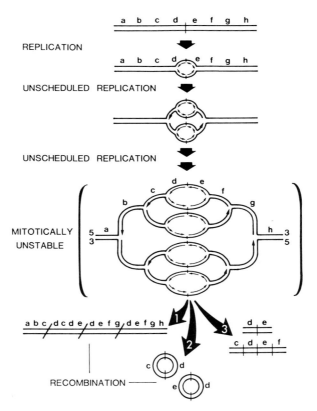

Fig. 1. A model for gene amplification. Unscheduled DNA replication is followed by recombination to generate intrachromosomal arrays of amplified DNA or extrachromosomal linear or circular DNA molecules. (20)

ble to study the structure of DNA coamplified along with the gene "CAD" in single-step mutants, in which the primary event of amplification leads to an increase in the number of CAD genes within a single chromosome from one to about four (20a). There are strong suggestions from this work that the amount of DNA coamplified with each CAD gene may be very large, perhaps 10 times more than had been estimated previously from studies of highly amplified CAD genes. It is possible that a major amount of a chromosome is amplified in the primary event and that the large amount of DNA coamplified with each copy of the CAD gene in this first step is reduced in subsequent steps of amplification.

Clearly, a better understanding of amplification is an important part of a better understanding of drug resistance and of the origin and progression of tumors. Progress at the basic level will come from a more detailed analysis of the phenomena underlying amplification and from further attempts to assess the involvement of amplification of specific genes in the genesis of specific tumors and in generating resistance to specific drugs or treatments. At a more practical level, attempts to deal with amplifications may lead to improvements in procedures now used in treating tumors.

For recent reviews on amplification, see Hamlin et al. (8), Schimke (16), and Stark and Wahl (20).

References

1. Alitalo, K., Schwab, M., Lin, C. C., Varmus, H. E., and Bishop J. M. (1983). Homogeneously staining chromosomal regions contain amplified copies of an abundantly expressed cellular oncogene (c-myc) in malignant neuroendocrine cells from a human colon carcinoma. Proc. Natl. Acad. Sci. U.S.A. 80, 1707–1711.
2. Beverley, S. M., Coderre, J. A., Santi, D. V., and Schimke, R. T. (1984). Unstable DNA amplifications in methotrexate-resistant Leishmania consist of extrachromosomal circles which relocalize during stabilization. Cell (Cambridge, Mass.) 38, 431–439.
3. Brison, O., Ardeshir, F., and Stark, G. R. (1982). General method for cloning amplified DNA by differential screening with genomic probes. Mol. Cell. Biol. 2, 578–587.
4. Brodeur, G. M., Seeger, R. C., Schwab, M., Varmus, H. E., and Bishop, J. M. (1984). Amplification of N-myc in untreated human neuroblastomas correlates with advanced disease stage. Science 224, 1121–1124.
5. Collins, S. J., and Groudine, M. T. (1983). Rearrangement and amplification of c-abl sequences in the human chronic myelogenous leukemia cell line K-562. Proc. Natl. Acad. Sci. U.S.A. 80, 4813–4817.
6. Flintoff, W. F., Livingston, E., Duff, C., and Worton, R. G. (1984). Moderate-level gene amplification in methotrexate-resistant Chinese hamster ovary cells is accompanied by chromosomal translocations at or near the site of the amplified DHFR gene. Mol. Cell. Biol. 4, 69–76.
7. George, D. L., Scott, A. F., Trusko, S., Glick, B., Ford, E., and Dorney, D. J. (1985). Structure and expression of amplified cKi-ras gene sequences in Y1 mouse adrenal tumor cells. EMBO J. 4, 1199–1203.
8. Hamlin, J. L., Milbrandt, J. D., Heintz, N. H., and Azizkhan, J. C. (1984). Sequence amplification in mammalian cells. Int. Rev. Cytol. 90, 31–82.
9. Kavathas, P., and Herzenberg, L. A. (1983). Amplification of a gene coding for human T-cell differentiation antigen. Nature (London) 306, 385–387.
10. Lee, W.-H., Murphree, A. L., and Benedict, W. F. (1984). Expression and amplification of the N-myc gene in primary retinoblastoma. Nature (London) 309, 458–460.
11. Libermann, T. A., Nusbaum, H. R., Razon, N., Kris, R., Lax, I., Soreq, H., Whittle, N., Waterfield, M. D., Ullrich, A., and Schlessinger, J. (1985). Amplification, enhanced expression and possible rearrangement of EGF receptor gene in primary human brain tumors of glial origin. Nature (London) 313, 144–147.
12. Riordan, J. R., Deuchars, K., Kartner, N., Alon, N., Trent, J., and Ling, V. (1985). Amplification of P-glycoprotein genes in multidrug resistant mammalian cell lines. Nature (London) 316, 817–819.

13. Roninson, I. B., Abelson, H. T., Housman, D. E., Howell, N., and Varshavsky, A. (1984). Amplification of specific DNA sequences correlates with multi-drug resistance in Chinese hamster cells. *Nature (London)* **309,** 626–628.
14. Saksela, K., Bergh, J., Lehto, V.-P., Nilsson, K., and Alitalo, K. (1985). Amplification of the c-*myc* oncogene in a subpopulation of human small cell lung cancer. *Cancer Res.* **45,** 1823–1827.
15. Schimke, R. T. (1984). Gene amplification, drug resistance, and cancer. *Cancer Res.* **44,** 1735–1742.
16. Schimke, R. T. (1984). Gene amplification in cultured animal cells. *Cell (Cambridge, Mass.)* **37,** 705–713.
17. Shibuya, M., Yokota, J., and Ueyama, Y. (1985). Amplification and expression of a cellular oncogene (c-*myc*) in human gastric adenocarcinoma cells. *Mol. Cell. Biol.* **5,** 414–418.
18. Shiloh, Y., Shipley, J., Brodeur, G. M., Bruns, G., Korf, B., Donlon, T., Schreck, R. R., Seeger, R., Sakai, K., and Latt, S. A. (1985). Differential amplification, assembly, and relocation of multiple DNA sequences in human neuroblastomas and neuroblastoma cell lines. *Proc. Natl. Acad. Sci. U.S.A.* **82,** 3761–3765.
19. Srivastava, A., Norris, J. S., Shmookler, R. J., and Goldstein, S. (1985). c-Ha-*ras*-1 proto-oncogene amplification and overexpression during the limited replicative life span of normal human fibroblasts. *J. Biol. Chem.* **260,** 6404–6409.
20. Stark, G. R., and Wahl, G. M. (1984). Gene amplification. *Annu. Rev. Biochem.* **53,** 447–91.
20a. Stark, G. R., Giulotto, E., and Saito, I. (1986). *EMBO J.* **5,** (in press).
21. Turner, D. R., Morley, A. A., Haliandros, M., Kutlaca, R., and Sanderson, B. J. (1985). *In vivo* somatic mutations in human lymphocytes frequently result from major gene alterations. *Nature (London)* **315,** 343–345.
22. Wahl, G. M., de Saint Vincent, B. R., and DeRose, M. L. (984). Effect of chromosomal position on amplification of transfected genes in animal cells. *Nature (London)* **307,** 516–520.

A Molecular Genetic Approach to the Problem of Drug Resistance in Chemotherapy

DAVID HOUSMAN

Center for Cancer Research
Massachusetts Institute of Technology
Cambridge, Massachusetts 02139

JAMES CROOP

Dana-Farber Cancer Institute
Boston, Massachusetts

TAKETO MUKAIYAMA

Cancer Chemotherapy Center
Japanese Foundation for Cancer Research
Tokyo, Japan

HERBERT ABELSON

Department of Pediatrics
University of Washington School of Medicine
Seattle, Washington

IGOR RONINSON

Center for Genetics
University of Illinois at Chicago Circle
Chicago, Illinois

PHILIPPE GROS

Department of Biochemistry
McGill University
Montreal, Quebec, Canada

I. The Problem of Drug Resistance in Chemotherapy

The utility of chemotherapeutic agents for the induction of an initial remission has been demonstrated for a variety of forms of cancer. However, when relapse occurs following an initial remission induced by chemotherapy, further response to chemotherapy is often limited. Understanding the altered response of tumor cells to chemotherapeutic agents in relapse versus response at initial presentation represents a fundamental issue in the development of more effective chemotherapy protocols (7,8,17). We have taken an approach to this problem which involves the use of a variety of laboratory techniques which we believe will ultimately provide fundamental insight into the reasons for resistance to chemotherapy in relapse. Our objective in these studies is to eventually provide a theoretical basis for improved modalities in chemotherapy which overcome the difficulties just cited. The approach we have taken involves the application of molecular genetic techniques to identify and characterize genes which are associated with resistance to agents commonly used in chemotherapy. Our studies have been carried out initially using Chinese hamster and mouse cells grown in tissue culture. Recent studies using DNA probes derived in this work indicate that analogous mechanisms to those described here operate in human cells as well.

II. Application of Molecular Genetic Techniques to Multidrug Resistance

A. Rationale

The course of chemotherapy can be viewed as a genetic selection on the tumor cells present in the body of the patient. The emergence of drug-resistant cells can be viewed as the outcome of this selection process. To gain insight into this process, the response of cultured mammalian cells to analogous selection procedures *in vitro* has been studied by a number of laboratory groups (2,5,13,16). Two basic findings relevant to our approach to the problem were made in these studies. First, cells selected in culture for resistance to a single agent exhibit cross-resistance to a wide variety of other agents which act by very different cellular targets to produce cytotoxicity. Cells exhibiting this pattern of cross-resistance are termed multidrug resistant. Thus cells selected for resistance to colchicine exhibit cross-resistance to Adriamycin and vice versa, despite the fact that the primary target for colchicine is the microtubule apparatus, while the primary cytotoxic effects of Adriamycin are thought to involve binding to DNA. These results have led investigators to postulate the involvement of cellular uptake or efflux mechanisms in the mechanism of multidrug resistance (12,14). The second key finding which relates to our approach to the problem is the demonstration of homogeneously staining regions or double minute chromosomes in cell lines exhibiting multidrug resistance (1,11). These karyotypic observations are strongly indicative of gene amplification. We therefore initiated our analysis of multidrug resistance with the goal of identifying and characterizing the gene or genes amplified in multidrug-resistant cell lines. In the discussion which follows, we will describe techniques which we developed to assist in the identification and characterization DNA sequences encoding a gene family involved in the expression of multidrug resistance and the development of DNA probes for an mRNA species which we believe is central to the expression of the multidrug resistance phenotype.

B. Identification of Amplified DNA Sequences in Multidrug-Resistant Cells

To identify amplified sequences in mammalian cells, a technique which permits the direct visualization of such sequences was developed (15). The procedure which we developed was based on the following consider-

ations. If an amplified DNA sequence represents a sufficiently high proportion of the DNA content of an organism and the sequence contains
within it two or more recognition sites for a particular restriction endonuclease, then the digestion of DNA of the organism with this restriction
endonuclease will permit direct visualization of the amplified DNA sequence. Agarose gel electrophoresis of the digested DNA followed by
staining of the fractionated DNA with ethidium bromide results in the
appearance of a discrete band representing the amplified sequence over
the background of other DNA fragments present in the genome of the
organism. In order for a sequence to be visualized in this way it must
represent at least 1% of the DNA content of the organism. For mammalian genomes, a DNA sequence present once per genome (single-copy
DNA) which is 1 kilo-base-pair (kb) in length represents less than 0.001%
of the DNA in the genome. Thus sequences amplified even 100 times in a
mammalian genome cannot be visualized directly, because they represent
less than 1% of the DNA. The technique we have utilized is applicable for
amplified sequences which occur in a range between 0.01 and 1% of the
DNA content of mammalian cells. Our approach involves the following
steps:

1. Digest DNA with a restriction endonuclease.
2. Label DNA with ^{32}P by replacement synthesis with incorporation of
$[^{32}P]$deoxynucleotide triphosphates in a reaction catalyzed by T4 DNA
polymerase.
3. Fractionate DNA by agarose gel electrophoresis.
4. Denature DNA *in situ* by treatment of the gel with dilute alkali.
5. Neutralize alkali and adjust salt concentration to permit renaturation
in gel of homologous DNA sequences.
6. Digest unrenatured DNA in the gel with the single stranded endonuclease S1.
7. Wash gel to remove products of DNA digestion.
8. Steps 4–7 are then repeated to improve resolution.

Using this approach, DNA sequences which are amplified are present
at a higher local concentration in the gel than DNA sequences present
once per genome. The amplified DNA sequences renature more rapidly,
because they are present at a higher local concentration in the gel than the
single-copy DNA sequences. For this reason the amplified DNA sequences are protected from the effects of the S1 nuclease. Visualization of
the amplified DNA sequences is accomplished by autoradiographic exposure of the gel.

We applied this technique to Chinese hamster cell lines LZ and C5,
which had been selected for resistance to the drugs Adriamycin and col-

chicine, respectively. The results of an in-gel renaturation experiment on cell line LZ are shown in Fig. 1. A large number of well-resolved bands corresponding to amplified DNA sequences are observed. To determine which of these amplified DNA sequences are specific for the multidrug resistance phenotype, the pattern of amplified DNA sequences observed in the drug-sensitive parental cell line V79 was compared to the pattern observed in LZ. As we have discussed previously (16), a series of DNA fragments can be identified which are specifically amplified in LZ and therefore are likely to represent the genetic domain within which the multidrug resistance gene or genes are located. Comparison of these DNA sequences to the DNA sequences amplified in another multidrug-resistant cell line C5 has allowed us to identify a series of DNA fragments which are apparently amplified in both cell lines. To further characterize these DNA sequences we initiated the isolation of these DNA sequences by molecular cloning techniques.

C. Isolation of Cloned DNA Sequences Derived from the Amplified DNA Domain of Multidrug-Resistant Cell Line LZ

1. Use of in-Gel Renaturation to Characterize the Amplified Domain

The initial steps in the isolation and cloning of a DNA segment from the amplified domain involved a modification of the in-gel renaturation procedure described in the preceding section. We carried out steps 1–5 as described above on *Bam*HI-digested DNA from cell line LZ but omitted step 6 the S1 nuclease digestion. Instead, we isolated renatured DNA molecules from a region of the gel known to contain a *Bam*HI fragment (1.1 kbp in length) amplified in both LZ and C5 and cloned them into *Bam*HI-cleaved pBR322. Twenty-four independent clones were isolated initially, and their sequences compared by restriction mapping. Of the 24 clones, 6 had identical restriction maps. Hybridization of the DNA fragment isolated in one of these clones (designated pDR1.1) demonstrated that sequences homologous to the isolated DNA fragment were indeed amplified in drug-resistant cell lines LZ and C5. As expected, amplification of sequences homologous to this segment was not observed in drug-sensitive parental cell lines V79 and CHO. The isolation of a 1.1-kbp segment of the amplified domain of cell line LZ provided a point of entry which allowed us to initiate the cloning and characterization of a domain of DNA amplification which we estimated to be greater than 100 kbp in length (16).

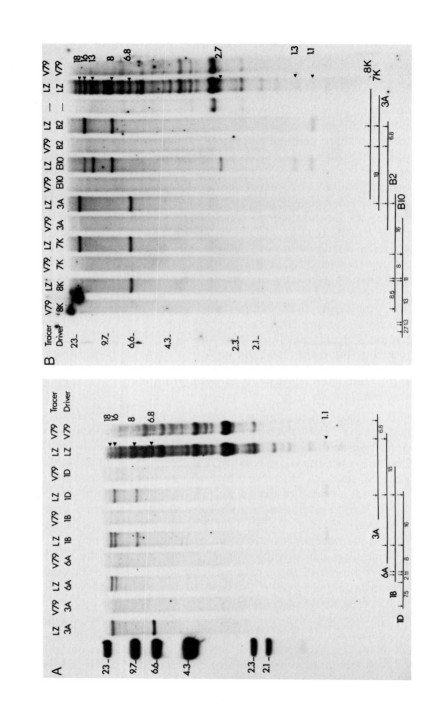

2. Isolation of Over 100 kbp of Contiguously Amplified DNA Sequences

Genomic libraries from LZ cell DNA were constructed in bacteriophage and cosmid vectors in order to isolate and characterize the amplified DNA in this cell line. High-molecular-weight DNA was isolated from these cells and was initially used to construct a library in bacteriophage lambda EMBL (4). Thirty thousand recombinant phages were screened using plasmid pDR1.1 as a hybridization probe. Six phage clones hybridizing to pDR1.1 were identified, purified, and characterized. The six clones proved to represent overlapping DNA fragments, each of which included a 1.1-kb *Bam*HI segment homologous to pDR1.1. The restriction map of two informative clones spanning 35 kb of DNA is presented in Fig. 1 (lambda DRG2 and lamda DRZ3). Phage DNA was digested with various restriction enzymes, and the digestion products were separated on agarose gels. The gels were transferred to nitrocellulose, and the filters hybridized to nick-translated total V79 DNA. A 7.8-kb *Eco*RI fragment free of highly repeated sequences was identified and subcloned into the *Eco*RI site of vector pUC18. After this initial cloning step cosmid libraries were used to expand the size of the cloned region. LZ DNA was used to construct a genomic library in cosmid vector pSAE (10). Gel-purified insert DNA from pDR7.8 was used as a hybridization probe to screen 50,000 recombinant clones from this library; 18 positive clones were identified, their restriction map established, and fragments free of repeated sequences were again isolated (pDR9.7, pDR2.9). Four successive rounds of screening using left-side probes pDR2.9 and pDR2.7 and right-side probes pDR9.7, pDR1.6, and pDR2 were performed, and a total of 75 cosmids were isolated. The restriction map of DNA inserts from these cosmids was obtained using enzymes *Bam*HI, *Kpn*I, *Xba*I, and *Bgl*II either alone or in combination. The position and orientation of cosmid

---

Fig. 1. In-gel hybridization of LZ, V79, and cloned DNA sequences. Tracer DNA was digested with *Bam*HI and was P[32]-labeled with T4 DNA polymerase. Genomic driver DNAs were digested with *Bam*HI (LZ and V79; A,B), while cosmid driver DNAs, were digested with *Bam*HI alone (A) or *Bam*HI in combination with *Sal*I (B). For each lane, both tracer and driver DNA are identified at the top of the gel. Cloned *Bam*HI fragments in cosmid driver DNA hybridize to a corresponding *Bam*HI fragment in LZ DNA and V79 DNA, but only the amplified fragments of LZ tracer DNA are detectable against the background. This homologous set of *Bam*HI fragments amplified in LZ DNA and contained within the cosmid clones analyzed is identified by a series of arrowheads in the LZ tracer/LZ driver control lane. The size of these homologous fragments is indicated and was derived by comparison with the *Hin*dIII fragments of lambda DNA. To facilitate reading of the autoradiogram, the *Bam*HI restriction map of each of the cosmid insert DNA used is presented.

cloning arms was determined using the unique *Cla*I and *Sal*I sites present in the vector. The position of 7 relevant overlapping cosmids is presented in Fig. 1, along with the composite *Bam*HI and *Kpn*I restriction map of the entire cloned domain. After five rounds of screening approximately 125 kb of contiguous chromosomal DNA was isolated from adriamycin-resistant LZ cells. The number of clones identified in cosmid cloning varied considerably depending on the hybridization probe used. Probes from the right end of the amplified unit (pDR9.7, pDR1.6) detected five to seven times more clones than left-end probes (pDR2.9, pDR2.7). Also, a significant number of clones obtained from the left side showed independently rearranged insert fragments: cosmids 1D (Fig. 2a) and B2 (Fig. 2b) show insert fragments rearranged in the region left of the 1.1-kb fragment, while only cosmid 1A shows the correct configuration. These rearrangements either could have occurred during the amplification process, therefore representing minor components of the amplified domain, or could have been generated during the cloning procedure (6).

3. Assignment of Cloned Sequences to Amplified Fragments in the DNA of LZ cells

The isolation of the set of cosmid clones posed the following questions: first, whether the entire cloned region was amplified in LZ DNA, and second, whether the set of clones constituted an accurate representation of the complete amplified unit. The usual approach to an analysis of this type involves the use of single-copy fragments, obtained from the cloned genomic region, as probes for Southern hybridization to DNA of the parental and drug-resistant cell lines. This approach has two major disadvantages: (1) the presence of highly repeated DNA sequences in certain regions of DNA makes it difficult to gather single-copy fragments for analysis of the entire cloned region; (2) artifacts involving rearrangements of the DNA after insertion in the cloning vector can result in isolation of single-copy fragments that would confound the analysis. A new method was developed based on the in-gel renaturation process, which circumvents both of these difficulties [see (15)]. Briefly, cloned DNA fragments from the cosmids (driver DNA) are used to protect the corresponding ^{32}P-labeled genomic DNA (tracer DNA) from digestion with S1 nuclease following electrophoresis and in-gel denaturation. Two representative examples of such gels are presented in Fig. 2, and the *Bam*HI restriction map of individual cosmids is presented to facilitate reading of the gel. In these experiments 10 ng of cosmid DNA digested with *Bam*HI was used as driver DNA. This amount is grossly equivalent to approximately 50–100 copies of an arbitrary 10-kb fragment present in 10 μg of genomic DNA. This should mimic experimental conditions present when total ge-

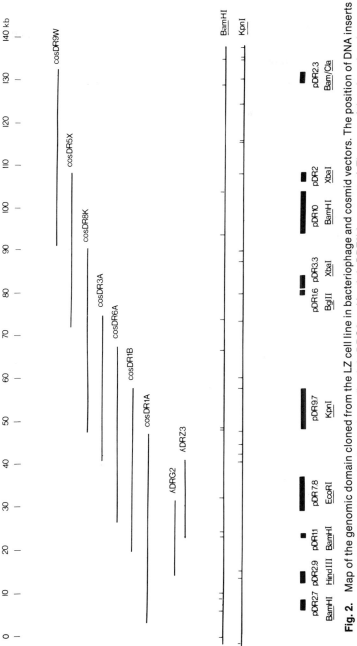

Fig. 2. Map of the genomic domain cloned from the LZ cell line in bacteriophage and cosmid vectors. The position of DNA inserts from the two initially isolated bacteriophage clones (lambda DRG2 and lambda DRZ3) is presented. The map of the cloned region was then expanded using cosmid libraries constructed in cosmid pSAE, and the position of DNA inserts from 7 overlapping cosmid clones (cosDR1A to cosDR12W) is presented immediately above the bacteriophage clones. A composite restriction map of the cloned domain for restriction endonucleases *Bam*HI and *Kpn*I obtained after analysis of a total of 75 independent clones is also presented; the size of the edge *Bam*HI and *Kpn*I fragments was deduced from Southern blotting data. Various repeat-free plasmid subclones of these bacteriophages and cosmids were used to isolate overlapping cosmids or in Southern or Northern analyses. The position of these subclones within the cloned region (pDR2.7 to pDR2) is shown at the bottom of the figure as dark boxes along with the restriction enzyme used for cloning. The scale is in 10 kb, and the orientation of the DNA region (0–130 kb), referred in the text as left and right sides, is chosen arbitrarily.

nomic DNA is used as driver. Driver cosmid DNA is combined with both tracer DNA and 10 μg of heterologous human carrier DNA digested with *Eco*RI prior to electrophoresis. This allows reproduction of the same DNA concentrations present in the LZ and V79 tracer/driver control lanes. Results show that when LZ DNA digested with *Bam*HI is used both as tracer and driver, the characteristic pattern of amplified fragments appears over the background fragments present in the V79 tracer/V79 driver control lane. When *Bam*HI-digested cosmid DNA is used as driver DNA, it protects the homologous genomic fragments both in LZ and V79 DNA from S1 degradation. The intensity of the signal, however, is directly proportional to the fragment copy number in tracer DNA, and since the corresponding DNA sequences are amplified 60-fold in LZ relative to V79 DNA (16), the corresponding bands are clearly detectable against the background in lanes containing LZ but not V79 tracer DNA. In the experiments of the type shown in Fig. 2, it was possible to directly assign eight *Bam*HI fragments, present in independent cosmids and spanning 65 kb, to the corresponding set of fragments amplified in LZ cells (LZ tracer/LZ driver lane). These results show that this procedure can be used advantageously as a mapping tool for DNA amplified to 30–50 copies. Control experiments, using 77A as tracer DNA, demonstrated that 7 copies of the gene cannot be detected by this approach (data not shown).

This procedure was also very valuable for the identification of cosmid clones carrying rearranged insert DNA. Two examples of such clones are presented in Figs. 2a and 2b. Cosmid 1D (Fig. 2a) has five internal *Bam*HI fragments of size 16, 8, 7.5, 2, and 1.1 kb. When used as driver in combination with LZ tracer DNA, only three of these segments (16, 8, and 1.1 kb) protected LZ tracer DNA against S1 nuclease digestion. The two other fragments (7.5 and 2 kb) are therefore rearranged and not representative of the amplified domain in LZ. Another rearranged fragment was identified in cosmid B2 (Fig. 2b, 8.5-kb fragment) using the same approach. The correct restriction map of this area of the amplified region was obtained from cosmic B10 (Fig. 2b), which carries contiguous 13-, 1.3-, and 2.7-kb *Bam*HI fragments, all of which hybridize to LZ tracer DNA.

During these experiments, it was discovered that potential artifacts might arise: as long as the fragments comigrate in the gel, a fragment of driver DNA showing partial but continuous homology to its homolog present in the tracer can protect it from S1 digestion. Cosmid B10 (Fig. 2b) shows a 16-kb *Bam*HI fragment which contains both a piece of vector DNA plus a flanking sequence homologous to the 16-kb fragment amplified in LZ with which it happens to comigrate. This partial homology is, however, sufficient to produce a band at 16 kb (Fig. 2b, B10.1 driver/LZ tracer). Similarly, the 18-kb band protected by cosmid 1B (Fig. 2a, 1D driver/LZ tracer) reflects only partial homology between the cloned fragment and the genomic fragment.

D. Characterization of a Major Transcription Unit within the Amplified Domain

1. RNA Hybridization Experiments

Once we had established the structure of the amplified DNA domain associated with the multidrug resistance phenotype, our next objective was to identify and characterize the mRNA encoded by this DNA region. To address this issue we isolated cellular RNA from drug-sensitive V79 cells, as well as drug-resistant 77A, LZ, and C5 cells. In order to identify the mRNA encoded by the amplified domain we hybridized DNA probes isolated from this domain to these RNA samples. Prior to hybridization, the RNA was separated by electrophoresis in denaturing formaldehyde gels and transferred to a solid support. Three subclones spanning 75 kb of cloned DNA (Fig. 3a, pDR 7.8; Fig. 3b, pDR 1.6; Fig. 3c, pDR 2) were used as hybridization probes to detect the presence of transcribed sequences. All three probes detected the presence of a large mRNA species transcribed at high levels in the two multidrug-resistant cell lines C5 and LZ. Probes pDR 9.7 and pDR 10 also identified the same RNA species in LZ cells but produced a much weaker signal. Probes mapping to the left of pDR7.8 and to the right of pDR10 (Fig. 2) did not hybridize to this mRNA. The size of this mRNA was estimated to be approximately 5 kb, using 28 S and 18 S ribosomal RNA species as reference markers. Also, the 77A cells (low level of Adriamycin resistance) show a small but significant increase of the level of this mRNA above the almost undetectable background level of V79 cells (Fig. 3b). This amplified region, therefore, seems to contain a gene that spans at least 75 kb and that encodes an mRNA species whose level of expression correlates with the relative level of multidrug resistance of each cell line. Cross-hybridization between individual cosmids overlapping this region could not be detected, suggesting that this region contains a single copy of the gene encoding this mRNA rather than a cluster of related sequences.

2. Isolation of cDNA Clones: The Potential Existence of a Multigene Family

To further characterize the nature of the transcript encoded by the amplified domain of LZ cells, we isolated cDNA clones using DNA probes which showed homology to the 5-kb mRNA in Northern blotting

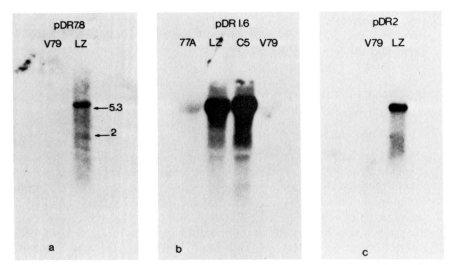

Fig. 3. Characterization of sequences transcribed from the genomic domain amplified in LZ and C5 cells. Northern blotting analysis of total cellular RNA (b) prepared from V79, 77A, LZ, and C5 cell lines and poly A RNA (a,c) from V79 and LZ cells. Twenty micrograms of total cellular RNA (b) or 1 μg of poly A RNA (a,c) were electrophoresed on 1% agarose–formaldehyde gels, transferred to hybridization membranes, and hybridized to P^{32}-labeled insert DNA from plasmid overlapping 75 kb of the cloned domain: pDR7.8 (a), pDR1.6 (b), and pDR2 (c). The size of the hybridizing band (approximately 5kb) was estimated from 2- and 5.3-kb ribosomal RNA markers. Autoradiograms were exposed for 16 hr.

experiments. Screening a cDNA library constructed from a drug-sensitive cell, we identified two classes of cDNA molecules. The structure of these molecules is indicated in diagrammatic form in Fig. 4. We interpret the identification of two discrete classes of cDNA molecules as an indication that the drug resistance gene may be part of a multigene family. Support for this view can also be obtained from a more detailed analysis of hybridization of DNA probes from the amplified domain to genomic DNA from drug-resistant cell lines. In Fig. 5, each probe identified a set of weakly cross-hybridizing bands in the DNA of drug-resistant cell lines LZ and C5, as well as the set of strongly hybridizing bands. These sets of cross-hybridizing bands are identified on each of the autoradiograms with small arrows (Fig. 5b, pDR2.9 detects a 17-kb fragment; Fig. 5e, pDR 10 detects multiple bands). These homologous fragments follow a pattern of amplification similar to the pattern observed for the intensely hybridizing bands in cell lines V79, 77A, and LZ. We interpret these DNA fragments to represent another member of a multigene family with homology to the region we have already characterized. Should this interpretation prove

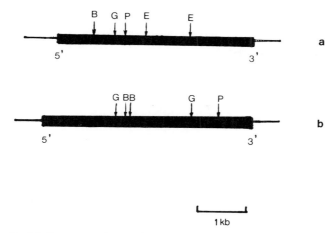

Fig. 4. Restriction map of two cDNA clones homologous to multidrug-resistant genes. A mouse cDNA library selected for DNA inserts of size greater than 2.3 kb was constructed from a drug-sensitive mouse cell line. This library was then screened with single-copy subcloned fragments isolated from the cloned domain amplified in LZ and C5 multidrug-resistant cell lines. Thirty thousand independent clones were screened and 6 positive clones were plaque-purified. Restriction analysis of these positive clones revealed that they could be separated into two groups, both hybridizing to the hamster genomic probes. The preliminary restriction map of two representative clones of these families (a and b) was established for enzymes *Eco*RI (E), *Bam*HI (B), *Pst*I (P), and *Bgl*II (G).

correct, it would be of interest to determine whether the expression of this DNA domain plays a significant role in multidrug resistance.

III. Prospects for Future Work on Multidrug Resistance

The isolation and characterization of DNA probes which identify the amplified mRNA species characteristic of multidrug-resistant cells open the door to a wide variety of functional studies. Detailed analysis of the structure of the cDNA for the multidrug resistance gene could provide immediate clues to its mode of action. It will also be very important to determine whether drug-resistant cells in patients undergoing chemotherapy exhibit increased levels of expression of this gene compared to drug-sensitive cells. Finally, should this mechanism prove to be operative in human tumors (3), then the availability of the gene and cells expressing it could prove to be valuable reagents in designing strategies to overcome the drug resistance problem in chemotherapy.

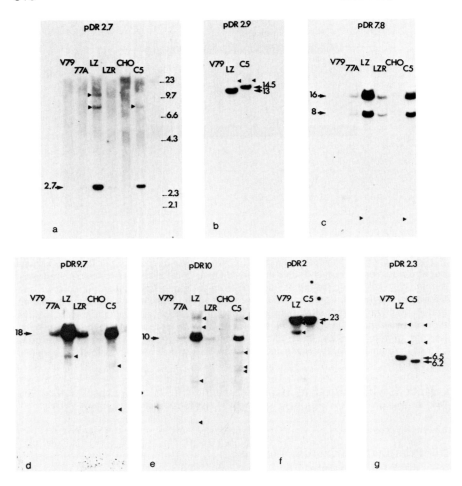

Fig. 5. Characterization of the genomic domain commonly amplified in LZ and C5 cell lines. Southern blotting analysis of *Bam*HI-digested DNA from V79 and CHO AuxB1 parental cell lines along with their respective Adriamycin-resistant derivatives 77A, LZ, and LZR (V79 derived) and colchicine-resistant derivative C5 (CHO derived). Five or 10 μg of DNA was digested to completion, electrophoresed on 1% agarose gels, transferred to a hybridization membrane, and hybridized to ³²P-labeled insert DNA from plasmid subclones overlapping the entire cloned region: pDR2.7 (a), pDR2.9 (b), pDR7.8 (c), pDR9.7 (d), pDR10 (e), pDR2 (f) (see Fig. 1). Amplified DNA fragments exhibiting strong hybridization are identified by arrows with the fragment size in kilobases. DNA fragments exhibiting weak hybridization are identified by small arrowheads. Size markers are the *Hin*dIII fragments of lambda DNA. Autoradiograms were exposed for 2–8 hr.

References

1. Baskin, F., Rosenberg, R. N., and Vaithilingham, D. (1981). Correlation of double-minute chromosomes with unstable multidrug cross-resistance in uptake mutants of neuroblastoma cells. *Proc. Natl. Acad. Sci. U.S.A.* **78,** 3654.
2. Beck, W. T., Mueller, T. J., and Tanzer, L. R. (1979). Altered surface membrane glycoproteins in vinca alkaloid resistant human leukemic lymphoblasts. *Cancer Res.* **39,** 2070.
3. Bell, D. R., Gerlach, J. H., Kartner, N., Buick, R. N., and Ling, V. (1985). Detection of p-glycoprotein in ovarian cancer: A molecular marker associated with multidrug resistance. *J. Clin. Oncol.* **3,** 311.
4. Benton, W. D., and Davis, R. W. (1977). Screening lambda recombinant clones by hybridization to single plaques *in situ. Science* **196,** 180.
5. Biedler, J. L., Chang, T., Meyers, M. B., Peterson, R. H. F., and Spengler, B. A. (1983). Drug resistance in Chinese hamster lung and mouse tumor cells. *Cancer Treat. Rep.* **67,** 859.
6. Federspiel, N. A., Beverly, S. M., Schilling, J. W., and Schimke, R. T. (1984). Novel DNA rearrangements are associated with dihydrofolate reductase gene amplification. *J. Biol. Chem.* **259,** 9127.
7. Goldie, J. H., and Coldman, A. J. (1983). Quantitative model for multiple levels of drug resistance in clinical tumors. *Cancer Treat. Rep.* **67,** 923.
8. Goldin, A. (1978). Basic cancer chemotherapy: Obstacles and future pharmacologic aspects and selective toxicity. *Cancer Chem. Trials* **58,** 119.
9. Gros, P., Croop, J., Roninson, I., Varshavsky, A., and Housman, D. (1986). Isolation and characterization of DNA sequences amplified in multidrug resistant hamster cells. *Proc. Natl. Acad. Sci. U.S.A.* (in press).
10. Grosveld, F. G., Lund, T., Murray, E. J., Mellor, A. L., Dahl, H. M., and Flavell, R. A. (1982). The construction of cosmid libraries which can be used to transform eukaryotic cells. *Nucleic Acids Res.* **10,** 6715.
11. Howell, N., Belli, T. A., Zaczkiewics, L. T., and Belli, J. A. (1984). *Cancer Res.* **44,** 4023.
12. Inaba, M., Kobayashi, H., Sakurai, Y., and Johnson, R. K. (1979). Active efflux of daunorubicin and adriamycin in sensitive and resistant sublines of P388 leukemia. *Cancer Res.* **39,** 2200.
13. Ling, V., and Thompson, L. H. (1974). Reduced permeability in CHO cells as a mechanism for resistance to colchicine. *J. Cell. Physiol.* **83,** 103.
14. Ramu, A., Shan, T., and Glaubiger, D. (1983). Enhancement of doxorubicin and vinblastine sensitivity in anthracycline resistant P388 cells. *Cancer Treat. Rep.* **67,** 895.
15. Roninson, I. B. (1983). Detection and mapping of homologous, repeated and amplified DNA sequences by DNA renaturation in agarose gels. *Nucleic Acids Res.* **11,** 5413.
16. Roninson, I. B., Abelson, H. T., Housman, D. E., Howell, N., and Varshavsky, A. (1984). Amplification of specific DNA sequences correlates with multidrug resistance in Chinese hamster cells. *Nature (London)* **309,** 626.
17. Skipper, H. E. (1978). Reasons for success and failure in treatment of murine leukemia with the drugs now employed in treating human leukemias. *Cancer Chemother.* **1,** 166.

Index

A

M